# XIIIᵉ CONGRÈS INTERNATIONAL DE MÉDECINE. PARIS 1900

*COMPTES RENDUS*

Publiés sous la direction de A. CHAUFFARD, Secrétaire général

# SECTION

DE

# CHIRURGIE URINAIRE

## COMPTES RENDUS

PUBLIÉS PAR

## E. DESNOS

SECRÉTAIRE DE LA SECTION

PARIS

MASSON ET Cⁱᵉ, ÉDITEURS

LIBRAIRES DE L'ACADÉMIE DE MÉDECINE

120, BOULEVARD SAINT-GERMAIN

XIII<sup>e</sup> CONGRÈS INTERNATIONAL DE MÉDECINE. PARIS 1900



# SECTION

DE

# CHIRURGIE URINAIRE

*Les Comptes rendus des Travaux des Sections du XIII[e]
Congrès international de Médecine sont publiés en 17 volumes
ainsi répartis :*

1. Anatomie descriptive et comparée. — Histologie et Embryologie. —
   Physiologie physique, Chimie biologique.
2. Pathologie générale, Pathologie expérimentale.
3. Anatomie pathologique. — Bactériologie, Parasitologie.
4. Pathologie interne.
5. Médecine de l'enfance. — Chirurgie de l'enfance.
6. Thérapeutique, Pharmacologie, Matière médicale.
7. Neurologie.
8. Psychiatrie.
9. Dermatologie et Syphiligraphie.
10. Chirurgie générale.
11. Chirurgie urinaire.
12. Ophtalmologie.
13. Laryngologie, Rhinologie. — Otologie.
14. Stomatologie.
15. Obstétrique. — Gynécologie.
16. Médecine légale.
17. Médecine et Chirurgie militaires : Sous-sections de Chirurgie, d'Épi-
    démiologie et Hygiène, de Médecine navale, de Médecine coloniale.

*Chaque volume est vendu séparément 5 fr. — On peut
souscrire pour l'ensemble des 17 volumes au prix de 50 fr*

---

*Chaque congressiste reçoit gratuitement le volume de la
section à laquelle il a été inscrit. Il peut se procurer les
volumes des autres sections au prix de 4 fr et souscrire à
l'ensemble au prix de 45 fr.*

41150. — Imprimerie Lahure, 9, rue de Fleurus, à Paris.

XIIIᵉ CONGRÈS INTERNATIONAL DE MÉDECINE. PARIS 1900

*COMPTES RENDUS*

Publiés sous la direction de A. CHAUFFARD, Secrétaire général

# SECTION

DE

# CHIRURGIE URINAIRE

## COMPTES RENDUS

PUBLIÉS PAR

## E. DESNOS

SECRÉTAIRE DE LA SECTION

PARIS

MASSON ET Cⁱᵉ, ÉDITEURS

LIBRAIRES DE L'ACADÉMIE DE MÉDECINE

120, BOULEVARD SAINT-GERMAIN

# XIIIᵉ CONGRÈS INTERNATIONAL DE MÉDECINE

## PARIS, 2-9 AOUT 1900

### SECTION

#### DE

# CHIRURGIE URINAIRE

## BUREAU ET COMITÉ D'ORGANISATION DE LA SECTION DE CHIRURGIE URINAIRE

*Président :* M. le Professeur GUYON.

*Vice-Présidents :* MM. ALBARRAN, POUSSON (Bordeaux).

*Secrétaire :* M. DESNOS.

*Secrétaire adjoint :* M. MICHON.

*Membres :* MM. BAZY, CARLIER (Lille), CHEVALIER, DELAGENIÈRE (Tours), DUCHASTELET, ERAUD (Lyon), ESCAT (Marseille), ESTOR (Montpellier), FORGUE (Montpellier), GUIARD, GUILLET (Caen), HALLÉ, LEGUEU, MALHERBE (Nantes), CH. MONOD, PONCET (Lyon), ROUTIER.

*Secrétaires des séances :* MM. PASTEAU, ALGLAVE, AUFRET, BARBIN, BRÉCY, DUVAL, HANOTTE, JAVAL, RAVASINI (Trieste), SACCO.

### Présidents d'honneur :

MM. D'ANTONA (Naples); BOTTINI (Pavie); M. T. CABOT (Boston); FARKAS (Buda-Pest); FENGER (Chicago); FINGER (Vienne); VON FRISCH (Vienne); GUISY (Athènes); REGINALD HARRISON (Londres); ISRAEL (Berlin); KEYES (New-York); KÜMMELL (Hambourg); KÜSTER (Marbourg); LAMBOTTE (Bruxelles); LLURIA (Madrid); NICOLICH (Trieste); POSNER (Berlin); G. REVERDIN (Genève); SAXTORPH (Copenhague); SEPP (Amsterdam); SEVEREANU (Bucarest); SINITZINE (Moscou); ED. DE SMETH (Bruxelles); Henry THOMPSON (Londres); ZAMBACO-PACHA (Constantinople).

### LIEU DES RÉUNIONS :

**Hôpital Necker.**

# PREMIÈRE SÉANCE

## VENDREDI 3 AOUT

*A 10 heures du matin.*

---

### Présidence de M. le professeur GUYON

---

#### ALLOCUTION D'OUVERTURE

#### par M. le professeur GUYON.

MESSIEURS,

C'est la première fois que, dans un Congrès international, se réunit une section de chirurgie urinaire. Le Président et le Comité exécutif du XIII<sup>e</sup> Congrès ont pensé que la chirurgie urinaire méritait cet honneur, nous leur en sommes reconnaissants.

Ils nous fournissent l'occasion d'associer dans une action commune nos confrères de l'étranger et nos compatriotes, afin de poursuivre ensemble la réalisation de plus en plus complète de nos progrès. Semblable collaboration ne peut pas ne pas être efficace, et, nous nous félicitons qu'elle s'établisse à Paris. C'est un véritable privilège dont nous sentons tout le prix. Je suis certain d'être l'interprète de tous les chirurgiens français en témoignant, à ceux qui sont venus de tant de pays différents se réunir à nous, notre désir de nous solidariser avec eux dans la lutte obstinée que nous avons à soutenir contre notre même et seul ennemi, contre la maladie. Ils sont les bienvenus, nous les saluons cordialement et nous prions nos confrères Italiens de nous permettre de joindre nos sentiments douloureux aux leurs.

L'union des chirurgiens assure la possibilité d'étendre le pouvoir déjà si grand de la chirurgie. Les brillants succès obtenus par les opérations dans les maladies des viscères naguère inaccessibles aux efforts de cette thérapeutique audacieusement bienfaisante, s'affirment dans la chirurgie urinaire. Ils deviennent la règle, là, où peut-être, plus encore que dans toute autre attaque opératoire, se multipliaient les désastres.

La persistance de ces échecs eût été d'autant plus pénible, que l'antisepsie et l'asepsie n'en auraient pas conjuré le retour, si les méthodes et les procédés mis en œuvre dans les opérations et explorations, ne s'étaient pas modifiés et perfectionnés. Le choix de l'opération, ainsi que la manière de l'exécuter, sont l'une des conditions indispensables de nos succès. Les résultats obtenus légitiment notre confiance dans « la bonne technique ».

Pour peu que l'on se demande d'où nous sont venus les éléments de ces transformations tutélaires, les noms de leurs auteurs se présentent en nombre à notre esprit. Il n'est pas besoin de les citer. Est-il nécessaire, par exemple, de rappeler les services rendus à la chirurgie urinaire par les leçons de Sir Henry Thompson, dont les clartés nous montrent tant de vérités, et par sa pratique merveilleusement habile : l'influence de la révolution profonde accomplie dans la lithotritie par Bigelow, qui a placé pour toujours cette belle opération au rang des plus utiles et des plus sûres de la chirurgie ; l'importance des initiatives hardies de Simon qui ont fait naître la chirurgie rénale et assuré son remarquable essor ; celles des recherches de Petersen qui, après tant de fortunes diverses, ont enfin fait rentrer dans la pratique la taille sus-pubienne ; ne constatons-nous pas chaque jour, aussi bien pour le diagnostic que dans le traitement, les conséquences de l'éclairage de la vessie porté par Nitze au point de perfection qu'il fallait atteindre. Ces belles acquisitions de la chirurgie urinaire datent d'hier, on pourrait dire d'aujourd'hui ; elles sont déjà définitives.

Les rapports qui vont être lus, les communications annoncées, les discussions qui vont naître, prouveront que la marche en avant ne s'est pas ralentie et que nos richesses augmentent. Nous aurons une satisfaction particulière à les entendre dans cet hôpital Necker où Civiale créa la lithotritie, et qu'il a désigné à ceux qui devaient s'occuper des maladies de l'appareil urinaire. Le souvenir de votre savante réunion ne sera pas oublié ; il donnera à ceux qui ont coutume de travailler ici une raison de plus de vouloir y poursuivre assidûment leurs recherches.

Messieurs, je déclare ouverts les travaux de la Section de chirurgie urinaire du Congrès international de 1900.

*Première question mise à l'ordre du jour :*

# LES OPÉRATIONS CONSERVATRICES DANS
# LES RÉTENTIONS RÉNALES

*Rapporteurs* : MM. KUSTER (Marbourg), CHRISTIAN FENGER (Chicago), BAZY (Paris).

## DIE CONSERVATIVEN OPERATIONEN BEI STAUUNGSGESCHWÜLSTEN DER NIERE.

VON

### Professor ERNST KÜSTER

in Marburg (Hessen).

Meine Herren. Es ist mir die Ehre zu Theil geworden als erster über einen Gegenstand berichten zu dürfen, welcher in den letzten Jahren innerhalb des Gebietes der Nierenchirurgie eine immer steigende Bedeutung gewonnen hat; und nicht zum Wenigsten durch die Bemühungen und Arbeiten unsers sehr verehrten Vorsitzenden, des Herrn Professors *Guyon* und seiner Schule. Aber bevor ich auf das Thema « Die conservativen Operationen bei Stauungsgeschwülsten der Niere » eingehe, liegt es mir am Herzen, um allen Missverständnissen vorzubeugen, zunächst eine Erklärung abzugeben, bei welcher ich allerdings eine gewisse Polemik gegen zwei von mir sehr hoch verehrte Männer, die Herren *Guyon* und *Albarran* nicht vermeiden kann.

Wie wohl den meisten von Ihnen bekannt sein wird, habe ich in einer im Jahre 1888 erschienenen kleinen Arbeit vorgeschlagen die Hydronephrose und Pyonephrose unter dem gemeinsamen Namen der Sackniere, Cystinephrosis zusammen zu fassen. Gegen diesen Vorschlag haben sich die genannten Herren in aller Schärfe ausgesprochen; *Albarran* nennt ihn sogar « une confusion regrettable ».

Wenn ich bisher gezögert habe diese Angriffe zu beantworten, so kann ich doch nunmehr nicht umhin ihnen Rechnung zu tragen. Zunächst muss ich freilich zugeben, dass ich damals, den überall herrschenden Anschauungen entsprechend, die *secundäre* Stauung nicht genügend scharf von der *primären* Stauung unterschieden habe; allein hiervon abgesehen muss ich euch heute noch an den Ausführungen jenes Aufsatzes durchaus festhalten. Es ist doch ganz unmöglich ein Krankheitsbild nur aus dem Grunde zu zerreissen, weil eine eitrige Form vorkommt; würden wir in gleicher Weise z. B. beim Nierenechinococcus verfahren, so würden gleichfalls zwei gänzlich verschiedene Kranheiten herauskommen. Und bei den zwei Formen der Hydro- und Pyonephrose ist man nicht einmal stehen geblieben. *Guyon* und *Albarran* haben bereits eine dritte, eine Intermediärform, die Uropyonephrose, anerkannt; und wenn wir auf dem Wege fortfahren die Krankheiten nur nach dem Sackinhalte zu scheiden, so würden, je nachdem der Sack Blut, oder einen schmierigen, oder trockenen Brei enthält, noch weitere 3 bis 4 Formen mit besondern Namen aufgestellt werden müssen. Das ist offenbar ein durchaus falscher Weg, der in Gestrüpp und Dornen endigt, ein Weg, der weitab liegt von einer pathologisch-anatomischen Auffassung der Dinge.

Wir unterscheiden, abgesehen von der Tuberkulose, zwei Gruppen der Niereneiterungen :

1. Die Pyelonephritis, welche gelegentlich zu einer secundären Stauung, aber dann immer mit gleichzeitiger Zerstörung der Niere führt und die wir *Empyem des Nierenbeckens* oder, bei vorwiegender Betheiligung des Nierenparenchyms, *Nierenabscess* nennen.

2. Die Pyonephrose, welche aus der Infection eines durch primäre Stauung entstandenen Nierensackes hervorgeht. Da hier die Eiterung nur als ein neues Symptom zu dem bisherigen Krankheitsbilde hinzutritt, so haben wir alle Berechtigung das Gesammtleiden als *Sackniere, Cystinephrosis* zu bezeichnen. Nur diese kommt für unsere Besprechung in Betracht, da bei dem Empyem des Nierenbeckens und dem Nierenabscess erhaltende Methoden nur ganz ausnahmsweise am Platze sind.

Die Hindernisse, welche zur Aufstauung eines aseptischen Urins im Nierenbecken führen, haben ihren Sitz fast ausschliesslich im Harnleiter; denn wenn auch Erkrankungen der Blase und der Harnröhre gelegentlich zu Stauungen Anlass geben, so führen diese doch viel häufiger, fast ausschliesslich zur Pyelonephritis und nicht zur Hydronephrose. Aus diesem Grunde werden wir die Abflusshindernisse an der Einmündungsstelle des Harnleiters in die Blase bei unserer Besprechung übergehen. Im übrigen Theile des Harnleiters ist es vorwiegend der Uebergang von diesem zum Nierenbecken, in welchem die Hindernisse gelegen sind; und zwar ist diese Stelle sowohl bei angeborenen, als bei erworbenen Sacknieren bevorzugt. Bei angeborenen Sacknieren tritt das Hinderniss in Form von ringförmigen Narben und klappenartigen Falten auf. Hierzu kommen bei

erworbenen Sacknieren, zumal für die grosse Gruppe der durch
Wandernieren erzeugten, die Biegungen und winkligen Knickungen
des Canals. Endlich sind hierher die im Harnleitereingang und im
Harnleiter eingeklemmten Steine zu rechnen. Alle diese so sehr verschiedenen Hindernisse erfordern zu ihrer Beseitigung sehr verschie-
denartige Eingriffe, wie sie in der immer noch nicht erheblichen
Anzahl von Krankengeschichten verzeichnet sind, welche uns über
plastische Operationen wegen renaler Verhaltungen zu Gebote
stehen.

Die Zeit ist freilich noch kurz, seit man zum ersten Male dem
Gedanken Raum gab durch einen Eingriff am Harnleiter die ent-
sprechende Niere zu erhalten. Die erste derartige Operation machte
*Trendelenburg* im Jahre 1888; und zwar drang er auf transperitone-
alem Wege gegen die Niere vor. Seine Kranke erlag indessen an
Ileus. Den ersten glücklichen und zwar lumbalen Eingriff unternahm
*ich* im Jahre 1891; dann folgen *Fenger*, *Weller van Hook* (beide 1893),
*Kelly* und *Bardenheuer* (1894). In neuester Zeit hat sich an dem
Ausbau dieses Verfahrens ganz besonders lebhaft die französische
Chirurgie betheiligt.

Die 21 Operationen, welche, mit Ausschluss der zur Beseitigung
von Steinen im Harnleiter unternommenen, bis jetzt veröffentlicht
worden sind, wurden nach sehr verschiedenen Grundsätzen ausgeführt. Nur bei dreien derselben kam der transperitoneale Schnitt zur
Anwendung (*Trendelenburg*, *Helferich-Enderlen* und *Bazy*), von denen
nur 1 Fall heilte, während die andern beiden starben; von den
übrig bleibenden 18 Fällen, die auf lumbalem Wege operirt wurden,
heilten 17 vollständig und bei einem (*Weller van Hook*) wurde nach
vollendeter Plastik sofort zur Nephrectomie übergegangen, weil eine
vorher übersehene zweite Striktur des Harnleiters entdeckt worden
war.

Wenn wir uns zunächst mit den nicht durch Steine hervorgerufenen
Hindernissen beschäftigen, so können wir folgende 5 Gruppen von
Operationen unterscheiden, welche bisher zu deren Beseitigung in
Anwendung gezogen sind :

### A. *Operationen zur Veränderung der Form des Nierenbeckens.*

Es handelt sich fast ausschliesslich um Sacknieren, welche durch
*Verlagerung des Organs* erzeugt worden sind und welche in den
meisten Fällen die Form der intermittirenden Hydronephrose angenommen haben. Hier gehört es zu den gewöhnlichen Erscheinungen,

dass einzelne Theile des Nierenbeckens sich erheblich stärker erweitern als andere, so dass dieselben sich blindsackartig aus ihrer Umgebung hervorheben.

Die Verfahren zur Beseitigung dieses Zustandes sind folgende :

1. Die Nephropexie, von *Guyon* im Jahre 1889 vorgeschlagen, gestattet den verbogenen Harnleiter zu strecken und die Hindernisse für den Urinabfluss zu beseitigen.

2. Die Harnleiterstreckung im engern Sinne, die Ureterolysorthosis nach Rafin (Verrière) besteht in der operativen Lösung des in seiner Verkrümmung angewachsenen Harnleiters, welcher demnächst durch Nephropexie in normaler Stellung festgehalten wird.

3. Die Beckenfaltung (Pyeloplicatio, besser Pyeloptyxis) nach *J. Israel.* Das eröffnete und genau abgetastete Nierenbecken wurde durch mehrere Nahtreihen geschlossen in der Weise, dass zunächst die erste Nahtreihe, ohne die Schleimhaut zu betheiligen, die äussern Sackflächen nach Art *Lembert*'scher Nähte aneinander zog. Die folgenden Nahtreihen brachten weiter ausgreifend immer neue Theile der Sackwand in Berührung, so dass die Ausbuchtung aussen verschwinden, dafür aber innen ein Vorsprung entstehen musste. Zugleich wurde auch die Umgebung der Harnleitermündung durch einige Nähte beeinflusst.

In ähnlicher Weise verfuhr *Albarran*; er nennt sein Verfahren Capitonnage, Unterpolsterung. In einem zweiten Falle schnitt er ein grösseres Stück des Nierenbeckens aus und vernähte den Schnitt.

Diese verschiedenen Operationsweisen sind zwar alle verwendbar, aber doch in sehr verschiedenem Umfange. Die einfache Nephropexie ist am wichtigsten; sie heilt eine grössere Zahl beginnender, oder bereits ausgeprägter Sacknieren, bei denen wenigstens der Harnleiter noch leicht durch Zug gestreckt werden kann. Ist Letzterer aber bereits auf der Unterlage, oder mit der Sackwand verwachsen, so gewährt *Rafin's* Verfahren noch die Möglichkeit eine Streckung vorzunehmen. Ob diese allein einen Erfolg erzielen kann, das lässt sich bei starker Erhebung der Niere mit einiger Wahrscheinlichkeit beurtheilen; denn die Heilung kann nur erfolgen, wenn nach der Streckung der Inhalt des Nierenbeckens vollkommen abfliesst. Geschieht das nicht, so ist zur Beseitigung des Hindernisses eins der später zu nennenden Verfahren in Betracht zu ziehen.

Was die Beckenfaltung anbetrifft, so kann diese für sich allein in nur wenigen Fällen etwas nützen. Denn bleibt ein Hinderniss bestehen, so wird das Becken bald genug sich von neuem dehnen; und besteht kein Hinderniss, so wird die Harnleiterstreckung für sich allein genügen, um eine allmähliche Zusammenziehung des Sackes zu bewirken. Nur wenn die Ausbuchtung bereits sehr alt ist und wenn in Folge dessen die Sackwandmusculatur Schaden gelitten hat, selbst vollständig zu Grunde gegangen ist, kann die Verkleinerung des Beckens durch Faltung oder Ausschneidung der Wand in Frage kommen.

Die Ausschneidung des Sackes ist auch bei der Hydronephrose in Hufeisennieren in Betracht zu ziehen. Ich operirte einen solchen Fall im Jahre 1895 auf lumbalem Wege mit vollem Erfolge so, dass der ganze Sack bis auf zwei kleine Lappen ausgeschält und abgetragen, die Lappen aber miteinander vernäht wurden. *Duret* verfuhr in ähnlicher Weise, nur mit transperitonealem Vorgehen. Sein Kranker starb und die Section deckte einen Blasenkrebs auf.

B. *Anastomosenbildung.*

Auch hier haben wir drei Unterformen zu unterscheiden :

1. Anastomosenbildung zwischen zwei Bezirken desselben Harnleiters, *Uretero-Ureterostomie* nach *Kelly*. Nach *C. Fenger* wurde die Operation im Jahre 1892 in folgender Weise ausgeführt : Bei Gelegenheit einer Hystero-Myomectomie war der eine Harnleiter unterbunden und durchschnitten worden. *Kelly* suchte die beiden Stümpfe auf, schlitzte den untern Stumpf ein wenig, führte das obere in das untere Ende ein und verband sie durch einige Nähte, welche nur die Adventitia durchdrangen.

2. Anastomosenbildung zwischen Harnleiter und Nierenbecken, *Ureteropyelostomie* nach *Trendelenburg* kommt bei zu hoher Einmündung des Harnleiters in das Nierenbecken mit gleichzeitiger Anlötung des Harnleiters an die Sackwand in Frage. Mittels eines geknöpften Messers spaltet man vom Innern des Hohlraumes aus Sackwand und Harnleiter zugleich, und zwar von der Einmündungsstelle des letztern bis auf den tiefsten Punkt des Sackes. Sodann vernäht man an den Schnitträndern mittels einer Nahtreihe jeder Seits die Schleimhaut des Harnleiters mit derjenigen der Sackwand. Es bleibt ein weit offener Trichter, durch welchen aller Harn bequem abfliesst.

Operationen dieser Art machten *Trendelenburg, Bardenheuer, Helferich* und *Albarran*.

3. Anastomosenbildung zwischen Nierenbecken und Blase, *Cystipyelostomie, Nephrocystanastomose (Reisinger)*.

Auf dem Chirurgencongresse von 1900 zu Berlin machte *Reisinger-*

*Mainz* Mittheilung über einen Fall von Hydronephrose in einer vor dem Promontorium und dem Kreuzbein gelegenen, also fötal verlangerten Niere. Die Diagnose wurde erst nach Eröffnung des Leibes gestellt, zunächst eine abdominale Nierenbeckenfistel angelegt, später aber eine Verbindung zwischen der letztern und der nur 5 Centimeter entfernten Blase mittels einer Doppelnaht angelegt. Die Heilung erfolgte und der Kranke war fortan frei von allen Beschwerden.

Für diese Gruppe von Operationen ist zu bemerken, dass sie überall da gerechtfertigt sind, wo man im Stande ist, die Bildung todter Räume zu vermeiden; ist das aber nicht möglich, so ist der Eingriff verwerflich, weil er unfehlbar zur Ablagerung von Harnsalzen und zur Steinbildung führen muss.

C. *Plastische Operationen mit und ohne Harnleiterresection.*

Auch hier lassen sich wiederum mehrere Formen unterscheiden :

1. Durchschneidung des verengernden Gewebes in der Längsrichtung und Naht in der Richtung des Schnites. Gewöhnlich handelt es sich um Klappenbildung und spaltförmige Verziehung der Harnleitermündung; nur in einem Falle scheint *Fenger* auch eine *narbige* Harnleiterverengerung in gleicher Weise behandelt zu haben.

Der freie Rand der Klappe wird mit dem geknöpften Messer bis zur Wiederherstellung der Lichtung eingeschnitten. *Gerster* wiederholte diesen Einschnitt an drei verschiedenen Stellen. Dann wurde nach der für den Magen erdachten Methode von *Heinecke-Mikulicz* die Wunde von oben nach unten vernäht, so dass Nierenbeckenschleimhaut an Harnleiterschleimhaut gefügt wurde. Nach dieser Methode operirten *Bardenheuer, Israel, Küster, Gerster* und *H. Morris* je einmal, *Fenger* dreimal.

2. Resection des Harnleiters und Vereinigung der Stümpfe durch die Naht. In dieser Form ist die Operation noch nicht gemacht worden, wahrscheinlich aus Furcht vor einer später eintretenden Verengerung. Immerhin sind Fälle denkbar, in welchen kaum etwas Anderes übrig bleibt, falls man nicht die Niere opfern will z. B. bei zweifacher Striktur des Harnleiters. Man würde dann aber die Resectionsschnitte schief auf die Längsachse des Canals zu legen haben, um eine etwa später wiedereinsetzende Verengerung auf verschiedene Ebenen des Harnleiterquerschnittes zu vertheilen und dadurch unschädlich zu machen.

3. Resection des Harnleiters und Einfügung des untern Stumpfes in das Becken, *Pyeloneostomie* nach *Küster*. Die Methode ist nur auf hochgradige Harnleiterverengerungen anwendbar, welche ihren Sitz dicht unterhalb des Nierenbeckens haben. Der enge Theil des Harn-

leiters wird quer resecirt, der untere Stumpf soweit gelockert, dass
er bequem durch eine Schnittöffnung in das Nierenbecken hinein-
gezogen werden kann, dann an der Vorderseite 1 bis 1 1/2 Centimeter
lang geschlitzt, der Stumpf auf der Hinterfläche des Nierenbeckens
ausgebreitet und durch Nähte befestigt. Ebenso wird die behufs
Durchtrittes des Harnleiters angelegte Oeffnung im Nierenbecken
wieder geschlossen und mit der Harnleiterwand vernäht. Die trichter-
förmige Harnleiteröffnung liegt dann am tiefsten Punkte des Nierenbeckens. Zur Lendenwunde wird ein Drain nach aussen geführt.

Die Operation ist nach dem Vorgange *Küster's* von *Bazy*, *Delbet*,
*Bardenheuer* und *Weller van Hook* ausgeführt worden, von letzterem
allerdings nur so, dass er unmittelbar an die Vollendung der Plastik
die Nephrectomie anschloss. Die übrigen vier Fälle wurden geheilt.


Nach ausführlicher Darlegung der Operationen, welche durch
Narben, Klappen und Knickungen im Harnleitereingange und im
Harnleiter selber nothwendig werden, können wir uns über die viel
einfacheren Verhältnisse, wie sie durch einen im Harnleiter festsitzen-
den Stein geschaffen werden, erheblich kürzer fassen. Ist einmal der
Sitz des Steines festgestellt worden, so bleibt nur übrig ihn entweder
nach unten in die Blase, oder nach oben ins Becken zu verschieben,
oder ihn durch einen Schnitt in die Harnleiterwand freizulegen und
herauszuziehen. Ersteres, die Verschiebung des Steines nach unten
ist meines Wissens bisher noch niemals gelungen, auch dürfte dies
wohl nur in seltenen Ausnahmsfällen zu erwarten sein. Dagegen ist
es nach *J. Israel's* Vorgange einige Male geglückt den Stein einfach
den Weg wieder zurücklegen zu lassen, den er vom Becken her
bereits gemacht hatte. Zu diesem Zwecke, wie auch für die nachfol-
gende Operation ist die Anlegung eines langen Schnittes durch die
seitliche und vordere Bauchwand nothwendig, um das Bauchfell
weithin ablösen und den Harnleiter in seinem Verlaufe übersehen zu
können. Unterhalb des sicht- und fühlbaren Steines umfasst man
dann den Canal von beiden Seiten und sucht jenen vorsichtig und
ohne Gewalt nach oben zu verdrängen. Weicht er, so fährt man mit
den Druck- und Schiebebewegungen so lange fort bis der Stein im
Nierenbecken erscheint, dort mit einer Zange erfasst und ausgezogen
werden kann. — Ist derselbe aber zu fest eingeklemmt, so spannt
man die Harnleiterwand mit linkem Daumen und Zeigefinger, schnei-
det zwischen diesen in der Längsrichtung ein, bis der Stein freiliegt,
und drückt oder zieht ihn aus. Es darf dann niemals versäumt werden
durch Einführen einer Sonde nach der Blase hin sich davon zu über-

zeugen, ob der Weg nach dieser Richtung frei ist. Wäre dies der Fall, so würde man den Längsschnitt sofort wieder durch einige Knopfnähte schliessen können, welche aber die Schleimhaut nicht mit umfassen dürften.

Nach einer mir von *H. Morris* mündlich gemachten Mittheilung hat derselbe einen im untern Ende des Harnleiters fest eingeklommene Stein auf sacralem Wege zugängig gemacht und ausgezogen.

Eine der grössesten Schwierigkeiten für die Durchführung der vorstehend geschilderten Operationen liegt in den Hindernissen, welche sich der Auffindung der Einmündungsstelle des Harnleiters in das Becken widersetzen. Nun hat nach *Boccard* im Jahre 1896 *Jaboulay* eine eigenartige Nephrotomie gemacht der Art nämlich, dass er den eröffneten Sack von innenher packte, nach aussen hervorzog, also völlig umstülpte und in dieser Lage durch einige Nähte festhielt. Die Heilung erfolgte bis auf eine feine Fistel. So wenig nachahmungswerth uns dies Verfahren an sich erscheint, so zeigt es doch in der leichten Umstülpbarkeit des Hydronephrosensackes den einzuschlagenden Weg.

Im Jahre 1899 hat denn auch *Fenger* ein Verfahren zur Aufsuchung des Harnleiters mitgetheilt, welches der Operation *Jaboulay's* im Principe vollkommen gleicht. Man soll, so lehrt er, nach dem Lendenschnitte den Sack schrittweis hervorziehen und umdrehen; insbesondere, so fügen wir hinzu, wird man an der medialen Sackwand zu suchen haben. Bei diesem schrittweisen Vorgehen ist die Harnleitermündung nicht leicht zu übersehen. Schlimmsten Falles würde man versuchen können sich den Harnleiter von hintenher freizulegen, ihn bis ins Nierenbecken zu verfolgen und dadurch den Punkt zu bestimmen, an welchem man auf der Innenseite zu suchen hätte. In die gefundene Harnleitermündung ist eine Sonde einzuführen, welche Sitz und Art des Hindernisses feststellt.

Meine Herren. Es brauchen heutigen Tages keine Worte darüber verloren zu werden, dass die Nephrectomie gegenüber der Sackniere nur als ein nach Möglichkeit einzuschränkender Nothbehelf angesehen werden muss; beträgt doch die Sterblichkeit bei Nephrectomie meinen Zusammenstellungen nach 29 %, bei Nephrotomie oder besser Pyelotomie nur 8 %. Freilich wird den Vertretern der Nephrotomie mit Recht die ungeheure Zahl der Fistelbildungen entgegengehalten, welche in mehr als der Hälfte der Fälle hinterbleibt. Die Vertheidigungsstellung derjenigen Chirurgen, welche die Nephrotomie bevorzugen, würde deshalb eine ungünstige sein, wenn ihnen nicht durch die conservativen Operationen am Harnleiter eine ausserordentliche Unterstützung zu Theil geworden wäre. Wir stehen erst im Beginne der Entwickelung derselben; aber schon heute darf es ausgesprochen werden, *dass die Harnleiteroperationen die typischen Operationen der Zukunft für jede Form der Sackniere darstellen, auf welche unter allen Umständen in erster Linie zurückgegriffen werden muss.*

Und so dürfte denn auch für die Nierenchirurgie es mehr und mehr in die Ueberzeugung der Aerzte eindringen, dass es erhebender und verdienstvoller ist ein gefährdetes Glied zu erhalten, als durch seine Wegnahme den Körper zu verstümmeln.

---

## CONSERVATIVE OPERATIONS FOR RENAL RETENTION

*RAPPORT*

### by Dr. CHRISTIAN FENGER,

de Chicago.

It is only in the last decade that this new branch of surgery has come into existence, and as it is still very young and not well developed, the technique of the methods of operation is not yet well defined. The number of operations already performed, however — and there are about thirty on record — permits us to form and idea, not only as to the justifiability of the object aimed at; namely, the salvation of the kidney, doomed to removal, which may be considered as firmly established, but also as to the general direction in which the different methods of operating, which are already well grouped, must be developed for further perfection.

This subject has already been made accessible to the profession at large by the articles in the larger modern hand-books — in France by Albarran[1] and Tuffier[2] and in the English literature by Henry Morris[3] and Fenger[4].

1. J. ALBARRAN. Maladies du rein. *Traité de Chirurgie*, par Le Dentu et Delbet, vol. VIII, p. 805.

2. TUFFIER. Appareil urinaire. *Traité de Chirurgie*, par Duplay et Reclus, vol. VII.

3. Henry MORRIS. Hunterian Lectures on the Surgery of the Kidney. *British Medical Journal*, March 26, 1898, p. 809.

4. C. FENGER. Surgery of the Ureter. American Text-Book of Genito-Urinary Diseases, Philadelphia, 1898, p. 470.

The field for this group of operations has thus far been limited to the kidney and the upper portion of the ureter and it is this territory that has been the object for direct operative attacks in renal retention. This has naturally come to pass because it is accessible and the operations are reasonably safe and easy, and because the majority of the unilateral retentions are located in this region.

Unilateral obstruction to the flow of secreted urine may be located from the kidney downward :

*a*) In the neck of a calyx;

*b*) In one branch of the ureter;

*c*) At the exit of the ureter from the renal pelvis, and

*d*) In the course of the ureter.

It will be seen from the tabulated statement of cases that the exit of the ureter from the renal pelvis was by far the most common location for the obstruction : 26 operations for obstruction in this locality are recorded as against 1 in a branch of the ureter and 5 in the ureter below the pelvis.

There have been excluded from this consideration :

*a*) Nephrotomy and drainage;

*b*) Nephropexy, to correct and straighten a bend in the upper end of the ureter caused by descent of the kidney;

*c*) Catheterization of the ureter from below to overcome retention from stricture or bending.

These procedures have been excluded, not because they do not deserve earnest consideration, as they are in some cases sufficient for cure, but because this paper must be limited to operations which directly attack the place of obstruction. I shall also leave out of consideration those cases of obstruction in which renal calculus is the cause of the retention, which is relieved by the removal of the stone.

I. — *Obstruction located in the kidney; namely, in the calyces or in one branch of the ureter, partial cystonephrosis.* — The operation to relieve this condition is bisection of the kidney and division of the partition walls between the sacs and the pelvis, thus making an unilocular, out of a multilocular cavity or sac. If no obstruction be found at the exit of the pelvis or in the ureter, no further operation is required as in removal of stones from the calyces or pelvis of the kidney. If no stones are found, it is probable that there is obstruction below this point in one of the locations mentioned, and this must be overcome by one or another of the operations which have been devised for the relief of obstruction in these localities.

Hæmorrhage from the division of voluminous partition walls may be overcome by the Paquelin cautery, ligation or continuous suture.

Only one case of this variety has been recorded : by Fenger (n° 9).

II.   *Obstruction located at the exit of the ureter from the renal pelvis.*
— This variety possesses naturally the greatest practical interest as
it is the most frequent site of non-calculous obstruction. Twenty-six
of the operations collected were for obstruction at this point and the
methods of operation were quite varied.  The condition found was
either valve-formation without stricture of the ureter, from unilateral
dilatation of the pelvis and consequent oblique insertion of the ureter
on the side of the dilated pelvis rather than at its lowest point, or
stricture of the ureter at its exit with insertion either at the lowest
part of the pelvis or on the side higher up.

The operations to re-establish free passage of the urine through the
place of obstruction have varied with the existence or non-existence
of stricture of the ureter, and with the point from which the valve-
formation is attacked, either from within through an opening in the
pelvis or the bisected kidney — transpelvic operation, — or from
without — extrapelvic operation.

Finally, the distorted shape of the pelvis has been made the object
of operation — pyeloplication and capitonnage.

*Transpelvic operation on valve — section of uretero-pelvic spur; —
amelioration of ureteral orifice.* —  This is the oldest of the plastic
operations in this locality and was first done by Trendelenburg in 1886.
Nine cases are on record, operated upon by Trendelenburg, Fenger,
Mynter, Bardenheuer, Fenger, Helferich, Israel, Gerster and Fenger,
in chronological order.

Valve-formation from oblique implantation of the ureter was first
seen through the divided pelvis or kidney (cystonephrotic sac); it was
natural, therefore, that the first attempts at widening the opening into
the ureter should be made from inside the pelvis.

The valve formed by the oblique implantation of the ureter into the
side of the dilated pelvis is seen through an incision in the dilated
pelvis or through the bisected kidney, and the valve; that is, the wall
of the pelvis and ureter in contact with each other, divided. This is done
either by one incision sufficiently long to secure an amply wide opening
into the ureter or, better, to the bottom of the pelvis, or by multiple
incisions of the valve (which was incised in three places by Gerster).

In all the cases the incision was closed transversely by sutures, one
of which united the upper and lower ends of the incision and others
which united the divided walls of the ureter to those of the pelvis
throughout the whole extent of the divided surface.

This operation was performed in nine cases : two patients died, one from ileus (Trendelenburg N° 1) and one from uremia in a case of bilateral disease (Helferich N° 12). In two cases the operation was not successful : in one, where obliteration of the ureter at the seat of operation followed (Fenger, N° 23), and one in which the operation was temporarily successful as the ureter remained open for about one year, after which relapse occurred, the ureter closed and a second operation became necessary (Gerster, N° 15).

In five cases the operation was successful (Fenger, N° 5; Mynter, N° 7; Bardenheuer, N° 8; Fenger, N° 10, and Israel, N° 14).

*Extrapelvic Operations.* — 1. Resection of ureter and reimplantation in renal pelvis, uretero-pyelo-neostomy (Küster). Six resections have been made by Küster, Van Hook, Bardenheuer, Bazy, Bazy and Morris. A stricture in the upper end of the ureter led Küster to excise the strictured part of the ureter although he had planned to make a transpelvic division of the valve. Resection and reimplantation proved successful in Küster's case (N° 2), Bardenheuer's (N° 6) and in one case of Bazy's (N° 17.) Bazy's second patient, a case of calculous anuria (N° 18), died from sepsis : iodoform poisoning. In Van Hook's case (N° 3), the result was uncertain, as an extensive stricture in the ureter below necessitated immediate nephrectomy. In Morris's case (N° 22), the operation was planned but the operator abandoned his plan and made an immediate nephrectomy which he considered to be demanded by the extreme atrophy of the ureter.

It will thus be seen that resection and reimplantation of the ureter in the pelvis proved successful in three and was abandoned for nephrectomy in two cases. It was followed by death in one case from sepsis, a result that cannot be considered as attributable to the operation as such.

2. Operation on ureter and pelvis at the seat of the valve or stricture (Fenger). It was the same condition that obtained in Küster's case; namely, a stricture in the pelvic end of the ureter, that caused Fenger to abandon an intended transpelvic operation and to resort to extrapelvic division of the ureter from below the stricture up into the pelvis, followed by transverse union of the longitudinal wound.

This operation has been performed in eleven cases and none of the patients has died. In some of the cases there was stenosis of the pelvic end of the ureter and in others the obstruction was caused solely by the oblique implantation of a normal ureter. In one case, (Fenger, N° 20), the operation was unsuccessful and was followed by nephrectomy. In the other ten cases (Fenger, N°s 4, 9, 30; Albarran, N°s 25, 26; Bardenheuer, N° 16; Richardson, N° 19; Delbet, N° 24;

Kelly, N° 21 ; Morris, N° 28), the operation was followed by successful functional results. In one of Albarran's cases (N° 25), the operation was combined with partial excision of the dilated pelvis — capitonnage — to re-establish the normal shape of the pelvis.

In one case only (Bazy, N° 17), was the kidney approached through the peritoneal cavity by lateral laparotomy; in the other ten cases extraperitoneal lumbar incision was made.

3. Pyeloplication. — Plastic operation on the renal pelvis (Israel) ; capitonnage (Albarran). In lateral implantation, when the ureteral orifice is of normal caliber, the passage of urine would be free were the ureter inserted at the lowest part of the pelvis or if the normal shape of the pelvis were re-established. This has been accomplished by the following operations on the pelvis :

*a*) Shortening the excess of pelvic wall by folding it in toward the lumen of the pelvis and uniting the folds by sutures — (pyeloplication of Israel; pelvioplication of Albarran).

*b*) Excision of part of the wall of the dilated pelvis and closure of the defect by sutures (capitonnage of Albarran).

In Israel's case (N° 15) the operation sufficed to re-establish the flow of urine and effect a cure. In the case of Albarran (N° 26), pelvioplication was made and in case N° 25, the same operator made a partial excision of the superabundant portion of the sac-wall with a portion of the kidney, but in both of these cases the operation was combined with extrapelvic operation on the valve.

Israel's case is the only one in which pyeloplication alone was effective in relieving the obstruction.

III. — *Obstruction located in the Ureter.* — 1. Ureterolysorthosis. This operation, first performed by Rafin and reported by Verrière, consists in loosening the adhesions around a bend in the ureter. The upper end of the ureter below the renal pelvis is made impervious by a bend due to descent of a floating kidney. In Rafin's case the bend was double and S-shaped. The bend was buried in connective tissue adhesions which prevented the straightening of the ureter. After division of these adhesions without opening the ureter, it was straightened and remained straight and permeable after the kidney had been replaced and retained by nephropexy. One successful case (N° 27) is reported by Rafin.

2. Plastic operation on the ureter (Fenger). Longitudinal division of the strictured or obliterated ureter through the stricture into the normal ureter above and below it, followed by transverse union of the ureteral incision by folding the ureter upon itself has been performed

by Fenger in two cases and was effective in both. In one (Nº 11), a valve was excised from the inside of the opened ureter at the point of occlusion; in the other (Nº 29), complete occlusion of the ureter had followed a plastic operation on a stricture caused by a stone in the ureter. The second plastic operation through the then obliterated ureter was successful notwithstanding that great tension was made on the ureter after folding and suture. This case demonstrated that an operation for re-opening a closed ureter may be successful after an unsuccessful attempt has been made, and this justifies even repeated attempts to re-establish the patency of the ureter and thereby save the kidney from removal.

**Conclusions.** — 1. *Choice of operation.* — The choice of operation comes into question only in the cases of obstruction at the pelvic orifice of the ureter (unilateral implantation with or without stricture of the ureter at this point), and lies between transpelvic plastic operation, extrapelvic incision and plastic operation, and pyeloplication.

Transpelvic plastic operation may be the operation of necessity in large cystonephrotic sacs because of the difficulty in reaching the ureter outside of the pelvis (in nine cases, two were followed by obliteration). In smaller sacs with moderate dilatation of the pelvis, I consider extrapelvic plastic operation preferable to transpelvic plastic operation and to resection and reimplantation of the ureter (ureteropyelo-neostomy). Resection was practised in six cases. In two, the operation was incomplete and was followed by nephrectomy. It was successful in three cases and functionally successful in one. One patient died from iodoform poisoning or sepsis. Thus it proved effective in all the four cases in which the operation was completed.

Extrapelvic plastic operation was chosen by most of the operators. It was performed eleven times, was successful in ten cases with good functional results and was unsuccessful in one case. It would thus seem that this should be the operation of choice by reason of the results obtained and because its technique is relatively simple.

2. *Danger to life.* — The risk to life from this entire group of conservative operations for renal retention is small. Three of the thirty patients died, but in none of them was death due to the operation per se; in Trendelenburg's case, the patient died from ileus and both Helferich's and Bazy's patients had bilateral disease and could not have been saved by nephrectomy.

3. *Effect of the Operations.* — The result of the operations to reestablish evacuation of urine and thus save the kidney were as follows :

## Chronological Table of Operations for Renal Retention.

| No. | OPERATOR | DATE | OPERATION | RECOVERY | DEATH | MUCOUS FISTULA | NEPHRECTOMY FOR URINARY FISTULA |
|---|---|---|---|---|---|---|---|
| 1 | Trendelenburg. | 1886. | Transpelvic division of valve. | | Ileus. | | |
| 2 | Küster. | July 14, 1891. | Resection of ureter. Implantation in pelvis. Uretero-pyelo-neostomy | » | | | |
| 3 | Fenger. | May 31, 1892. | Transpelvic plastic operation in valve. | » | | | |
| 4 | Fenger. | Nov. 26, 1892. | Extrapelvic plastic operation. Stricture of upper end of ureter. | » | | | |
| 5 | Van Hook | 1892. | Resection. | | | | » |
| 6 | Bardenheuer. | March 24, 1893. | Resection. Uretero-pyelo-neostomy. | » | | » | |
| 7 | Mynter. | Aug. 14, 1893. | Transpelvic plastic operation. | » | | | |
| 8 | Bardenheuer. | Jan. 28, 1894. | Transpelvic plastic operation. | » | | » | |
| 9 | Fenger. | Sept. 17, 1894. | Extrapelvic operation on valve at exit of pelvis. | » | | | |
| 10 | Fenger. | Nov. 17, 1894. | Transpelvic plastic operation on valve. | » | | | |
| 9* | Fenger. | April 13, 1895. | Bisection of kidney. Division of valve in lower branch of ureter. | » | | | |
| 11 | Fenger. | Aug. 6, 1895. | Plastic operation on ureter. Excision of valve. | » | | | |
| 12 | Helferich | Nov. 13, 1895. | Extrapelvic plastic operation. Bilateral disease. | | Uremia 9th day. | | |
| 13 | Israel | 1896. | Pyeloplication. | » | | | |
| 14 | Israel | 1896. | Transpelvic plastic operation on valve. | » | | | |
| 15 | Gerster | Feb. 6, 1896. | Transpelvic plastic operation on valve. | » | | » | |
| 16 | Bardenheuer. | Feb. 17, 1896. | Extrapelvic plastic operation. | » | | | |
| 17 | Bazy. | July 27, 1896. | Resection-uretero-pyelo-neostomy | | Sepsis, or iodoform poisoning. | | |
| 18 | Bazy. | Oct. 13, 1896. | Resection-uretero-pyelo-neostomy. | | | | |
| 19 | Richardson. | Nov. 11, 1896. | Extrapelvic operation. | » | | | |
| 20 | Fenger. | March, 1897. | Extrap. operat. Unpublished. | | | | |
| 21 | Kelly | 1897. | Extrapelvic operation. | » | | | |
| 22 | Morris. | 1897. | Resection attempted. | » | | | » |
| 23 | Fenger. | Feb. 22, 1898. | Transpelvic operation on valve. Obliteration of ureter at place of operation. | | | | » |
| 24 | Delbet. | 1898. | Uretero-pyelo-neostomy. | » | | | |
| 25 | Albarran. | 1898. | Uretero-pyelo-neostomy. | » | | | |
| 26 | Albarran. | 1898. | Pyeloplication. | » | | | |
|  | Albarran. | 1898. | Extrapelvic plastic operation. | » | | | » |
| 27 | Rafin (Verrière). | Nov. 12, 1898. | Ureterolysorthosis. | » | | | » |
| 28 | Morris. | 1898. | Extrapelvic plastic operation. | » | | | |
| 29 | Fenger | May 23, 1899. | Extrapelvic plastic operation on ureter. Unpublished. | » | | | |
| 30 | Fenger. | July 9, 1899. | Extrapelvic plastic operation on pelvis and ureter. Unpublished. | » | | | |

## Table of Operations for Renal Retention.

| CHRONOLOGICAL NUMBER | OPERATOR | DATE | AGE | SEX | DISEASE | OPERATION | RESULT | | | | | BIBLIOGRAPHICAL NUMBER |
|---|---|---|---|---|---|---|---|---|---|---|---|---|
| | | | | | | | RECOVERY | DEATH | MUCOUS FISTULA | NEPHRECTOMY FOR URINARY FISTULA | | |
| | | | | | **I. Branch of Ureter.** | | | | | | | |
| 9 | Fenger . . . ⓑ | April 13, 1895. | 22 | M | Gonorrhea. Renal colic. Lumbar nephrotomy. Passage of stones hrough fistula. Intermittent obstruction of ureter. Operation for oblique implantation and stricture of pelvic end of ureter. Urinary fistula. Pyelitis. Sacculated kidney. | Incision through fistula and old cicatrix into sacculated kidney. Could not find entrance to ureter. Bisection of kidney and division of partition walls between calyces. Ureter patent. Plastic operation on ureteral entrance; incision with transverse union of wound. Four months later reunion of bisected kidney. Five months thereafter fistula closed spontaneously. . . . . . . . . . . . . . | » | | | | » |

**II. Ureter and Pelvis for Valve Formation or Oblique insertion with or without Stenosis of upper End of Ureter.**

*a. Transpelvic Operation on Valve.*

| CHRONOLOGICAL NUMBER | OPERATOR | DATE | AGE | SEX | DISEASE | OPERATION | RECOVERY | DEATH | MUCOUS FISTULA | NEPHRECTOMY FOR URINARY FISTULA | BIBLIOGRAPHICAL NUMBER |
|---|---|---|---|---|---|---|---|---|---|---|---|
| 1 | Trendelenburg, | 1886. | » | » | Large hydronephrosis. . . . | Anterior wall of sac opened by lateral laparotomy. Division of ureter to lower part of sac. Suture of divided borders of ureter to inner wall of sac. Displacement of ureteral opening to bottom of sac. | | Ileus. | | | |
| 5 | Fenger. . . . | May 31, 1892. | 28 | F | Valvular stricture or stenosis of pelvic orifice of ureter in somewhat floating kidney. Intermittent hydronephrosis for 8 years. . . | Nephrotomy in interval between attacks. No stone in pelvis. Pelvic origin of ureter not found. Incision of pelvis. Valvular opening seen. Plastic operation on valve. Fixation of floating kidney. . | » | | | | » |
| 7 | Mynter . . . . | Aug. 14, 1893. | 25 | M | Intermittent hydronephrosis for 12 years . . . . . . . | Lumbar incision. Valve formation. Transpelvic operation on valve through incision one inch long, prolonged downward through valvular stricture. | » | | | | » |
| 8 | Bardenheuer . | Jan. 28, 1894. | 45 | F | Right pyonephrosis. . . . | Bisection of kidney. Intrapelvic division of ureter and sac to bottom of sac. Union of ureter to sac. | » | | » | | » |

## Table of Operations for Renal Retention (continued).

| CHRONOLOGICAL NUMBER | OPERATOR | DATE | AGE | SEX | DISEASE | OPERATION | RECOVERY | DEATH | MUCOUS FISTULA | NEPHRECTOMY FOR URINARY FISTULA | BIBLIOGRAPHICAL NUMBER |
|---|---|---|---|---|---|---|---|---|---|---|---|
| | | | | | | II. *a. Continued.* | | | | | |
| 10 | Fenger . . . | Nov. 17, 1894. | 28 | F | Large, aseptic remittent cystonephrosis in movable kidney for 7 months. . . . . | Lumbar nephrotomy and drainage. Two months later sac retracted one half. Transpelvic operation on valve. Division of valve of ureter and pelvis to bottom. Suture . . . . . . . . . . . | » | | | | » |
| 12 | Helferich. . . | Nov. 13, 1895. | 25 | F | Intermittent left hydro-or pyonephrosis. . . . . . . | Bisection of kidney. Division of ureter. Implantation in lower end of divided sac. Uremia. Bilateral disease. | | Uremia 9th day. | | | » |
| 11 | Israel. . . . . | 1896. | 11 | M | Right intermittent hydro-or pyonephrosis, colic, etc., for 2 years. . . . . . . . | Lumbar incision. Kidney double ordinary size. Lateral implantation and bend at origin of ureter. Adhesions. Incision in posterior wall of pelvis. Valve divided with scissors. Ureteral mucosa united to pelvic mucosa. No permanent catheter. . | » | | | | » |
| 15 | Gerster. . . . | Feb. 6, 1896. | 9 | M | Traumatism (rupture of kidney or ureter) in 1895. Hematuria. 6 months later tumor in right hypochondrium containing 2 quarts of urine. Large aseptic cystonephrosis for 6 months oblique implant. and strict. of pelvic end of ureter . . | Transpelvic operation. Division of valve and stricture in 3 places, and partial excision of valve. Lumbar fistula closed after 6 months, remained closed for 6 months, when it re-opened, necessitating a second operation. . . . . . . . . . . . | » | » | » | » | » |
| 25 | Fenger . . . . | Feb. 22, 1898. | 25 | F | Right intermittent hydro-nephrosis for 5 years . . . | Lumbar incision. Multilocular hydronephrosis. Incision of sac. Eversion of its inner side. Division of partition walls between dilated calyces. Intra-pelvic division of exit or valve of obliquely inserted ureter and corresponding wall of pelvis to bottom. Suture of ureter to pelvis. Fistula 3 months later. Extrapelvic plastic operation. Ureter completely obliterated. Valve in lower end of ureter persisting. Urinary fistula, 1899, nephrectomy. | | | | » | » |

## Table of Operations for Renal Retention (continued).

| CHRONOLOGICAL NUMBER | OPERATOR | DATE | AGE | SEX | DISEASE | OPERATION | RESULT | | | | BIBLIOGRAPHICAL NUMBER |
|---|---|---|---|---|---|---|---|---|---|---|---|
| | | | | | | | RECOVERY | DEATH | MUCOUS FISTULA | NEPHRECTOMY FOR URINARY FISTULA | |
| | | | | | *II. b. Resection and Re-implantation of Ureter. Extrapelvic.* | | | | | | |
| 2 | Küster . . . . | July 19, 1891. | 11 | M | Left open hydronephrosis. Lumbar nephrotomy. Vesical anuria and fistula. One year later, dilatation of fistula. Catheterization of ureter impossible. Septic pyelitis . . . . . . . | Lumbar extraperitoneal incision. Ureter not found. Incision of dilated pelvis. Ureter in or on posterior wall of sac. Division of pelvic wall of ureter prevented by stricture of ureter 2 cm. below pelvis. Division of ureter to stricture. Resection of ureter. Divided end of ureter unfolded and sutured to opening in sac. Five months later fistula was closed by curettting and dilating. Canal closed by sutures. . . . . . . | » | | | | » |
| 5 | Van Hook . . . | 1892. | 19 | » | Infected cystonephrosis. Nephrotomy-urinary fistula. Oblique implantation of valve . . . . . . . | Resection of ureter. Reimplantation in pelvis. Exploration of ureter below. Ureter obliterated for several inches. Nephrectomy . . . . . . . | | | » | ● | » |
| 6 | Bardenheuer . | May 24, 1893. | 49 | M | Right cystonephrosis . . . . | Lumbar operation. Unilateral oblique implantation for 5 cm. Resection of ureter. Implantation in deepest part of sac. Small fistula 6 months later. | » | | » | | » |
| 17 | Bazy . . . . . | July 27, 1896. | 40 | M | Non-intermittent hydronephrosis . . . . . . . | Transperitoneal operation. Median incision. Ureter inserted at middle of sac. Resection of 4 cm. of ureter. Implantation in lower portion of sac. Resection of portion of pelvic sac. Catheter from ureter through pelvis and out through abdominal wound. . . . . . . | » | | | | » |
| 18 | Bazy . . . . . | Oct. 13, 1896. | 48 | M | Hematuria. No pain. Large right kidney. Calculous anuria for 5 days. . . . . | Lumbar incision. Bilobate kidney. Stone and old coagulum in pelvis. Ureter very hard and dilated. Resection and implantation. Death. Operation a mechanical success. . . . . . . | | Iodoform poisoning or sepsis. | | | » |
| 22 | H. Morris . . . | 1897. | 56 | F | Intermittent hydronephrosis. Extrapelvic operation unsatisfactory . . . . . . | Küster's operation, uretero-pyelo-neostomy. Ureter thin and small. Operator dissatisfied with result. | | | | » | » |

## Table of Operations for Renal Retention (continued).

| CHRONOLOGICAL NUMBER | OPERATOR | DATE | AGE | SEX | DISEASE | OPERATION | RESULT — RECOVERY | RESULT — DEATH | RESULT — MUCOUS FISTULA | RESULT — NEPHRECTOMY FOR URINARY FISTULA | BIBLIOGRAPHICAL NUMBER |
|---|---|---|---|---|---|---|---|---|---|---|---|
| | | | | | | II. c. *Extrapelvic Operation on Valve and Stricture.* | | | | | |
| 4 | Fenger . . . . | Nov. 6, 1892. | 17 | M | Traumatic stricture of ureter close to pelvis of kidney. Intermittent pyonephrosis for 4 years. . . . | Nephrotomy Sacculated kidney. No stone found. Ureteral entrance not found. Incision of pelvis. Longitudinal ureterotomy showed stricture. Longitudinal incision of stricture and plastic operation on ureter and pelvis. . . . . . . . . . . | » | | | | » |
| 9 | Fenger . . . . | Sept. 17, 1894. | 21 | M | Gonorrhea. Renal colic. Lumbar nephrotomy. Passage of stones through fistula. Intermittent obstruction of ureter . . . . . . | Operation for oblique implantation and stricture of pelvic end of the ureter . . . . . . . . . . . | » | | | | » |
| 16 | Bardenheuer . | Feb, 17, 1896. | 52 | F | Intermittent hydronephrosis for 5 years. Movable kidney. . . . . . . . . . | Incision from pelvis through spur into ureter below. Transverse union of longitudinal wound. . . . . . | » | | | , | » |
| 19 | Richardson . . | Nov. 11, 1896. | 29 | F | Intermittent hydronephrosis for 8 or 10 years. Gall-stone suspected. Celiotomy. Gall-bladder normal. Retroperitoneal tumor in region of kidney . . . . . . . . | Ureteroplasty. Lumbar incision. Ureter found inserted in minor convexity of dilated pelvis, collapsed and flattened. Lifting kidney straightened ureter. Change of pelvic outlet of ureter into funnel-shaped mouth. Operation on principle of pyloroplasty . . . . . . . . . . . | » | | | | » |
| 20 | Fenger . . . . | March, 1897. | 58 | F | Remittent infected cystonephrosis in floating kidney. Renal stone passed per urethram. Stricture of ureter. . . . . . . . . | Extrapelvic operation. Kidney small. Pelvis dilated. Incision of pelvis. Stricture of ureter below exit. Division of stricture into pelvis. Pyelitis and cystitis persisted. One year later, nephrectomy . . . . . . . . | » | | | • | » |
| 21 | Kelly. . . . | 1897. | 35 | F | Stricture of ureter. Hydronephrosis 5 years, close to pelvis, probably calculous. . . . . . . . . . | Stricture close to pelvis. Strictured portion of ureter divided longitudinally and sutured transversely to pelvis. . . . . . . . . . | » | | | | » |

## Table of Operations for Renal Retention (continued).

| CHRONOLOGICAL NUMBER | OPERATOR | DATE | AGE | SEX | DISEASE | OPERATION | RESULT | | | | BIBLIOGRAPHICAL NUMBER |
|---|---|---|---|---|---|---|---|---|---|---|---|
| | | | | | | | RECOVERY | DEATH | MUCOUS FISTULA | NEPHRECTOMY FOR URINARY FISTULA | |
| | | | | | | II. c. *Continued.* | | | | | |
| 24 | Delbet . . . . | 1898. | 33 | F | Intermittent hydronephrosis for 15 years . . . . . . . | Lumbar incision. Stenosis and oblique insertion of ureter. Division of ureter through stricture from pelvis (uretero-pyelo-neostomy). . . . . . . . . | » | | | | » |
| 25 | Albarran . . . | 1898. | 22 | F | Left pyonephrosis. Nephrotomy. Permanent ureteral catheter. . . . . . . . . | Lumbar incision. Extrapelvic division of spur. Extirpation (capitonnage) of lower portion of sac. Suture of borders of ureter to pelvis. . . . . . . . | » | | | | » |
| 26 | Albarran . . . | 1898. | 22 | F | Hydronephrosis, stricture and oblique insertion of ureter. Stone in bladder. Nephrot. Removal of stone. | Extrapelvic operation. Ureter incised. Opening in ureter united to opening in lowest part of pelvis. . . . . . . . . . . . . . . . . . | » | | | | » |
| 28 | Morris . . . . | 1898. | 29 | F | Stricture and valvular obstruction in upper end of ureter. Normal insertion. | Longitudinal ureterotomy. Division of stricture. Transverse union of ureter to pelvis. . . . . . . | » | | | | » |
| 30 | Fenger . . . . | July 9, 1899. | 41 | F | Intermittent infected hydronephrosis for ten years. Left floating kidney . . . | Lumbar incision. Kidney large and elongated. Pelvis dilated. Oblique insertion of ureter. Upper end bent. Incision of pelvis. Division of exit of ureter and pelvis. Transverse union. . . . . . . . | » | | | | » |
| | | | | | | II. d. *Pyeloplication.* | | | | | |
| 15 | Israel. . . . . | 1896. | 59 | F | Intermittent hydronephrosis for 6 months. Pelvis so dilated that ureter originated from lateral side of wall. Ureter bent upward for 15 cm. then bent downward. . . . . . . . | Incision of posterior wall of pelvis in direction of axis. No stone, no fold. Folding in and suturing of medial side of pelvis (pyeloplication). Ureteral bend straightened by similar folding in of another part of the pelvis. Nephropexy . . . . . . | » | | | | » |
| 26 | Albarran . . . | 1898. | 22 | F | Hydronephrosis. Stricture and oblique implantation of ureter. Stone in pelvis. | Nephrotomy. Removal of stone. Pelvioplication. Two months later extrapelvic operation. . . . . . | » | | | | » |

## Table of Operations for Renal Retention (concluded)

| CHRONOLOGICAL NUMBER | OPERATOR | DATE | AGE | SEX | DISEASE | OPERATION | RESULT | | | | BIBLIOGRAPHICAL NUMBER |
|---|---|---|---|---|---|---|---|---|---|---|---|
| | | | | | | | RECOVERY | DEATH | MUCOUS FISTULA | NEPHRECTOMY FOR URINARY FISTULA | |
| | | | | | **III. Ureter.** | | | | | | |
| | | | | | *a. Ureterolysorthosis.* | | | | | | |
| 27 | Rafin (Verrière). | Nov. 12, 1898. | 32 | F | Left movable kidney, 1890. Intermittent left hydronephrosis, 1895. Nephropexy, April, 1896. Relief then relapse. . . . . . . | Lumbar incision. Kidney small, lobulated. Pelvis dilated. S. shaped bend of ureter. Insertion in lower part of pelvis. Adhesion S separated and bend straightened. Nephropexy, Nov. 12, 1899. No swelling of kidney since operation. . . . . . | » | | | | » |
| | | | | | *b. Plastic Operation.* | | | | | | |
| 11 | Fenger. . . . | Aug. 6, 1894. | 32 | F | Probable traumatic right floating kidney, 1880. Remittent attacks of pain reawakened after pregnancy in 1885, but returned in 1893, after miscarriage. Pyonephrosis. Tumor in region of right kidney. . . . . . . . . . | Pelviotomy. Removal of four stones from above valvular stricture. Longitudinal ureterotomy over and excision of stricture. Plastic operation on ureter . . . . . . . . . . . . . . . | » | | | | » |
| 29 | Fenger. . . . | May 23, 1899. | » | M | Large left pyonephrosis, 1897. Lumbar nephrotomy. Ureterotomy. Removal of stone inch long from upper end of ureter. Lumbar urinary fistula. Fenger's plastic operation on strictured ureter by D. W. H. Allport. Fistula persisted. | Isolation of kidney. Bisection. Stricture 2 inches below pelvis. Ureter isolated and found to be completely obliterated for 1 cm. Longitudinal ureterotomy 1 inch through stricture. Transverse union. Considerable tension on ureter. Bougies from kidney into ureter below stricture. Reunion of bisected kidney. Lumbar urinary fistula closed Jan. 1900 Osteomyelitis. Fistula remains closed. . . . . . . . . . . . . . . . | » | | | | » |

*a*) Non-effective. The operation was non-effective in five cases, in four of which nephrectomy was performed (Van Hook, N° 5; Fenger, N° 20; Morris, N° 22; Fenger, N° 25), with no deaths. In one case, Gerster, N° 15), a urinary fistula returned.

*b*) Functionally effective. The operation was functionally effective in twenty-two of the thirty cases; that is to say, twenty-two out of thirty kidneys, or 75 per 100 have been saved from nephrectomy. In a few of these cases a mucous fistula still remained at the time of publication, but an almost dry mucous fistula, leading probably to a suture or ligature, will close in time and will never necessitate the removal of a kidney, the urine from which passes into the bladder.

## Bibliographie.

1. ALBARRAN (J.). Maladies du rein. *Traité de Chirurgie*, par Le Dentu et Delbet, t. VIII, p. 805.

2. TUFFIER. Appareil urinaire. *Traité de Chirurgie*, par Duplay et Reclus, t. VII.

3. MORRIS (Henry). Hunterian Lectures on Surgery of the Kidney. *British Medical Journal*, March 26, 1898, p. 809.

4. FENGER (C.). Surgery of the Ureter. *American Text-Book of Genito-Urinary Diseases*. Philadelphia, 1898, p. 470.

5. FENGER (C.). Conservative operative Treatment of Sacculated Kidney Cystonephrosis. *Annals of Surgery*, June 1896, p. 637.

6. TRENDELENBURG (F.). *Volkmann's Sammlung klinischer Vorträge*, n° 335, 1890, p. 3578.

7. FENGER (C.) Operations for the Relief of Valve-Formation and Stricture of the Ureter in Hydro or Pyonephrosis. *Journal of the American Medical Association*, March 10, 1894, p. 355.

8. MYNTER (H.). Case of Acute Intermittent Hydronephrosis from Valvular Stricture of the Ureter. *Annals of Surgery*, December 1895, p. 658.

9. BARDENHEUER. Zur konservativen Behandlung der Hydro resp.-Pyonephrose von J. Cramer, Assistant. *Centralblatt für Chirurgie*, November 24, 1894, n° 47, p. 1145.

10. HELFERICH. Ein Beitrag zur Ureterchirurgie von D' Enderlen. *Deutsche Zeitschrift für Chirurgie*, Band XXXIV, heft 3, 1896, p. 323.

11. ISRAËL (J.). Ueber einige neue Erfahrungen auf dem Gebiete der Nierenchirurgie. *Deutsche medicinische Wochenschrift*, n° 28, 1896, p. 345.

12. GERSTER, ARPAD (C). A Contribution to the Surgery of the Kidney and of the Ureter. *American Journal of the Medical Sciences*, june 1897, p. 677.

13. FENGER (C.). Eversion or Turning Inside out of the Sac of a Cystonephrosis as and Aid in Operating upon the Renal End of the Ureter and upon the Partition Walls between dilated Calyces. *American Journal of the Medical Sciences*, july 1899, p. 48.

14. KÜSTER. Ein Fall von Resection des Ureter. *Archiv für klinische Chirurgie*, Band XLIV, heft 4, 1893, p. 850.

15. VAN HOOK (W.). The Surgery of the Ureters; a Clinical, Literary and Experimental Research. *Journal of the American Medical Association*, t. XXI, 1894, p. 911 et 965.

16. BARDENHEUER. Eine operative Behandlungsweise der hydronephrotischen Wanderniere, von D' K. Cramer, Assistant. *Centralblatt für Chirurgie*, n° 21, May 21, 1897, p. 586.

17. BAZY. Contribution à l'étude de la chirurgie de l'urétère. Urétero-pyélonéostomie. *Revue de Chirurgie*, 1897, p. 400.

18. MORRIS (Henry). *Loc. cit.*, p. 814.

19. FENGER (C.). Unpublished.

20. Fenger (C.). *Loc. cit.*, n° 7, p. 19.

21. Fenger (C.). *Loc. cit.*, n° 5, p. 12.

22. Albarran (J.). *La Presse médicale*, 1898.

23. Albarran (J.). Mémoire et présentation du malade, capitonnage de la poche. Anastomose latérale de l'uretère.

24. Bardenheuer. *Loc. cit.*, n° 16, p. 586.

25. Richardson (H.-H.). A Successful Case of Ureteroplasty for intermittent Hydronephrosis. *Transactions of the American Surgical Association*, t. XV, 1897, p. 555.

26. Delbet. Présentation d'un malade, urétero-pyélo-néostomie. Acad. de Méd., decembre 29, 1898. *La Presse médicale*.

27. Kelly (H. S.) and Ramsey (O.). De l'usage du cathéter rénal dans le diagnostic et le traitement des maladies des reins et des uretères. *Revue de Gynécologie et de Chirurgie abdominale*, n° 5, october 1897, p. 834.

28. Verrière (A.). Contribution à la chirurgie conservative dans le traitement des rétentions rénales, bassinet et extrémité supérieure de l'uretère. *Thèse de Lyon*, 1899, p. 56.

29. Fenger (C.). An operation for Valvular Stricture of the Ureter. *American Journal of the Medical Sciences*, december, 1896.

---

## DES OPÉRATIONS CONSERVATRICES DANS LES RÉTENTIONS RÉNALES

*RAPPORT*

### par M. BAZY

(de Paris).

La sécurité que donne l'emploi raisonné des méthodes aseptique et antiseptique devait amener forcément à modifier la thérapeutique d'un certain nombre de lésions chirurgicales.

Elle nous a conduit à faire des opérations qui eussent été jugées autrefois impossibles ou dangereuses.

De ce nombre sont les opérations autoplastiques et anaplastiques qu'on fait sur l'appareil urinaire.

Un certain nombre de ces opérations ont besoin d'une réunion par première intention et par conséquent ne pouvaient être faites, pour pouvoir réussir, que sous le couvert de l'asepsie.

Ces opérations sont celles qui portent sur les canaux excréteurs dont le faible calibre est facilement rétréci et oblitéré par le tissu cicatriciel pour peu qu'il s'en forme, et il s'en forme quand la réunion primitive n'est pas obtenue.

En chirurgie urinaire, comme, du reste, dans bien d'autres branches de la chirurgie, l'expérimentation a précédé et guidé la clinique et la thérapeutique opératoire, et il n'est que juste de rappeler ici les noms de Novaro, de Paoli et Busachi, de Bardenheuer et Harvey Reed pour tout ce qui touche à la chirurgie urétérale.

La chirurgie urétérale est, en effet, la chirurgie des rétentions rénales dont nous avons à nous occuper.

On dit qu'il y a rétention rénale, quand de l'urine séjourne d'une façon constante dans le bassinet et les calices, par suite d'un obstacle à son écoulement.

Où commence la rétention rénale ? En d'autres termes quand peut-on dire qu'il y a rétention, c'est-à-dire état pathologique ? Où cesse l'état physiologique ?

La démarcation est très difficile et, du reste, peu importante en clinique.

Si l'on voulait établir une limite, on serait bien vite arrêté par cette considération que la forme et les dimensions du bassinet sont variables avec les individus et tel bassinet qui peut contenir un certain nombre de grammes d'urine est normal, alors que tel autre qui en contiendrait la même quantité serait dilaté.

Au reste, la quantité de liquide contenu dans un bassinet n'est pas proportionnelle à l'altération du parenchyme rénal. Nous savons, en effet, que beaucoup de rétentions rénales ne s'accompagnent pas de dilatation du bassinet, ni d'augmentation de volume du rein et il n'est pas rare de trouver, à l'autopsie des cancers de l'utérus ayant comprimé l'uretère, le rein complètement atrophié sans augmentation de volume de l'organe.

Quand on dit donc rétention rénale, on emploie ce mot dans son sens clinique, c'est-à-dire quand la rétention est cliniquement appréciable, qu'il y a augmentation de volume de l'organe.

La rétention rénale est la conséquence de tout obstacle à l'écoulement de l'urine depuis le prépuce jusqu'au bassinet.

Nous ne nous occuperons pas des obstacles qui siègent dans la vessie et en aval d'elle, ce serait faire l'histoire de presque toute la chirurgie urinaire.

Au demeurant, ces lésions entraînent des rétentions presque toujours doubles et nous ne nous occuperons que des lésions unilatérales.

Or celles-ci siègent dans l'uretère.

C'est surtout aux extrémités qu'on les observe, rarement dans son parcours.

Ces obstacles sont constitués soit par des rétrécissements, soit par des coudures ou insertions vicieuses, soit par des calculs.

1º Les coudures siègent, en général, sinon exclusivement, à l'extrémité supérieure de l'uretère.

Leur étude se confond avec celle du rein mobile et avec celle des insertions vicieuses de l'uretère sur le bassinet.

2º Les calculs peuvent siéger dans tous les points de l'uretère, mais on les rencontre le plus souvent à l'extrémité supérieure et à l'extrémité inférieure.

5° Les rétrécissements peuvent siéger dans tous les points de l'uretère, mais leur lieu d'élection est soit l'extrémité supérieure, soit l'extrémité inférieure.

Ce rétrécissement peut être dû à une lésion des parois du conduit par un corps étranger ou toute autre cause, plaie, etc., ou. à des lésions inflammatoires des organes avoisinant ce conduit (périmétrite, périnéphrite) et donnant lieu à la production d'un tissu cicatriciel enserrant ce conduit et le rétrécissant.

Je considère comme un point important d'indiquer que ce rétrécissement existe toujours dans le cas de fistules urétéro-vaginales.

Les rétentions rénales peuvent être temporaires ou intermittentes, rémittentes et enfin continues.

Les deux premières formes appartiennent aux deux premières catégories de causes : coudure, insertion vicieuse, rein mobile d'une part, calculs du bassinet de l'autre.

Les rétentions continues ou permanentes, ou progressives sont quelquefois causées par des calculs, mais surtout par les rétrécissements dont l'action est progressive et permanente : le dernier terme en est l'hydronéphrose fermée ou la pyonéphrose fermée.

Mais il faut établir une distinction autrement importante et qui va commander la thérapeutique : les rétentions sont *septiques ou aseptiques*.

Les *aseptiques* constituent les *hydronéphroses*. Les *septiques* comprennent les *hydronéphroses infectées* et les *pyonéphroses*.

Cette distinction est importante, dis-je, parce qu'on peut faire pour les rétentions aseptiques des opérations qu'il ne serait peut-être pas prudent, ni indiqué de faire en cas de rétention septique.

Ces opérations conservatrices ne sont indiquées en effet que quand le rein n'est pas une source de dangers et ne contient pas d'abcès dans le parenchyme. C'est là la condition *sine qua non*.

Il faut en outre que ce rein puisse être utile : car ces opérations conservatrices sont longues, elles sont plus délicates et peuvent être plus dangereuses qu'une néphrectomie.

L'indication de la conservation est *nette* dans le cas d'hydronéphrose simple pour peu que le rein fonctionne encore ; elle est *beaucoup moins nette* dans les cas d'hydronéphrose infectée, elle est *absolue* dans les cas du rein unique, quel que soit, au demeurant, l'état de ce rein.

Je n'ai pas besoin de développer longuement ces idées : il me semble qu'elles sont conformes aux doctrines généralement acceptées.

Le pouvoir utile du rein peut être apprécié par l'analyse chimique de l'urine qu'il sécrète comparée à celle que sécrète le rein opposé, par la façon dont il élimine le bleu de méthylène ou la phloridzine.

Cette constatation et cette comparaison n'ont d'application réelle que dans les cas de lésions de l'extrémité inférieure de l'uretère et en particulier de fistules urétéro-vaginales.

Il s'agit de savoir, en effet, si on devra agir sur cette fistule pour l'aboucher dans la vessie ou, au contraire, si on s'adressera directement à l'extrémité opposée, c'est à dire si on fera la néphrectomie.

*A priori* une fistule urétéro-vaginale récente devra être traitée par la conservation ; même quand elle date d'un certain temps, elle doit être traitée de la même manière, s'il n'y a pas des phénomènes d'infection sérieuse.

L'étude du mode de sécrétion du rein sera cependant utile.

Quant aux lésions de l'extrémité supérieure de l'uretère, c'est surtout l'examen de l'état du rein au moment de l'opération qui devra guider le chirurgien.

L'examen de la sécrétion urinaire, dans ces cas, peut être utile et pourra et devra être fait s'il ne comporte pas de manœuvres ennuyeuses, pénibles ou dangereuses, comme le serait le cathétérisme de l'uretère par exemple.

Pour citer un exemple de cette manière de voir, je dirai qu'ayant eu dernièrement à intervenir pour tarir une fistule urinaire rénale consécutive à une néphrotomie pour hydronéphrose infectée, ayant trouvé un uretère oblitéré sur une étendue de 4 centimètres environ à partir du bassinet, j'ai pensé que le rapprochement de l'uretère et du bassinet ne pourrait se faire, j'ai fait la néphrectomie.

C'est donc la constatation d'un fait inattendu qui, pendant l'opération, a guidé mes déterminations opératoires. Permettez-moi d'ouvrir ici une parenthèse et de dire que cette oblitération me paraît avoir été traumatique et consécutive à la présence d'une bougie que j'avais, suivant mon habitude, placée dans l'uretère après avoir ouvert le rein.

C'est là un des nombreux faits sur lesquels je me suis appuyé pour me méfier du cathétérisme urétéral et qui me rendra désormais circonspect dans l'application du procédé.

L'opération conservatrice dont est justiciable la rétention rénale varie avec l'espèce considérée.

Les calculs seront enlevés soit par néphrotomie, soit par urétérotomie directe ou urétérotomie transvésicale ou transvaginale : celle-ci doit être exceptionnelle.

Les rétrécissements, situés par le trajet de l'uretère, s'ils étaient diagnostiqués pourraient être traités par la dilatation, soit de bas en haut, soit de haut en bas ou par l'urétérotomie oblique ; mais leur diagnostic, en dehors de la constatation directe par la vue et le toucher restera toujours problématique.

Il nous reste à étudier la classe la plus importante des rétentions rénales, celles qui sont dues à des lésions de l'extrémité supérieure, et celles qui ont pour causes des lésions de l'extrémité inférieure.

Les coudures temporaires, donnant lieu à des rétentions temporaires, intermittentes, peuvent guérir spontanément ; j'en ai vu un exemple très net : une femme chez laquelle j'avais constaté la rétention temporaire et intermittente liée à un rein mobile et avec des dimensions telles qu'aucun doute n'était permis, d'autant qu'elle était maigre, cette femme, dis-je, a vu ses crises disparaître ; et leur disparition datait de 3 ans, quand je l'ai vue pour la dernière fois (actuellement elle date de 4 ans).

Comment s'est effectuée ici la guérison ? Est-ce par fixation naturelle de son rein mobile ? Est-ce par atrophie de l'organe ? Je ne saurais le dire.

J'incline toutefois à admettre la première hypothèse, parce qu'un rein, qui est susceptible de donner lieu à une grosse hydronéphrose, me paraît peu apte à subir l'atrophie.

Il est donc très probable que le rein s'est fixé, réalisant ainsi un procédé de guérison employé par la chirurgie, la néphropexie, qui paraît avoir donné des succès depuis que M. Guyon l'a indiqué.

Les abouchements anormaux et les rétrécissements de l'extrémité supérieure de l'uretère sont justiciables d'opérations anaplastiques auxquelles j'ai donné le nom d'urétéro-pyélo-néostomie, qui paraît être entré dans le langage.

Cette opération a pour but, comme son nom l'indique, d'établir une nouvelle communication entre l'uretère et le bassinet pour suppléer à l'abouchement naturel, devenu insuffisant ou mal placé.

Cette opération a été faite pour la première fois par Trendelenburg, mais sa malade est morte. Le premier succès est dû à notre co-rapporteur, le professeur Küster (de Marburg) ; elle a été répétée un assez grand nombre de fois depuis, par notre co-rapporteur Fenger, par Israël, Cramer, etc.; en France, en suivant l'ordre chronologique, par Bazy, puis Albarran, Delbet, etc.

Cette opération peut se faire soit par voie transpéritonéale, soit par voie lombaire.

Je crois être le premier et peut-être le seul à avoir employé la voie transpéritonéale qui convient bien dans le cas d'*hydronéphrose* volumineuse et qui permet de ne pas toucher au rein ou du moins le permet mieux.

La voie transpéritonéale est contre-indiquée dans les cas où le bassinet est infecté, et c'est à la voie lombaire qu'il faut alors avoir recours.

Il est évident que cette voie peut être employée aussi dans les cas d'hydronéphrose non infectée, mais elle me paraît moins commode.

L'abouchement peut se faire de beaucoup de manières, et je n'y insisterais pas, n'attachant à la manière d'unir l'uretère au bassinet qu'une importance secondaire si, notre distingué co-rapporteur, M. Küster n'avait attribué à Albarran la paternité d'une manœuvre opératoire qui m'appartient, à savoir la résection du bassinet.

En effet, dans ma communication à l'Académie, et plus tard dans mon mémoire paru dans la Revue de chirurgie (10 mai 1897), je dis (page 404), à propos de ma première opération : « j'achevai, *après avoir réséqué une partie de la poche,* la suture du bassinet. » Je vais du reste m'expliquer sur cette résection de la poche hydronéphrotique. Mais auparavant, disons que l'urétéro-pyélo-néostomie peut être primitive ou secondaire.

Elle est dite *primitive*, quand c'est la première opération qu'on pratique sur le rein. Elle est *secondaire*, quand elle est faite sur un rein déjà néphrotomisé antérieurement, et pour tarir une fistule urinaire.

L'opération primitive ne convient qu'aux hydronéphroses simples ; en cas de pyonéphrose, il convient de se borner tout d'abord à la simple néphrotomie destinée à évacuer le pus et à parer aux accidents d'infection, remettant à plus tard, quand l'état général sera redevenu bon et si l'état du rein le permet, l'opération complexe qu'est l'urétéro-pyélo-néostomie.

Dans les opérations primitives, il est bon et nécessaire de réduire la poche par résection.

Dans les opérations secondaires, la résection ou le capitonnage de la poche est inutile.

On sait, en effet, avec quelle rapidité reviennent sur elles-mêmes les cavités purulentes des pyonéphroses et telle poche, qui avait le volume d'une mandarine au moment de l'incision, se trouve être du volume d'une noix quand le pus a été évacué. De même, j'ai vu des poches pyonéphrotiques, contenant un litre de pus, réduites au volume d'un petit œuf au moment de l'intervention secondaire.

Donc résection et capitonnage sont inutiles pour préparer une intervention secondaire.

Je dirai de même que la résection du rein est inutile, parce qu'on peut toujours insérer l'uretère dans un point déclive, de plus, il me paraît irrationnel de restreindre le champ d'épuration d'un rein qui n'est plus vaste et qu'il faut conserver aussi grand que possible.

Au demeurant, j'ai employé, suivant les circonstances, les différents modes d'abouchement, et il serait quelquefois difficile de dire les différences qui séparent ce qu'on appelle les procédés de tel ou tel chirurgien.

La suture de l'uretère au bassinet s'est faite soit en dehors du rein, soit à travers le rein largement incisé : j'estime que ce dernier mode est mauvais ; il est inutile et par suite nuisible de faire subir à un rein malade un traumatisme qui en réduira encore le pouvoir excréteur.

Les opérations pratiquées sur l'extrémité inférieure de l'uretère sont les urétéro-cysto-néostomies : elles ont été faites dans les cas de fistules utéro-vaginales.

Ces fistules s'accompagnent toujours de rétrécissements de l'uretère et par suite de rétention rénale.

Cette rétention rénale a pu être nettement constatée trois fois par mois avant l'opération sur les 4 malades que j'ai opérées et elle est la conséquence du rétrécissement. Il faut donc détruire ce rétrécissement et l'empêcher de se reproduire.

Pour cela, une suture muqueuse à muqueuse de l'uretère à la vessie et une réunion par première intention sont indispensables.

Toute opération qui ne détruira pas ce rétrécissement est frappée de stérilité ; ce sera une néphrectomie lente, si je puis ainsi parler et ainsi que je l'ai dit à la Société de chirurgie, au lieu d'une néphrectomie instantanée qu'on fera subir à la malade.

Or les opérations vaginales ne me paraissent pas pouvoir aboutir à la destruction de ce rétrécissement, en raison des difficultés excessives de l'opération, de l'impossibilité d'isoler l'uretère, de bien placer les fils.

C'est dire qu'il faut repousser toutes les opérations plastiques faites par la voie vaginale.

C'est donc à la voie abdominale qu'il faut avoir recours.

On peut faire l'opération sous-péritonéale ou transpéritonéale.

L'opération transpéritonéale est celle qui me paraît préférable : c'est celle que nous avons employée, Novaro et moi, dans nos premières opérations et les chirurgiens qui nous ont suivis ont adopté la même voie.

Les divergences se montrent dans la manière de se comporter vis-à-vis du péritoine après la suture de l'uretère.

Certains chirurgiens ont conseillé de drainer depuis la ligne de suture jusqu'à l'incision de la paroi en mettant une mèche sous-péritonéale. J'aime mieux renforcer la suture vésico-urétérale par une suture péritonéale et drainer l'intérieur de la cavité péritonéale. On prévient ainsi mieux l'écoulement de l'urine par la plaie abdominale.

Un point que je considère comme important, c'est de protéger la suture contre le contact de l'urine par une sonde urétérale en caoutchouc sortant par l'urètre à travers la vessie.

Je repousse, au contraire, cette sonde comme inutile, parce qu'elle ne protège rien, et même comme nuisible, dans les opérations d'abouchement de l'uretère au bassinet.

J'ai fait l'urétéro-cystonéostomie 4 fois et dans 2 cas l'uretère et le bassinet étaient infectés.

Dans un cas même, il s'est écoulé par la sonde que j'avais mise dans l'uretère du pus pur. J'insiste sur cette particularité.

Or mes 4 malades ont guéri de l'opération et la fistule a été tarie. Chez ma dernière opérée, la fistule vaginale a continué à couler après l'opération, mais de moins en moins, et aux dernières nouvelles que j'en ai eue et qui remontent à 6 mois, elle était complètement guérie.

Mais il importe de savoir si l'opération a été utile, chez ces malades. En d'autres termes, l'opération destinée à conserver le rein, l'a-t-elle conservé, ou bien ce rein ne s'est-il pas, quand même, atrophié ?

L'étude des malades infectées est, à ce point de vue, très instructive. Si l'abouchement n'était pas resté large et si l'écoulement des produits septiques n'avait pas pu se faire facilement, il en serait résulté une pyonéphrose qui eût forcé à intervenir.

Or les 2 malades ne se sont jamais mieux portées que depuis l'opération ; or pour l'une, l'opération date de 7 ans, pour l'autre de 2 ans, et pour l'une et l'autre leur santé a été en s'améliorant tous les jours.

Chez les malades non infectées et chez lesquelles j'avais constaté cliniquement la rétention rénale, c'est-à-dire une notable augmentation de volume du rein, je n'ai plus retrouvé cette augmentation et il n'y a pas de raison pour que, si le rétrécissement s'était reproduit, la rétention et par suite la tumeur ne se fussent pas reproduites.

Or j'ai pu suivre ces malades pendant un certain temps après l'opération et je n'ai rien constaté d'anormal.

J'en dirai autant pour les malades opérés d'urétéro-pyélo néostomie ; pour l'un, l'opération date de 4 ans : j'ai vu ce malade bien des fois depuis, et jamais il n'a rien senti d'anormal ; jamais je n'ai rien constaté qui pût me faire supposer que l'hydronéphrose se fût reproduite.

Chez ma dernière malade infectée, l'opération date de 8 mois et elle se porte très bien.

Donc toutes ces opérations conservatrices sont justifiées.

Pourrait-on en dire autant des opérations d'urétéro-colostomies faites dans les mêmes conditions ? Ce serait difficile à dire : on ne sait pas quel a été le sort du rein en pareil cas, il faut donc être très réservé.

Enfin, permettez-moi d'ajouter à cette liste des opérations conservatrices, dans les rétentions rénales, la *néphrotomie précoce* que j'ai préconisée, il y a 2 ans. Cette néphrotomie est vraiment conservatrice, d'abord parce qu'elle évite au parenchyme rénal des destructions qui résultent de la présence du pus, et puis parce qu'elle peut dispenser des autres opérations dont nous venons de parler.

Mais c'est un point que je me réserve de développer ultérieurement.

---

## OPÉRATIONS CONSERVATRICES DANS LES RÉTENTIONS RÉNALES

### par M. J. ALBARRAN,

de Paris.

Je limite ma communication aux variétés de rétentions rénales dont les lésions causales se trouvent dans le bassinet ou dans la portion initiale de l'uretère. L'obstacle au libre écoulement de l'urine par l'uretère, variable suivant les cas, exige des traitements différents lorsqu'on se propose de conserver le rein et d'empêcher la formation de fistules rénales.

Dans les cas les plus simples, il suffit d'enlever un calcul ou de redresser, par la néphrorrhaphie une coudure encore peu fixée, pour que l'urine reprenne son cours normal. Je n'insiste pas sur ces faits et je me limite à indiquer qu'il est indispensable, même dans ces cas simples, de s'assurer que des lésions secondaires déterminées par la rétention elle-même n'ont pas donné naissance à un nouvel obstacle surajouté. On s'épargnera bien des surprises désagréables en pratiquant dans ces cas le cathétérisme urétéral pour s'assurer de la liberté de ce conduit.

Dans d'autres cas, il existe des lésions, cause primitive de la rétention, ou consécutives à la rétention elle-même, qui exigent des procédés particuliers de traitement. Ces lésions siègent dans la poche rénale elle-même ou dans la partie initiale de l'uretère.

Dans la poche rénale, les *cloisons intérieures* incomplètement détruites pendant la néphrostomie peuvent être cause de la persistance des fistules; il est nécessaire de détruire ces cloisons pour que la poche de rétention ne présente pas de diverticules.

Les *lésions urétérales* sont les plus importantes. On peut distinguer : 1° l'insertion trop haute de l'uretère dans le bassinet dilaté; la partie de la poche de rétention située au-dessous de l'uretère ne peut se vider par ce conduit; 2° l'insertion oblique de l'uretère dans la poche avec formation d'une valvule empêchant l'urine de s'écouler; 3° des rétrécissements perméables ou non de la portion initiale de l'uretère, avec ou sans coudures du conduit.

Souvent ces différentes variétés se combinent de manière diverse : parfois encore on trouve plus bas dans l'uretère, loin du rein, d'autres rétrécissements.

*Indications des opérations dites plastiques.* — Il serait aujourd'hui banal d'insister sur l'utilité de conserver, dans la plupart des cas, les reins atteints de rétention : la néphrostomie a gagné dans ces cas tout le terrain que la néphrectomie a perdu, mais, souvent, à la suite de la simple incision du rein il persiste une fistule.

Les opérations plastiques, ayant pour but de rétablir le libre cours des urines dans l'uretère peuvent être pratiquées d'emblée, lorsqu'on intervient sur la rétention elle même, ou secondairement pour guérir une fistule déjà constituée.

Lorsqu'on pratique la néphrostomie pour une rétention rénale septique ou aseptique, on peut souvent reconnaître au moment même de l'opération, le plus souvent à l'aide du cathétérisme urétéral, plus rarement par l'examen direct, que les conditions anatomiques sont telles que l'ouverture du rein restera définitivement fistuleuse. Logiquement on pourrait en conclure qu'il faudrait, d'emblée, au moment même de la néphrostomie, avoir recours à une opération rétablissant en même temps le cours normal de l'urine par l'uretère. Il faut pourtant distinguer soigneusement, au point de vue des indications opératoires, les uro-néphroses simples des uropyonéphroses et des pyonéphroses vraies. Cette distinction que nous avons établie, M. Guyon et moi en 1898 dans notre rapport au Congrès français de chirurgie, est généralement acceptée.

Lorsque la rétention rénale n'est pas infectée, ou lorsque le liquide de la poche n'est pas franchement purulent, mais simplement trouble, on peut souvent procéder d'emblée à une opération plastique. Dans ces cas, les conditions générales du malade sont presque toujours assez bonnes pour lui permettre de subir une opération plus longue

que la simple ouverture de la poche et les conditions locales permettent de pratiquer sans trop de peine l'opération dans un milieu aseptique ou peu infecté.

En cas de pyonéphrose, au contraire, nous nous trouvons souvent
en présence de malades chez qui il serait dangereux de pratiquer une
longue opération. Dans beaucoup de cas, il existe en outre des conditions locales défavorables : les lésions inflammatoires ont déterminé
des adhérences qui gênent les manœuvres opératoires, et le milieu
infecté dans lequel on opère est peu favorable à la réussite des
sutures. Pour mon compte, je n'ai pratiqué qu'une fois une urétérotomie au moment même de l'ouverture d'une pyonéphrose et j'ai eu
à déplorer la mort de ma malade; depuis, je préfère attendre et pratiquer ultérieurement, pour guérir la fistule déjà constituée, l'opération complémentaire qui vise au rétablissement du cours des urines.

Dans des cas exceptionnels, on pourra, avant d'opérer, modifier suffisamment le contenu de la poche rénale pour permettre de pratiquer
d'emblée, avec chances de succès, une opération plastique, même en
cas de pyonéphrose vraie. C'est ainsi que j'ai pu, grâce au cathétérisme
urétéral et à des lavages répétés du bassinet, transformer une pyonéphrose en uropyonéphrose, ce qui m'a permis de pratiquer d'emblée
l'urétéro-pyelo-anastomose.

Lorsque le malade est porteur d'une fistule consécutive à la
néphrostomie, on sait que la guérison peut survenir spontanément;
certains chirurgiens attendent cette guérison pendant des mois et
des années, d'autres se décident à enlever le rein. Pour que la guérison survienne, il faut ou que la lésion causale soit capable de rétrocéder, comme les rétrécissements par urétérite, ou que le rein, finissant par se détruire, cesse de sécréter de l'urine.

En cas de rétrécissement par urétérite, la guérison spontanée sera
toujours longue à obtenir, souvent même elle manquera, les lésions
inflammatoires ayant déterminé des modifications définitives. Il est
donc logique, dans ces cas, d'intervenir, aussi bien que dans les autres
lésions urétérales plus haut énumérées, mais il est utile de ne pas
trop se presser pour opérer et d'attendre que l'état général du malade
et les conditions locales du rein se soient modifiés.

Localement, la transformation du liquide qui s'écoule par la fistule
est un des meilleurs guides : la quantité de pus diminue progressivement et l'urine que le rein sécrète devient de plus en plus claire. En
même temps que l'urine devient plus limpide et plus riche en matériaux excrémentitiels, il se passe du côté du rein et de l'uretère des
modifications anatomiques qui rendent l'opération plus aisée dans

son exécution et plus sûre dans ses résultats : les phénomènes inflammatoires de périnéphrite et péri-urétérite diminuent en même temps que la poche rénale revient sur elle-même et se rétrécit grandement.

J'ajoute enfin, sans insister sur ce point que je développe dans une autre communication, qu'à mon avis *une opération plastique ne se trouve indiquée que lorsqu'il est bien démontré que la sonde urétérale à demeure ne peut empêcher la formation d'une fistule ou se montre impuissante à la guérir.*

PROCÉDÉS OPÉRATOIRES.

Certains procédés opératoires ne s'appliquent qu'à des cas particuliers, tels la section de l'éperon pyélo-urétéral, le capitonnage de la poche et la résection orthopédique du rein : d'autres peuvent être appliqués dans la plupart des cas, tels l'urétéro-pyélostomie de Kuster et l'anastomose néphro-urétérale.

La *section de l'éperon pyélo-urétéral*, employée d'abord par Bardenheuer, trouve son indication lorsque l'uretère s'insérant trop haut dans la poche rénale, se trouve en même temps accolé à cette poche pendant une partie de son trajet, avec ou sans implantation oblique et formation valvulaire à l'ouverture du bassinet. Dans ces cas, la section de l'éperon, formé par l'accolement des parois du bassinet et de l'uretère, avec suture isolée des deux lèvres de la plaie, a non seulement pour résultat de faire disparaître la valvule, si elle existe, mais encore d'abaisser le point d'abouchement de l'uretère de toute la longueur de l'éperon sectionné.

Lorsque l'uretère se sépare à angle aigu de la poche, lorsque, avec ou sans couture de son extrémité supérieure, ce conduit se trouve rétréci au delà du point où ses parois sont accolées à la poche rénale, la section de l'éperon ne peut permettre le parfait écoulement de l'urine par l'uretère et on se trouve forcé d'avoir recours à d'autres opérations, qui peuvent d'ailleurs n'être que complémentaires et parfaire le résultat incomplet du procédé de Bardenheuer.

Le *capitonnage de la poche* rénale n'a été employé, que je sache, que par Israël et par moi. Israël obtint un succès; je dus intervenir secondairement par une anastomose urétérale pour guérir ma malade. Dans l'opération du capitonnage, on plisse la partie de la poche rénale qui se trouve au-dessous de l'embouchure urétérale, de manière à rétrécir la cavité et empêcher les liquides de s'accumuler dans les parties déclives, sous-urétérales. Pour que l'opération soit possible, il est nécessaire que la poche rénale soit assez mince pour pouvoir être plissée dans la portion où elle doit être capitonnée : c'est là une condition préalable qui ne sera pas souvent rencontrée.

Je dois dire aussi que, lorsque le capitonnage peut être fait, il constitue une bonne ressource opératoire. J'ai été très frappé de voir, chez la malade dont je viens de parler, combien en quelques semaines la poche capitonnée avait diminué de volume : les plis que j'avais suturés avaient disparu en même temps que la poche s'était rétrécie considérablement.

*Résection orthopédique.* — Lorsque l'uretère se sépare à angle aigu de la poche rénale ou lorsque la portion de cette poche qui se trouve au-dessous de son embouchure est constituée par une portion du rein encore épaisse, on ne peut songer aux procédés déjà décrits de section de l'éperon ou de capitonnage. Dans ces cas, l'uretère tout en ayant un calibre convenable et ne présentant pas de coudures, peut être raccourci ou difficile à détacher, comme cela est nécessaire dans l'urétéro-pyélostomie ou dans l'anastomose urétéro-rénale. Chez une malade, je trouvai réunies ces conditions et je pratiquai la résection partielle de toute la portion de la poche rénale qui se trouvait au-dessous de l'embouchure urétérale : c'est l'opération que j'ai nommée résection orthopédique du rein.

*L'urétéro-pyélostomie* typique consiste à sectionner l'uretère et à le suturer à la partie la plus déclive de la poche. Ce procédé peut être appliqué aussi bien aux cas d'insertion haute de l'uretère, avec ou sans obliquité, qu'à ceux de rétrécissements coudés ou non coudés de la partie supérieure de l'uretère. Dans certains cas pourtant, le procédé de Küster est inapplicable ; toujours il est d'une exécution délicate.

La difficulté opératoire vient de ce que l'uretère sectionné en travers, privé de son attache rénale, peut être difficile à bien suturer, même lorsqu'on fait la section du conduit en bec de flûte ou lorsqu'on ajoute à la coupe transversale une incision longitudinale.

Dans les cas d'uronéphrose la manœuvre peut être assez aisée : lorsque l'uretère est raccourci par l'inflammation, lorsque le rein lui-même est très adhérent, comme dans un bon nombre de pyonéphroses, on peut se voir obligé d'opérer au fond de la plaie ; les difficultés sont grandes et le résultat thérapeutique incertain.

*L'anastomose urétéro-rénale* est d'exécution beaucoup plus facile et je crois qu'elle peut, avec avantage, être substituée dans tous les cas à l'urétéro-pyéostomie. J'ai pratiqué sept fois cette opération que j'exécute ainsi.

*Manuel opératoire.* — Je commence par introduire dans l'uretère au moyen du cathétérisme cystoscopique, une petite sonde à bout arrondi n° 6 Charrière. Je me propose ainsi : 1° de trouver facilement l'uretère pendant l'opération ; 2° de pouvoir constater, si la sonde pénètre dans le bassinet, dans quel endroit de la poche se trouve l'ouverture de l'uretère : si la sonde ne pénètre pas dans le bassinet, de savoir jusqu'à quel niveau l'uretère est libre : je ne suis pas ainsi exposé à faire une opération inutile au-dessus d'un rétrécissement non senti ; 3° enfin, la sonde urétérale n° 6 me permet de guider sur elle la grosse sonde que je laisse à demeure après l'opération.

La sonde urétérale se trouvant placée, je fais dans la région lombaire une longue incision très oblique, commençant sur la dernière côte au niveau du bord externe de la masse sacro-lombaire, se dirigeant en bas et en avant pour passer à un large travers de doigt au-dessus de la crête iliaque et se prolongeant plus ou moins loin vers le muscle droit de l'abdomen.

Lorsque le rein est intact, en cas d'uronéphrose par exemple, je commence par inciser largement la poche et si le rein est fistuleux, j'agrandis la fistule de manière à bien détruire toutes les cloisons intérieures et à voir, si la sonde urétérale a pénétré dans son intérieur, quelle est la disposition de l'ouverture urétérale dans le bassinet et quel est le meilleur procédé à suivre. Je fais ensuite l'isolement de la portion supérieure de l'uretère.

La décortication de la partie inférieure du rein étant faite, j'arrive toujours facilement à sentir avec le doigt le conduit urétéral, grâce à la sonde qui se trouve dans son intérieur : je n'ai jamais eu de difficulté à l'accrocher avec le doigt et à l'attirer du côté de la plaie. Je place alors une anse de fil de soie plate sous l'uretère pour le maintenir facilement à l'endroit voulu.

En introduisant un doigt dans l'intérieur de la poche rénale je cherche alors quel est son point le plus déclive et je choisis, pour l'incision de la bouche anastomotique, un point aussi mince que possible. Le mieux, quand on le peut, est de prendre une portion du bassinet et non du rein lui-même parce que les sutures seront plus faciles et tiendront mieux.

Le point où portera l'incision de la poche étant choisi et la partie supérieure de l'uretère décortiquée le mieux possible, je cherche le niveau où l'uretère sera incisé en amenant ce conduit au contact du point rénal et en constatant qu'il n'y a pas de tiraillement.

On procède ensuite à l'incision de la paroi de la poche rénale dans l'étendue de 1 1/2 centimètres : on incise aussi longitudinalement l'uretère dans une étendue semblable, au niveau du point choisi pour établir la bouche anastomotique.

Si elle n'y pénétrait déjà, la sonde urétérale est alors introduite dans la poche rénale à travers les deux ouvertures de la poche et de l'uretère et on la fait sortir par la plaie lombaire. L'extrémité arrondie de cette sonde (n° 6) est alors introduite dans l'intérieur d'une autre sonde urétérale plus grosse, (n° 10 à 12), à laquelle elle va servir de mandrin pour être passée de haut en bas, de la plaie vers la vessie. En poussant la grosse sonde de haut en bas et en tirant doucement au niveau du méat sur la petite sonde-mandrin, on voit bientôt apparaître au niveau du gland ou de la vulve la grosse sonde qui servira à drainer le rein. Cette grosse sonde a une extrémité rénale coupée en bec de flûte et qui présente quatre ou cinq yeux latéraux : dans l'œil le plus supérieur on passe un fil de soie en anse qui sera fixé au bord cutané de la plaie lombaire avec une aiguille lorsque, après avoir suturé les lèvres de l'anastomose, on aura bien placé la portion supérieure de la sonde dans la cavité de la poche rénale. Cette précaution a pour but de mieux assurer la fixité de la sonde pour bien établir le drainage. Le fil fixateur permettrait en outre, s'il en était besoin, de tirer la sonde par la plaie lombaire.

Lorsque la grosse sonde urétérale a été placée, on suture, avec de fins fils de soie, les deux lèvres des incisions pratiquées à la poche rénale et à la paroi de l'uretère et on vérifie que la suture est bonne en constatant que la sonde joue librement dans la nouvelle bouche urétérale.

Il est encore plus commode de faire cette suture en deux temps : les deux lèvres postérieures sont suturées alors que la petite sonde urétérale a été introduite de bas en haut dans le rein, tandis que les deux lèvres antérieures sont suturées lorsque déjà la grosse sonde définitive se trouve en place. Les sutures urétéro-rénales sont, dans ce procédé, généralement très faciles parce que la continuité du conduit urétéral persiste malgré l'incision longitudinale faite à sa paroi.

Lorsque l'abouchement urétéro-rénal est fini il ne reste plus qu'à bien placer la sonde et à la fixer à la peau comme je l'ai dit. On ferme ensuite l'incision de la néphrotomie. En cas d'uronéphrose on peut faire une suture complète : lorsque la poche rénale est infectée il est plus prudent de laisser un drain intra-rénal de sûreté. La plaie des parties molles sera elle-même plus ou moins complètement fermée.

*Soins consécutifs.* — Dans les jours qui suivent l'opération j'ai l'habitude de pratiquer, par la sonde urétérale et par le drain rénal, un ou deux lavages par jour. Ces lavages sont faits avec de l'eau boriquée simple si l'urine sécrétée par le rein est claire et avec une solution de nitrate d'argent au 1/1000, lorsque cette urine contient du pus.

Le drain placé directement dans le rein par la plaie lombaire est généralement supprimé le 6ᵉ ou le 8ᵉ jour et à partir de ce moment on voit la sonde urétérale donner passage à presque toute, souvent même à toute l'urine du rein malade.

Lorsque toute l'urine s'écoule par la sonde urétérale depuis 5 ou 6 jours sans que le pansement lombaire soit mouillé, on coupe le fil de soie qui attachait à la peau de la région lombaire la partie supérieure de la sonde et on laisse encore cette sonde en place pendant 6 ou 8 jours. La sonde urétérale qui a été mise pendant l'opération peut ainsi rester en place pendant une vingtaine de jours sans aucun inconvénient ; souvent j'ai laissé la même sonde plus de 20 jours. Lorsque la sonde s'altère et ne fonctionne pas bien, on peut facilement la changer sans avoir besoin de recourir à la cystoscopie : il suffit de placer dans l'intérieur de la sonde un de mes longs mandrins, de la retirer ensuite et de glisser à nouveau, sur ce mandrin, la nouvelle sonde qui doit remplacer l'ancienne.

Il peut arriver que lorsque la sonde urétérale est définitivement retirée, le malade souffre et présente même de l'élévation de température : ces phénomènes sont dus à ce que le nouvel orifice urétéral ne fonctionne pas bien. Lorsque pareil accident arrive il ne faut pas croire immédiatement à un échec ; j'ai pu, dans un cas, obtenir un résultat définitif parfait en replaçant une nouvelle sonde par le cathétérisme urétéral et en la laissant à demeure pendant deux semaines.

J'ai pratiqué 6 opérations urétéro-rénales avec succès pour des rétentions aseptiques et septiques ou pour des fistules consécutives à la néphrostomie. Ma plus ancienne opération date de 27 mois ; la malade reste guérie.

Dans un cas où le rein avait été fixé à la paroi abdominale antérieure par une néphrostomie transpéritonéale, j'eus un échec. Chez une malade atteinte de pyonéphrose grave je fis, en même temps que l'incision du rein, l'urétérotomie externe : la malade mourut.


## DISCUSSION.


M. Kuster (de Marbourg). — M. Albarran préconise sa méthode d'urétéro-pyélo-anastomose ; mais je crains qu'elle ne produise des espaces morts, favorables pour le dépôt de cristaux urinaires. Probablement une partie de ses opérés de cette manière ne restera pas longtemps guérie.

Enfin, je ne suis pas de son avis eu égard au drainage des uretères après les opérations plastiques. Si l'on a opéré pour une pyonéphrose, on verra bientôt disparaître la suppuration, pourvu que la suture soit bonne et l'écoulement de l'urine sans empêchement; par contre, un corps étranger, comme un drain, maintiendra la suppuration plus longtemps, et il va sans dire que cela pourrait présenter des inconvénients.

M. ALBARRAN. — Les objections de M. Kuster ne me paraissent pas excessives. La portion de l'uretère comprise au-dessus de l'anastomose est presque toujours oblitérée et ne livre plus passage à l'urine; par conséquent, elle ne peut être le lieu de formation des calculs. D'ailleurs, si on le craignait, il serait facile, l'anastomose faite, de réséquer la partie de l'uretère qui se trouve au-dessus d'elle et qui est devenue inutile. L'anastomose conserverait toujours ce grand avantage sur l'abouchement de l'uretère complètement sectionné, que l'opération est plus facile et plus sûre dans ses résultats.

La sonde urétérale à demeure après les opérations uretéro-rénales a les mêmes avantages que la sonde uréthrale qu'on laisse après les résections de l'urèthre : elle empêche l'urine d'être en contact avec les sutures, avantage surtout important dans les cas infectés. Ce drainage urétéral permet en outre de pratiquer des lavages modificateurs de la poche. Parmi mes malades guéris par ce procédé, plusieurs ont été opérés il y a plus d'un an; il en est un opéré depuis vingt-sept mois et qui reste guéri.

J'ajoute que la sonde urétérale permet pendant l'opération de trouver facilement l'uretère, ce qui peut être fort difficile en cas de pyonéphrose et que grâce à elle on peut, si l'uretère est encore perméable, voir dans l'intérieur de la poche rénale le point d'abouchement de l'uretère et le meilleur procédé à employer.

---

## UN CAS DE RÉTENTION D'ORIGINE RÉNALE, GUÉRIE PAR LE CATHÉTÉRISME DE L'URETÈRE

par M. le docteur P. HAMONIC,

de Paris.

Voici un petit fait qui m'a paru assez intéressant pour être relaté.

Un homme de 50 ans, vigoureux, n'ayant jamais eu de maladie, est pris tout à coup d'une rétention absolue d'urine avec besoin violent, douleurs lombaires, langue sèche et tendance à l'hypothermie.

Quand je fus mandé près du malade, je m'attendais à trouver un rétrécissement de l'urèthre, d'autant qu'il avait eu une blennorrhagie violente dans sa jeunesse.

Mais le canal fut trouvé sain, et un gros cathéter parvenait facilement dans la vessie qui ne contenait pas une goutte d'urine.

La palpation abdominale m'a permis de constater une certaine résistance dans la région rénale gauche; mais cette palpation était rendue très difficile par l'état de contracture des muscles de la paroi.

Je me décidai à pratiquer le cathétérisme de l'uretère en commençant par le côté gauche.

Le cystoscope étant mis en place, je trouvai la vessie absolument saine. J'introduisis alors un long cathéter mince dans l'uretère gauche et après avoir rencontré une certaine résistance, j'arrivai jusqu'au rein.

Comme mes manœuvres avaient déterminé l'écoulement par l'uretère d'une certaine quantité de sang, je n'insistai pas davantage et fis mettre dans un bain le malade qui affirmait être sensiblement soulagé.

Quelques instants après il commençait à évacuer dans le bain une certaine quantité d'urine. Dans la journée ce fut une vraie débâcle. Le malade évacua environ 4 litres de liquide.

Très rapidement, il reprit son équilibre normal, et l'analyse de l'urine faite ultérieurement ne décéla que de l'exagération des urates et quelques cristaux d'oxalates.

Faut-il admettre ici que la rétention, qui était évidemment d'origine urétérale, était due à une coudure de ce conduit? Ce n'est pas probable car je ne découvris pas trace de ptose rénale dans les jours qui suivirent.

Faut-il invoquer un spasme urétéral? A coup sûr ce spasme existait pour le côté droit et il devait être la conséquence d'un réflexe. Ce qui le démontre, c'est que ce côté droit qui ne fonctionnait pas plus que le gauche a récupéré sa perméabilité dès que ce dernier a eu subi l'action du cathétérisme. Donc le côté droit, soit le rein, soit l'uretère, était privé de ses fonctions parce que le gauche était altéré.

L'explication qui me paraît la plus vraisemblable c'est l'existence dans l'uretère gauche d'un petit amas de sable urique ayant donné lieu à une anurie complète en raison de la réaction nerveuse du sujet. Le cathétérisme urétéral en déplaçant ce léger obstacle, cause première des accidents, a rétabli l'état normal et ramené l'urine.

## A PROPOS DES OPÉRATIONS CONSERVATRICES
## DANS LES RÉTENTIONS RÉNALES

### par M. F. LEGUEU,
de Paris.

De plus en plus la chirurgie doit s'efforcer d'être conservatrice : déjà pour d'autres organes ces tendances se sont accentuées, la chirurgie des annexes, la thérapeutique des fibromes ont orienté leur direction vers des tendances nettement conservatrices. Pour le rein, il n'y a pas de raisons pour qu'il n'en soit pas de même; il est au contraire beaucoup de raisons pour qu'il en soit ainsi. Le rein a dans l'économie une fonction vitale à remplir, et tout ce que l'on conserve de son parenchyme même altéré continue à sécréter et à éliminer les poisons de l'organisme.

Aussi bien je me déclare nettement partisan des opérations, qui en présence d'une rétention rénale ont pour but et pour effet la conservation du rein.

Mais dans l'application de ce principe, il est des réserves à formuler : ces opérations conservatrices ont des *indications*, dont il ne faut pas se départir, sous peine de les voir donner un mauvais résultat.

D'une façon générale, pour être efficaces, ces opérations conservatrices doivent être précoces; elles doivent être faites de bonne heure, et je dirai même volontiers que leur résultat fonctionnel est proportionnel à la précocité de leur application. Les rétentions rénales doivent être traitées, qu'elles soient aseptiques ou septiques, avant la désorganisation totale du rein. Quand le rein est totalement transformé et détruit, quand son parenchyme est fort aminci, je ne crois plus guère à l'efficacité des opérations conservatrices, malgré le capitonnage de la poche. J'ai bien eu moi-même à traiter une hydronéphrose de trois litres de contenance par l'urétéronéphrostomie, mais je ne me sens pas pour l'instant décidé à recommencer, et lorsque j'aurai affaire à une poche aussi volumineuse, je l'enlèverai comme je l'ai fait à plusieurs reprises, et d'autant plus volontiers que l'autre rein est dans ces cas généralement intact.

Je crois donc à l'utilité des opérations conservatrices, quand elles seront précoces. A cette époque, la suppression de la cause permettra au rein de revenir à l'état normal, quelle que soit la nature septique ou aseptique de la rétention. C'est ce que nous voyons souvent se réa-

liser spontanément dans les rétentions de la grossesse : dès que la
cause de compression est supprimée, le rein se vide, reprend son
volume, la rétention cesse, malgré que les urines restent quelque
temps encore légèrement troubles.

Au début, il est tout naturel de traiter ces rétentions par le cathétérisme de l'uretère : j'y ai eu recours souvent, et il m'est arrivé à plusieurs reprises, d'évacuer et de faire disparaître de petites rétentions
aseptiques dans l'hydronéphrose intermittente au début, par coudure
de l'uretère. Mais le cathétérisme de l'uretère ne me paraît un moyen
de traitement que dans les petites rétentions, dans celles qui sont
observées tout à fait au début. Plus tard, le cathétérisme n'est plus
qu'un moyen de diagnostic excellent pour préciser et définir le siège
de l'obstacle et formuler l'indication opératoire ; mais je ne crois
guère qu'on puisse compter sur lui, pour drainer la poche, évacuer
la collection et lui permettre de revenir sur elle-même. Ce résultat
ne serait obtenu que par le cathétérisme à demeure : celui-ci a l'inconvénient de réaliser presque à coup sûr l'infection de la poche.

J'y ai eu recours sur un malade qui portait dans le flanc gauche
une énorme hydronéphrose : le cathétérisme était facile, bien que
l'opération pratiquée plus tard nous ait montré un rétrécissement
large ; et par la sonde j'évacuai jusqu'à 5 litres et quelques cents
grammes d'urine. Après avoir répété à plusieurs reprises cette évacuation, je voulus laisser une sonde à demeure pour permettre à la
poche de revenir sur elle-même. Mais au bout de trois jours les urines
se troublèrent, la fièvre s'éleva et je fus obligé de renoncer au cathétérisme et de pratiquer l'urétéropyélostomie que j'aurais bien mieux
fait de pratiquer de suite. L'opération eut lieu à travers le péritoine,
par la voie transpéritonéale, et l'infection de la poche se propagea à
la séreuse ouverte, et le malade mourut de péritonite au bout de
quelques jours.

Dans ces rétentions aseptiques, d'un certain volume, alors même
que le cathétérisme de l'uretère semble devoir amener la guérison, il
vaut mieux recourir d'emblée à l'opération sans courir le danger d'infecter la rétention aseptique par un drainage à demeure. Dans les
rétentions septiques au contraire, il y a avantage ou à utiliser le
cathétérisme de l'uretère, s'il est praticable, ou à pratiquer la néphrostomie tout d'abord pour recourir ensuite dans un second temps à
l'opération anaplastique sur l'uretère. C'est ce que je me propose de
faire sur un malade que j'ai opéré il y a deux mois et à qui je vais d'ici
peu pratiquer la restauration de l'uretère pour traiter une fistule
urinaire.

J'en arrive maintenant à envisager la *technique* et la *nature* de ces opérations. Elles sont multiples, ne s'adressent pas toutes à la même lésion : mais quelles qu'elles soient, elles se pratiquent par la voie lombaire ou par la voie abdominale. J'ai suivi ces deux voies, j'ai dit comment dans l'opération que j'ai faite abdominale, j'avais vu la péritonite emporter mon malade en quelques jours. J'avais choisi la voie antérieure pour aborder plus directement la poche très volumineuse, pour trouver et explorer plus facilement l'uretère, et à ce point de vue je n'ai pas eu à le regretter. Mais de ce côté la gravité de l'acte opératoire est augmentée, les risques sont plus grands : et si chez mon malade j'avais choisi la voie lombaire, il est probable que malgré l'infection de la poche je n'aurais pas eu d'accident mortel. Depuis lors j'ai eu recours une autre fois pour une uropyonéphrose de volume beaucoup moins considérable il est vrai, à la voie lombaire et j'ai pu me rendre compte combien de ce côté les manœuvres se faisaient faciles, simples et expéditives.

La voie d'accès étant déterminée, le choix de l'opération reste subordonné à la nature et surtout au siège de la lésion. D'une façon générale je préfère l'anastomose latérale à la résection de l'uretère et à l'abouchement terminal. Dans les deux opérations que j'ai eu l'occasion de pratiquer j'ai eu recours à cette anastomose latérale : dans un cas, dans cette grosse hydronéphrose dont j'ai parlé, l'uretère n'était pas précisément rétréci, mais son calibre semblait un peu diminué au-dessous de son attache rénale. Y avait-t-il là des adhérences périurétérales qui effaçaient son calibre en partie? Je ne le saurais dire. Je me contentai de faire au-dessous de cet obstacle relatif une fente à l'uretère et je l'abouchai à la partie déclive de la poche rénale, faisant ici une urétéronéphrostomie.

Dans un autre cas, il s'agissait d'une hydronéphrose intermittente très nette dans un rein mobile : à l'origine de l'uretère, il y avait un rétrécissement dû à la transformation d'une de ces valvules mobiles, que j'ai montré être la cause de l'hydronéphrose du rein mobile. J'ai abouché l'uretère au-dessous de la valvule au bassinet légèrement épaissi, et j'ai fait ainsi une urétéropyélostomie. Le résultat a été très bon : la réunion a été obtenue par première intention, et depuis, les accidents de douleurs et de distension qui avaient été la raison de mon opération ne se sont pas reproduits.

La résection de l'uretère, que je n'ai pas eu l'occasion de pratiquer me paraît plus difficile à réaliser, et je n'y aurais recours que si l'obstacle urétéral siégeait à une distance telle du rein, que l'abouchement au bassinet fût difficilement réalisable.

Dans la dernière opération que j'ai pratiquée, je n'ai pas mis de sonde à demeure, au niveau de l'abouchement urétéro-pyélique : et je crois cette pratique préférable, si la suture au catgut a été bien faite, c'est-à-dire si l'affrontement a été bien réalisé par deux plans de suture, l'un pour les muqueuses et l'autre de renforcement pour les parois conjonctives.

## DISCUSSION.

M. ALBARRAN. — Dans les grosses hydronéphroses, la néphrostomie, aidée dans certains cas du capitonnage, diminue beaucoup le volume du rein, et permet de faire secondairement l'anastomose urétéro-rénale qui conserve le rein. J'ai agi ainsi avec succès et je ne me déciderais à la néphrectomie qu'après l'échec de ces procédés.

Je répéterai encore qu'on ne doit rechercher par le cathétérisme urétéral la guérison complète des grosses hydronéphroses ou des pyonéphroses que dans des cas exceptionnels; dans les rétentions rénales, la sonde urétérale sert au diagnostic précis et facilite les manœuvres opératoires. Après l'opération elle est surtout utile dans les cas infectés, comme le démontrent mes observations.

# DEUXIÈME SÉANCE

## VENDREDI 3 AOUT

*A deux heures et demie.*

Présidence de M. le Professeur KUSTER (Marbourg).

*Communications diverses :*

## REIN ET URETÈRES

---

### DIE BEDEUTUNG DES GEFRIEPRUNCTSBESTIMMUNG DES BLUTS UND DES URINS VOR OPERATIVEN EINGRIFFEN AN DEN NIEREN

#### von Dr HERMANN KÜMMEL,

Chirurg-oberarzt der Neuen Allgem-Krankenhauses.

Die bedeutenden Fortschritte in der Therapie und vor Allem der Diagnose der Nierenkrankheiten während der letzten Jahre, verdanken wir zum grossen Teil dem Ureterenkatheterismus. Dieser gestattet uns fast ausnahmslos den Nachweis, ob beide Nieren vorhanden sind, ferner ob eine oder beide Nieren secerniren ; er gestattet uns ferner, das Secret jeder einzelnen Niere gesondert aufzufangen und auf seine Beschaffenheit in den verschiedenen Richtungen hin (in chemischer, physikalischer, bacteriologischer u. a. m.) eingehender zu untersuchen und eventuell die ungefähre Menge des von jeder einzelnen Niere in einer gewissen Zeit ausgeschiedenen Urins festzustellen. Wie wichtig und notwendig es ist, das Vorhandensein einer functionsfähigen Niere vor einem geplanten operativen Eingriff an der erkrankten festzustellen, wissen wir Alle und bedarf keiner Erwähnung. Dass man oft mit Sorge nach vorgenommener Exstirpation der einen Niere die erste Nierenentleerung erwartet und sich erleichtert fühlt, wenn die Functionsfähigkeit sich als ausreichend erweist, haben wir wohl Alle mehr oder weniger erfahren, und Manchem von uns wird das traurige Factum nicht erspart geblieben sein, dass die Urinausscheidung nicht eintrat und dass der Operirte zu Grunde ging; sei es, dass nur eine Niere vorhanden war, sei es, dass, was weit häufiger ist, die nicht operirte Niere ebenfalls nicht intact war; wissen wir doch, beispielsweise, dass gerade die Nierensteine häufig in beiden Nieren zugleich vorkommen, oder dass endlich die andere Niere,

auscheinend gesund, doch nicht in der Lage war, die Function der
fehlenden Niere mit zu übernehmen und die im Organismus zurück-
gehaltenen Stoffe in vollständiger Weise auszuscheiden. Dass die
« falsche Niere », wenn ich so sagen darf, die weniger oder kaum
erkrankte exstirpirt wurde, da jeder örtliche Anhaltspunkt, Schmerz,
Schwellung, Tumorbildung u. a. m., fehlten und nur die Beschaffenheit des Urins bei normalen Blasenverhältnissen auf die ernste Erkrankung der einen Niere hinwies, gehört nicht zu den seltenen Vor-
kommnissen. Vor diesen erwähnten Irrtümern und Gefahren wird uns
meistenteils der Ureterenkatheterismus schützen können.

Immerhin wird es Fälle geben, welche nur mit grosser Schwierigkeit oder garnicht den Katheterismus der Harnleiter auszuführen
gestatten. Diese Vorkommnisse werden natürlich um so seltener sein,
je mehr Uebung der Untersuchende erlangt hat ; doch können beispielsweise Schrumpfblasen, wie sie bei der Tuberculose des Harn-
organs öfter beobachtet werden, eigentümliche hagerungen der Urete-
renmündungen, trüber Inhalt der Blase u. a., ausnahmsweise und in
gewiss seltenen Fällen den Katheterismus unmöglich machen. Die
schwer erkrankte tuberculöse Niere zum Beispiel soll exstipirt werden. Dürfen wir es wagen, wird das eine nicht ganz intacte Organ die
Function des anderen sicher kranken übernehmen können oder nicht?
Hier blieb uns der Ureteren Katheterismus bis jetzt die Antwort
schuldig. Wir hatten derartige Fälle zu behandeln und die Entscheid-
ung zu treffen.

Es handelte sich zum Beispiel um einen circa 55 jährigen, sonst gut-
genährten kräftigen Mann, der über heftige Kolikartig auftretende
Schmerzen in der linken Seite klagte. Die Anfälle traten fast täglich
auf, der Urin war trüb, eitrig. Eine Gonorrhoe war vor einigen Jahren
vorhanden gewesen, Tuberkelbacillen wurden nicht im Urin gefunden.
Bei der cystoscopischen Untersuchung war die linke Ureterenmündung sehr weit, eine gelockerte ectropionirte Schleimhaut zeigend,
wie wir sie bei der auf den Ureter übergegangen Nierentuberculose
meist zu sehen pflegen. Der Ureterenkatheterismus war nur schwierig
auf dieser Seite auszuführen, da sich das Instrument leicht in der
faltenreichen Schleimhaut fing. Der Urin dieser Seite enthielt sicher
viel Eiterkörperchen, keine Tuberkelbacillen ; der mit dem Ureterenkatheterismus der anderen Niere entnommene Urin war ebenfalls
etwas trüb, wenn auch bei weitem nicht so wie der der anderen Seite,
er enthielt Epithelien und einige Eiterkörperchen, die Ureterenmündung war normal. Die Diagnose wurde auf Tuberculose der linken
Niere gestellt, hauptsächlich nach der Beschaffenheit der Ureteren-

mündung; die Möglichkeit einer Pyelonephritis mit secundärer Steinbildung, worauf die heftigen Koliken deuten konnten, wurde nicht
ausgeschlossen. Durch die physikalische Untersuchung des Urins,
sowie des Blutes, auf die ich gleich zu sprechen komme, konnten wir
die Functionsfähigkeit der rechten Niere feststellen, es war keine
Insuffisienz der rechten Niere vorhanden. Die linke Niere wurd exstirpirt, sie erwies sich als vollkommen tuberculös erkrankt, die Urinens-
scheidung der rechten Niere ging in normaler Weise von statten.

In einem anderen Falle von tuberculoser rechtseitiger Wanderniere
bei einem 24 jährigen Mädchen, bei der auch die andere Ureterenmündung ein nicht normales Aussehen darbot, und der Urin der als
gesund angenommenen Seite trüb entleert wurde, konnte die Functionsfähigkeit der linken Niere festgestellt werden. Nach der Exstirpation der erkrankten Nieren functionirten die anderen normal, ob-
wohl der Urin auch später noch trüb blieb.

Eine andere 45 jährige Patientin wurde uns als Nierensteine oder
als Pyelonephritis der linken Seite überwiesen. Das im Urin enthaltene
spärliche Albumen wurde für Eiteralbumen gehalten. Vor der Kysto-
scopie stellten wir in der gleich zu schildernden Weise durch Untersuchung des Blutes und des Urins fest, dass eine Insufficienz der
Nieren vorhanden war, dass eine Exstirpation der angenommenen
kranken linken Niere unter allen Umständen nicht vorgenommen
werden konnte. Der Katheterismus der Ureteren ergab, dass aus
beiden Nieren ein spärlicher, Niereneiweis enthaltender Urin, links
mehr als rechts entleert wurde; später wurden auch Cylinder konsta-
tirt. Hier handelt es sich um eine beginnende Nephritis mit Niereninsufficienz. Der weitere Verlauf bestätigte unsere Diagnose.

Der Ureterenkatheterismus giebt uns wohl über die Beschaffenheit
des Secrets der einzelnen Nieren in chemischer und microscopischer
Beziehung Aufschluss, darüber aber, ob die Functionsfähigkeit und
Arbeitsleistung der Nieren überhaupt eine genügende ist, ob von
vornherein eine Niereninsufficienz besteht, welche einen erfolgreichen chirurgischen Eingriff ausschliessen muss, gab uns bisher der
Harnleiterkatheterismus keinen Aufschluss.

Die neueren Untersuchungen und Erfahrungen haben jedoch
gezeigt, dass auch in dieser Beziehung dem Ureterenkatheterismus
eine sehr wesentliche Bedeutung zukommt. Die Gefahren, welche mit
dem Ureterenkatheterismus verknüpft sind und welche mir vielfach
übertrieben zu sein scheinen, halte ich für sehr gering. Wir haben
bei unserm in recht zahlreichen Fällen ausgeführten Katheterismus
der Harnleiter bis jetzt noch niemals irgend einen Nachteil erleb

und ebenso haben Albarran, Casper, Rovsing u. A. nach ihren Berichten in weit mehr als 1000 Fällen niemals eine Infection beobachtet. Dass eine solche bei aller Vorsicht ausnahmsweise, ebenso wie bei dem Katheterismus der Blase einmal vorkommen kann, bezweifele ich nicht. Hier beweisen Thatsachen und Erfahrungen mehr als theoretische Erwägungen.

Um nun die Functionsfähigkeit der Nieren oder ihre Insufficienz genauer festzustellen, hat man einen neuen Weg eingeschlagen und physiologische Methoden zu Hülfe genommen. Die Physiologie und die innere Medicin haben sich, wie Ihnen bekannt, in letzter Zeit eingehend mit der Frage der Niereninsufficienz und dem osmotischen Druck der Flüssigkeit unseres Organismus beschäftigt; jedoch auch die Chirurgie, vor Allem die Nierenchirurgie, welche wohl am meisten practischen Nutzen zu ziehen berufen ist, sollte diese Anregung nicht ungenutzt vorüber gehen lassen und alle Momente berücksichtigen, welche die Insufficienz der Nierenleistung vor chirurgischen Eingriffen feststellen helfen.

Es sind verschiedene Momente, deren Feststellung uns einen Fingerzeig für die Leistungsfähigkeit oder Insufficienz der Nieren geben.

1) Die Bestimmung des Harnstoffs.

2) Die Bestimmung des Gefrierpunktes des Blutes.

3) Die Bestimmung des Gefrierpunktes des Urins, besonders des jeder einzelnen Niere durch den Ureterenkatheterismus entnommenen.

Es sind das Methoden, die zum Teil in relativ einfacher Weise bei einiger Uebung von Jedem rasch ausgeführt werden können, ohne besondere chemische Kenntnisse zu verlangen.

Die Feststellung der innerhalb 24 Stunden ausgeschiedenen Harnstoffmenge ist wohl die einfachste, jedoch auch die am wenigsten zuverlässige Methode. Immerhin giebt sie uns einen Fingerzeig und einen vorläufigen Anhaltspunkt über die eventuelle Insufficienz der Leistungsfähigkeit der Nieren und hat auch schon oft Anwendung gefunden. Wenn man annimmt, dass normal arbeitende Nieren eine bestimmte Menge Harnstoff ausscheiden müssen, so liegt es nahe aus dem Unvermögen, diese Stoffwechselprodukte in genügender Menge aus dem Körper auszuscheiden, einen Rückschluss auf eine mangelhafte Arbeitsfähigkeit der Niere zu ziehen. Leider ist nun die unter normalen Verhältnissen ausgeschiedene Harnstoffmenge eine ungemein schwankende und Tagesmengen von 20 bis 55 Gr. gelten im Allgemeinen als Durchschnittszahlen. Man nimmt nun an, dass ein Heruntergehen der innerhalb 24 Stunden ausgeschiedenen Harnstoffmengen unter die Hälfte, unter etwa 15 bis 16 Gr. auf eine Insufficienz der Nieren schliessen lasse, welche einen schweren operativen Eingriff, die Entfernung der einen Niere nicht ausführbar erscheinen lässt. Wir haben in einer grösseren Anzahl von Fällen diese Harnstoffbestimmung vor jeder Nierenoperation in Anwendung gezogen. Die Resultate stimmten im Grossen und Ganzen mit den zuverlässigen Methoden der Gefrierpunktbestimmung überein. In allen Fällen, in welchen wir eine Entfernung der Niere vornahmen, betrug die tägliche Harnstoffausscheidung mehr als 15 Gr. und in allen Fällen erwiess sich die zurückbleibende Niere als functionsfähig.

Natürlich wird die Bestimmung der einmaligen Tagesmenge des ausgeschiedenen Harnstoffs nicht zu verwerten sein; sondern die in einer Reihe aufeinanderfolgender Tage bei genügender Nahrungsaufnahme annähernd gleichen Zahlen werden erst einen einigermassen sicheren Schluss auf die Sufficienz der einen Niere gestatten.

Zur Feststellung der Menge des Harnstoffs bedienen wir uns des sehr genau arbeitenden Esbach'schen Apparates, welcher durch einfaches Ablesen von der Scala eines Glascylinders und Nachlesen in der aufgestellten Tabelle die Harnstoffmenge direct in Procenten angiebt und danach die Gesammtmenge nach der innerhalb 24 Stunden ausgeschiedenen Urinmenge leicht feststellen lässt.

Wesentlich genauere Resultate giebt die Bestimmung des Gefrierpunktes der Flüssigkeit des menschlichen Körpers, vor Allem des Blutes.

Schon auf dem diesjährigen Congress der deutschen Gesellschaft für Chirurgie berichtete ich über die Bedeutung der Gefrierpunktsbestimmung des Blutes und Urins für die Feststellung der Functionsfähigkeit der Nieren. Wir haben unsere Untersuchungen festgesetzt und unsere Beobachtungen in allen Fällen, es sind über 70, bestätigt gefunden, so dass wir nun mehr die *Gefrierpunktsbestimmung* als ein *wichtiges diagnostisches Hilfsmittel zum Nachweis der Functionsfähigkeit der einen Niere von operativen Eingriffen ansehen zu dürfen lauben.*

Es ist aus der Physik und Physiologie bekannt, dass zwischen zwei chemisch gleichen Lösungen von verschiedener Concentration Wechselbeziehungen stattfinden, indem sich bei Berührung der Flüssigkeiten die Concentrationsunterschiede durch Strömung der gelösten Stoffe nach der Seite der schwächeren Concentration hin auszugleichen streben. Sind die Lösungen durch eine Scheidewand getrennt, die nur das Lösungsmittel, aber nicht die gelösten Stoffe, hindurch lässt, so strömt das Lösungsmittel von der Seite der stärkeren Concentration zu der der schwächeren, bis der Unterschied ausgeglichen ist. Dieser Vorgang heisst bekanntlich Osmose, die Anziehungskraft derartiger Lösungen der osmotische Druck. Von den Flüssigkeiten des menschlichen Körpers sind das Blut und der Harn als Lösungen gedacht, den Gesetzen der Osmose unterworfen. Der osmotische Druck ist proportional der Menge der in einer Flüssigkeit gelösten Moleküle. Die Menge der gelösten Molecüle wird gemessen durch die Erniedrigung des Gefrierpunktes. Enthält nämlich eine Lösung wenig gelöste Molecüle, so ist ihr Gefrierpunkt nur wenig tiefer als der des Wassers. Je grösser die Zahl der gelösten Moleküle, desto tiefer liegt ihr Gefrierpunkt, desto stärker ist also die Gefrierpunktserniedrigung.

Diese Beobachtung, auf welche van t'Hoff u. A. zuerst aufmerksam gemacht haben, hat A. v. Korányi in eingehender Weise studirt und zahlreiche Gefrierpunktsbestimmungen von Blut und Harn an gesunden und kranken Menschen ausgeführt. Ihm folgten Lindemann, Dreser und andere. In Berlin sind sowohl in der Senator'schen Klinik von Richter und Roth sehr interessante experimentelle Studien über die Niereninsufficienz, als auch auf der Renvers'schen Abteilung von M. Senator eingehende klinische Beobachtungen über den osmotischen Druck angestellt. Näher auf diese interessanten Arbeiten einzugehen, würde zu weit führen; die Beobachtungen stimmen im Grossen und Ganzen mit den Korányi'schen überein.

Nach den Untersuchungen von A. v. Koranyi und andere, sowie durch *unsere eigenen zahlreichen Beobachtungen ist als feststehend zu betrachten, dass der Gefrierpunkt, also die molecülare Concentration des menschlichen Blutes unter physiologischen Bedingungen eine constante Grösse mit nur ganz unerheblichen Schwankungen darstellt.*

*Das normale menschliche Blut hat einen Gefrierpunkt von — 0,56° Cels. unter dem des destillirten Wassers.* Schwankungen von — 0,55°-0,57°, also von 2/100°, sind noch als physiologisch anzusehen. Eine Zunahme der Gefrierpunktserniedrigung auf — 0,58°-0,60° und darüber zeigt an, dass beide Nieren mangelhaft functioniren, dass eine Niereninsufficienz vorhanden ist. Von einem operativen Eingriff ist so lang Abstand zu nehmen, bis der Gefrierpunkt von annähernd —0,56° erreicht ist.

In den zahlreichen Fällen (über 70), in denen wir die Functionsfähigkeit der Nieren nachweisen konnten, fanden wir den constanten Blutgefrierpunkt von 0,56; nur selten die erwähnten geringen Schwankungen.

*Findet die Elimination der Gesammtheit der Stoffwechselproducte in der genügenden Weise statt, so ist stets der normale Blutgefrierpunkt*

*von —0,56° als Zeichen jedenfalls einer genügend arbeitenden Niere
vorhanden.*

*Sobald die Nierenfunction im Verhältnis zum Stoffwechsel unzu-
reichend wird, vermehren die aufgespeicherten Zersetzungsstoffe die
moleküläre Concentration und dem entsprechend wird die Gefrier-
punkterniedrigung mehr als 0,56 betragen.*

Diese Beobachtung konnte in allen von uns untersuchten und operirten Fällen bestätigt werden. Bei Tumoren, Pyelitis und Pyelonephritis, bei Tuberculose der Nieren und bei internen Nierenleiden
(parenchymatöser, interstitieller Nephritis, Schrumpfniere u. a.).

In 16 Fällen von doppelseitiger Nierenaffection (Schrumpfniere,
doppelseitiger Cystenniere, Anurie nach Laparotomie in Folge gleich-
zeitigen Nierencarcinoms, Amyloid, renalen Blutungen) betrug der
Gefrierpunkt 0,60-0,65 in einem Falle sogar bis 0,71. In zwei Fällen
renaler Blutungen, in denen durch den Ureterenkatheterismus aus
der einen Niere blutiger, aus der andern klarer Urin ohne Eiweis und
Cylinder entleert wurde und bei denen anfangs die Annahme eines
einseitigen Nierentumors nahe lag, wurde ein operativer Eingriff
unterlassen, weil der Gefrierpunkt des Bluts über 0,60 betrug ; später
wurde bei beiden Kranken eine interstitielle Nephritis mit Blutungen
festgestellt.

Eine Niere mit genügender Arbeitsleistuug hat stets den normalen
Gefrierpunkt von 0,56.

In 11 Fällen, in denen die Nephrectomie vorgenommen werden
musste (wegen Tuberculose, Tumoren, Steinniere, Nierenvereiterung
u. a.), betrug der Gefrierpunkt vor der Operation 0,56. als sicheres
Zeichen der Functionsfähigkeit des einen Organs.

Nach der Operation functionirte in allen Fällen das zurückbleibende
Organ in normaler Weise und behielt der Gefrierpunkt seine normale
Höhe von 0,56. Nur in einem Falle eines linksseitigen paranephri-
tischen Abscesses, bei welchem sich nach der Incision eine Nieren-
fistel gebildet hatte, betrug der Gefrierpunkt 0,59. Erst allmählich
nach Kräftigung des Patienten übernahm die gesunde Niere nach
circa 4 Wochen die Arbeitsleistung der Kranken. Der Gefrierpunkt
stieg allmählich auf 0,57. Die Extirpation der Fistelniere verlief nunmehr ohne Zwischenfall ; die zurückbleibende functionirte in normaler
Weise. Gefrierpunkt 0,57.

Noch einfacher als die Bestimmung des Gefrierpunktes des Blutes
ist die des Urins selbst. Indess erscheint mir die Metode nicht so zu-
verlässig, da die physiologischen Schwankungen nach den Untersuchungen der einzelnen Autoren sehr gross sind. Während der

Gefrierpunkt des normalen Harns nach Lindemann bei mittlerer Harnmenge zwischen —1,5° und —2,5°, nach Korányi zwischen —1,5° und —2,0°, nach Albarran zwischen —1,50° und —2,0° schwankt, fanden wir Erniedrigungen zwischen —0,9° und —2,0°. Gefrierpunktserniedrigungen unter —0,9° deuten auf Nierenerkrankungen, resp auf Insufficienz der Nieren hin. Tritt bei Cystitis oder Pyelitis eine Verminderung der Concentration des Harns, eine Gefrierpunktserniedrigung unter 0,9° ein, so ist ein Uebergreifen des Krankheitsprocessen auf die Nieren sehr wahrscheinlich.

Bei schweren Nierenerkrankungen — doppelseitigen Cystennieren, Schrumpfnieren, u. s. w., wie ich sie erwähnte — tritt eine bedeutende Gefrierpunktserniedrigung des Harns ein, sodass derselbe dem des Blutes näher kommt, ihn sogar übertrifft.

Einen weit sicheren Anhaltspunkt giebt die Gefrierpunktsbestimmung des Urins, wenn derselbe durch den Ureterenkatheterismus jedem Organ gesondert entnommen und vergleichend gegenübergestellt wird. Hierauf haben Casper und Albarran zuerst aufmerksam gemacht.

Bei Pyelitis und anderen Erkrankungen ohne Mitbeteiligung der Nieren war der Gefrierpunkt des jeder einzelnen Niere entnommenen Urins annähernd gleich.

zum Beispiel R. 0,56 — L. 0,42
—        R. 1,70 — L. 1,72
—        R. 1,01 — L. 1,02

War eine Niere erkrankt, was durch die spätere Exstirpation bestätigt wurde, so war der Unterschied des Gefrierpunktes des Urins ein sehr grosser. Zum Beispiel in drei Fällen von Pyelonephritis ·

kranke — gesunde Niere
0,19    —    1,75
0,13    —    1,05
0,57    —    ' 1,53

Der Ureterenkatheterismus gestattet uns ausserdem noch das Secret jeder einzelnen Niere nach den verschiedensten Richtungen hin zu untersuchen. Er hat uns gezeigt, dass jede Niere für sich, unabhängig von der andern, functionirt.

Ich habe Ihnen nur in kurzer Skizze die Resultate unserer Untersuchungen mitgeteilt, um bei dem noch vorliegenden reichen und interessanten Material die Zeit nicht zu sehr in Anspruch nehmen. In einer baldigst erscheinenden ausführlichen Arbeit werden für diejenigen welche sich für den Gegenstand interessiren, unsere Versuche und Erfahrungen eingehender niedergelegt.

Wenn ich das Gesagte noch einmal kurz zusammen fassen darf, so ,würde sich folgendes ergeben :

Die mit dem Beckmann'schen Gefrierapparat unschwer auszuführende Gefrierpunktsbestimmung des Blutes genügt zur Feststellung der Functionsfähigkeit der Nieren. Zur weiteren Sicherung der Diagnose, welches die erkrankte Niere, und welcher Art die Erkrankung ist, wird die Untersuchung des jedem einzelnen Organ durch den Ureterenkatheterismus entnommenen Urins nach den verschiedensten Richtungen hin, sowie die Gefrierpunktsbestimmung desselben anzuwenden sein.

---

## LE INDICAZIONI DELLA NEFRECTOMIA E SPECIALMENTE PER TUMORI MALIGNI

par M. A. D'ANTONA, .

prof. di clinica ghirurgica Propedeutica nella R. Università di Napoli.

Della chirurgia degli organi delle grandi cavità la renale ed ureterica sono certamente tra quelle che hanno più progredito in questi due ultimi decennii.

I successi pratici sempre migliori sono dovuti ai progressi delle conoscenze patogeniche, anatomo-patologiche, e specie della diagnostica e tecnica operativa.

Nel rene tanto esposto ai processi infettivi in via ascendente dalla vescica, e per via ematica, ed ai processi neoplastici, perchè è in esso che si compie la più complicata formazione embriologica, concorrendovi tutti i foglietti blastodermici, e perci più facili le aberrazioni, si ha in compenso nella sua forte capsula una ragione di circoscrizione dei processi.

La rimozione di un rene infetto, o con neoplasia, premunisce l'altro rene, il quale iperfunzionando è meno disposto ad essere infettato.

La nefrectomia nei suoi risultati operativi e curativi non è più una gravissima operazione, grazie al miglioramento dei mezzi diagnostici e della tecnica.

La nefrotomia preparatoria in alcuni casi di pielonefriti piogeniche riesce curativa, in altri prepara condizioni migliori locali e generali per la migliore riuscita della nefrectomia.

I risultati variano nelle idronefrosi, nelle pielonefriti, nei tumori. Ecco uno specchietto delle mie nefrectomie.

Statistica.

| | NUMERO DEI CASI | MORTI | GUARITI | PERCENTUALE DELLA MORTALITA | OSSERVAZIONI |
|---|---|---|---|---|---|
| Per tuberculosi. | 2 | 1 | 1 | 50 0/0 | La prima operata del 1882 vive ancora, ed è madre di 5 figli viventi. |
| Per pielonefrite (dal 1884 al' 87). | 5 | 4 | 1 | 80 0/0 | Il guarito mori atassico dopo 10 anni. |
| Id. (dal 1888 al' 99) | 19 | » | 19 | » | Per lo più metodo lombare. In 9 casi la nefrectomia fu preceduta dalla nefrotomia preparatoria. Tutti godo..o presentemente buona salute. |
| Per tumori renali (del 1888 al 1900). | 6 | 2 | 4 | 55 0/0 | Una operata segnita per 2 anni; poi mancarono sue notizie. — Una sta bene dorpo circa 50 mesi dall'operazione. — Una sta bene da 16 mesi. Uno dopo 15 mesi riproduzione; adesso sta bene dopo la seconda operazione che data da 10 mesi. |
| Tumori perirenali (dal' 1893 al' 95). | 2 | » | 2 | 00 0/0 | |

Come si rileva, il metodo lombare è preferibile, e pratico il mio a curva posteriore, resecando l'estremo della dodicesima costola, ed eventualmente resecando anche l'undicesima con speciale riguardo alla pleura. Quando è necessità, allora procedo col mio metodo addomo-estraperitoneale.

Dei sei casi di nefrectomie per tumori, in cinque ho potuto fare uno studio istogenetico accurato, dal quale ho ottenuto rilievi importanti per contribuire con osservazioni proprie allo intendimento genetico e strutturale dei tanto discussi tumori renali e perirenali.

Nel 1° caso operato nel 1888 trattavasi di *carcinoma peri-pelvico da tessuto tubolare renale aberrato*. Il tumore era tutto sviluppato nel connettivo peri-pelvico posteriore, ed appena nel polo superiore renale il tumore prendeva aderenze ed infiltrava il tessuto renale.

Nelle quattro figure della Tavola I, si possono seguire tutte le fasi iperplastiche dell' epitelio dei tuboli renali sino alla sua completa trasformazione ed infiltrazione disseminata nel tessuto connettivo interstiziale, quindi la origine adenomatosa renale e percio ecto, e mesodermica, sino alla fase carcinomatosa.

Della donna s'ebbero sempre per due anni buone nuove, e dal'90 in poisnunaes.

Il 2° caso di *liposarcoma* è del 1898. I molti lobi lipomatosi sono separati da quello sarcomatoso fusicellulare. I primi erano di antichissima data e probabilmente da blocchi grassosi pericapsulari inclusi nel rene, ed il sarcoma derivava certamente dal connettivo, e percio tumori mesenchimali.

La donna gode tuttora buona salute.

Il 5° caso è tipo di *ipernefroma papillare intracanalicolare cistico primitivo surrenale*, ed è un esemplare nel quale si riscontrano le note sommarie di un tumore da germi surrenali, cioè : 1° la multiplicità. — Ed è singolare che vi siano noduli parenchimali, ma e pochi sono più piccoli e più giovani, altri sotto-capsulari più grandi, ed altri extra-capsulari più grandi ancora, numerosi e più evoluti.

2° Il perfetto incapsulamento, e non pure di quelli intra ma altresi degli extra-capsulari.

5° La consistenza molle, sino al punto che la massa di uno è ridotta ad una poltiglia.

4° L'aspetto uniforme, spongioso, cribrato, granuloso e giallo-arancio o zolfo, come le ovaie degli echini.

5° Molto vascolare, con degenerazione grassa jalina degli elementi delle pareti vasali ; manca solamente il glicogeno e l'amiloide.

All'esame istologico potrebbe sorgere la quistione di un adenoma da tubi uriniferi. Pero la speciale struttura dello stroma e disposizione degli elementi, e specie la somiglianza con quell'adenoma primitivo della capsula ([1]), confortano nella idea della genesi addirittura surrenale primitiva, che poi ha in vaso il rene (vedi fig. 1, 2, 5, 4, 5, 6 e 7 della Tav : II e III.)

Difatti in questo caso mai disturbi urinarii, non albumina, mai sangue.

Il 4° caso è di tipico *ipernefroma intrarenale maligno*.

Uomo di 59 anni : — da un anno disturbi renali, ematurie ricorrenti ed abbondanti ; varicocele pronunziatissimo a sinistra e prolungantesi nel canale inguinale, e più oltre ancora.

11 Luglio operazione. — Metodo addomo-estraperitoneale ; emorragie secondarie da tutto il campo operativo ; suppurazione ; guarigione. Riproduzione dopo 14 mesi ; seconda operazione. Adesso sono trascorsi 10 mesi ed il signore sta bene.

Il tumore siede nel polo inferiore e nel corpo del rene ; resta libero

1. Vedi T. V. fig. 1 e 2.

il solo polo superiore. Il tumore è tutto intrarenale, ed è costituito da una grossa massa con molti noduli attorno, incapsulati. La sostanza di essi è molto vascolare, molle; aspetto spongioso, qua che punto di rammollimento.

Al taglio microscopico di un nodulo a piccolo ingrandimento si rileva una struttura adenoide cistica (Tav : IV, fig. 1), e civoè tubi dilatati più o meno ridotti a cavità di diversa larghezza, irregolari, e coverti di epitelio, e cordoni pieni degli stessi elementi; e tutti circondati ed intermezzati da tessuto connettivo. — Nelle figure successive 2 e 5 gli elementi assumono un carattere chiaramente epiteliale, ed alcuni con incipiente degenerazione ialina. — Nella fig. 5 la struttura si accentua come alveolare carcinomatosa, quindi con spazii più o meno piccoli ed alveolari e con elementi più piccoli e giovani.

Nella fig. 4 vi ha una papilla tagliata longitudinalmente con grosso epitelio da rivestimento e con stroma connettivale alquanto infiltrato di elementi giovani. Dette papille sporgono nella cavità, come si puo rilevare dalla fig. 1 a più forte ingrandimento.

Nella fig. 6, Tav. V, la struttura si fa atipica ed irregolare. — Setti connettivali fibrosi intersecano in vario senso il tumore e circoscrivono degli spazii irregolari, ripiedi di giovani cellule epiteliali, delle quali alcune in degenerazione, e che quasi isolatamente o a due infiltranoli connettivo interstiziale. — È una vera struttura carcinomatosa.

Nella fig. 7, è riportato un taglio del tessuto renale prossimo alla periferia del tumore, e che è in istato di cronica nefrite con sclerosi.

Nella Tav. V, fig. 1 e 2 sono riprodotte le immagini, a piccolo e forte ingrandimento, di un *piccolo tumore iniziato in una capsula surrenale*, rinvenuto in un cadavere sezionato dal professor Maffucci, e che riproduce perfettamente le immagini dei due preparati precedenti.

Il 5° caso è *d'ipernefroma maligno intrarenale*. — Signora di 40 anni e di costituzione debole, con petecchie emorragiche cutanee. — Rene sinistro mobile per molti anni, ma con poche molestie. — Nel 1896 (tre anni prima dell'operazione) dolori al fianco sinistro e vescica urinaria; emissione di un fiocco giallo-nerastro, e poi sangue nelle urine durato otto giorni. — Nel'99 ricomparve l'ematuria.

Grosso tumore, lobato, in parte molle, in parte duro, mobile, occupa tutta la metà sinistra dell'addome.

Urea 22 gr. per litro.

Emoglobina 47 (Fleischl.)

22 giugno 1899 operazione; — metodo addomo-estraperitoneale. — Asportazione piuttosto facile. — L'ampia ferita viene riunita per

prima. — Al 5° giorno gravi fatti tossicemici — s'apre la ferita e vien fuori molto prodotto sanguinolento putrido e con sviluppo di gas.

Si coltiva un corto bacillo capsulato, anerobio, gassogeno in sommo grado.

Largo uso di acqua ossigenata e tintura di iodo. Cessa la tossicemia e l'albuminuria, e la signora guarisce rapidamente. La guarigione si mantiene ancora, e sono sedici mesi.

Esame anatomico. Il tumore è incapsulato : è di centim : 15 per 13 e 10. Il solo polo inferiore del rene è conservato : il resto è costituito da un aggregato di grossi e piccoli noduli incapsulati : qualcuno sporgente nella pelvi renale.

Al microscopio, a piccolo ingrandimento si osservano noduli più o meno grandi, circondati da tessuto connettivo fibroso, che li delimita nettamente, come una capsula, dalla quale partono delle gittate connettivali che penetrano nei noduli.

Ad un ingrandimento più forte gli elementi cellulari che costituiscono la massa del nodulo sono distribuiti a cordoni, hanno aspetto di cellule epitéliali, poligonali, stivate ed addossate fra di loro, con protoplasma chiaro, omogeneo od appena granuloso, a nucleo centrale, grosso, vescicoloso, di cui alcuni sono ricchi di granulazioni cromatiche.

Questi cordoni sono limitati allo esterno da un sottile strato di elementi endoteliali e da vasi.

In alcuni punti nello stroma connettivale del tumore si notano abbondanti sezioni di vasi sanguigni neoformati a tipo embrionale.

Questo è il tipo di tumore che più si avvicina alla struttura istologica della parte corticale della capsula surrenale.

Le figure relative ai preparati di questo 5° caso non si sono riportate, perchè ripetono perfettamente lo schema di quelle del 4° caso precedente (Tav ; IV e V, fig. 1 à 7.)

Il 6° caso è di *antica pielonefrite suppurativa* e consecutivo sviluppo d'*ipernefroma maligno intrarenale*.

Nobile signora, poco meno di 60 anni, di costituzione gracile e consumata da lunga malattia : — pielonefrite suppurata portata da più di tre lustri. — Ematuria nell'agosto'99. Moltissimo pus nelle urine — cronica tossicemia subfebbrile — gravi disturbi digestivi.

Tumore grosso che occupa tutto il lombo, ipocondrio e fossa iliaca dritta, in grande parte solido, in basso molle.

Nel febbraio 1900 operazione, con taglio obliquo; — operazione spedita : — collasso durante la narcosi, che si ripete dopo due ore e dopo tre ore muore.

Il grosso tumore è costituito dal rene che verso il polo inferiore è trasformato insieme alla pelvi in una sacca purulenta. Il tumore spaccato presenta le solite apparenze a lobi incapsulati, una sporgenza nella sacca pelvica purulenta.

Un nodulo fu estirpato dal connettivo perirenale superiore.

Il tumore ando smarrito.


Dallo studio dei miei casi e consimili mi sono convinto che nessuna teoria unilaterale sulla natura e genesi di quei tumori degli adulti è esatta, ed invece sta che nel più dei casi è :

1° o da germi aberrati nel parenchima renale (Grawitz e compagni);

2° o dalla stessa capsula surrenale in sito o da porzione succenturiata di essa ed il rene viene invaso secondariamente (caso 5° riportato sopra);

3° o dagli epitelii preesistenti dei canalicoli uriniferi in sito (Sudek);

4° o da canalicoli uriniferi succenturiati estrarenali (1 caso riportato sopra);

5° o dagli endotelii dei vasi o del connettivo (Hildebrandt.).

Adunque nel rene si riscontrano tutti i tipi di tumori connettivali mesenchimali (fibroma, lipoma, angioma, endotelioma) o mesodermici (rabdomioma, adenoma), e tumori epiteliali derivanti dall'ectoderma o dall' entoderma (papilloma, epitelioma, cancro).

Da una parte il fatto della speciale disposizione del rene, della capsula e loro dintorni a poter divenir sede di sviluppo di tumori di derivazione ora ectodermica, ora entodermica, ora mesodermica, ed infine mesenchimale; dall'altra il fatto che non raramente si trovano tumori di varia origine combinati insieme da costituire dei veri tumori misti, oltre a creare difficoltà di ricognizione e distinzione delle diverse entità morbose, rendevano il loro intendimento difficilissimo, e percio si sono avuti tanti studii e conclusioni incerte e spesso contradditorie.

Invero la ragione di tutte quelle incertezze è di ordine generale, e sta appunto nella singolare e speciale costituzione anatomica normale, e nel complicato sviluppo embrionale degli organi genito-urinarii.

Se l'embriologia non vedeva chiaro nel modo di sviluppo del corpo e canale di Wolff, se tutti gli organi e tessuti derivati da quelli non avevano una natura ben definita e riconoscibile, come si poteva intendere la patogenesi e la natura dei tumori di quelle sedi?

Gli studii modernissimi d'embriologia comparata e sviluppo filogenetico degli organi genito-urinarii hanno fatto un gran passo, ed i primi ad approfittarne siamo stati noi patologi e chirurgi.

Cosi pare si sia oggi di accordo tutti :

1° Che il canale segmentario, venturo condotto di Wolff e suoi derivati, e di origine chiaramente ectodermica ;

2° Che dall'ectoderma deriva il mesoderma, e quindi il celoma ;

5° Che dal fondo di questo, e propriamente dal seno posteriore comincia a formarsi e svilupparsi l'epitelio germinativo, i cui prodotti formativi affondandosi vanno ad incontrarsi e mischiarsi coi prodotti del canale segmentario ; e tutti insieme compenetrano e si lasciano compenetrare da tessuti mesenchimali (connettivo dei vasi).

Sicchè nella costituzione di quegli organi contribuiscono prodotti dei due foglietti primitivi (ecto ed entoderma) e secondarii (mesoderma e mesenchima) non solo, ma essi si compenetrano, ed a loro volta si modificano a vicenda, e sino ad un punto che non è facile apprezzare, ond'è che la loro differenziazione in alcuni punti à difficile determinare.

Questo che accade nel normale sviluppo si ripete nella quistione dei tumori, specie in quelli a sviluppo rapido embrionale e maligno. Come conseguenza ed espressione di questa facile compenetrazione e modificazione scambievole tra i tessuti di diversa derivazione, si ha il fatto frequente che zolle adipose, o blocchi di sostanza surrenale vengano ad includersi nel rene ; altra volta ed è il caso più raro, isole di sostanza renale si trovano o nel connettivo perirenale o a distanza vengono incluse nelle capsule surrenali ; e sono queste specialmente che danno occasione a neoformazioni a sviluppo spesso embrionale.

------

**SPIEGAZIONE DELLE TAVOLE**

par M. le docteur D'ANTONA,

## TAVOLA I.

### CASO I°.

FIG. I. — Una sezione del tumore guardata a debole ingrandimento (obb. I oc. II Seibert). La massa neoplastica è fatta da grossi accumuli cellulari con scarso intermezzo di tessuto connettivo fibroso.

   *a* - masse cellulari ;

   *b* - capsula del tumore.

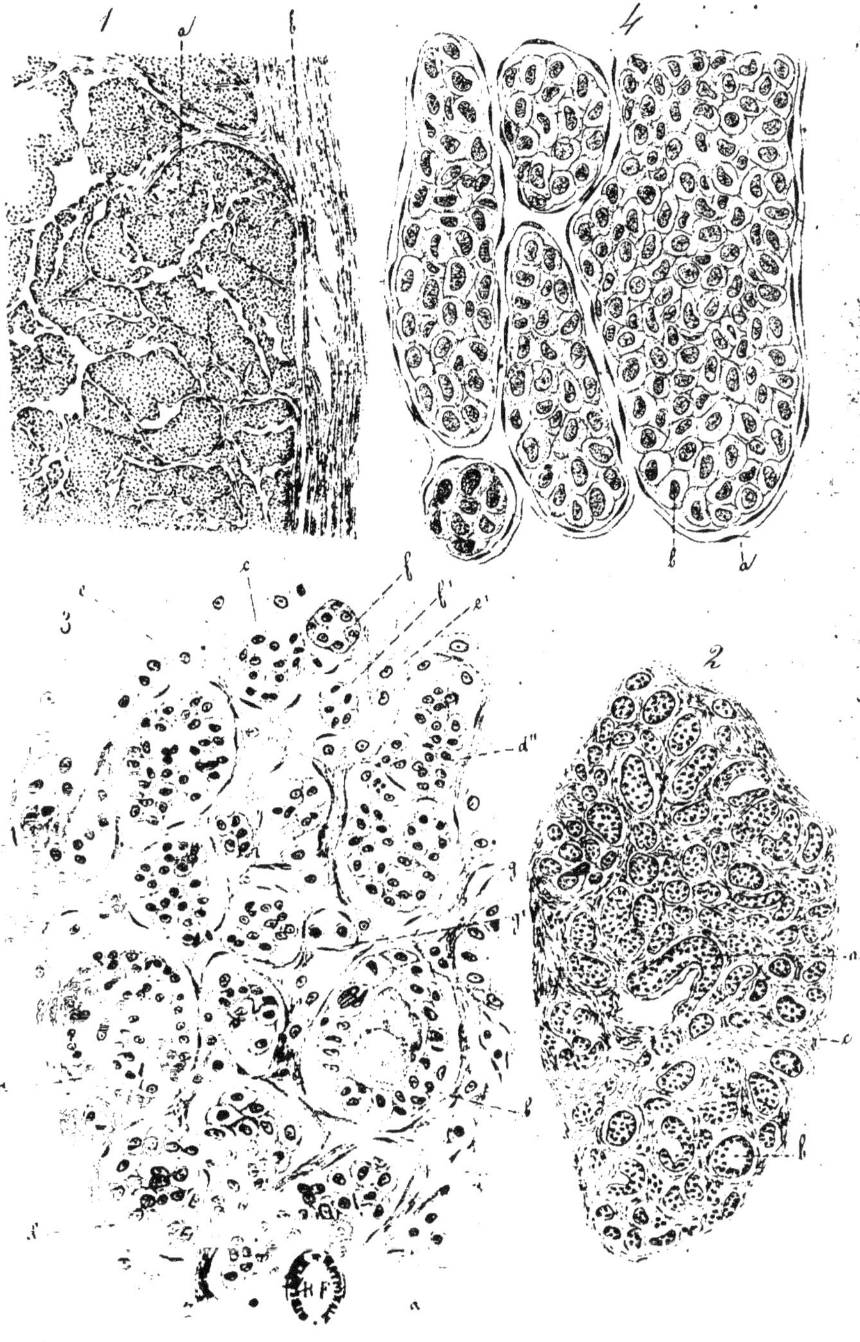

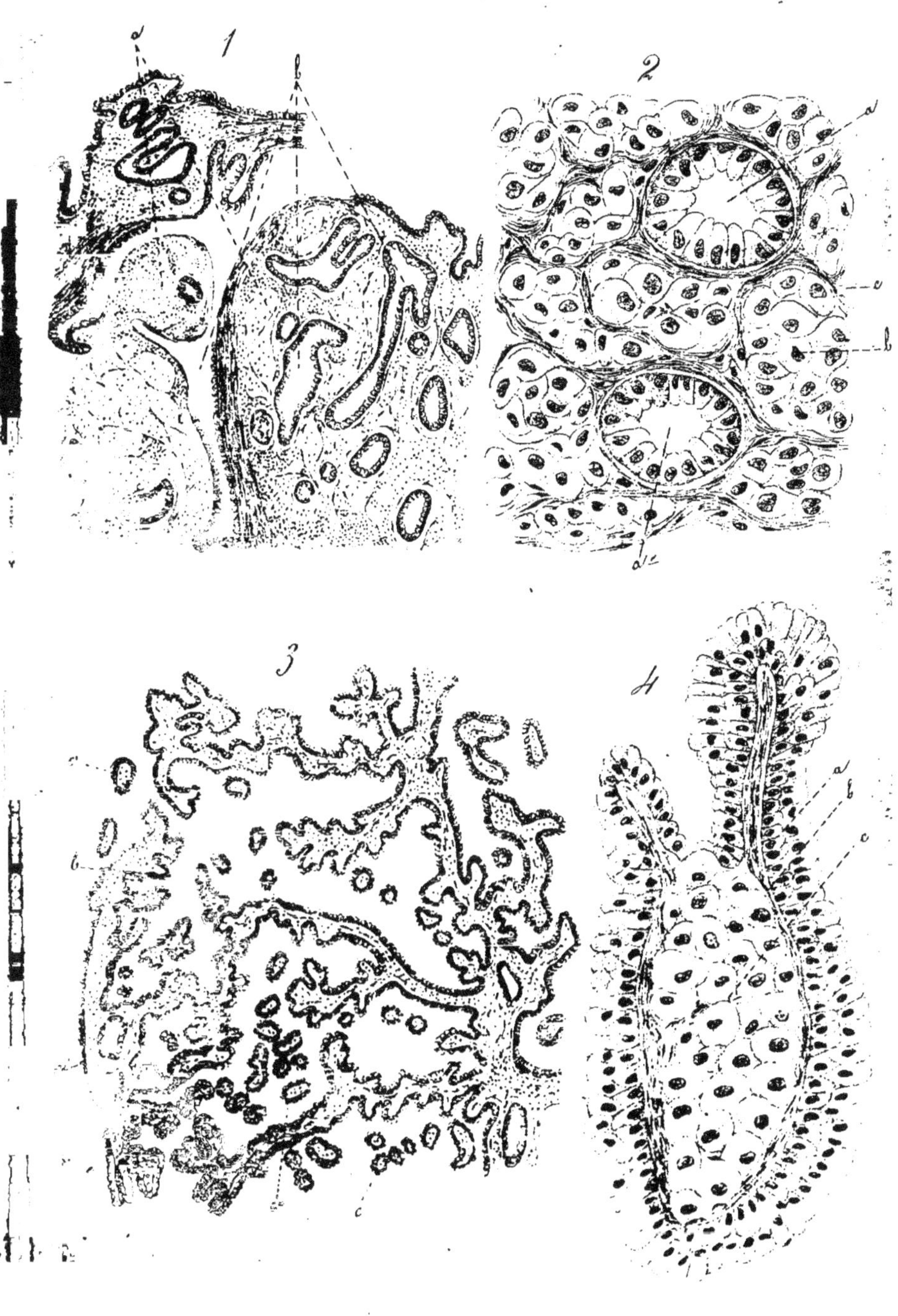

FIG. II. — *a-b-* cordoni e tubi epiteliali renali;

> *c* - tessuto connettivo fibroso fra i nidi epiteliali (oc. 5, obb. A Zeiss).

FIG. III. — *a* - connettivo interstiziale;

> *b* - tubolo renale dilatato con epitelio proliferato e cilindro amorfo.
>
> *c, c'* - tuboli renali di aspetto normale ;
>
> *d, d' d''* - trasformazione dei tuboli renali in massa neoplastica per rigogliosa formazione epiteliale;
>
> *e, e'* - cellule epiteliali infiltrate nel connettivo interstiziale ;
>
> *g, g'*-vasi sanguigni.

FIG. IV. — Enorme sviluppo degli alveoli con scarso tessuto connettivo fibroso intermedio.

> *a* - tessuto connettivo;
>
> *b* - alveoli epiteliali (ocul. 5, obb. *D* Zeiss).

## TAVOLA II.

### CASO 5°.

FIG. I. — Massa della neoplasia, in alcuni punti esistono residu i di

1. Del 2ᵉ caso non vi sono figure.

> sostanza renale.
>
> *a* - tessuto e sostanza del tumore ;
>
> *b* - tubi, e cavitâ o spazii irregolari con rivestimento epiteliale Di quâ della grande fessura si vede un' arteria (oc. 5, obb. *A* Zeiss).

FIG. II. — Sezione del tumore nei suoi punti iniziali.

> *a - a'* lume dei tubuli renali residuali tagliati trasversalmente ;
>
> *b* - elementi del neoplasma, fatto di cellule epiteliali con scarso protoplasma e leggiermente granuloso;
>
> *c* - tessuto connettivo fibroso, che circonda le masse epiteliali del tumore (obb. *D* oc. 5 Zeiss).

FIG. III. — La neoplasia prende uno sviluppo fortemente papillare intracanalicolare, alcune papille sono tagliate trasversalmente, altre in senso longitudinale.

> *a* - epitelio di rivestimento delle papille;
>
> *b* - tessuto centrale delle papille (obb. *A* oc. I Zeiss).
>
> *c, c', c''* - papille tagliate trasversalmente.

FIG. IV. — Sezione trasversale di una papilla.

> *a* - epitelio cilindrico della papilla ;

    *b* - stroma connettivale della papilla ;

    *c* - tessuto centrale della papilla costituito da elementi epiteliali immigrati ed infiltrati, e che si differenziano da quelli epiteliali del rivestimento della papilla (oc. 5. obb. *D* Zeiss).

## TAVOLA III.

### SEGUITO DEL CASO 3°.

**FIG. V.** — Le papille del tumore sono numerosissime, assottigliate e variamente anastomizzate fra loro.

    *a-a'* - spazii che intercedono fra le singole papille da costituire in alcuni punti delle piccole cavità cistiche ;

    *b-b'* - Stroma delle papille ;

    *c* - vaso sanguigno dello stroma delle papille (oc. 5, obb. *A* Zeiss).

**FIG. VI.** — Un punto più centrale della figura precedente, in cui si vedono spazii interpapillari rivestiti di epitelio e divisi da tessuto connettivo fibroso molto lasso.

    *a-a'* - rivestimento epiteliale ;

    *b* - tessuto connettivo fibroso.

**FIG. VII.** — Una papilla tagliata in senso longitudinale, nella quale si vedono gli elementi centrali in fase degenerativa.

    *a* - elementi epiteliali in degenerazione ialina con alcuni nuclei residuali ;

    *b* - capillare sanguigno ;

    *c* - epitelio di rivestimento della papilla (obb *A* oc. 5 Zeiss).

## TAVOLA IV.

### SEGUITO DEL CASO 4°.

**FIG. I.** — Nodulo neoplastico circondato da capsula fibrosa, costituito da formazioni papillari a spazii irregolari, ora ripieni, ora tapezzati da epitelio.

    *a* - capsula del nodulo ;

    *b* - cavità rivestite da epitelio ;

    *c* - spazii riempiti da epitelio ;

    *d-d'* - setti fibrosi intermedii (obb. *aa* oculare 5 Zeiss).

**FIG. II.** — Sezione del tumore, in cui si vedono gli spazii con epitelio degenerato.

    *a* - cordoni con epitelio degenerato ;

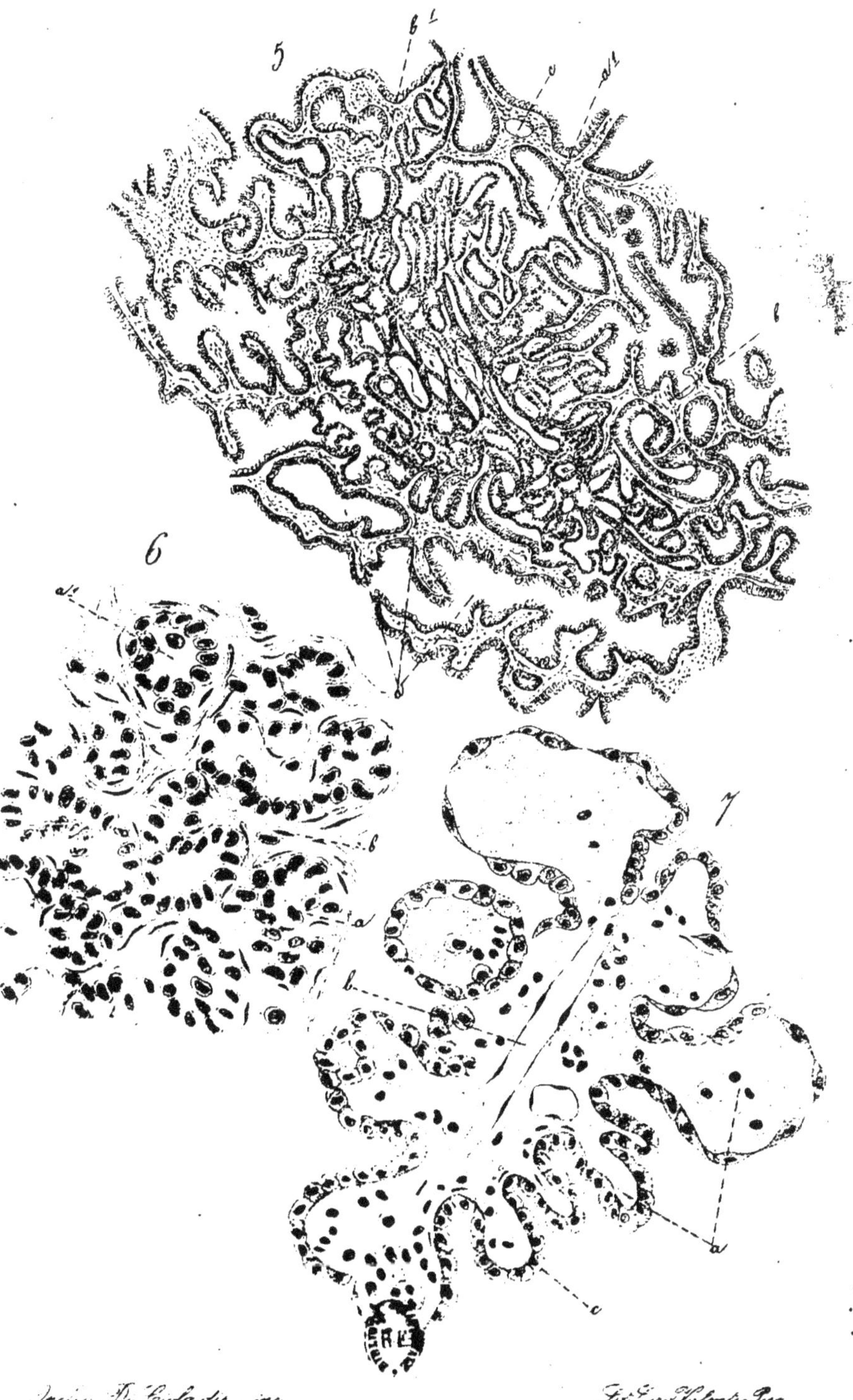

5
6
7

D'Antona — Tumori Primarii del Rene
Tav: IV
1
2
3
4
5
a
b
c

*b* -connettivo, che li divide ;

*c* -vaso sanguigno (oculare 5 obb. *D* Zeiss).

Fɪɢ. III. — Massa del tumore fatto da epitelio ben conservato, con scarso protoplasma e leggermente granuloso, qui non vi sono nè papille nè cavità, ma estesi strati epiteliali irregolarmente attraversati quà e là da vasi sanguigni circondati da tessuto connettivo.

    *a* -.massa epiteliale;

       *b-b'-b''*-v si sanguigni (obb. *D* oculare 5 Zeiss).

Fɪɢ. IV. — Una papilla del tumore tagliato in senso longitudinale.

     *a* - stroma fibroso della papilla ;

     *b* - epitelio di rivestimento della papilla, polimorfo con scarso protoplasma e leggermente granuloso (obb. *D* ocul. 5 Zeiss).

Fɪɢ. V. — Sezione del tumore, in cui si vedono una serie di vasi sanguigni e fra essi la neoplasia epiteliale.

     *a'-a-a''* - vasi sanguigni con struttura embrionale ;

     *b-b'-b''* - epitelio palimorfo con scarso protoplasma e leggermente granuloso (obb. *D* ocul. 4 Zeiss.)


## TAVOLA V.

### SEGUITO DEL CASO 4º.

Fɪɢ. VI. — Sezione del tumore in cui si vedono gli spazii del connettivo infiltrati da elementi epiteliali,

     *a-a'-a''* - masse epiteliali abbondanti ;

     *b-b'-b''* - setti connettivali, che dividono le masse epiteliali ;

     *c* - vaso sanguigno ;

     *d- d'* - setti connettivali divisi da scarse cellule epiteliali infiltrate (obb. *D* ocul. 5 Zeiss).

Fɪɢ. VII. — Sezione residuale del rene, in cui si nota una nefrite interstiziale cronica.

     *a-a'* -glomeruli di Malpighi, nei quali l'epitelio di rivestimento del gomitolo vascolare è in proliferazione.

     *b-b'* - tubuli renali, nei quali si vede ben conservato l'epitelio ;

     *c-c'* - tubuli renali con epitelio in atrofia e necrosi;

     *d* -connettivo renale fortemente ispessito (oculare 5 obb. *D* Zeiss).

## Tumore primario di una capula surrenale, trovato in un' autopsia dal professore Maffucci.

### TAVOLA V.

Fig. I. — Incipiente adenoma cistico.

  *a* - capsula dell'organo;

  *b*-cavità cistiche;

  *c* - tubi della sostanza corticale della capsula surrenale (obb. *aa* oculare I Zeiss.)

Fig. II. — Taglio di una sezione del tumore della capsula surrenale.

  *a* - stroma fibroso del tumore, che si continua nello stroma delle papille della neoplasia.

  *b*-*b'*-*b''* - epitelio di rivestimento delle papille e delle cavità esistenti fra le papille, l'epitelio è cilindrico, in alcuni punti polimorfo, con scarso protoplasma e leggermente granuloso (obb. *D* ocul. 5 Zeiss).

---

## DE LA NÉPHROSTOMIE DANS L'ANURIE CAUSÉE PAR LE CANCER DE L'UTÉRUS

### par M. G. NANU,

de Bucharest.

On sait qu'à peu près la moitié des femmes atteintes de cancer de l'utérus succombent avec des phénomènes de rétention rénale, causés par la compression des uretères. Le symptôme le plus inquiétant est l'anurie et c'est contre elle qu'il faut lutter, pour prolonger la vie de ces malheureuses.

Tout dernièrement ayant eu l'occasion d'observer un cas d'anurie de cette espèce, à l'exemple de Jayle, Labbé et Picqué, j'ai fait une néphrostomie.

La femme avait un cancer avancé du col; le corps de la matrice était très volumineux et avait une surface irrégulière; depuis quelque temps, oligurie, céphalalgie, nausées, etc. Enfin, bientôt elle eut une anurie complète qui a persisté pendant 10 jours. Du côté des reins, il n'y avait pas de phénomènes appréciables de rétention.

J'ai décidé de lui faire une fistule rénale lombaire et j'ai choisi le côté gauche pour opérer, parce que la tumeur de l'utérus s'était développé surtout de ce côté.

Tav: V

J'ai trouvé le rein gros, hyperémié et long de 15 centimètres ; mais, en le sectionnant jusqu'au bassinet, je n'ai pas trouvé la moindre rétention urinaire ; il n'y avait pas de dilatation des calices et du bassinet.

Vers le soir, on retira de la vessie 40 grammes d'urine sanguinolente.

Depuis lors, elle n'a plus eu la moindre goutte d'urine par l'urètre ; mais, dès le lendemain, les phénomènes urémiques ont disparu. La malade se sentait mieux et elle aurait été très contente si elle n'avait pas eu les douleurs causées par le néoplasme de l'utérus.

On voit que, contrairement à ce qu'on aurait dû s'attendre, il n'y avait pas de rétention rénale, c'est-à-dire d'hydronéphrose : Cependant l'obstruction n'a pu être rapide, mais lente. Cela serait en accord avec l'opinion de Donnadieu qui prétend qu'au début il n'y aurait pas d'hydronéphrose mais une simple dilatation des tubuli.

J'ai suivi cette femme pendant 115 jours à partir de l'opération. Après ce laps de temps, des phénomènes de rétention auraient dû se montrer du côté du rein non opéré ; or je n'ai rien observé de semblable. Le rein a conservé son volume normal et il n'était pas douloureux.

On le voit, en dehors de l'intérêt que cette néphrostomie peut avoir au point de vue de l'opportunité du traitement palliatif de l'anurie, elle a la valeur des expériences qu'on a faites pour élucider la pathogénie des rétentions rénales.

---

## ZUM URETER-XATHETERISMUS

### von Dr. LEOPOLD CASPER

Privatdocente, Berlin.

MEINE HERREN !

Fünf Jahre sind eine kurze Zeit wenn es gilt, eine neue Untersuchungsmethode in die wissenschaftliche und practische Medicin einzuführen und zu propagiren.

In Anbetracht dessen dürfen wir zufrieden sein mit dem, was wir in fünf Jahren mit dem Harnleiter-Katheterismus erreicht haben. Dies moderne Kind, in Deutschland zur Welt gebracht, hat Frankreich liebevoll aufgenommen und gepflegt. Brüderlich haben Frankreich und Deutschland zusammen gearbeitet, um diese glänzende Untersuchungsmethode für die leidende Menschheit nutzbar zu machen. In den heissen Kämpfen, die ich für diese Methode zu bestehen hatte, wurde ich auf das Wirksamste unterstützt durch meinen Freund Albarran und heute haben wir zwei neue Lobredner des Ureter-Katheterismus hören dürfen, die Herren *Kümmel* und *Mankiewicz*. Der Werth ihrer Mittheilungen wird niemand entgehen, der die Wichtigkeit und Schwierigkeit einer genauen Nierendiagnostic zu würdigen versteht.

Diese begnügt sich nicht damit, die Erkrankung einer Niere zu erkennen; sondern sie will auch erforschen, wie steht es in einem solchen Fall mit *der Beschaffenheit der andern*, eine Frage deren Bedeutung zu sehr bekannt ist, als dass hier darüber gesprochen werden brauchte.

Diese Frage zu lösen ist der Ureter-Katheterismus berafen.

Hatte man sich bisher darauf beschränkt, den Harn jeder Niere gesondert aufzufangen, ihn auf abnorme Bestandtheile (Albumen, Cylinder) zu untersuchen, die Quantität an Salzen und Harnstoff zu bestimmen, so sind wir jetzt noch einen Schritt weiter gegangen. Es st uns gelungen, aus dem Secret jeder Niere einen Schluss auf die funktionelle Kraft derselben zu ziehen. Und das ist das punctum saliens.

Wenn wir an einer als krank erkannten Niere eine Operation vornehmen wollen, so werden wir gewiss an erster Stelle erforschen, ob die andere albumenhaltigen Harn absondert. Da aber ein Mensch mit Albumenharn bekanntlich noch lange leben kann, so erscheint es uns von grösserer Wichtigkeit zu erfahren : Funktionirt diese Niere, gleichviel ob sie gesund oder krank ist, noch ausreichend, so dass bei Ausschaltung der andern sie allein die Arbeit des Organismus zu leisten vermag.

Doctor Paul Friedrich *Richter* und ich haben nun gestützt auf die vortrefflichen Untersuchungen von *Achard* und *Delamare* mit dem Phloridzin nach dieser Richtung hin Untersuchungen angestellt und sind zu folgenden interessanten Resultaten gekommen :

1. Wenn man Phloridzin *gesunden* Menschen injicirt, so scheiden beide Nieren die *gleiche Menge Zucker* in *gleichem Zeitraum zu gleicher* Zeit gemessen aus. Der *Entstehungsort* des Zuckers sind die Nieren.

2. Ist eine Niere erkrankt, die andre gesund, so zeigt sich auf der *kranken* Seite stets eine *geringere* Zuckerausscheidung als auf der gesunden.

5. Ist die Erkrankung derart, dass das *ganze Nierenparenchym* oder der grösste Theil zu *Grunde* gegangen ist, so *fehlt auf* dieser Seite

die Zuckerausscheidung gänzlich, beziehungsweise sind nur *Spuren* vorhanden.

Diese Thatsachen haben wir mit frappirender Regelmässigkeit constatiren können bei Nephritis, Pyelonephritis, Tuberculose der Niere, Pyonephrose, Calculose und Renaltumoren.

Wir haben auch umgekehrt aus der *Gleichheits-Grösse* der Zuckerausscheidung bei Kranken, die auf eine Nierenaffection verdächtig waren und an der Niere operirt werden sollten, vorhersagen können, dass hier eine *Nierenerkrankung nicht* vorliegt.

Wir hoffen, dass es auf diese Weise möglich sein wird, in jenen dunklen Fällen von Nephralgie, manche unnöthige Nephrotomie oder auch Bloslegung der Niere zu vermeiden.

Wir können heut auf die Details der Methode nicht eingehen, auch hier nicht erörtern, welche Consequenzen sich für die Nierenchirurgie daraus ergeben werden; wir wollten heut nur die Thatsachen mittheilen, damit unsere Collegen schon jetzt im Stande sind mitzuarbeiten an diesem Gebiet, das uns ebenso interessant wie wichtig erscheint.

---

## LA SONDE URÉTÉRALE A DEMEURE DANS LE TRAITEMENT PRÉVENTIF ET CURATIF DES FISTULES RÉNALES

### par M. J. ALBARRAN,
de Paris.

Les fistules rénales urinaires consécutives à la néphrostomie sont exceptionnellement dues à ce que le tissu rénal malade cicatrise difficilement (tuberculose, certains reins lithiasiques). Dans presque tous les cas la persistance de la fistule est due à ce que l'urine ne peut s'écouler librement par l'uretère, et la fistule ne guérit que lorsque ce conduit est devenu facilement perméable.

La guérison spontanée des fistules consécutives à la néphrostomie pour pyonéphrose se fait presque toujours attendre des mois et même des années; elle est la conséquence, en dehors de la destruction totale du rein, d'un mécanisme complexe. Du côté du rein, la poche ouverte se rétrécit et le liquide qu'elle contient devient plus fluide; du côté de l'uretère les phénomènes inflammatoires diminuent et le calibre du canal se rétablit en partie.

La persistance définitive des fistules sera due à des rétrécissements avec ou sans courbure, perméables ou non de l'uretère, ou à des vices d'insertion de l'uretère dans la poche rénale.

Je crois qu'on peut, par le cathétérisme urétéral à demeure, empêcher la formation ou hâter la guérison des fistules qui guériraient spontanément après un délai variable. Je crois encore qu'un certain nombre de fistules, qui ne guériraient pas spontanément et qui sont dues à des rétrécissements perméables de l'uretère, peuvent guérir par ce même moyen, et je réserve les opérations urétéro-rénales pour les cas où le drainage urétéral se montre impuissant.

*Traitement préventif.* — Il consiste, au moment où l'on pratique la néphrostomie, à introduire dans l'uretère une large sonde dont l'extrémité supérieure draine le bassinet et dont l'extrémité inférieure sort par le méat. Avant d'inciser le rein, je place, par le cathétérisme cystoscopique, une petite sonde dans l'uretère en la faisant pénétrer jusqu'au rein : lorsque la poche rénale est ouverte, je me sers de cette sonde mince pour faire passer, de haut en bas, une grosse sonde n° 10 ou 11.

Lorsque le cathétérisme urétéral n'a pu être pratiqué, on peut parfois réussir à trouver dans la poche rénale l'orifice de l'uretère et à y introduire une sonde jusque dans la vessie : avec un lithotriteur on prend ensuite la sonde dans la vessie pour la faire sortir par le méat. Deux fois j'ai opéré ainsi avec succès.

La sonde urétérale mise en place reste à demeure et la poche rénale est en outre drainée, comme à l'ordinaire, par la plaie lombaire. Les jours suivants, on pratique par la sonde et par les drains des lavages boriqués et nitratés.

Le drainage lombaire est supprimé après une semaine en moyenne et, peu de jours après, toute l'urine s'écoule par la sonde qui sert toujours à faire des lavages et qu'on retire définitivement quelques jours après que l'urine ne passe plus par la plaie.

J'ai opéré par ce procédé six pyonéphroses et j'ai obtenu la guérison complète sans fistule dans un délai de trois à quatre semaines.

*Traitement curatif.* — Lorsque la fistule rénale urinaire est déjà constituée, j'introduis, par le cathétérisme cystoscopique, une sonde n° 6 ou 7 dans le bassinet. Souvent, dès le premier jour, toute l'urine s'écoule par la sonde et le malade n'est plus mouillé. Quelques jours après, la sonde est remplacée par une autre plus grosse que j'introduis sur un mandrin de bas en haut (de l'urètre vers le rein) et j'arrive de suite, ou après un nouveau changement, au n° 11 ou 12. Lorsque la plaie lombaire est bien cicatrisée on retire la sonde.

J'ai réussi ainsi chez deux malades à guérir complètement la fistule en quinze ou vingt jours. Chez deux autres malades la fistule se ferma bien, mais les accidents de rétention rénale, qui revenaient dès que la sonde était enlevée, m'obligèrent à pratiquer une opération urétéro-rénale pour déplacer l'insertion supérieure de l'uretère.

Le drainage urétéral par la sonde à demeure ne peut être pratiqué lorsqu'on ne réussit pas à faire pénétrer la sonde dans l'intérieur du bassinet. Il échoue encore lorsque l'uretère s'insère trop haut par rapport au point le plus déclive de la poche.

L'échec de la sonde à demeure justifie l'emploi des procédés opératoires sanglants.

## UEBER NIEREN OPERATIONEN BEI MANGEL ODER ERKRANKUNG DER ZWEITEN NIERE

### par von MANKIEWICZ[1],

de Berlin.

Es ist nicht gar so selten, dass der Mensch nur eine Niere besitzt; auf 3000 bis 4000 Autopsieen kommt der Fund einer Solitärniere. Bei Durchsicht von 254 Fällen dieser Art machten wir uns folgende bemerkenswerthe Notizen. Die Niere fehlte 127 Mal auf der linken Seite, 97 Mal auf der rechten Seite. Beim männlichen Geschlecht kam der Nierendefekt 76 Mal links, 47 Mal rechts zur Beobachtung; beim weiblichen Geschlecht wird er gleich oft links und rechts gefunden. Doppelt so oft wurde er bei Männern wie bei Weibern constatiert, doch kommen weniger Frauen zur Autopsie. Das Lebensalter spielt dabei keine Rolle. Die Nierengefässe fehlen regelmässig, nur selten fand man Rudimente derselben. Der Ureter fehlt meist, nur 17 Mal war er auffindbar; wahrscheinlich war in diesen Beobachtungen ein Nierenrudiment übersehen worden. Eine Ureterenöffnung in der Blase war einige Male 1 bis 2 Centimeter sondierbar; weiterhin war der Harnleiter obliteriert; in wenigen anderen Fällen war nur eine kleine Ausstülpung der Blasenschleimhaut vorhanden. In vierundsiebenzig Fällen war auf der dem Nierenmangel entsprechenden Seite keine Spur einer Ureterenmündung vorhanden. Viermal fehlte die linke Trigonumhälfte der Blase völlig; die rechte Trigonumhälfte fehlte niemals. Zweimal fand sich ein Blasendivertikel, viermal mündete der einzige Harnleiter in der Mitte der Blase, zweimal endete der Harnleiter zugleich mit dem Samenleiter in einer Cyste unter der Blasenschleimhaut. In ungefähr einem Drittel der Fälle

---

1. Die ausführliche Veröffentlichungmit Litteraturnachweis erfolgt in Casper — Lohnstein's Monatsberichten über die Gesammtleistungen auf dem Gebiehe des Harn und Sexual-apparates. September 1900.

macht uns daher die Cystoscopie auf den Nierenmangel aufmerksam.
Von den fünf zur Operation gelangten Fällen ist nur einer am Leben
geblieben. Nach *Beumer* erkranken ungefähr die Hälfte aller Jäger
von Solitärnieren, und ungefähr ein Viertel davon an Calculose.

Fälle mit einer normalen und einer rudimentären Niere, ferner
Hufeisen und Kuchennieren stehen der erst erwähnten Categorie der
Solitärnieren klinisch gleich. Von den bisher bekannt gewordenen
Fällen dieser Art sind nur wenige zur Operation gekommen und nur
zwei gerettet worden (Socin, König).

Zweiunddreissig Fälle von beiderseitiger Erkrankung der Nieren,
welche ich aus den letzten Jahren gesammelt habe, bieten mancherlei
Interessantes. An 17 Frauen und 8 Männern, 13 Mal rechts, 11 Mal
links, wurde eine chirurgische Behandlung der Niere gewagt. 11 Mal
bot eine Steinniere, 6 Mal die Tuberculose die Indication zum Eingriff, 2 Mal Nierenkrebse, 2 Mal Hydronephrose, je einmal Pyelitis,
cystische Entartung der Niere, Ureterfistel, Nierencyste, Struma
suprarenalis, Nierenabscess, Steatose. Am häufigsten fand sich die
Calculosis, dann die Tuberculosis beiderseits (50%). Von 19 Patienten
mit Nephrectomie blieb nur eine Patientin noch vier Monate am
Leben, von 15 Nephrotomierten lebten nur 3 Patienten länger als
2 Monate und zwar mit Fisteln. Selbst nach Abzug von etwa durch
Carbol oder Sublimatvergiftung (5) zu Grunde gegangenen, müssen
wir leider constatieren, dass von 52 Operierten 25 *ad exitum* kamen,
weil der Operateur nicht im Stande war, die Functionsunfähigkeit
der zweiten Niere nachzuweisen. Ist die Statistik auch nicht überall
so schlecht (siehe König), so müssen wir doch berücksichtigen, wie
viele unglücklich verlaufene Fälle überhaupt nicht veröffentlicht
werden.

Mancherlei Mittel besitzen wir, den Mangel oder die Vergrösserung
einer Niere nachzuweisen. Die *Inspection* des Rückens, besonders in
der Kniecllenbogenlage, ferner der Harn und Genitalorgane auf Missbildungen, wie solche bei Nierenmangel vorkommen und die *Per-
cussion* der Nieren sind von geringem Wert; die *Palpation* in Rücken-
lage, in Halbseitenlage und als Ballotement rénal, eventuell mit
Schmerz verbunden, giebt nur relativ selten sicher verwertbare Resultate und nur dann, wenn die Nieren sehr gross oder herabgesunken
sind oder die Kanten und Oberflächen derselben starke Veränderungen aufweisen.

Die *Röntgendurchstrahlung* leistet hier bisher noch gar nichts. Die
*Abtastung* der Nieren nach Freilegung derselben durch Laparatomie
oder Lendenschnitt beweist nur die Anwesenheit eines Körpers,

allenfalls dessen Grösse und Consistenz, aber nichts über seine Funktion, seine Verbindung mit der Blase, über seine eventuelle Erkrankung. *Wahren Wert hat nur die Untersuchung der Funktion der Niere*, d. h. die Untersuchung des gesonderten Secretes einer jeden Niere für sich. Versuche die Ureteren zu catheterisieren machten *Simon* und *Pawlik*; sie scheiterten aber an dem Mangel der Beleuchtung und kamen nur einige Male bei Frauen zum Ziel. *Grünfeld*, *Neumann* und *Kelly* haben bei reflectiertem Licht einige Male den Ureter catheterisiert. Andere Autoren haben durch Abklemmung eines Ureters den Harn aus dem anderen Ureter allein aufzufangen versucht; ein Theil der Forscher suchte durch Aufrichtung von Zwischenwänden in Blase, Darm oder Vagina dieses Ziel zu erreichen; eine dritte Gruppe ligierte den Ureter temporär oder nahm den Ureterencatheterismus nach vorbereitenden Operationen (Sectioalta, etc.) vor. Erst mit der Schaffung der intravesicalen Beleuchtung durch *Nitze's Cystoscop*, welches schon den aus dem Ureter kommenden Strudel zu beobachten erlaubte kam man weiter. Nach vielen Versuchen namhafter Autoren glückte es *Casper* ein Instrument für den Ureterencatheterismus unter Beleuchtung in die Praxis einzuführen, welches mutatis mutandis allen neueren derartigen Apparaten zum Vorbild diente. Die mit dem Uretercatheter getrennt aufgefangenen Nierensecrete müssen nun einer eingehenden physicalischen und chemischen Untersuchung unterzogen werden : Specifisches Gewicht, Farbe, Durchsichtigkeit, Reaction, Eiweiss, Eiter anderweitige morphologische Bestandtheile, Chloride, Harnstoff müssen gesucht und bestimmt werden. Auf Tuberkelbacillen, Gonococcen und andere Bacterien ist zu fahnden, eventuell mit dem Thierversuch. Mit dieser Untersuchung kann man die Krankheit der einen Niere feststellen, zur Funktionsfähigkeit der anderen Niere kann man noch nichts aussagen. Um diese zu prüfen haben viele deutsche und französische Forscher durch subcutane Injection oder Eingeben per os von Farbstoffen und Chemicalien (Methylenblau, Rosanilinsulfonatrium, Urobilin, Iodkalium) und Bestimmung der ausgeschiedenen Farbstoffmengen für jede Niere die Funktion derselben prüfen wollen; abgesehen davon, dass das meist verwandte Methylenblau im Körper leicht zum Methylenweiss oxydiert wird, beweisen diese Experimente nur die Durchlässigkeit der Niere, aber nichts für ihre Function. Viel näher kommt *A. von Koranyi* dieser Forderung, wenn er durch Gefrierpunktsbestimmung des Harns beziehungsweise des Blutes die moleculare Concentration der Flüssigkeit nachweisst; je *niedriger* die moleculare Concentration des *Harns*, desto weniger feste Bestandtheile werden ausgeschieden, desto functionsunfähiger ist die Niere, desto mehr nähert sich der Gefrierpunkt des Harns dem des destillierten Wassers; umgekehrt, je *höher* die moleculare Concentration des *Blutes*, desto weniger Harnbestandtheile werden ausgeschieden, desto functionsfähiger ist die Niere, desto weiter entfernt sich der Gefrierpunkt des Blutes von dem des destillierten Wassers. Die Methode bedarf noch der klinischen Ausgestaltung, theoretisch ist sie richtig.

Durch Bestimmung der Brechungsexponenten von Urin und Blut durch den Pulfrich'schen Eintauchrefractometer glaubt *Strubell* eine neue Methode für die Untersuchung der Nierenfunction gegeben zu haben, insbesondere da für die Untersuchung minimale Mengen Secret ausreichen.

*Casper* und *Richter* haben die *Achard* und *Delamarre*'sche Arbeit fortgesetzt und durch Injection von 5 Milligramm Phloridzin einen renalen Diabetes erzeugt; die dann mit Hülfe des Ureterencatheterismus vorgenommene Untersuchung der gesonderten Nierensecrete hat ergeben, dass die kranke Niere weniger (oder gar keinen) Zucker basondert als die gesunde Niere und dass die Grösse der Zuckerausscheidung mit der Grösse der Harnstoffenscheidung und mit der molecularen Concentration parallel geht.

So gelangen wir nicht nur zu einer anatomischen sondern auch zu einer functionellen Diagnose der Nierenerkrankung und können die Sätze aufstellen :

1. Die Chirurgie der Nieren muss möglichst conservativ sein.

2. Ein chirurgischer Eingriff an einer Niere darf niemals stattfinden, wenn der Operateur sich nicht mit allen Mitteln bemüht hat, die Anwesenheit und Functionstüchtigkeit der anderen Niere festzustellen. Im Zweifelfalle darf niemals die Exstirpation der kranken Niere vorgenommen werden, sondern primär nur die Nephrotomie (oder Nephrostomie), welcher später, nachdem man sich von der genügenden Function der anderen Niere überzeugt hat, die Nephrectomie folgen kann.

3. Die bisher sicherste Methode die Funktionsfähigkeit der Nieren zu prüfen, besteht in der Untersuchung der durch den Ureterencatheterismus getrennt aufgefangenen Nierensecrete, besonders nach der durch subcutane Injection von Phloridzin hervorgerufenen Glycosurie.

## NÉPHRONÉVROSE VASO-MOTRICE ET SÉCRÉTOIRE

POLYURIE, ANURIE AVEC LITHIASE ET MIGRATIONS CALCULEUSES PENDANT 80 JOURS.
NEPHROSTOMIE. CRISES D'AZOTURIE ET DE LIPURIE. GUÉRISON COMPLÈTE MAINTENUE
DEPUIS 5 MOIS,

par le docteur J. ESCAT,

de Marseille.
Chargé de cours des maladies génito-urinaires à l'École de Médecine.

Voici une observation bizarre comme la pathologie nerveuse nous
en offre parfois. La complexité des phénomènes observés, leur allure
déconcertante, je dirai même paradoxale, offre plus cependant qu'un
intérêt de physiologie pathologique. La gravité des accidents et l'inefficacité des moyens médicaux m'ont obligé à intervenir chirurgicalement. A quelques mois de distance j'ai pratiqué deux fois la néphrostomie chez la même malade pour des accidents que je n'ai pu rattacher
à une lésion organique primitive. Je considérerai ces troubles jusqu'à
nouvel ordre comme liés à une néphronévrose qui a vicié le fonctionnement vasculaire et sécrétoire du rein.

Les accidents d'anurie ont ici dominé la scène, ils se sont présentés
avec tous les caractères de l'anurie hystérique bien qu'accompagnés
de migrations calculeuses quotidiennes. La tolérance de l'organisme
a dépassé les plus longs délais relevés dans l'anurie calculeuse.
L'anurie aurait été bénigne sans la lithiase carbonatée calcaire qui
a évolué parallèlement. Le calcul a paru être ici à la fois agent provo-
cateur et effet de l'anurie, c'est lui, en somme, qui a déterminé l'intervention. La lithiase rendait la situation sans issue, et l'urémie devenait fatale. Je vais brièvement résumer cette observation et les
réflexions qu'elle m'a inspirées. Il s'agit d'une jeune fille de 20 ans
qui a déjà été opérée par moi pour des accidents d'anurie calculeuse
à forme anomale (*Association française d'urologie*, 1899). Les phénomènes qui ont suivi cette première intervention ont éclairé la nature
de ces premiers accidents et je puis aujourd'hui les interpréter dans
un sens plus précis. Dès le début les accidents d'anurie ont eu le
caractère de l'anurie hystérique. Après avoir été précédés de polyurie,
ils ont duré plus d'un mois sans urémie; toutefois l'émission de calculs
quotidiens, les douleurs néphralgiques et surtout la cachexie menaça-
çante, perte de poids de 14 kilogrammes, imposèrent une première
néphrostomie. La jeune malade fut guérie en 17 jours, mais un mois
après elle récidive; les coliques néphrétiques, la contracture lombo-
abdominale, l'anurie jointe à la rétention des quelques grammes

d'urine sécrétée, l'expulsion quotidienne des calculs de carbonate de chaux avec milieu urinaire aseptique, les vomissements aqueux et finalement sanglants font prévoir la nécessité d'une nouvelle intervention. La tolérance générale était cependant extraordinaire et contraire à toutes les données physiologiques acquises. Les précautions les plus rigoureuses furent toujours prises pour éviter toute supercherie. Deux chloroformisations amenèrent une débâcle éphémère de quelques heures. L'anurie et les migrations calculeuses reprirent ensuite et durant plus de 80 jours émission de 10, 20, 30, 50 grammes d'urine en 24 heures, l'anorexie, la cachexie, les gastrorragies, l'expulsion quotidienne et bi-quotidienne des calculs qu'il faut extraire de l'urètre imposent une seconde néphrostomie. Comme la première fois aucun calcul ne fut trouvé dans le bassinet; je ne pus faire pénétrer une sonde de haut en bas. Il y avait cependant des graviers dans la partie inférieure de l'uretère, car la malade était en pleine colique néphrétique quand je l'opérai. Tous les accidents cessèrent et, quelques semaines après, 5 calculs à facettes furent expulsés, mais cette fois la migration calculeuse fit tomber la malade en léthargie, je la tirai de cet état par la compression ovarienne. Une autre migration calculeuse produisit l'anurie du rein (500 grammes) non ouvert, et du côté ouvert toutes les urines passèrent par la fistule. Je pus ainsi faire l'analyse des deux urines recueillies et constater que le rein ouvert était azoturique, émettant 24 grammes d'urée tandis que l'autre n'en rendait que 7 grammes par litre. Les urines eurent bientôt repris les voies naturelles. Quelques jours après, subitement polyurie de 4 litres avec urines graisseuses analogues à du lait, débâcles phosphaturiques et uratiques 40 grammes d'urée en 24 heures, puis débâcle de carbonate de chaux. Ces accidents cessèrent brusquement par un simple changement de drain. Voulant maintenir le rein ouvert je le drainai, avec un drain en argent doré, pendant un mois. Un jour, pendant les règles, les urines ont passé entièrement par le drain, comme si l'ovaire congestionné avait comprimé l'uretère; les règles finies l'urine a repris la voie naturelle. Le 2 mai 1900, trois mois après l'opération, enlèvement du drain par la malade. Guérison parfaite et urines normales.

Cette observation complexe m'a paru remarquable :

1° Comme type d'anurie réflexe et comme exemple d'hystérie interne provoquée ou entretenue par la migration calculeuse.

2° La lithiase carbonatée calcaire, inexplicable ici par l'état des urines et de l'appareil urinaire, a été à la fois l'effet et plus tard la cause des troubles de la sécrétion rénale.

3° L'azoturie, la lipurie ont évolué parallèlement aux phénomènes d'excitation rénale, elles ont cessé avec les causes de cette excitation, elles laissent entrevoir des rapports physiologiques entre la fonction rénale éliminatrice de l'urée et les fonctions uropoiétiques.

4° Cette observation semble fournir quelques arguments à l'existence de nerfs sécrétoires du rein et d'une fonction régulatrice de la sécrétion rénale, enfin à la possibilité d'une sécrétion interne du rein, sécrétion antitoxique telle que Brown-Séquard l'a démontrée en 1875.

5° Le bon effet, malheureusement transitoire, de la chloroformisation sur l'anurie, fait indiqué déjà par Israel de Berlin, confirme la nature réflexe de l'anurie.

6° Le fait principal de cette observation est que tous les accidents ont cessé dès que le rein a été ouvert, la suppression de la tension intra-rénale n'a agi ici que par la suppression des réflexes vaso-moteurs et sécrétoires, elle a entraîné la guérison de la lithiase et de l'anurie. Ce titre de néphronévrose vaso-motrice appliqué à ces accidents complexes nous paraît ainsi légitimé.

---

## HÉMATURIE PSEUDO-ESSENTIELLE; DIAGNOSTIC CYSTOSCOPIQUE; NÉOPLASME RÉNAL; NÉPHRECTOMIE TOTALE; GUÉRISON COMPLÈTE

par M. le docteur HENRY REYNÈS,
de Marseille.

Membre des Associations françaises de Chirurgie et d'Urologie. Ex-chef de clinique chirurgicale
à la Faculté de Médecine de Montpellier.

Les observations d'hématuries essentielles, ou mieux soi-disant essentielles, deviennent de plus en plus rares, au fur et à mesure que les examens cystoscopiques se multiplient, que les cathétérismes urétéro-rénaux sont plus fréquents, que la chirurgie rénale est devenue plus hardie non seulement dans des interventions curatives, mais même dans des néphrotomies exploratrices.

Aussi, après avoir soumis à un rigoureux contrôle toutes les observations d'hématuries dites essentielles, Malherbe et Legueu[1] n'admettent comme hématuries pouvant être dites essentielles que cinq cas dus à Schede, Klemperer, Broca, Loumeau (de Bordeaux) et Debesarques. Dans tous les autres cas il s'agissait d'hématurie due à de discrètes lésions de lithiase, de tuberculose, de sclérose, de néoplasme, etc.

---

1. MALHERBE ET LEGUEU. Rapport présenté au 4° Congrès d'Urologie; 19 octobre 1899.

L'observation, que j'ai l'honneur de présenter au Congrès, est intéressante, à plusieurs points de vue :

1° Parce que cliniquement il s'agissait d'une hématurie dont l'indolence, la continuité, l'absence de cortège symptomatique, tant du côté vésical que du côté rénal, semblaient indiquer le type « essentiel » ;

2° Parce que le diagnostic clinique hésitait à déterminer le siège de l'hémorrhagie : vessie, rein droit, rein gauche ;

3° Parce que la cystoscopie seule m'a permis de localiser l'origine de l'hématurie dans le rein droit ;

4° Parce que l'opération, pour être efficace, a dû consister en une néphrectomie totale ;

5° Parce que, le rein ouvert, on a vu qu'il s'agissait d'un très gros néoplasme intra-rénal ;

6° Parce que la guérison a été parfaite, et qu'elle se maintient intégrale, *depuis dix mois* que j'ai pratiqué la néphrectomie.

OBSERVATION. — Un homme de trente-deux ans était depuis *plus d'un an* atteint d'hématuries continuelles ; ni le jour, ni la nuit, ni le repos, ni la marche, ni les médications les plus variées n'ont d'influence sur cette hémorragie qui ne cesse pas, colore uniformément l'urine au commencement, au milieu, à la fin de la miction, et qui est absolument indolente. Progressivement affaibli par cette continuelle perte de sang, le malade était dans un état de complète cachexie hémorragique.

Jamais il n'avait eu de coliques néphrétiques ; pas d'antécédents tuberculeux ou vénériens ; pas de traumatisme. Aucun symptôme vésical ou rénal : la palpation lombo-abdominale la plus attentive ne montre ni augmentation sensible des reins, ni douleur à la pression.

Le malade avait été vu par divers confrères et non des moins compétents, notamment par les D\rs Vincent et Acquaviva qui voulurent bien m'adresser ce cas intéressant.

Les avis différaient beaucoup ; les uns avaient cru à une hématurie essentielle, d'autres à une tuberculose vésicale au début. Sur ce dernier point j'examinai le malade, mais ne trouvant aucune lésion concomitante dans les testicules, les épididymes, la prostate, ou les vésicules séminales, j'avais éliminé l'idée de tuberculose. Ne trouvant dans les reins aucun symptôme objectif ou subjectif, il n'y avait qu'à pratiquer la cystoscopie qui seule pouvait mettre sur la voie du diagnostic.

*L'examen cystoscopique* me montra : 1° l'intégrité absolue de la vessie dont la paroi était parfaitement saine ; 2° de l'uretère du côté droit, au milieu du liquide clair qui remplissait la vessie[1], je vis, en un mince

1. Ce liquide était, comme je fais toujours, une solution de *sulfi-benzoate de*

et rouge filet, le sang couler lentement. J'avais sous les yeux la reproduction exacte des figures classiques qui représentent, dans le champ
du cystoscope, une hémorragie qui sourd par l'orifice urétéral[2]. Du
côté urétéral gauche tout était sain, rien ne troublait la limpidité du
liquide intra-vésical, et, en faisant sur le ventre le long du trajet urétéral
une compression expressive, rien ne sortit de l'uretère.

Le diagnostic topographique était donc précisé; la vessie était hors
de cause, et le rein gauche aussi. J'avais affaire à une *néphorragie
droite*. A la vérité, je pensai que l'uretère était sain, et qu'il s'agissait
d'une hémorragie rénale; pourtant, pour en être sûr, il eût fallu faire
le cathétérisme urétéral : je ne l'ai pas fait, et volontairement; car les
renseignements que ce mode d'exploration aurait pu me fournir
n'étaient pas absolument nécessaires, et, malgré toutes mes mesures
de désinfection, j'aurais risqué peut-être d'apporter dans ce milieu,
aseptique jusque là, quelque germe de contamination.

Tel était l'état de mon diagnostic lorsque j'ai publié une partie de
l'observation de mon malade, dans un précédent travail[3].

Ce diagnostic était simplement topographique; en l'absence de tout
autre symptôme il était impossible de préciser davantage : pas de
tumeur, pas de douleur; aucune maladie antérieure à détermination
rénale ne m'autorisait à penser à une de ces hématuries liées à
certaines formes de néphrite chronique, récemment étudiées dans le
travail de Michaux[4]. Je me demandai aussi si je n'avais pas affaire à
une de ces hématuries dites angioneurotiques dont on a signalé des
cas[5].

Les remèdes les plus divers ayant déjà été vainement essayés,
j'essayai, sans espoir, une médication dont le repos, l'ergotine et
l'iodure de potassium firent la base : ce traitement fut entièrement
négatif.

En l'état, malgré l'incertitude de la cause hémorragique, vu l'anémie progressive, et la situation de plus en plus compromise du malade,
je proposai une intervention.

*Mon plan opératoire* comprenait d'abord une néphrotomie explo-

souke à 4 gr. pour 1000; j'ai complètement abandonné l'acide borique; depuis
trois ans, je n'emploie plus que le sulfi-benzoate, beaucoup plus antiseptique
que l'acide borique, et nullement irritant. Voir Heckel fils : *Du Sulfi-benzoate de
soude*. Thèse de Toulouse, 1896-1897.

2. Voir fig. dans Fenwick. *Urinary surgery*, p. 124, fig. 20. London, 1894.

3. H. Reynès. Études de chirurgie urinaire. Les hématuries essentielles. *Marseille médical*, 1er novembre 1899, p. 645.

4. Georges Michaux. Les néphrites chroniques hématuriques. Thèse Paris,
1900; analysé par Reynès in *Presse médicale*, n° 53, 4 juillet 1900.

5. Poljakoff. Hématurie rénale d'origine angioneurotique. *Deutsch medicin.
Wochenschr.*, 2 nov. 1899.

ratrice, par voie lombaire; cette opération me permettait de constater
la présence et la nature des lésions, si lésion il y avait : dans ce cas je
me serais comporté suivant les circonstances : grattage d'une pyramide
incrustée (cas de Abbe), curage d'un petit tubercule (Routier, Reynier,
Albarran), ablation de papilles (Fenwick[1]). Le cas échéant, j'aurais pu
être amené, en l'absence de lésions visibles, à croire à une néphrite
chronique hématurique, contre laquelle la simple néphrotomie, par la
décongestion qu'elle provoque, a une très heureuse influence[2]. En cas
de lésions bénignes suffisamment limitées et permettant une conservation partielle de l'organe, j'aurais pu faire une néphrectomie partielle[3].
Enfin, comme ultime ressource me restait la néphrectomie totale, dont
l'analyse des urines me permettait l'exécution.

C'est à cette dernière opération que j'ai dû arriver.

*Opération*. Après anesthésie à l'éther, dont je préfère souvent
l'emploi à celui du chloroforme, je pratiquai la néphrectomie totale, le
11 octobre 1899, aidé par les D[rs] Acquaviva et Bartoli. Je fis l'incision
lombaire classique, mais le rein, dont le volume était normal, était trop
caché par les côtes; je réséquai la douzième côte, ce qui élargit suffisamment le champ opératoire; au cours de cette résection, malgré
les précautions usuelles, le sinus pleural fut légèrement ouvert, je le
fermai immédiatement par trois points de catgut, et l'incident n'eut
aucune suite.

J'attirai le rein au dehors, il paraissait tout à fait sain, sauf vers le
tiers inférieur du bord convexe où on voyait une plaque de couleur
feuille morte, correspondant à une zone très amincie, et qui n'eût
pas tardé sans doute à s'ulcérer.

Je fendis le rein sur son bord convexe avec le bistouri : un flot de
liquide séro-hématique brunâtre s'échappa violemment, témoignant
qu'il était inclus sous pression dans le rein; j'agrandis l'incision et vis
apparaître de nombreuses végétations dont mes doigts détachèrent
quelques morceaux; au fur et à mesure que je poursuivais mon exploration intra-rénale, j'acquis la certitude que les lésions étaient tellement étendues que la conservation de l'organe était impossible. Le
bassinet lui-même quoique sain extérieurement était très agrandi, et
avait le volume d'une grosse noix.

---

1. FENWICK. Deux cas de papillectomie rénale pour hématurie indolente provenant d'un seul rein chez l'adulte *British medic. Journ.*, 5 février 1900.

2. ISRAEL. Influence de la néphrotomie dans les processus aigus et chroniques
du parenchyme rénal. *Mitteb. a. d. Grenzg. der Mediz. und Chir.*, 1899. Analysé in
*Gaz. hebd. de Med. et Chir.*, n° 46, 10 juin 1900. Voir également G. Michaux, *loc. cit.*

3. G. DE ROUVILLE. Néphrectomies partielles. Thèse de Paris.

Sans préjuger de la nature tuberculeuse ou épithéliale de ces végétations, mais considérant que le tissu rénal n'était plus réduit qu'à une mince coque, considérant également l'envahissement du bassinet, l'uretère étant d'ailleurs sain, je me résolus à pratiquer la *néphrectomie totale*.

La ligature du pédicule étant impossible, tant à cause de l'abondance de la graisse périrénale qu'à cause de l'obstacle apporté par l'augmentation de volume du bassinet, je pinçai le pédicule avec une solide pince courbe, et coupai tous les éléments du pédicule, laissant la pince à demeure. L'uretère seul put être lié séparément, et je touchai sa surface de section avec une goutte de Zn Cl².

Le rein et le bassinet enlevés, je mis une gaze iodoformée dans la loge rénale, rétrécis la plaie par quelques sutures et appliquai un pansement *aseptique*.

Les suites opératoires furent parfaites : le lendemain, une rétention réflexe d'urine étant survenue, je sondai le malade et évacuai un litre d'urine et de sang noirâtre mélangés : ce sang était celui qui était dans la vessie avant l'opération et celui qui coula du rein pendant les manœuvres opératoires.

Le lendemain la rétention avait cessé, et les urines reprenaient la coloration jaune paille, qu'elles n'ont jamais plus quittée.

La pince placée sur le pédicule fut retirée le troisième jour, sans incident ; la gaze fut progressivement retirée ; la cicatrisation se fit ; un mois après le malade était entièrement guéri ; une légère fistule se ferma au deuxième mois.

*Après l'opération*. Après deux mois de repos, le malade, parfaitement guéri, put reprendre ses travaux comme employé d'octroi ; il ne ressent aucune espèce de fatigue ; il est dans un excellent état de santé générale ; et, quoique monorénale, le taux de son excrétion urinaire, au point de vue des éléments azotés, est supérieur à la moyenne normale, ainsi qu'en témoigne l'analyse suivante, faite par M. le Dr Jacquême, pharmacien, cinq mois après l'opération.

| | | | |
|---|---|---|---|
| Quantité | 1000 cc. | Mat. fixes. | 59.80. |
| Couleur | jaune citrin. | Mat. minérales | 14. |
| Aspect | transparent. | Mat. organiques | 25. |
| Dépôt | néant. | Urée | 24.70 au litre. |
| Consistance. | normale. | Acide urique | 0.90. |
| Densité. | 1025. | Chlorures. | 8.80. |
| Réaction | acide. | Acide phosphorique. | 1.70. |
| Acidité. | 1.10. | | |

Ni sucre, ni albumine. Au microscope, rien. Caractéristique des urines : excès des éléments azotés.

Au moment où j'écris cette observation, *il y a dix mois que j'ai enlevé le rein de mon malade*, et rien n'est venu troubler une santé qui s'est affirmée dès le lendemain de l'opération.

*Examen de la pièce.*

Macroscopiquement cette tumeur se présente sous la forme d'abondantes végétations occupant à la fois l'intérieur du rein et l'intérieur du bassinet; elle a la forme d'une production en chou-fleur ramifié.

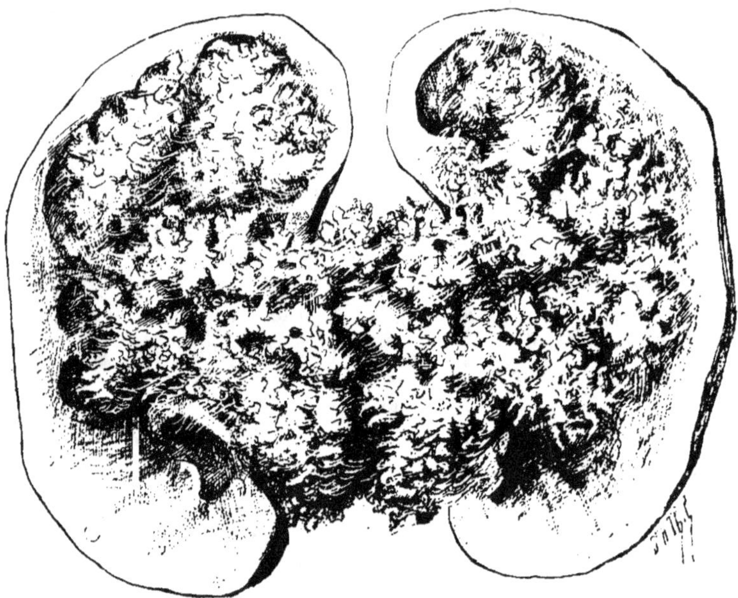

Il est impossible de dire si ce néoplasme a commencé par le rein pour verser dans le bassinet ou si l'inverse s'est produit.

Histologiquement, la tumeur paraît bénigne : il n'y a pas d'infiltration de cellules épithéliales dans le tissu qui soutient les végétations; quant aux végétations elles sont formées par de fines arborisations plus ou moins contournées : l'axe central en est formé par de minces tractus conjonctifs et vasculaires; cet axe est revêtu par de nombreuses cellules épithéliales embryonnaires. Parfois on observe des sortes de kystes dans lesquels des végétations arborescentes dessinent leurs contours : on dirait un kystome végétant.

La tumeur ne poussait aucun prolongement vers l'uretère et je n'ai, nulle part, perçu de ganglion suspect. Il s'agit en somme, très probablement, d'une prolifération *papillomateuse.*

Quant au tissu rénal lui-même, le microscope montre qu'il est à peu près indemne à part un peu de congestion due à la compression produite par les masses végétantes ; cette congestion va même jusqu'à avoir produit par places quelque infiltration sanguine, se traduisant dans la préparation par de nombreuses hématies. Les tubes épithéliaux et les glomérules sont sains.

Il est fâcheux que l'opération n'ait pas été faite plus tôt ; car, si ces lésions avaient été moins étendues, j'aurais pu me contenter de gratter, de curetter toutes les végétations, en conservant un rein dont le microscope montre l'intégrité parenchymateuse.

## DU ROLE PATHOGÉNIQUE DU RÉFLEXE RÉNO-RÉNAL

par le docteur A. POUSSON,
de Bordeaux.

La suppléance d'un rein, supprimé chirurgicalement ou détruit à la suite d'une altération pathologique, par son congénère demeuré en place, est bien connue. La survie des opérés de néphrectomie fournit un frappant exemple de cette hypertrophie compensatrice, qui pour être moins évidente n'en est pas moins réelle dans les diverses affections chirurgicales et médicales du rein partiellement destructives du parenchyme. Ce processus providentiel, d'abord étudié dans les parties saines d'un même rein malade par Korster, Golgi, Nauverk, et constaté ensuite sur le rein sain dans les cas de lésions unilatérales par Berckmann, Perl, Lancereaux et autres, est loin de se réaliser d'une façon constante.

Ma communication a précisément pour objet d'attirer l'attention sur es perturbations qu'un rein malade peut apporter d'abord du côté des fonctions de son congénère et ensuite du côté de son état anatomique.

1° *Perturbations fonctionnelles déterminées du côté d'un rein sain par un rein malade.* — Le retentissement, qu'un rein pathologique peut avoir sur les fonctions de son adelphe anatomiquement sain, est le résultat d'un réflexe réno-rénal, réflexe sur l'importance duquel le professeur Guyon a depuis longtemps insisté. Le type de ce réflexe se trouve dans l'anurie calculeuse, qui survient alors même que le rein opposé à l'uretère bloqué est dans un état d'intégrité parfaite, ainsi que le prouvent péremptoirement les cas de Bourgeois, de Chapotot, de Godlee, d'Israel où l'autopsie a été faite, et avec eux un grand nombre d'observations cliniques. L'oligurie de la colique néphrétique est encore la conséquence de l'action inhibitrice que l'irritation d'un uretère détermine non seulement sur le rein correspondant mais aussi sur celui du côté opposé. Comme autres exemples des effets de ce réflexe citons l'oligurie ou même l'anurie consécutive à la contusion rénale unilatérale. Bien que les crises douloureuses d'étranglement dans le rein mobile peuvent exceptionnellement s'accompagner de suspension réflexe dans l'autre rein non ectopié, Albarran et Picqué en ont rapporté des exemples. Dans l'hydronéphrose commune l'anurie, rare au dire d'Albarran, existe incontestablement et j'en ai relaté une observation au 10ᵉ Congrès français de chirurgie. Dans les néoplasmes du rein, dans la tuberculose, dans les pyonéphroses unilatérales la suspension de la sécrétion urinaire, à ce que je sache, n'a pas été signalée, mais ce que l'on trouve souvent noté dans les observations, c'est une diminution de la quantité d'urine émise, qui se relève après l'opération.

L'existence d'un réflexe inhibitoire réno-rénal dans les néphrites médicales est assurément beaucoup plus exceptionnelle, mais elle ne fait aucun doute pour moi. Avant de rapporter les quelques exemples indiscutables que j'ai relevés dans les auteurs ou que j'ai observés par moi-même, je me permettrai de porter atteinte à ce dogme pathologique d'après lequel les néphrites parenchymateuses ou interstitielles, aiguës ou chroniques, seraient toujours bilatérales.

Assurément si l'on s'en tient aux seules autopsies des sujets succombant tardivement, les lésions infectieuses des reins portent dans l'immense majorité des cas sur ces deux organes. Mais en est-il de même au début de l'infection ? À l'exemple des autres organes pairs comme les yeux, les parotides, les testicules, les plèvres, les reins également irrigués par un sang chargé de micro-organismes ou de leurs produits de sécrétion ne peuvent-ils pas ne pas s'infecter simultanément ? La réponse à cette question a d'autant plus de chance d'être affirmative qu'il est surabondamment démontré par les expériences de Cornil et Brault, Philipoviez et Finkler Prior, Conheim, Trambusti et Maffuci, que les bactéries sont susceptibles de filtrer à travers le rein sain sans y déterminer de lésions, et qu'elles ou leurs toxines ne deviennent nocives que s'il existe certaines conditions de réceptivité du parenchyme rénal. Ces conditions sont multiples, et si un grand nombre comme les refroidissements, les brûlures étendues, les états constitutionnels et les grandes diathèses, les affections de la vessie, de la prostate et de l'urètre exposent également les deux reins à l'infection, il en est encore beaucoup d'autres, qui ne sont menaçantes que pour un seul, telles sont les tumeurs des organes de l'abdomen et du bassin susceptibles de comprimer seulement un des uretères.

Sans doute, pour les raisons invoquées précédemment, je n'ai pu trouver dans la littérature d'exemples de néphrite chronique, dont l'unilatéralité ait été constatée à l'autopsie, mais les mémoires de Goodhart[1] et de Robert Weir ne laissent aucun doute relativement à la possibilité de l'unilatéralité de l'infection aiguë. Le premier de ces auteurs, sur 150 cas de pyélonéphrite reconnue *post mortem*, a trouvé un seul rein atteint dans 19 cas, soit 14, 5 pour 100, et le second, sur 71 cas, a relevé l'unilatéralité dans 19 cas, soit 14 pour 100.

A défaut de constatations nécropsiques, je puis produire un certain nombre de faits cliniques montrant que des malades, chez lesquels l'examen du rein enlevé pour des accidents divers a révélé des lésions de néphrite, ont pu vivre ensuite dans un état de santé parfaite. Ces faits prouvent tout au moins que, si des altérations existaient dans l'autre rein, elles étaient minimes, et qu'elles n'ont été nullement aggravées par le surcroit de travail, peut-être même ont-elles été enrayées ?

OBS. I. — SENATOR (*Klin. Woch.* 5 *janv.* 1900. *t.* XXVI). Femme 19 ans. Hématuries rénales abondantes du côté droit depuis 3 ans, attribuées à l'hémophilie. Néphrectomie par Sonnenburg. Guérison se maintenant 9 mois après. Examen du rein par Israel montre des ilots profonds et limités de *néphrite interstitielle.*

OBS. II. — DE KEERMAEKER. (*Ann. de la Soc. belge de chir.*, *déc.* 1897.) Femme 43 ans. Hématuries permanentes du rein gauche depuis 3 ans. Néphrectomie. Guérison. Examen du rein : *néphrite mixte à type hémorragique.*

OBS. III. — DEMONS. (*Associat. franç de chir.* XII<sup></sup> *Congrès* 1898.) Femme 24 ans. Hématuries, précédées de vives douleurs dans le côté gauche persistant depuis 2 mois. Néphrectomie. — Guérison se maintenant 10 mois après. Examen du rein, *sclérose* avec prédominance des lésions dans les glomérules et le long des tubes collecteurs.

OBS. IV —. PÉAN (*De l'interv. chir. dans affections du rein. Brodeur, th. Paris* 1886). Homme 40 ans. Douleurs rénales excessives à gauche, amaigrissement considérable, tendance au suicide. Néphrectomie. — Guérison persistait 5 ans après. Examen du rein par Cornil : *glomérulite* et altération des tubes urinifères comme dans la néphrite albumineuse peu avancée.

OBS. V. — ROBERT J. WEIR (*Medical Record, vol.* 46, p. 324). Homme 25 ans. — Néphrite et uréthrite gonococciques avec température variant de 39°4 à 40°5 : pyurie. Le rein droit volumineux incisé est criblé d'abcès miliaires : néphrectomie d'urgence. La température tombe aussi-

1. GOODHART. *Guy's hospital Report*, 1874. — 2. Robert WEIR. *Medical Record*, 1894.

tôt à 37°5 et le malade sort trois semaines après avec des urines presque normales.

Obs. VI. — Israel (*Cité par Albarran* in *Traité de chirurgie de Le Dentu et Delbet*). Signes de néphrite infectieuse aiguë. Néphrectomie. - Guérison. — A l'examen du rein : *abcès miliaires*.

Obs. VII. — Max Jordan. (*Cité par Albarran loc. cit.*) Infection rénale hématogène aiguë. Néphrectomie. Guérison.

Obs. VIII. — Pousson (*Bull. de la Soc. de chir. de Paris*, 7 juin 1898). Femme 25 ans. Hématuries profuses provenant du rein droit. Néphrectomie. Guérison se maintenant depuis plus de deux ans. *Néphrite interstitielle*.

Obs. IX. Pousson (*Bulletin de la Soc. de chir. de Paris*, 12 juin 1900.) Homme 65 ans. Hématuries très abondantes depuis 2 mois. Néphrectomie. Guérison. *Néphrite infectieuse aiguë* avec nombreux abcès miliaires.

· A ces 9 faits d'infection très vraisemblablement unilatérale chronique ou aiguë du rein dans lesquels l'examen du rein extirpé a pu être pratiqué, je pourrais en joindre 6 autres publiés par Broca (*Ann. des mal. des org. génito-urin., décembre* 1894), Mac Lane Tiffany (*Ann. of. surg.*, 1889), Harrison 4 observations (*Brit. med. Journ.*, 1896), dans lesquels la simple incision de l'un des reins ayant fait cesser les symptômes, il y a tout lieu de croire que les lésions n'affectaient que l'un de ces organes.

Toutes ces observations prouvent péremptoirement l'unilatéralité des lésions rénales d'ordre médical, mais, faute de renseignements urologiques, elles ne peuvent servir à démontrer le retentissement fonctionnel d'un rein enflammé sur son congénère sain. Bien que ces renseignements aient été encore incomplètement relevés dans les deux faits suivants que je résumerai, je crois qu'ils sont de nature à confirmer la thèse que je soutiens.

Obs. XVI. — Sabatier. (*Rev. de chir.*, t. IX., *Paris* 1889). Femme 5 ans, présente depuis l'âge de 22 ans, en même temps que des troubles du côté de la sécrétion et de la composition chimique des urines (oligurie 450 à 750 grammes dans les 24 heures; diminution de l'urée 5 à 10 grammes; albuminurie 1 à 2 grammes; hématurie); tous les phénomènes de l'urémie (céphalée, dyspnée, état nauséeux et vomissements, coma). Pour remédier aux hémorragies devenues très abondantes et aux douleurs très vives, on pratique la néphrectomie. Immédiatement tous les symptômes s'amendent et disparaissent; (la quantité des urines se relève à 1000 à 1500 grammes; le taux de l'urée remonte à 20 à 22 grammes; l'albumine diminue considérablement). Un an après, la guérison se maintenait, la malade rendait 1000 grammes d'urine dans les 24 heures, avec 19 grammes d'urée et quelques légères traces d'albumine; l'état général était excellent, à part quelques troubles comateux, attribuables à des phénomènes nerveux.

Obs. XVII. — *(Cette observation, qui m'est personnelle, a été rapportée
in extenso à l'Académie de médecine, séance du 20 mars 1900.)* Une femme
atteinte de néphrite hématurique unilatérale, avec diminution de la quantité des urines (700 grammes), du taux de l'urée (4 à 6 grammes), de
l'acide phosphorique (0,52), de chlorure de sodium (1gr. 90) et avec
albuminurie (0 gr. 25), offre tout le cortège des symptômes de l'urémie. Je
pratique la *néphrotomie.* Dès le 5ᵉ jour la quantité des urines se relève
(200 grammes), leur teneur en urée (15 gr. 60), en acide phosphorique
(0 gr. 77), en chlorure de sodium (5 grammes), augmente parallèlement,
l'albumine reste dans les mêmes proportions, mais tous les accidents
urémiques disparaissent. Cette amélioration se maintient pendant 15 jours
durant lesquels l'incision du rein reste béante. A peine est-elle fermée, qu'on
voit se reproduire les modifications de quantité et de qualité des urines et
réapparaître les phénomènes d'urémie. Le volume des urines étant descendu à 500, l'urée à 5,25, l'acide phosphorique à 0,59, le chlorure de sodium
à 0,54, et la proportion d'albumine étant de 0,52, je me décide à extirper
le rein. Les signes de l'empoisonnement urémique disparaissent immédiatement après la néphrectomie et dès le 4ᵉ jour, le volume des urines est de
115 grammes, 1 gr. 24, le chlorure de sodium de 1 gr. 70, l'urée est remontée
à 16 gr. 20, l'acide phosphorique à 1 gr. 70, l'albuminurie est descendue à
0 gr. 12. A sa sortie de l'hôpital, 56 jours après l'opération, l'analyse donnait : volume des 24 heures, 1600 gr. urée 10 gr. 40 (par litre), acide phosphorique 1 gr. 20, chlorure de sodium 8 gr. 80, albumine traces légères,
plus de céphalée, ni dyspnée, ni vomissements.


2° *Modifications anatomiques déterminées du côté d'un rein sain par
un rein malade.* — Bien que l'innervation des reins soit encore très
obscure, on sait depuis Cl. Bernard et Brown Séquard que l'excitation des nerfs rénaux fait pâlir le parenchyme de l'organe correspondant et suspend sa sécrétion. L'excitation de la muqueuse de l'uretère
du bassinet et de la substance rénale elle-même produit les mêmes
effets et détermine l'arrêt de la sécrétion même du côté opposé, d'où
anurie. Que si au lieu d'exciter les nerfs du plexus rénal on les sectionne, le rein se congestionne et devient rouge, turgescent, pulsatile,
sans que pour cela sa sécrétion soit augmentée, bien au contraire.
Ces données de la physiologie permettent de comprendre comment
un grand nombre d'affections chirurgicales du rein mettant en jeu
sa sensibilité à la pression et surtout à la distension réalisent en clinique les excitations, points de départ du réflexe inhibitoire, agissant
soit sur un seul rein, soit sur les deux à la fois. Il est plus difficile
d'interpréter le retentissement du rein malade sur le rein sain dans
les affections lentes et chroniques, et particulièrement dans les néphrites parenchymateuses ou interstitielles. Outre les poussées aiguës
et douloureuses qui, survenant encore assez souvent au cours de ces
néphrites du côté du rein principalement atteint, déterminent l'aug-

mentation de volume et de la douleur du rein opposé (Guyon), ne peut-on pas invoquer aussi l'irritation sourde et constante des nerfs du rein malade et l'existence de ces névrites du plexus rénal décrites par Klippel?

Ces phénomènes sont peut-être pendant longtemps insuffisants à modifier anatomiquement la structure du parenchyme rénal, mais il ne répugne nullement d'admettre qu'à la longue ils puissent déterminer des troubles susceptibles sinon d'engendrer *ipso facto* une affection du rein ou tout au moins de créer les conditions, qui le mettent en état de réceptivité morbide.

Si, comme nous osons l'espérer, l'hypothèse de l'existence d'une néphrite sympathique devenait une réalité, on comprend quelles conséquences pratiques en découleraient.

Non seulement les interventions chirurgicales hâtives par la néphrotomie et la néphrectomie dans les affections chirurgicales et peut-être même médicales d'un rein deviendraient la règle pour prévenir les lésions secondaires de l'autre, mais elles s'imposeraient pour enrayer les lésions débutantes. J'ai dit précédemment les résultats que la néphrectomie a fournis à Sabatier et à moi-même dans deux cas où une néphrite unilatérale influençait le fonctionnement de l'autre rein et y avait peut-être même déterminé des altérations anatomiques. Deux observations, succinctement rapportées par le professeur Guyon, il y a déjà longtemps dans un article sur la physiologie chirurgicale du rein, sont également démonstratives à la fois du retentissement anatomique d'un rein malade sur son congénère et des heureux effets de l'intervention sur l'arrêt et la rétrocession des lésions initiales sympathiques de ce dernier[1].

---

## DES PETITES RÉTENTIONS RÉNALES DANS LE REIN MOBILE

### par MM. E. MICHON et O. PASTEAU,

de Paris.

Laissant de côté les grandes rétentions des reins mobiles (hydronéphroses), nous ne voulons attirer l'attention que sur les petites rétentions. Nous en avons observé quinze cas. La rétention est peu abondante et varie de 40 à 7 centimètres cubes; le plus souvent nous l'avons trouvée de 50 centimètres cubes. Elle s'accompagne toujours d'une diminution assez notable des éléments solides de l'urine dans

1. *Annales des malad. des organes gén.-urin.*, 1888, p. 720.

le liquide de rétention. Par exemple 5 grammes d'urée du côté du rein malade au lieu de 10 grammes, 5 grammes au lieu de 15 grammes.

Abandonnées à elles-mêmes, ces rétentions persistent, laissant le rein dans un état d'infériorité sécrétoire; elles peuvent aussi aboutir aux grandes rétentions, à la sclérose rénale et à la néphrite. Traitées, elles peuvent guérir.

Le diagnostic ne peut être fait ni par l'augmentation de volume du rein, ni par le degré de mobilité, ni par la douleur. Le cathétérisme urétéral seul nous a permis de l'établir.

Il existe quelques causes de difficultés de cathétérisme spéciales à ce genre de maladie, ptose viscérale, valvules ostiales de l'uretère, coudure, et le cathétérisme doit être fait particulièrement ici avec beaucoup de douceur.

Quand il y a rétention, l'écoulement d'urine se fait d'une façon continue « par jet, ou goutte à goutte »; lorsqu'il n'y a pas de rétention l'écoulement se fait d'une façon intermittente par éjaculation. Pratiqué avec ces précautions le cathétérisme urétéral est absolument inoffensif et donne des résultats exacts.

Lorsque ces rétentions persistent, il faut les traiter. Le cathétérisme répété peut amener parfois la guérison, comme dans deux de nos observations. Mais, si ce résultat n'est pas obtenu, on doit avoir recours à la néphrorraphie; nous avons pu, en effet, constater dans trois cas que la rétention avait disparu à la suite de cette opération.

Comme conclusion pratique, nous dirons donc que l'existence d'une petite rétention dans le rein mobile, persistant malgré le cathétérisme urétéral, est à elle seule une indication de la néphropexie.

---

### LE REIN MOBILE CHEZ LES ARABES

par M. le docteur TREKAKI,

d'Alexandrie.

La présente note a pour but l'étude d'un des chapitres non le moins controversés de l'histoire de la néphroptose.

L'utilité de cette étude ressort de ce que, chez les Arabes dont le genre de vie, les habitudes et la tempérance sont autrement simples et différentes de l'Européen, la diversité des lésions doit être aussi complexe.

La pathogénie de la néphroptose encore si discutée tirerait, croyons-nous, de l'étude de ces faits un grand profit et permettrait d'expliquer certains côtés pathologiques de la question.

Ce qui a rendu si obscure cette pathogénie, c'est que, à tort, chaque cause a été prise isolément et considérée comme seule capable d'expliquer la genèse de la néphroptose. C'est là une erreur. Si parfois une cause isolée peut à elle seule produire le déplacement rénal, rarement on peut dire que cette même cause peut, chez un autre individu, produire la néphroptose. C'est même l'exception et une foule de circonstances s'associeront la plupart du temps pour occasionner la chute du rein ou du moins son facile déplacement. Témoin ce qui arrive chez les Arabes chez lesquels, dans les neuf dixièmes des cas sinon dans tous, un faisceau des causes est le point de départ d'une mobilité rénale.

L'Arabe femme en effet, sur laquelle ont porté toutes mes observations a un genre de vie absolument différent de l'Européenne en si basse classe sociale que cette dernière puisse se trouver. L'Égyptienne vit misérablement et surtout sous un ciel qui conserve une foule de préjugés. De là à avoir des habitudes et une tempérance spéciale, il n'y a qu'un pas. De plus, la femme arabe de la classe inférieure et même de toutes les classes travaille beaucoup et se nourrit peu, conditions éminemment favorables pour le développement d'une altération des tissus. L'Égyptienne surtout, et j'y insiste, a un mode spécial d'habillement. Aucun lien constricteur ne sert à soutenir cet habillement. Si quelques-unes d'entre elles se servent d'un lien constricteur au ventre, celui-ci est situé bien au-dessous de l'ombilic et n'exerce aucune gêne au fonctionnement de la sangle abdominale. De sorte que de ce côté rien à trouver comme cause de l'ectopie rénale. Ni corset, ni ceinturon, ni vêtements lourds, rien de tout cet accoutrement pouvant être incriminé. C'est donc, pour toutes ces raisons, que l'étude que j'entreprends aujourd'hui est intéressante à plus d'un titre, étant donné le champ d'observations auquel je me suis placé qui, je l'espère doit servir comme contribution à l'étude de la néphroptose.

Il faut donc chercher ailleurs la vraie cause.

J'ai examiné à cet effet 100 femmes arabes prises au hasard. J'ai trouvé 42 fois le rein mobile et 58 fois où on ne sentait aucune mobilité. Donc les 2/5$^{mes}$ de femmes arabes ont un rein mobile.

Vous savez que cette proportion est loin de celle de Kustner et Lindner qui prétendent qu'on observe la néphroptose une fois sur 5 à 6 femmes européennes prises au hasard.

Parmi mes 42 femmes néphroptosiques chez 31 on sentait le tiers inférieur du rein, chez 9, les 2/5 inférieurs, et chez 2 la totalité du rein. Et parmi ces reins mobiles il y a eu 58 femmes avec grossesses, deux sans grossesse et deux vierges.

Poursuivant mon investigation plus loin, j'ai voulu savoir l'état de la sangle abdominale chez mes 42 néphroptosiques. C'est là une donnée extrêmement importante qui va nous servir à plus d'un enseignement. Or, chez mes néphroptosiques les parois abdominales étaient tendues et non relâchées 20 fois, et souples et relâchées 22 fois. Quant à la relation qu'il y a entre le degré de tension de la paroi abdominale et le degré de la ptose rénale, mes observations n'en donnent aucune : car il peut se faire que des ventres très tendus et nullement lâches puissent contenir un rein mobile à un degré considérable. Le contraire est encore possible. Il en est de même de l'épaisseur des parois abdominales qui ne présente, elle aussi, aucun effet fâcheux sur les liens d'attache du rein. Voilà pour le contenant.

Quelle relation y a-t-il maintenant entre le contenu de l'abdomen et la ptose rénale ?

Rien ne semble influencer la chute ou plutôt la mobilité du rein. Les ptoses viscérales en particulier ne paraissent pas être une cause de néphroptose. Sur mes 42 observations de rein ptosique 11 fois seulement des ptoses viscérales accompagnaient la ptose rénale et 15 fois où malgré les ptoses telles que l'entéroptose, l'hépatoptose, l'entéroptose ou vaginoptose, le rein ne quittait pas sa place. C'est un fait d'observation qui présente de l'intérêt, étant donné le rôle que jouent certaines ptoses viscérales sur la mobilité rénale. Je puis citer même à cet effet une observation extrèmement intéressante où il s'agissait d'une femme arabe neurasthénique de 60 ans, très maigre, à ventre flasque ayant eu six grossesses chez laquelle on constatait manifestement une entéroptose avec dilatation considérable de l'estomac et une hépatoptose assez accusée et chez laquelle il n'y avait pas la moindre néphroptose. D'autres observations semblables viennent s'ajouter à celle-ci.

Il ressort donc en matière de conclusion générale de cette courte note qu'étant donné le champ d'observation auquel je me suis trouvé, c'est à-dire chez des femmes qui ont un genre de vie absolument différent de celui sur lequel ont porté les nombreuses observations de l'étude de néphroptose jusqu'ici citées, étant donnée donc cette considération, nous devons admettre que l'ensemble des faits plaident en faveur d'une étiologie multiple de la mobilité du rein, celle-ci n'étant pas, dans la majorité des cas, sous la dépendance d'une seule et unique cause, mais relevant plutôt d'une foule de circonstances qui convergent toutes vers un but unique, à savoir l'altération des tissus qui doit entraîner comme conséquence ultime la détérioration des liens naturels de la glande rénale. Car, en fait de cause unique, mais seulement prédisposante, nous n'avons rencontré, chez les Arabes qui ont un genre de vie spécial, que la déchéance physiologique qui peut seule être invoquée comme facteur sérieux dans l'étiologie de la néphroptose.

## DE LA NÉPHRECTOMIE DANS LES TUMEURS MALIGNES DU REIN

### par M. le professeur GUILLET,

de Caen.

Depuis 1888, époque à laquelle a paru ma thèse sur les tumeurs malignes du rein, j'ai eu l'occasion d'observer un certain nombre de ces tumeurs et de pratiquer quelques interventions, bien que les occasions d'intervenir soient assez restreintes dans la pratique, les malades venant le plus souvent consulter le chirurgien trop tardivement ou n'acceptant pas l'opération qu'on leur propose.

Je n'ai eu que quatre fois à intervenir en présence d'une tumeur maligne du rein : dans deux circonstances, j'ai dû me contenter d'une laparotomie exploratrice ; deux autres fois, j'ai fait une néphrectomie transpéritonéale, avec une récidive au bout de six mois et une guérison qui se maintient encore d'une façon absolue depuis un an et demi. Je serai très bref pour les deux premiers cas.

Dans la première observation, il s'agissait d'un homme de 55 ans, qui depuis dix-huit mois s'était affaibli et se plaignait d'une douleur assez vive dans l'hypocondre gauche. Il n'avait eu aucune hématurie mais il portait une tumeur ayant environ le volume de deux poings ; elle paraissait encore mobile et était accompagnée d'un varicocèle gauche très développé. Je portai le diagnostic de carcinome du rein gauche ; mais, les dimensions de la tumeur m'effrayant un peu, j'envoyai le malade consulter mon maître, le professeur Guyon ; ce dernier fut d'avis que la néphrectomie devait être tentée. Une incision menée le long du bord externe du muscle droit me permit d'aborder facilement la tumeur après avoir récliné en dedans le côlon ; mais je m'aperçus en ce moment qu'il existait un gros paquet ganglionnaire en dedans du hile et adhérent aux organes voisins. Je dus refermer le ventre sans pousser plus loin l'opération. Le malade se remit de cette laparotomie et ne succomba que deux ans plus tard aux progrès de la généralisation.

Dans le deuxième cas, que j'observai au mois de février dernier, il s'agissait d'une jeune fille de 20 ans qui portait une volumineuse tumeur de l'abdomen, occupant l'hypocondre droit, l'épigastre, le flanc droit et la région ombilicale. Cette tumeur, qui s'était développée en l'espace d'un an et demi sans aucune manifestation urinaire, paraissait fluctuante et je pensai à un kyste hydatique du foie. Mais l'incision de la paroi abdominale me fit reconnaître que j'avais commis une erreur de diagnotic et que je me trouvais en face d'un très volumineux sarcome du rein droit absolument inopérable. Je me contentai de refermer le ventre ; la jeune fille succomba trois mois plus tard.

Dans les deux autres cas, je pus intervenir dans de meilleures conditions et faire l'ablation de la tumeur.

Dans l'un d'eux, il s'agissait d'une vieille demoiselle de 60 ans, que j'observai au mois de mars 1899. Cette malade avait éprouvé les premiers symptômes de son mal au mois d'octobre de la même année ; à ce moment, elle fut prise, à la suite d'un voyage, d'une violente hématurie qui dura huit jours. Depuis cette époque, les hématuries reparurent de plus en plus abondantes à trois ou quatre reprises ; elles s'accompagnaient de douleurs dans le rein droit qui était notablement abaissé et mobile dans l'abdomen. Comme la malade était très émaciée et avait des parois très flasques, il me fut facile de reconnaître sur la face antérieure du rein droit un noyeau induré du volume d'une prune, situé près du hile. Je portai le diagnostic de carcinome du rein droit et je proposai la néphrectomie qui fut acceptée. L'opération fut des plus faciles ; incision le long du bord externe du muscle droit, réclinaison du côlon en dedans, énucléation du rein, suture du pédicule en masse, suture des deux feuillets viscéral et pariétal du péritoine, suivant le procédé de Terrier, tout fut exécuté en trois quarts d'heure. Suites opératoires bonnes, mais six mois après la malade succombait à la généralisation. Il s'agissait bien, ainsi que le démontra l'examen de la pièce, d'un carcinome du volume d'une prune, développé près du hile. En apparence, j'étais intervenu dans d'excellentes conditions, ce qui n'empêcha pas la généralisation de se produire.

Dans le dernier cas, enfin, je fus plus heureux ; car au bout d'un an et demi, mon malade vit et se porte bien. Je vous demande la permission de rapporter cette observation en détail.

Le nommé R..., peintre, âgé de 45 ans, m'est adressé par le D<sup>r</sup> Bagourd, d'Argentan, pour une tumeur du flanc droit. Rien à signaler comme antécédents : le père est bien portant ; la mère est morte à 62 ans d'une affection du cœur ; il existe cinq frères en bonne santé. Le malade n'a jamais eu de maladie grave antérieurement, si ce n'est, en 1882, une bronchite qui dura six semaines environ.

Il y a deux ans, R... a commencé à ressentir certains troubles du ventre ; il éprouvait après les repas du gonflement avec oppression. Plus tard, il perdit l'appétit ; il éprouva des coliques et des vomissements. Un médecin appelé en consultation crut à l'existence de coliques de plomb. Les douleurs augmentant, le D<sup>r</sup> Bagourd fut appelé ; il reconnut l'existence d'une tumeur du flanc droit et m'adressa le malade. Ce dernier vint me consulter au mois d'août 1898. Je constatai qu'il était amaigri et émacié. Il se plaignait d'avoir perdu l'appétit et de souffrir beaucoup du ventre surtout après les repas. Comme trouble urinaire, il n'a eu qu'une légère hématurie, laquelle a consisté uniquement dans l'expulsion d'un petit caillot sanguin dont il ne peut me préciser la forme. Cette petite hématurie avait été précédée d'une crise douloureuse localisée au flanc droit. Ce dernier est d'ailleurs souvent le siège de douleurs spontanées qui jamais ne s'irradient du côté de la vessie. L'examen du ventre fait reconnaître facilement l'existence d'une tumeur située au-dessous des fausses côtes dans le flanc droit. Cette tumeur à surface irrégulière et bosselée est solide, elle se continue dans la région lombaire et donne très nettement la sensation du ballottement rénal. Elle a les dimensions d'un poing d'adulte. En avant d'elle existe une zone de sonorité et les mouvements du diaphragme ne lui sont pas transmis. Nous constatons l'existence d'un volumineux varicocèle droit. Les urines sont normales.

Je porte le diagnostic de tumeur solide du rein droit de nature maligne et je conseille une intervention immédiate. Le malade ne veut pas s'y soumettre et retourne chez lui.

Il vient me retrouver au commencement de février 1899, c'est-à-dire six mois plus tard ; les douleurs ayant augmenté, il se décide à accepter l'opération. Il a, du reste, beaucoup maigri depuis sa dernière visite et la tumeur a manifestement augmenté ; elle atteint maintenant les dimensions d'une tête de fœtus à terme ; elle a conservé tous ses caractères, y compris sa mobilité. Les troubles urinaires ont toujours fait défaut et il ne s'est produit aucune hématurie.

L'opération est faite le 15 février 1899 ; incision verticale le long du bord externe du muscle droit d'une longueur de 18 à 20 centimètres. Le côlon ascendant, qui passe au-devant de la tumeur très vasculaire, est récliné en dedans et le péritoine viscéral incisé le long du bord externe de l'intestin. La tumeur est libérée avec le doigt et amenée facilement entre les lèvres de la plaie ; le pédicule est lié en masse. Pas d'hémorragie. Suture des deux feuillets péritonéaux suivant la méthode de Terrier ; drainage antérieur et tamponnement léger à la gaze iodoformée. Suture de la paroi adominale dans le reste de l'étendue de l'incision. Durée de l'opération : une heure. Suites normales. Pas de fièvre. Le malade retourne chez lui au bout de trois semaines avec une petite fistule qui se cicatrise ultérieurement. Je l'ai revu depuis, il continue de bien se porter et n'éprouve plus aucune douleur. Il vient de prendre part dernièrement, m'écrit son médecin, aux épreuves d'un concours de pompiers sans en ressentir d'inconvénients.

L'examen de la pièce a montré qu'il s'agissait d'une tumeur, ayant à peu près les dimensions d'une tête de fœtus à terme, développée aux dépens de l'extrémité supérieure du rein droit. Cette tumeur molle, grisâtre, très vasculaire par place, avec de petits kystes, a l'aspect d'un encéphaloïde. L'examen microscopique a révélé qu'il s'agissait d'un épithélioma.

Bien qu'il puisse paraître téméraire de tirer des conclusions de ces quatre observations, je demande cependant la permission de les faire suivre de quelques remarques.

En 1888, dans ma thèse sur les tumeurs malignes du rein, j'avais insisté sur la gravité des interventions faites en pareil cas et j'étais arrivé à conclure que les résultats de la néphrectomie, pour cancer du rein, étaient loin d'être encourageants et qu'on pouvait être tenté de rejeter toute intervention chirurgicale. Il est vrai que plus loin j'adoucissais la sévérité de cette conclusion en disant :

« En résumé, il est difficile de se prononcer aujourd'hui d'une façon définitive sur la valeur thérapeutique de la néphrectomie dans les tumeurs malignes du rein ; jusqu'à présent, les résultats qu'a donnés cette opération sont peu encourageants, mais il faut reconnaître que le plus souvent cette opération a été pratiquée dans de mauvaises conditions, à une période beaucoup trop avancée de la maladie. Aujourd'hui les méthodes d'exploration du rein sont mieux connues, les symptômes auxquels donnent lieu les tumeurs rénales ont été mieux étudiés ; il est possible d'en faire le diagnostic à une période relativement peu avancée ; il est à supposer que la néphrectomie faite dans ces nouvelles conditions sera suivie de résultats plus favorables. »

La suite a démontré l'exactitude de mes prévisions. Depuis lors, en effet, les auteurs qui se sont occupés de cette question se sont prononcés d'une façon nette ; tous concluent à la nécessité et à la bénignité relative de l'intervention. A cet égard, l'opinion de Héresco (De l'intervention chirurgicale dans les tumeurs malignes du rein, thèse de 1899) mérite d'être rapportée. « La néphrectomie, dit-il, dans les tumeurs malignes du rein est une opération bénigne aussi bien chez

l'enfant que chez l'adulte, dans les conditions que nous avons déterminées et surtout lorsque le néoplasme est à une période d'évolution
voisine de son début. Dans les mêmes conditions, une longue survie
équivalant à une guérison est aujourd'hui presque la règle après
l'extirpation du néoplasme du rein. La néphrectomie ne doit être
rejetée que lorsqu'il y a généralisation ou des adhérences qui ne permettent pas l'extirpation. »

C'est actuellement l'opinion admise par tous et nous ne pensons pas
qu'il puisse y avoir désormais discussion sur ce sujet. Intervenir dès
qu'on le peut, telle doit être la règle ici comme dans toutes les
tumeurs malignes.

Pour ce qui est du manuel opératoire, nous avons eu recours à la
néphrectomie transpéritonéale à l'aide de l'incision de Langenbuck,
c'est-à-dire le long du bord externe du grand droit. Cette incision
nous a paru la plus convenable pour arriver sur la tumeur ; il peut se
faire cependant que dans des cas exceptionnels l'incision médiane soit
préférable. Quant à la méthode extra-péritonéale par l'incision lombaire, elle nous paraît devoir être réservée aux tumeurs de petit
volume. Quel est du reste l'avantage de la néphrectomie lombaire ?
L'ablation d'un néoplasme ne constitue-t-elle pas une opération asep=
tique qui n'a aucune chance d'infecter le péritoine? Pourquoi donc
redouter la voie péritonéale ? Ne permet-elle pas mieux que toute
autre une exploration minutieuse et directe des organes voisins du
ein dégénéré?

Nous pensons également que la ligature du pédicule doit se faire
séparément pour les vaisseaux et l'uretère et nous sommes d'avis que
le catgut doit être préféré à la soie qui entretient souvent des fistules.

La réunion des deux feuillets péritonéaux suivant le procédé de
Terrier nous paraît être indispensable, car il crée en dehors du péritoine une cavité qui peut être drainée soit en avant, soit en arrière,
par la région lombaire.

Ainsi comprise, la néphrectomie appliquée aux tumeurs malignes
du rein est une opération en général facile, relativement bénigne et
susceptible de donner de bons résultats éloignés, tel celui que nous
rapportons plus haut.

# TROISIÈME SÉANCE

## SAMEDI 4 AOUT 1900

*A 9 heures du matin.*

Présidence de M. le professeur NICOLICH,
de Trieste.

---

*Deuxième question mise à l'ordre du jour :*

# VALEUR DE L'INTERVENTION CHIRURGICALE DANS LES TUBERCULOSES URINAIRES

*Rapporteurs :* MM. Saxtorph (Copenhague); Hogge (Liège);
Poussox (Bordeaux).

---

## VALEUR DE L'INTERVENTION CHIRURGICALE DANS LA TUBERCULOSE VÉSICALE

### RAPPORT

par le professeur Sylvester SAXTORPH,

Chirurgien de l'hôpital communal à Copenhague.

Messieurs,

En mettant à l'ordre du jour la question de la valeur de l'intervention chirurgicale dans la tuberculose urinaire, le comité a sans doute estimé que l'heure est venue de soumettre à une critique rationnelle les interventions chirurgicales de ces dernières années, et de porter un jugement fondé sur les résultats obtenus. Sans doute le comité a été inspiré par l'espoir d'entendre des membres de cette assemblée apporter des preuves nouvelles et triomphantes de la possibilité de la guérison de cette maladie si terrible qui a défié les efforts des chirurgiens les plus illustres et les plus habiles. Et, cependant, la rédaction même de la question ne semble-t-elle pas prévoir qu'il pourrait s'élever des voix de cette assemblée pour dire que l'enthousiasme provoqué par les résultats obtenus est loin d'être en rapport avec l'énergie déployée par les chirurgiens et l'espoir qui les a guidés ?

La question du traitement de la tuberculose vésicale a déjà depuis nombre d'années vivement intéressé les chirurgiens, depuis les premières publications de notre illustre maître, M. le professeur Guyon, lesquelles publications, ainsi que tous les travaux ultérieurs, entrepris sous son inspiration par les élèves si renommés de l'école de Necker, sont connus de nous tous. Je passe donc sous silence tout l'historique de la question.

En parcourant la littérature de la tuberculose urinaire pour les dernières années, j'ai, bien entendu, rencontré un nombre très considérable de communications concernant le traitement de la tuberculose vésicale, de descriptions d'opérations les plus variées, de recommandations les plus enthousiastes de tel ou tel remède, de publications des cas d'amélioration et de guérison obtenus par telle ou telle méthode; d'un autre côté, des chirurgiens moins heureux proclament la nature presque incurable et l'issue presque toujours fatale de cette maladie.

Sans doute il serait possible, avec ces documents si nombreux de faire une statistique qui indiquerait les résultats de chacune de ces interventions et de chacun de ces traitements; mais, messieurs, je pense qu'une telle statistique n'aurait aucune valeur, et voici pourquoi. D'abord les documents sont de nature fort hétérogène, les mêmes interventions étant utilisées dans des cas d'origine et d'étendue très différentes. De plus les communications sont faites par de nombreux opérateurs, qui n'ont pas pu avoir eu les mêmes vues sur la maladie. Enfin il est évidemment impossible de comparer les résultats obtenus il y a quelques années, à ceux qu'on obtient maintenant, que l'expérience des chirurgiens, le développement de la technique, les conditions dans lesquelles le traitement se fait, ont provoqué de si grands progrès. Aussi je laisse de côté toute tentative pour faire une telle statistique.

Si nous voulons obtenir quelques résultats en discutant la valeur des interventions chirurgicales dans la tuberculose vésicale, il est donc de toute nécessité de nous représenter clairement les modifications pathologiques de la vessie et spécialement leur pathogénie, c'est-à-dire leur cause et leurs origines immédiates. Vous m'excuserez, messieurs, si je m'occupe avec quelque détail, de cette partie de pathologie générale, qui pourrait paraître un peu en dehors de la question; il n'en est rien, et je crois que la cause qui nous empêche de voir pour l'instant, avec assez de clarté, l'effet de nos interventions dans la tuberculose vésicale, est précisément d'avoir agi de façon trop empirique, sans nous être assez rendu compte des différentes formes des affections vésicales.

Sous quelles formes voyons-nous apparaître la tuberculose vésicale? Sous deux formes : l'une, la tuberculose miliaire, l'autre la tuberculose urinaire chronique et isolée.

Pour ce qui est de la première forme, elle est sans doute très rare. Dans tous les cas elle n'apparaît que comme une manifestation très minime de la tuberculose miliaire générale aiguë, dont les manifestations dans les autres grands organes attirent l'attention à ce point que l'affection insignifiante de la vessie — si elle existe réellement — passe presque inaperçue. En tout cas, elle n'est pas l'objet d'une intervention chirurgicale, elle n'a pour nous aucun intérêt, et je ne m'y arrêterai nullement.

Il ne s'agit donc que de la forme isolée et chronique de la tuberculose urinaire ou uro-génitale, qui se manifeste comme entité morbide bien caractérisée, soit comme tuberculose pure, soit comme tuberculose compliquée d'associations microbiennes pyogènes.

. D'après toutes les observations que j'ai faites personnellement au cours de nombreuses autopsies, et d'après des recherches faites avec beaucoup de soin par mon jeune et distingué collègue M. le docteur P.-N. Hansen, je suis arrivé à la certitude presque absolue que la tuberculose urinaire ou uro-génitale, dont il est question, a toujours pour première origine un foyer tuberculeux dans le poumon, foyer plus ou moins ancien, souvent très ancien resté inaperçu et qu'aucun symptôme n'a révélé pendant nombre d'années.

Provoqué par une occasion quelconque il se produit alors dans le voisinage de ce foyer une éruption miliaire; les bacilles tuberculeux qui, dans ce foyer d'une innocuité apparente, ont gardé toute leur virulence, comme le prouve la bactériologie, sont remis en liberté.

Dès ce moment l'infection de l'appareil uro-génital est donc devenu possible. Elle se produit d'une des deux façons suivantes :

*Premier cas:* Les bacilles tuberculeux sont entraînés par le courant sanguin jusqu'au rein, ils se fixent le plus souvent dans la substance corticale, dans les colonnes de Bertini, tout près des pyramides, qui sont vite envahies, probablement parce qu'elles sont moins riches en vaisseaux; les bacilles les transforment rapidement en foyers caséeux ou en cavernes, d'où ils descendent, avec l'urine, jusqu'à la vessie; celle-ci sera tôt ou tard infectée, les bacilles se greffant dans la muqueuse, le plus souvent dans le bas-fond, le trigone de Lieutaudii, mais pas toujours, comme on l'a voulu soutenir, dans le voisinage immédiat de l'orifice urétéral correspondant au rein malade. La tuberculose vésicale est donc dès à présent établie; et d'abord localisée à la surface interne de la vessie, elle se propage ensuite de la surface muqueuse, sous forme d'infiltrations tuberculeuses dans la profondeur de la paroi, formant plus ou moins rapidement, des ulcérations souvent entourées d'irruptions miliaires. C'est là sans doute la forme la plus fréquente de la tuberculose vésicale, la *forme descendante*, la *forme cavitaire*, dont l'origine première dans les organes urinaires est dans le rein.

*Second cas* : Les bacilles tuberculeux sont amenés par la voie circulatoire aux grands glands de l'appareil génital, la prostate, les vésicules séminales, les testicules et épididymes ; il se produit une tuberculose génitale : après avoir détruit la prostate et les tissus environnants par la formation des foyers caséeux ou d'abcès tuberculeux, les bacilles arrivent tôt ou tard par contiguitatem à la paroi de la vessie.

Les bacilles arrivent donc, soit par les interstices du tissu cellulaire, soit par l'ouverture spontanée d'un abcès tuberculeux, directement à la surface de la muqueuse vésicale. La tuberculose vésicale est donc encore ici établie, envahissant de même les parties profondes de la vessie. C'est la *forme ascendante*, la forme par propagation directe de la tuberculose vésicale, dont le foyer primaire est dans les organes génitaux. Bien entendu cette forme est beaucoup plus fréquente chez l'homme que chez la femme.

Autant que j'en puis juger, cette forme, qui paraissait autrefois plus fréquente que la forme rénale est actuellement la moins fréquente des deux. On en trouverait peut-être la raison dans l'exactitude moins grande des anciennes observations et dans la défectuosité des méthodes d'investigations antérieurement employées.

Reste à savoir si les bacilles de la tuberculose peuvent envahir la vessie par la voie circulatoire ; ceci est, bien entendu, de la plus grande importance, pour juger la valeur de nos interventions. *A priori* il semblerait aussi naturel que les bacilles soient amenés directement à la vessie, organe si vasculaire, qu'aux reins ou à la prostate ; cependant, mon opinion personnelle est que ce fait ne se produit jamais ou presque jamais.

Je sais bien que, sur ce point, je suis en contradiction avec les idées généralement admises, et soutenues spécialement par notre illustre maître et ses élèves de l'école de Necker ; je connais, bien entendu, l'opinion que M. Clado a émise depuis longtemps déjà sur l'origine sous-épithéliale de la tuberculose vésicale, les bacilles étant selon lui amenés directement par le sang jusqu'au-dessous de l'épithélium ; je sais même que M. le professeur Cornil a relaté deux cas de tuberculose vésicale primaire et isolée ; bien que je ne partage pas l'opinion de M. Albarran, dans l'explication qu'il en fournit, je cou-

nais le cas qu'il a publié, concernant une tuberculose vésicale primaire soi-disant ascendante, remontant jusqu'à la moitié d'un rein
pourvu de deux uretères; j'ai encore rencontré d'ailleurs, dans la littérature, les mêmes opinions; mais bien que je m'incline devant les
idées de ces distingués chirurgiens et pathologistes, je doute cependant beaucoup de la réalité de l'existence de cette forme primaire de
la tuberculose vésicale; dans tous les cas, elle doit être fort rare; par
conséquent, son importance au point de vue thérapeutique et opératoire est-elle beaucoup moins grande que celle des formes secondaires?

J'entends déjà les contradictions, les reproches. Mais je compte,
messieurs, pour me défendre, sur les observations que j'ai faites personnellement dans la salle d'autopsies, sur les recherches que j'ai
faites dans les registres de la salle d'autopsies et sur mes connaissances, basées sur l'expérience clinique.

. Voici donc les faits que j'ai recueillis, aidé par le docteur Hansen,
l'interne du service, et sur lesquels j'appuie mes opinions.

Pendant les seize dernières années, il a été fait à l'hôpital communal 10 016 autopsies dans lesquelles l'état des organes uro-géni-
taux a été soigneusement observé et noté. Sur ces 10 016 cas, il y en a
547 où la tuberculose uro-génitale a été trouvée. Parmi tous ces cas
on a relevé 542 cas de tuberculose miliaire aiguë des reins, et seulement 4 cas de tuberculose miliaire de la vessie, et encore ne s'agis-
sait-il dans tous ces quatre cas, que d'enfants au-dessous de 15 ans,
5 garçons et une fille. On comprendra donc mes doutes sur l'origine
hématogène de la tuberculose vésicale, puisque la vessie est si rarement attaquée par la tuberculose miliaire, cette forme que tout le
monde reconnaît comme la forme hématogène par excellence de la
tuberculose. Et comme il est démontré que les bacilles tuberculeux,
en cas de tuberculose miliaire rénale, peuvent passer par les reins, il
n'est pas absolument impossible que la tuberculose vésicale miliaire
dans les quatre cas mentionnés puisse avoir eu une origine cavitaire.
Restent 205 cas de tuberculose uro-génitale chronique. Parmi ces derniers, il y a 74 cas de tuberculose génitale pure (42 hommes, 32 femmes). Restent donc 131 cas, dont 42 cas de tuberculose urinaire chronique et 89 cas de tuberculose uro-génitale chronique (74 hommes et
15 femmes).

Il est, bien entendu, fort rare de rencontrer parmi ces cas un organe
unique, attaqué isolément; cependant on trouve des lésions isolées
dans les reins 23 fois, dans la prostate 9 fois, dans les vésicules séminales 2 fois, et dans les testicules et épididymes 10 fois. Au contraire

on n'a pas rencontré un seul cas où la vessie soit attaquée isolément par la tuberculose ; toujours un ou plusieurs des organes mentionnés s'est trouvé malade en même temps, ce qui est une nouvelle preuve de l'origine secondaire de la tuberculose vésicale.

Cette tuberculose vésicale a été observée 52 fois, chez 38 hommes (sur 6122 autopsies) et chez 14 femmes (sur 5894 autopsies), ce qui donne respectivement les proportions 0,6 et 0,4 pour 100. Chez les 38 hommes on a trouvé en même temps 52 fois la tuberculose des reins, 29 fois la tuberculose de la prostate, et 20 fois la tuberculose des vésicules séminales ; chez les 14 femmes on a trouvé en même temps 13 fois la tuberculose rénale, 2 fois la tuberculose génitale généralisée et une fois la tuberculose de l'ovaire. Ce dernier cas est le seul où, chez la femme, la vessie s'est montrée le seul des organes urinaires attaqué. La tuberculose vésicale n'était pas cependant d'origine hématogène puisque l'autopsie a montré un grand abcès tuberculeux collé à la paroi postérieure de la vessie, et une éruption tuberculeuse sur la partie correspondante de la muqueuse, l'éruption causée par la propagation directe du voisinage.

Il me semble bien évident, qu'en présence des faits que je viens de rapporter, il faille garder des doutes sérieux sur l'existence de la tuberculose vésicale primaire, qui, si elle existe, est certainement extrêmement rare et, par conséquent, ne saurait modifier les vues que j'expose sur la pathogénie de la tuberculose vésicale.

Dans les cas de tuberculose vésicale et rénale simultanée, ce qui a contribué à faire croire à l'origine primaire des lésions vésicales, c'est qu'il est souvent très difficile, même à l'autopsie, de se prononcer catégoriquement sur l'ancienneté respective des lésions. La lésion la plus étendue n'est pas toujours la plus ancienne ; un foyer tuberculeux dans le rein existe souvent très longtemps limité à une pyramide ou à un calyx, d'où les bacilles descendent continuellement jusqu'à la vessie, qui par des causes occasionnelles particulières est envahie très vite, avec une grande intensité et sur une grande étendue.

Dans ce dernier cas, on a souvent expliqué les faits en supposant une infection primaire vésicale, qui par la voie ascendante aurait attaqué le bassinet et le rein. Personnellement je ne crois pas beaucoup à cette extension anatomique, dans les affections dont il s'agit. D'abord et principalement à cause de mes opinions sur la pathogénie de la tuberculose vésicale. Ensuite à cause de l'invraisemblance de ce mode d'extension ; car le continuel courant descendant de l'urine et les mouvements péristaltiques de l'uretère vers le bas paraissent rendre l'ascension des bacilles fort difficile, pour ne pas dire impossible, en tout cas, quand l'uretère est sain. Encore faut-il se rappeler que les conditions physiques, — rétention de l'urine dans la vessie — qui causent l'infection ascendante ordinaire, n'existent nullement dans le cas de la tuberculose vésicale, la vessie se contractant sans cesse énergiquement et chassant son contenu jusqu'à la dernière goutte. De plus, on aurait dû, de temps à autre, rencontrer, en cas de tuberculose vésicale manifeste, une affection des parties inférieures des uretères, les bassinets et les reins étant complètement sains. Mais je ne connais pas de tels cas.

Sans aucun doute, il est possible qu'une tuberculose de la vessie, d'origine génitale, existe longtemps sans que les reins soient attaqués; ce n'est que pendant les dernières phases de la maladie que ceux-ci sont envahis à leur tour; cet envahissement ne se produit cependant pas nécessairement par la voie ascendante. La tuberculose peut, dans ces conditions, être due au transfert par le système circulatoire des bacilles, venant des foyers tuberculeux de la prostate, des vésicules séminales, de la vessie; amenés par le sang, les bacilles tuberculeux se fixent donc dans les reins, et y produisent, sur la fin de la vie du malade, une destruction plus ou moins grande et souvent très rapide, à cause de l'état d'affaiblissement extrême de l'individu.

Nous avons ici la tuberculose sous une forme pyohémique ou métastatique.

On pourrait encore expliquer cette dernière apparition de la tuberculose rénale, en admettant une nouvelle infection du foyer pulmonaire, comme celle qui a été cause de la tuberculose des organes génitaux de la vessie; cette nouvelle éruption cause donc la tuberculose rénale de la même façon que dans la tuberculose rénale primaire, mentionnée plus haut.

Enfin, d'une manière générale, on peut encore s'appuyer, pour démontrer l'origine secondaire et cavitaire de la tuberculose vésicale, sur la manière analogue dont l'infection tuberculeuse se produit dans d'autres organes. Tandis que la tuberculose envahit presque toujours les organes parenchymateux par la voie circulatoire, c'est un fait bien connu que les grandes muqueuses, comme celles des voies respiratoires et du canal intestinal, s'infectent toujours par les surfaces.

En résumé mon avis est donc celui-ci : la tuberculose vésicale n'a jamais une origine primaire. Toujours secondaire elle apparaît le plus souvent à la suite d'une infection descendante des reins, ou plus rarement à la suite d'une invasion bacillaire ascendante, venant des organes génitaux. Cette dernière forme est beaucoup plus fréquente chez l'homme que chez la femme. Jamais la tuberculose vésicale n'atteint les reins par une propagation ascendante par les uretères.

Je me suis arrêté longtemps, messieurs, à la pathologie et à la pathogénie de la tuberculose vésicale. Cependant, il importe certes d'avoir des idées claires et précises sur l'origine de cette affection, afin de pouvoir établir des indications ou contre-indications pour nos interventions chirurgicales; c'est la seule manière d'obtenir de bons résultats.

Dès lors, il nous sera facile de nous prononcer sur la question de la valeur des interventions chirurgicales dans la tuberculose vésicale; en nous appuyant sur ce qui précède, nous pouvons d'abord répondre ceci : aucune intervention opératoire, aucun traitement de la tuberculose de le vessie ayant un but curatif, ne doivent être entrepris avant que la cause de l'affection vésicale secondaire soit écartée complètement, ou que l'action de cette cause sur la vessie soit totalement supprimée. Au cas où ces opérations préliminaires n'ont pas eu lieu, ou ne peuvent pas avoir lieu, toute intervention ayant un but curatif est sans valeur, inutile, un coup d'épée dans l'eau, et par conséquent à rejeter.

Le diagnostic est donc le point capital, décisif dans nos interventions pour chaque cas donné de la tuberculose vésicale. L'infection, d'où est-elle venue? D'en haut ou d'en bas?

Dans le premier cas, et si la localisation limitée de l'affection vésicale et l'état général du malade font juger possible la guérison, le chirurgien doit donc, par une néphrectomie et une urétérectomie — si l'autre rein est sain — de prime abord éloigner la cause persistante de l'infection de la vessie.

Un des deux cas suivants peut alors se présenter :

Premièrement, l'affection vésicale peut être si superficielle, si peu étendue et l'état général du malade si peu compromis, que la tuberculose vésicale guérit spontanément sans aucune intervention chirurgicale, dès que l'infection continuelle qui en fut la cause n'existe plus. J'ai moi-même observé deux tels cas, sur deux femmes : avant la néphrectomie, la cystoscopie avait montré chez elles, d'une manière incontestable, des altérations tuberculeuses superficielles, mais évidentes, dans la vessie; ces altérations ont peu à peu, pendant de longs mois, disparu complètement sans aucun traitement; on trouve maintenant sur la muqueuse des cicatrices blanchâtres, rétractées en forme d'étoile ou d'éventail, là ou la muqueuse était autrefois rouge, enflée, veloutée, ulcérée par endroits, donnant l'image complète d'une affection tuberculeuse en plein développement. J'ajoute que j'ai observé ces deux cas à l'état pur: aucune des malades n'a été sondée avant mon examen, au moment duquel je n'ai trouvé aucune association microbienne étrangère à la tuberculose.

Bien entendu, il est trop tôt, les cas ne remontant qu'à un et deux ans, pour se prononcer au point de vue de la guérison définitive ; cependant les bacilles ont diminué de nombre peu à peu, jusqu'à leur disparition complète, ce qui parle en faveur de la possibilité de cette guérison.

Quelque paradoxal que paraisse le fait, le traitement de cette forme de la tuberculose vésicale est la néphrectomie : on ne touche pour ainsi dire pas à la vessie dont l'affection guérit spontanément, par la réaction naturelle de l'organisme, secondée par un des régimes hygiéniques ordinaires.

Mais il n'en est pas toujours ainsi : malgré la néphrectomie il se peut que la tuberculose vésicale persiste, parce que l'extension en profondeur et l'intensité de l'infection sont trop grandes pour que le processus puisse s'arrêter et guérir spontanément. L'intervention chirurgicale devient nécessaire. Mais, après la néphrectomie, elle peut se faire sur une affection localisée et isolée, dans les mêmes conditions où elle est pratiquée dans les cas de tuberculose des articulations, des os, des glandes et d'ailleurs.

La seule intervention chirurgicale qu'on puisse adopter est, bien entendu, la taille hypogastrique, la haute voie, quel que soit le sexe du malade. Je passe complètement tout ce qui appartient à la technique opératoire, déjà indiquée, dans tous ses détails, par M. le professeur Guyon, dont la méthode est universellement suivie par tous les chirurgiens.

La source de l'infection une fois écartée par la néphrectomie, les altérations pathologiques de la vessie enlevées par le bistouri et les ciseaux, autant que l'œil peut en juger, la destruction des parties malades assurée autant que possible par le thermo-cautère, la guérison de cette forme grave de la tuberculose peut avoir lieu ici encore. J'ai moi-même tout nouvellement traité, d'après cette méthode, une malade ayant une tuberculose rénale et vésicale très avancée. Le cas est trop récent pour qu'on puisse en prévoir les résultats, mais jusqu'à présent tout semble indiquer qu'il y a possibilité de guérison.

Les choses sont beaucoup plus graves quand la tuberculose de la vessie est produite par une tuberculose ascendante des organes génitaux. Si la vessie est envahie dans ces conditions, la malade est en réalité si avancée, la destruction du col de la vessie et de son entourage si étendue, que la guérison complète par l'intervention chirurgicale est des plus improbables. Dans toutes les circonstances, cette intervention est alors de la plus haute gravité ; car il faut non seulement extirper les foyers tuberculeux dans les organes génitaux proprement dits, mais encore fendre et curetter la prostate, les abcès et les tissus environnants ; à cela s'ajoute encore l'intervention directe sur la muqueuse de la vessie, cette intervention se faisant dans la plupart dés cas par la taille hypogastrique. Très souvent il est nécessaire de répéter ces opérations ; la partie prostatique de l'urètre en est considérablement affectée et des fistules urinaires très gênantes peuvent en résulter ; bref, sous peine de faire une chirurgie brouillonne, il faut certainement s'avancer aussi peu que possible sur un si mauvais terrain. Souvent même on trouve chez ces malades des affections tuberculeuses aiguës dans les poumons, qui enlèvent tout espoir de guérison.

Les résultats de tout traitement de cette forme de la tuberculose vésicale sont, d'après mes expériences personnelles et autant que je le puis voir d'après les expériences des autres chirurgiens, des moins encourageants.

Nos interventions chirurgicales dans cette affection consisteront donc, aussitôt que possible, dès que le moindre symptôme de l'attaque de la vessie se produit, avant même, à pratiquer les opérations sur les organes génitaux, qui empêcheront le processus tuberculeux d'arriver à la vessie même. L'opération vraiment curative dans ces cas est celle qui précède l'envahissement de la vessie ; mais pour tout ce qui est de ce traitement et de sa valeur, il appartient à M. le D\u1d63 Hogge de nous en parler.

Vous voyez, messieurs, que je m'exprime d'une façon très peu enthousiaste pour ce qui concerne la possibilité d'obtenir la guérison complète et définitive de la tuberculose vésicale. Jusqu'à présent, les résultats de nos interventions sont certes assez médiocres. Nous pouvons sans doute espérer en obtenir de meilleurs à l'avenir si, en nous appuyant sur ce que nous savons sur l'origine et la nature de l'affection, nous parvenions à instituer une thérapeutique plus rationnelle, qui consisterait essentiellement à éloigner aussitôt que possible la cause même du mal.

Reste à indiquer en deux mots le traitement palliatif et les résultats qu'on en peut obtenir. Le but que nous poursuivons, c'est le soulagement des deux graves symptômes : la pollakiurie et la douleur, dont souffrent jour et nuit les malheureux tuberculeux urinaires. Nous savons tous que nous réussirons souvent à soulager ces symptômes par le simple drainage de la vessie ou par son curettage, celui-ci étant pratiqué soit par la haute voie, soit par l'urètre chez la femme ou par la taille périnéale chez l'homme. Quelquefois la néphrotomie ou la prostatomie sont indiquées comme soulagement des symptômes vésicaux d'ordre réflexe. Il est vrai qu'il faut souvent répéter plusieurs de ces interventions. Le résultat est plus ou moins bon, l'effet dure plus ou moins longtemps, mais souvent nous arrivons cependant à soulager nos malades d'une certaine partie de leurs souffrances.

Le traitement local, par tous les différents remèdes bien connus, ne doit, bien entendu, pas être oublié. Cependant, il faut remarquer que parmi ces remèdes il n'en est aucun qui soit particulièrement efficace et aucun qui soit plus spécifique que tout autre. Le principal c'est que le traitement local soit exécuté avec la plus grande douceur et que le remède employé soit aussi peu irritant que possible. Le meilleur de ces traitements est peut-être celui qui consiste en de simples lavages à l'eau boriquée dans le but de vider la vessie au cas où il y a quelque rétention d'urine purulente. Tout le monde sait que tout traitement au nitrate d'argent n'est pas supporté.

Je finis en rappelant que le traitement général, par tous les moyens, est, bien entendu, tout à fait nécessaire pendant toute la durée de la maladie pour toutes ces formes graves de la tuberculose.

## CONCLUSIONS

1º Les résultats obtenus jusqu'à présent par nos interventions chirurgicales sont, au point de vue de la guérison complète, assez mauvais ;

2º La tuberculose vésicale chronique est toujours secondaire, d'origine ou rénale ou génitale ;

3º La tuberculose miliaire de la vessie ne sera pas l'objet d'interventions chirurgicales ;

4º L'éloignement de la source continuelle de l'infection de la vessie est de la plus haute importance, de la plus grande nécessité dans le traitement de la tuberculose vésicale ;

5º Après l'extirpation du rein tuberculeux, la tuberculose vésicale secondaire d'origine rénale peut guérir spontanément ou être guérie par une intervention chirurgicale faite par une cystotomie suspubienne ;

6º La tuberculose vésicale secondaire d'origine génitale, une fois manifeste, est d'un pronostic beaucoup plus grave. Dans la plupart des cas, elle est inguérissable. Dès les premiers symptômes, elle doit être traitée par des opérations aussi étendues, aussi radicales que possible sur les organes génitaux ;

7° Le traitement palliatif multiple, varié et continu, secondé par un traitement général suivi, soulage souvent les principaux symptômes, la pollakiurie et la douleur.

---

## VALEUR DES INTERVENTIONS CHIRURGICALES DANS LA TUBERCULOSE URÉTRO-GÉNITALE

### *RAPPORT*

par le docteur **ALBERT HOGGE**,
ancien assistant à l'Université de Liège.

Messieurs,

La seconde question mise à l'ordre du jour des Congrès ne vise que les tuberculoses urinaires. A m'en tenir strictement aux termes du problème à la mise au point duquel je suis pour ma part très flatté de collaborer, je n'aurais pas besoin de vous parler des tuberculoses génitales.

Mais vous savez tous, messieurs, et des voix plus autorisées que la mienne vous le rappelleront au cours de cas discussions, que la phymatose urinaire succède, dans la grande majorité des cas, chez l'homme du moins, à la tuberculose génitale.

Les deux appareils urinaire et génital réunis anatomiquement au confluent urétro-prostatique sont, pour la tuberculose plus peut-être que pour les autres affections auxquelles ces appareils sont exposés, cliniquement inséparables. La pathologie de l'urètre postérieur, le seul en cause, peut-on dire, quand il s'agit de tuberculose urétrale, est si intimement liée à celle des voies génitales en général et de la prostate en particulier, qu'il m'a paru nécessaire d'étendre notre étude aux indications opératoires ressortissant à la tuberculose de la prostate, des vésicules séminales, du canal déférent, de l'épididyme et du testicule.

En ce qui concerne la tuberculose de la prostate et des vésicules, la chirurgie, dont elle est justiciable aux yeux de quelques-uns, est toute neuve encore, il est vrai, mais les résultats en sont extrêmement intéressants et, disons-le immédiatement, fort encourageants.

Le *traitement chirurgical non sanglant de l'urétrite postérieure* tuberculeuse se confond avec celui de la cystite de même nature qui, généralement, coexiste. Les antiseptiques qui, en applications locales, ont donné les meilleurs résultats sont : le sublimé (*Guyon, Luys, B n-zet, Condé*, etc.), au taux de 1/10 000e à 1/5 000e en instillations (20 à 100 gouttes, vessie vide, tous les jours ou tous les deux jours, long-temps continuées); l'iodoforme et le gaïacol (*Frey, Chaudelux, Collin, Pousson, Bazy, Reniac, Petit, Talayrach, Loquin*, etc.) au titre moyen de 5 pour 100 dans la glycérine, l'éther, l'huile d'olives ou de vaseline stérilisée, en petits lavages de 20 à 50 c.c. ou en instillations (2 pour 100); le carbonate de gaïacol 1 pour 100 (*Collin*), l'acide picrique (*Desnos et Guillon*) à la dose de 1/2 à 1 pour 100 en instilla-tions; l'ichtyol (1 à 5 pour 100) en instillations (*Noguès, Goldberg*).

D'autres topiques ont été vantés, insuffisamment éprouvés ou aban-donnés : le baume du Pérou et l'europhène (*Marwedel*), l'eau naphto-lée, l'eau de goudron, l'eau créosotée, l'acide borique, l'acide lactique (5 pour 100) (*Witzach*), le chlorure de zinc (1 à 5 pour 100), le sulfate de cuivre (2 à 4 pour 100), le formol (en lavages au 1/500e) (*Lamarque*), l'air stérilisée (*Ramon*) Le nitrate d'argent semble devoir être défini-tivement proscrit.

Cette médication topique, quand elle est indiquée et qu'elle agit favorablement, modifie dans l'ordre suivant les symptômes cardinaux de la tuberculose urétro-vésicale : 1° la fréquence et les douleurs des mictions; 2° l'hématurie; 3° la pyurie. Les petits lavages ou les instillations doivent être pratiqués d'une façon rigoureusement asep-tique pour parer aux dangers des infections mixtes ou secondaires. Au surplus, ces moyens doivent éventuellement céder le pas aux indi-cations visant l'état général (cure d'air, station thermale, etc.), le traitement médical et hygiénique, conservant ici, comme dans toutes les tuberculoses, son droit de priorité. L'urètre antérieur n'étant qu'exceptionnellement le siège de tubercules, les instillations doi-vent être faites immédiatement derrière le sphincter membraneux.

Le meilleur traitement des *lésions tuberculeuses de l'urètre anté-rieur*, si l'on avait de bonnes raisons de les soupçonner[1], consisterait à les modifier ou à les détruire à l'aide de l'endoscope[2]. Les lésions

1. Comme dans le cas de Langhans où il s'agissait d'une excroissance tuber-culeuse siégeant à quelques centimètres du méat.
2. On donne, dans beaucoup d'auteurs, comme signe prémonitoire de la tuber-culose uro-génitale un écoulement urétral; mais cet écoulement, surtout en dehors des cas où il y a des antécédents blennorragiques, n'implique pas l'urétrite : écoulement n'est pas synonyme d'urétrite, d'urétrite antérieure particulièrement. Les constatations anatomo-pathologiques d'urétrite tubercu-leuse antérieure (Ricord, Vetleesen, Langhans, Soloweitschnick, Guyon, Guel-liot, van Brown, Schuchardt, Englisch, Kraske, Ahrens, Rendu, Garin, Chenet, Nickaus, Marwedel, Michaud, Delfan, Steinthal, Dufour, etc.) se rapportaient

tuberculeuses de l'urètre pouvant amener des rétrécissements (*Ahrens*), on pourrait être justifié à pratiquer dans ces cas, avec beaucoup de prudence, la dilatation progressive.

La curette et le thermo feront les frais du *traitement chirurgical sanglant* de l'urétrite au cours d'une taille périnéale dirigée contre une cystite tuberculeuse chez l'homme (*Thompson, Guyon, Hartmann, Legueu, Greiwer*). Chez la femme, les instruments seront conduits par la voie urétrale préalablement dilatée. « Cette dilatation de l'urètre et du col vésical, dit *Legueu*, n'est plus jamais pratiquée aujourd'hui que pour permettre le curettage ». On pourrait aussi utiliser la colpocystotomie (*Emmet, Hartmann, Brun*) pour racler la partie de l'urètre voisine du col vésical. Chez l'homme il pourrait être enfin procédé à l'extirpation du segment prostatique de l'urètre par le fait d'une prostatectomie totale avec suture urétro-vésicale, comme l'a fait Doyen[1].

Les *ulcérations tuberculeuses de la verge* (fourreau, gland, prépuce[2]) sont justiciables de la cautérisation ou mieux de l'excision[3].

*La périurétrite et la cowpérite* (souvent connexes) doivent être traitées par l'incision, l'excision, le curettage, le drainage quand il se produit une fonte purulente de l'infiltration ou une fistule (*Englisch, Tapret, Coulliard, Feleki*).

Les tubercules crus de la *prostate*[4], alors même que la tuberculose

toutes à des urétrites antérieures secondaires à des tuberculoses de l'urètre postérieur, de la vessie, du rein, de la prostate, des glandes de Cowper, des vésicules séminales, etc., et avaient été généralement occasionnées par des lésions blennorragiques antérieures ou des traumatismes (cathétérismes). Il n'existe donc pas jusqu'ici d'observation de tuberculose primitive de l'urètre antérieur. La constatation de bacilles de Koch au sein de la sécrétion uréthrale (Tuffier et Girode, Babès et Cornil, Marwedel, Schuchardt) n'implique pas davantage l'urétrite, ces bacilles pouvant provenir d'un point quelconque des appareils urinaire ou génital. Bien plus, Jani aurait vu des bacilles de Koch dans le liquide prostatique, chez des phtisiques, sans tuberculose génitale. D'après Krziwicki, l'urètre s'entreprendrait dans 1 0/0 des cas de tuberc. uro-génitale et Pavel a réuni 7 cas de tuberc. urétrale sur 380 cas de tuberc. uro-génitale.

Rare chez l'homme, la tuberculose urétrale serait exceptionnelle chez la femme, puisque Ahrens n'a pu en réunir que 4 cas (ceux de Krziwicki, de Hermann, de Winkel et de Warfoinge. Pour Kœnig pourtant, elle serait assez fréquente chez les petites filles.

1. Opération proposée par Proust et Gosset contre l'hypertrophie de la prostate et pratiquée notamment par Leisrinck, Stein et Verhoogen pour tumeur maligne de la prostate.

2. Kraske, Gaston, Malecot, Michaud, Wickam, etc., ont décrit de ces lésions, et Debrowitz, Eve, Lehmann, Elsenberg, Hofmokl en ont observé après la circoncision rituelle.

3. Le même traitement est à appliquer aux ulcérations tuberculeuses de la peau des bourses, que ces ulcérations soient secondaires, ce qui est la règle, ou qu'elles soient primitives, ainsi que Rochette et Reclus en ont donné des exemples.

4. Certains auteurs indiquent la prostate comme point de départ de la tuber-

prostatique semblerait primitive et isolée, comme dans les cas de *Béraud, Claude, Broca, Robin, Vidal, Thompson, Kapsammer, Simmonds, Kriziwicki, Konitzer, Orth, Marwedel*, ne sont pas justiciables pour la grande majorité des chirurgiens d'une opération, laquelle serait d'ailleurs le plus souvent refusée par les intéressés. La médication topique par l'urètre ne doit être tentée que lorsque les foyers prostatiques communiquent avec le canal uro-génital (dans la forme urétro-cystique), encore n'en faut-il pas attendre de grands succès. Il en est de même, ou à peu près, au point de vue curatif, des antiseptiques, résolutifs ou calmants introduits par la voie rectale sous forme de lavements ou de suppositoires (créosote, iode, iodoforme, iodure, ichtyol, morphine, belladone, cocaïne, etc.). Le massage et l'électro-massage sont contre-indiqués dans la tuberculose prostatique.

*Les injections interstitielles*, en plein parenchyme prostatique, de liqueur de Villate, d'éther, de glycérine ou de gomme iodoformée (*Marwedel, Dittel, Berkeley-Hill, Horteloup*), de chlorure de zinc (méthode sclérogène de *Lannelongue*), par les voies vésicale (*Desnos*), rectale (*Hammonic*), périnéale (*Horteloup, Ozenne, Wickham*) n'ont donné que des résultats nuls ou peu marqués. Même en mettant la prostate à nu par l'incision périnéale (*H. Delagenière*) pour pratiquer ces injections, c'est un procédé aveugle, incertain.

*L'intervention sanglante* (incision, curettage, cautérisation au thermo ou au chlorure de zinc, éradication des nodules tuberculeux ou prostatectomies) a donné, par contre, de bons résultats, quelquefois durables, entre les mains de *Guyon, Bouilly, Dittel, Le Dentu, Albarran, Zuckerkandel, Marwedel, Meyer et Hanel, Gaudier, Conitzer, Baudet, Doyen, Audry*[1]. Dans tous ces cas, l'intervention pratiquée toujours par la voie périnéale[2] n'a pas été une opération de nécessité,

culose génitale ou génito-urinaire. Mais cette tuberculose isolée de la prostate, très rare d'ailleurs, pour peu qu'elle ne siège pas tout près de l'urètre, pour peu qu'elle soit circonférencielle et non péri-urétrale, a les plus grandes chances de passer inaperçue, puisque dans bien des cas elle évolue sans symptômes marqués. (Pour Marwedel dans 1/3 des cas.) D'autre part, *Thompson, Le Dentu, Dittel, Von Frisch, Bryson, Keyes, Fuller, Carrié* ont signalé des guérisons spontanées de prostate tuberculeuse par transformation fibreuse et Broca a même rapporté un cas de calcification de la prostate.

1. Voir le tableau de ces opérations, annexé à ce Mémoire.

2. La voie périnéale est toute indiquée et aujourd'hui très généralement suivie dans toutes les opérations dirigées contre les affections chirurgicales de la prostate (abcès, tumeurs, calculs, tuberculose, hypertrophie, etc.). De nombreux et bons travaux semblent avoir définitivement établi les avantages de cette voie d'accès vers les organes génitaux périnéaux profonds et vers la vessie. Dittel, et plus récemment Zuckerkandel, Roux, Guelliot, H. Delagenière, Proust, Gosset, Baudet, etc., en ont bien étudié la technique opératoire et fixé les différents temps. Dans les opérations sur la prostate, il est parfois utile d'ouvrir l'urètre quitte à le suturer après, de réséquer l'urètre (prostatectomie totale avec suture

comme s'il s'était agi d'ouvrir un abcès chaud prostatique ou périprostatique[1] dont la rupture vers le périnée, l'urètre, le rectum, aurait
été imminente, mais bien une opération décidée, systématique, dirigée contre un abcès froid, un foyer caséeux, une fistule, etc.

Comme dans les cas de fonte caséeuse de la prostate, *les vésicules
séminales*, *les déférents* et même les testicules et les épididymes parti-
cipent presque toujours au processus de tuberculisation, il fallait
s'attendre à ce que les chirurgiens conçussent des exérèses plus
larges et attaquassent les organes qu'ils savaient malades au même
titre que la prostate. C'est ainsi que, depuis 1889, *Ullmann, Villeneuve, Platon, Roux, Sick, Weir, Schede, Guelliot, Routier, Baudet et
Keudirzy, Doyen, Bolton, Moulin*, extirpèrent l'une ou les deux vésicules, l'un ou les deux déférents après la castration, uni ou bilatérale.
*Weir, Schede* et *Baudet* combinèrent à ces épididymo-déférento-sper-
matocystectomies des résections partielles (et totale pour *Doyen*), de
la prostate ; récemment *Baudet* (*Journal de médecine de Bordeaux,*
18 février 1900) a dit avoir pratiqué et conseillait de pratiquer toujours
non seulement l'ablation de la vésicule malade, mais aussi celle de la
vésicule paraissant saine avec l'extrémité correspondante du canal
déférent. Dans un travail[2] inspiré par Roux (de Lausanne) et paru
l'année dernière, se trouvent réunies vingt observations de spermatocystectomie combinées à des opérations sur le testicule, le
déférent, l'épididyme, la prostate (parfois). Parmi ces vingt cas[3],
on trouve six spermatocystectomies doubles et quatorze unilatérales. La technique opératoire varie à peu près avec chacun de ces
chirurgiens, les uns ne recourant pour l'excision du déférent et de
la vésicule qu'à la seule voie inguino-scrotale (*Villeneuve et Platon*[4]), les autres décomposant leur opération en deux temps : 1° recherche, libération, excision d'une partie ou de la totalité du déférent et de la vésicule par la voie inguinale ; 2° mise à nu et excision
d'une ou des deux vésicules et de ce qui reste du ou des déférents

urétro-vésicale), d'ouvrir la vessie par la voie hypogastrique, de prolonger l'incision périnéale d'un côté ou des deux côtés de l'anus, jusqu'au coccyx, jusqu'au
sacrum, de réséquer le coccyx et le sacrum. Doyen a fendu longitudinalement
la paroi rectale antérieure pour atteindre plus aisément la prostate et les vésicules.

1. Comme le firent *Reclus, Segond, Dittel, Bruns,* etc.

2. Princesse GUEDROYTS DE BELOSÉROFF. Excision de la vésicule séminale et du
canal déférent en totalité en cas de castration pour tuberculose primaire. *Revue
médicale de la Suisse Romande,* mars et avril 1899.

3. Dont 7 de Roux, 1 de Uhlmann, 1 de Villeneuve, 1 de Platon, 1 de Sick,
1 de Weir, 5 de Schede, 2 de Guilliot, 1 de Routier.

4. Incision unique que préconise aussi Poirier (*Bulletin de la Soc. de Chirurgie,*
mai 1899) qui toutefois n'a fait cette opération que sur le cadavre.

par la voie périnéale (prérectale), périnéo-circum-anale, périnéo-para-sacrée ou périnéo-sacrée.

Depuis le travail de Mme de Beloseroff ou en dehors des cas qui y sont relatés, existent les deux observations de Baudet, les deux observations de Doyen, celles de Bolton, de Moulin, de Chavanaz et une observation ultérieure de Roux[1]. Nous-même avons récemment pratiqué avec succès le raclage d'une vésicule séminale. En tout il existe donc une trentaine d'observations connues relatives à des opérations sur les vésicules séminales tuberculeuses.

Les résultats immédiats de toutes ces opérations furent tous bons; il n'y a eu aucun décès opératoire. Certains malades furent retrouvés en bon état longtemps après l'intervention. Il en fut ainsi de trois opérés de Roux : obs. II, 8 ans après, obs. V, 6 ans après, obs. XIV, 4 ans après, d'un opéré de Guilliot, obs. XVI, 8 ans après, des deux cas de Baudet (2 ans).

Trois malades succombèrent à la phtisie après un temps plus ou moins long (obs. de Ullmann, Guelliot), d'autres virent des récidives se produire du côté des voies génitales non opérées. Et c'est dans le but de prévenir ces récidives que Baudet a conseillé non seulement l'ablation du déférent et de la vésicule malades, mais aussi celle de la vésicule saine ou paraissant telle et de l'extrémité du déférent correspondant.

Malheureusement beaucoup d'observations sont récentes et pour quelques autres, anciennes déjà, les résultats éloignés sont inconnus.

En général, après les opérations sur la prostate et les vésicules, on observe des fistules périnéales (8 fois définitives et 4 fois passagères sur 21 cas). Il est également à remarquer que dans la plupart des cas publiés on parle peu de l'influence de l'intervention sur l'évolution ultérieure de la tuberculose urinaire là où l'affection n'était pas purement génitale, et que l'on s'est peu préoccupé de l'état de la prostate. A part *Schede*, *Weir*, *Baudet* qui combinèrent à la déférento-vésiculectomie des résections partielles ou des grattages de la prostate, on ne trouve rien à ce sujet dans les autres observations. Cette façon de faire compliquerait cependant peu l'acte opératoire. *Doyen*, dans deux cas, a enlevé la prostate en même temps que les vésicules.

La spermatocystectomie étant le complément d'une opération sur la glande génitale et son conduit excréteur, ce n'est pas d'après les préceptes et les tendances actuels de la chirurgie épididymo-testiculaire

1. Lettre personnelle due à l'obligeance du professeur Roux.

à la castration qu'il faudrait recourir en pareil cas, mais à l'une ou à l'autre des opérations économiques proposées et pratiquées surtout dans le cours de ces vingt dernières années.

Il résulte en effet de nombreux travaux[1], de discussions retentissantes[2] et de la pratique d'un grand nombre de chirurgiens que, dans *la tuberculose épididymo-testiculaire*, la glande génitale doit le plus possible être conservée, au moins en partie, et que la castration totale ne doit rester que comme méthode d'exception. De l'avis du plus grand nombre, pour la tuberculose du testicule et de ses voies d'excrétion, la thérapeutique de choix est donc la méthode conservatrice sanglante et cette méthode consiste en résections typiques et atypiques de l'épididyme (à l'aide du cautère, de la curette tranchante ou des ciseaux) (Kocher) et du déférent. *Malgaigne, Bardenheuer, Villeneuve, Tuffier, Humbert, Lejars, Quenu, Longuet, Pasteau, Angelesco, Pujol, Demoulin, Tillaux, Duplay, Legueu, Delbet, Dimitresco*, etc., furent les chirurgiens qui imaginèrent ou vulgarisèrent les funiculo-épididymectomies partielles ou totales. A ces procédés on a combiné parfois la résection de la vaginale, l'orchidotomie exploratrice (*Poncet, Villard et Curtillet, X. Delore, Lejars, André, Delbet*) et l'orchidectomie particlle.

Sans doute, cette méthode conservatrice n'échappe pas à certains reproches qu'elle partage, du reste, le plus souvent, avec la castration; elle a ses détracteurs et aussi ses contre-indications; mais si toutes les formes de tuberculose épididymo-testiculaire n'en sont pas justiciables, elles n'excluent pas, au moins à titre d'essai, certains modes de traitement qui à juste titre conservent leurs partisans ; tels sont parmi ces procédés l'emploi des caustiques, la cautérisation ignée (*Velpeau, Verneuil, Routier, Reynier, Bazy, Isch-Wall*), l'injection intra-nodulaire de naphtol camphré (*Michaud*), d'éther iodoformé, de chlorure de zinc; les injections périnodulaires de chlorure de zinc (*Lannelongue, Coudray, Ozenne, Desnos, Bourlier, Vessaux*); l'injection sous-cutanée au niveau de la tumeur ou dans l'abcès même d'une émulsion glycérinée d'euphorbe (*Penières-Toulouse*); le raclage suivi d'attouchement au chlorure de zinc (*Kocher, Volkmann, Quénu*), d'ébouillantement et de marsupialisation des poches caverneuses (*Quénu*), de résection de la membrane tuberculogène (*Duplay*), ces derniers moyens s'appliquant surtout aux abcès.

Enfin tout récemment *Mauclaire* a préconisé, pour traiter la tuber-

---

1. Lire entre autres les travaux de Dimitresco, de Longuet, de Pedebidou, etc.
2. Lire les *Bulletins de la Société de Chirurgie*, 1899.

culose épididymo-testiculaire, la ligature et la section des éléments
du cordon. Les faits qu'il rapporte, si encourageants qu'ils soient,
sont trop peu nombreux et surtout trop neufs encore pour être con-
cluants[1].

En somme, que l'on envisage la tuberculose de la prostate, de l'épididyme, du déférent, du testicule ou des vésicules, l'indication opératoire est formelle et admise par tous quand il s'agit d'abcès de ces
organes, que ces abcès soient en voie de formation, encore fermés, ou
qu'ils aient donné lieu par leur rupture spontanée à des fistules s'ouvrant à l'extérieur ou établissant une communication anormale entre
deux organes (fistule urétro-rectale par exemple). Les procédés opératoires peuvent varier selon les préférences de l'un ou de l'autre
chirurgien, selon aussi l'étendue des lésions et l'état des voies urinaires, mais dans ces cas (abcès, foyers caséo-purulents, fistules), à
de rares exceptions près relevant, par exemple, d'un état général très
grave, il faut opérer parce que, dans ces conditions, l'intervention
sanglante a sûrement une valeur curative plus grande et fait courir
moins de risques au malade que l'expectation armée et le traitement
purement médical.

Dans l'état actuel de nos connaissances relatives à la tuberculose
uro-génitale en particulier et à la tuberculose en général, ne faut-il
opérer que ces cas, comme le voulait Marwedel pour la tuberculose
de la prostate?

Les hésitations légitimes et la dissidence des chirurgiens commencent avec les autres formes ou, si l'on veut, avec les autres stades
de la tuberculisation de ces organes. Pour quelques-uns, l'on doit ou
du moins l'on peut intervenir dans les phases initiales de la maladie,
alors qu'on se trouve en présence de formes froides mono ou pauci-
nodulaires, ou de formes massives, froides ou ramollies (*Quénu, Longuet, Roux, Albarran*, etc.), tandis que, à l'heure actuelle, beaucoup
de chirurgiens, dans ces conditions, se tiennent dans l'expectation.

Où surtout se poursuivent les divergences de vue, l'opération étant
décidée, c'est quand se pose la question de savoir l'extension qu'il
faudra donner à l'acte opératoire et les organes qu'il faudra racler,
brûler ou enlever. Faudra-t-il se limiter à une castration uni ou bilatérale, ou à une déférento-épididymectomie, alors qu'on saura ma-

---

1. Il est à peine besoin d'ajouter que les applications médicamenteuses sur
les bourses (pommades, cuirasse d'emplâtre, enveloppements humides) et le port
du suspensoir ne peuvent être que des adjuvants du traitement, dénués de vertu
curative à proprement parler.

Tableau des opérations pratiquées pour tuberculose de la prostate.

| NUMÉROS | CHIRURGIENS | LÉSIONS | INTERVENTION | RÉSULTAT |
|---|---|---|---|---|
| 1 | F. Guyon (1885). *Thèse de Guillain*, 1 cas. | Abcès de la prostate, cystite, épididymite. | Incision, curettage (p. v. périnéale). | Amélioration notable, fistule périnéale persiste, plus d'hématurie. |
| 2 | Bouilly (1885). *Soc. de chir.*, 29 juill. *Ann. mal. gén. ur.*, 1885, p. 636, 1 cas. | Abcès de la prostate, avec fistule (loge prostat. réduite à un cloaque caséo-purulent ; castration unilatérale précédemment. | Incision, curettage (par voie périnéale). | Presque mourart lors de l'opération, a repris ses forces et son travail. |
| 3 | Dittel (1889). *Wien. klin. Woschenschr.*, p. 438, 1 cas. | Prostate grosse, élastique, sensible, pas d'abcès, pas de fistule. | Incision, curettage (par v. périnéale). | Guérison complète en 3 semaines. |
| 4 | Le Dentu (1889). *Congrès français de chirurgie, Semaine médicale*, p. 387, 1 cas (30 ans). | Abcès du lobe gauche de la prostate. précédemment incisé ; une fistule existait. | Curettage par la fistule périnéale agrandie. | Guérison (maintenue 1 an après). |
| 5 | Albarran (1891). *Thèse de Zinke*), 1 cas. | Cystite, fistule périnéale, vésiculite, épididymite double, léger rétrécissement. | Urétrotomie interne, incision, curettage par v. périnéale. | Guérison (sans fistule) maintenue 4 ans après. |
| 6 | Zuckerkandel (1891). *Wien. klin. Woch.*, p. 804, 1 cas. | Orchi-épididymite (castration), abcès central de la prostate. | Incision, curettage par v. périnéale. | Résultat général bon, fistule urétro-périnéale persiste. |
| 7 | Marwedel (1892). *Beiträge z klin. chir.* IX Bd, 1er cas. | Épididymite double, cystite, phtisie, nécrose de la prostate. | Prostatectomie par voie périnéo-urétrale. sonde à demeure, tamponnement. | Amélior. quant aux douleurs et la fréquence des mictions, cessation des hématuries. Mort 4 mois après. |
| 8 | Marwedel, *Id.*, 2e cas. | Cystite, spermato-cystite, abcès de la prostate. | Incision par voie rectale (au galvano-cautère). | Fistule prostato-rectale par laquelle se faisaient les éjaculations. |
| 9 | Marwedel, *Id.*, 3e cas. | Épididymite double suppurée, prostatite supp., fistule urétro-rectale. | Plusieurs opérations réglées par fistules. | Guérison relative après de longs traitements (3 ans). |
| 10 | Marwedel, *Id.*, 4e cas. | Épididymite fistuleuse et fistule urétro-périnéale, cystite. | Excision des trajets fistuleux, raclage de la prostate. | Amélioration de la cystite et de l'état général. |

## Tableau des opérations pratiquées pour tuberculose de la prostate.

(*Suite.*)

| NUMÉROS | CHIRURGIENS | LÉSIONS | INTERVENTION | RÉSULTAT |
|---|---|---|---|---|
| 11 | Meyer et Hanel (1893), *Nitze. Oberlander's Centralbl.*, p. 424. | Cystite, prostatite, etc. (pas de fistule, pas d'abcés. | Raclage de la prostate par voie hypogastrique (vésicale) et périnéale combinées. | Amélioration passagère (2 semaines). Mort 2 mois et demi après. |
| 12 | Gaudier (1895). *Ann. des mal. des org. g.-ur.*, p. 125. 1 cas (22 ans). | Cystite, prostate élastique (petit abcès central): rien aux testicules ni aux cordons. | Incis., curettage par v. périnéale, tamponnement. | Guérison sans fistule en 15 jours, maintenue plusieurs mois après, cystite améliorée (instillation de sublimé). |
| 13 | Conitzer (1897). *Nitze. Oberlander's Centralbl.*, 1 cas. | Cystite, prostatite (rien aux autres org. g.-u.), rétention d'urine. | Prostatectomie partielle et curettage par voie périnéourétrale. | Persistance d'une fistule. Mort moins de deux ans après (tuberc. rénale). améliorat. passagère, disparition de la rétention d'urine, diminution des douleurs. |
| 14 | Albarran (1900). *Traité de chirurg.*, 1900, p. 578, 2 cas. | Grosse caverne prostatique; fortes hémorragies. | Curettage, prostatectomie partielle, cystotomie. | Guérison. |
| 15 | Audry (mars 1900). Travail de Sarda. *Archives provinc. de chirurg.* | Abcès prostatique et périprostatique, épididym. double. | Incision, évidement des poches, cautérisation, tamponnement, déférentectomie. | Guérison, relèvement de l'état général, maintenue trois mois après. |
| 16 | Baudet (1899). *Gazette hebdomad.*, 6 avril, 1 cas, 55 ans. | Doute entre hypertrophie ou tuberculose, rétention d'urine. | Prostatectomie par morcellement, sans ouvrir l'urètre et sans sonde à demeure. | Rétablissement de la fonction vésicale : relèvement de l'état général. |
| 17 | Doyen (1899). *Association française de chir.*, p. 588, 1 cas, 20 ans. | Castrat. précéd. d'un côté, fistule urétro-rectale, prostatite, vésiculité déférentite tuberculeuse. | Prostatectomie par voie périnéo-urétrale, incision do l'urètre et du rectum qui furent suturés après. | « Le malade reprit au bout de quelques mois sa vigueur d'autrefois. » |
| 18 | Doyen. *Id.*, 1 cas, 33 ans. | Tuberculose de la prostate et des vésicules, rien aux testicules ni aux déférents. | *Id.* Suture urétro-vésicale. | « Succès. » |
| 19 | Albarran (1900). *Traité de chir.*, p. 579. | Caverne tuberc. sans fistule. | Prostatectomie par morcel' (voie périnéale) tampon'. | Guérison sans fistule. |

Tableau des opérations pratiquées pour tuberculose des vésicules séminales.

| NUMÉROS DES OBSERVATIONS | NOMS DES AUTEURS | AGE | DATE DES OPÉRATIONS | EXAMEN CLINIQUE | NATURE DE L'OPÉRATION | COMPLICATIONS | RÉSULTATS IMMÉDIATS | DATE DE SORTIE | AFFECTIONS ANTÉRIEURES AU DÉBUT | RÉSULTATS ÉLOIGNÉS |
|---|---|---|---|---|---|---|---|---|---|---|
| 1 | D' Ullmann, Cent. für chir., 1890, p. 337. | 17 | 17 juin 1889 27 juill. 1889 | Tub. épididyme dr., vésicule séminale droite 2 fois plus grande que la normale. Canal déférent infiltré. | Castration latérale droite, extirpation vésicale séminale. | Forte hémorragie soir de l'opération. | Très bon état général, fistule. | » | » | Mort tub. pulm. peu de temps après. |
| 2 | P' Roux, Congrès chirurg., 1891. | 44 | 20 mars 1890 | Tub. test. et vés. sém. gauche. | Castration gauche et extirpat. vés. sém. gauche. | » | Guérison. | 20 avril 1890 | Janvier 1890, influenza. | Revu en août 99, guérison complète. |
| 3 | P' Roux. | 50 | 2 févr. 1891 | Tub. du test. épididyme, etc. | Castration droite et extirpation. | Inoculation tub. Koch, troubles digestifs. | Réunion per primam. Bon état général. | Mai 1891 | Fin sept. 1890. | Mort 4 ans après. |
| 4 | Villeneuve, Marseille, Extrait Congrès Marseille, septembre 1891. | » | 7 sept. 1891 | Fistule tub. aboutis. à la tête de l'épididyme. | Castration et spermatocystectomie par voie inguinale. | » | » | » | » | » |
| 5 | P' Roux. | 62 | 14 juill. 1892 | Tub. test. et vésic. sém. gauche. | Castration gauche, extirpat. vés. sém. gauche. | » | Bon état général. | 20 août 1892 | Juin 1892. | Bon état général en 1898. |
| 6 | P' Roux. | 19 | 22 mars 1898 | Tub. test. dr. Cordon chapelet. | Castration droite, extirpat. de la sém. | Vésicule sémin. crève au cours de l'opération. | Réunion per primam. | 2 mai 1895 | 1891, Test. droit grossi, 1895, fistule. | » |
| 7 | P' Schede, Soc. m. Hambourg, janvier 1895. | » | 1895 | Tub. test. gauche. | Castration latérale gauche, spermatocystectomie. Méthode sacrée. | Dénudé canal déférent. | Rétablissement prompt, fistule sacrée. | » | » | » |
| 8 | P' Schede, Soc. m. Hambourg, janvier 1898. | » | 1893 | Tub. de 2 vés. sém. | Extirpat. des 2 vés. sém. (von Dittel), résect. prostatique partielle. | » | Guérison fistule fessière (tub. sacro-iliaque second. | » | Châtré des deux côtés. | » |

Tableau des opérations pratiquées pour tuberculose des vésicules séminales (*suite*).

| NUMÉROS DES OBSERVATIONS | NOMS DES AUTEURS | AGE | DATE DES OPÉRATIONS | EXAMEN CLINIQUE | NATURE DE L'OPÉRATION | COMPLICATIONS | RÉSULTATS IMMÉDIATS | DATE DE SORTIE | AFFECTIONS ANTÉRIEURES AU DÉBUT | RÉSULTATS ÉLOIGNÉS |
|---|---|---|---|---|---|---|---|---|---|---|
| 9 | D' Sick. | » | 1895 | Tub. vés. sém. gauc. | Incision von Dittel et incision parasacrée. | Récidive tub. dans région de la vés. extirpée | Bonne cicatrisation. | » | Châtré à gauche. | Fistule donnant beaucoup de pus. |
| 10 | P' Schede. | » | 1894 | Tub. épidid. gauche, vés. sém. agrandie. | Castration gauche, extirp. de Rydigier, voie parasacrée. | » | Guérison complète. | 5 sem. après opération. | Traumatisme. | |
| 11 | P' Schede. | » | 1894 | Tub. épididyme et vés. sém. droite. | Castration droite, extirpation droite de von Dittel, voie sacrée. | Fistule pendant convalescence. | Fistule. | | | |
| 12 | P' Schede. | » | 1895 | Tub. vés. sém. droite. | Extirpat. 2 vés. sém. pararectale. | » | Raie granulations sur périnée, | 2 mois après. | Depuis six sem. châtré. | |
| 13 | P' R. Weir. *Med. Record*, 1894, n° 46, p. 163. | 18 | 1892 | Épididyme gonflé, tub. droite. | Castration bilatérale. résection prostat. partielle. | Lésion du péritoine. | Irritabilité de la vessie. | » | Avril 1892. | |
| 14 | Roux. | 46 | 1895 | Tub. test. et cordon gauche et vésicules dures aux limites. | Castration et extirp. | Hémorragies. | Guérison, fistule. | 1" août 1895 | Castration droite | 1899. Excellent état. |
| 15 | D' Platon. | 33 | 17 janv. 1897 | Épididyme induré test. gauche douloureux, canal déférent en chapelet, résection : prostate volum. et vés. sém. gauche agrandie. | Épididymo-funiculo-vésiculectomie, Villeneuve. | Rupture canal déférent, partie vésic. sém. entraînée. | Guérison. | 1" mars 1897 | Septembre 1895. | Fin 1896. Guérison complète. |
| 16 | D' O. Guellot, *Presse médicale*, 20 avril 1898. | 20 | 17 juill. 1895 | Épididymite et vésiculite, tub. gauche vés. sém. dure et agrandie. | Castrat. latér. gauche et spermatocystectomie par incision prérectale, jusqu'à l'anus. | » | Plaie scrotale suppurée, début, puis guérison. | Nov. 1895. | 1894, épididymite à gauc., noyau à la queue. | Mars 1896. Guérison. |

Tableau des opérations pratiquées pour tuberculose des vésicales séminales (*suite*).

| NUMÉROS DES OBSERVATIONS | NOMS DES AUTEURS | AGE | DATE DES OPÉRATIONS | EXAMEN CLINIQUE | NATURE DE L'OPÉRATION | COMPLICATIONS | RÉSULTATS IMMÉDIATS | DATE DE SORTIE | AFFECTIONS ANTÉRIEURES AU DÉBUT | RÉSULTATS ÉLOIGNÉS |
|---|---|---|---|---|---|---|---|---|---|---|
| 17 | D' O. Guellot. | 34 | 4 nov. 1896 | Tub. test., épididyme et vés. sém., vés. sém. volumineuse. | 1° Cast. latér. droite. 2° Épidid. et curet. à g. 3° Spermatocystectomie droite par incision prérectale prol. et extirpat. vés. par morcell. 4° Prothése test. | » | Guérison petite fist. périnéale. | » | 10 oct. 1896, tub. génit. | 28 janv. 97. Mort rapide, tuberc. pulm. aiguë. |
| 18 | Routier. | » | » | Rétr. rectum par compr. vés. volum. | Résect. part. vés. par op. sacrée de Krashe. | » | Guérison du rétrécissement. | » | » | » |
| 19 | P' Roux. | 18 | 23 mai 1898 | Tub. épidid. du canal défér. et vés sém. gauche dure. | Extirpation vés. sém. gauche Roux, puis castrat. gauche. | » | Bon état général, petite fist. | 17 juin 1898 | Janv. 1898, sans cause connue. | Août 1892. Guérison sans fist. |
| 20 | P' Roux. | 53 | 6 août 1897 | Tub. test., épidid., canal défé . et vés. sém. gauche. | Castr. gauche et extirpation vés. sém. gauche par procédé Roux. | Convalescence, écoulement purulent par plaie pararectale, température élevée. | État général bon, petite fistule, pus. | 29 nov. 1897 | 14 ans, suite traumatisme, tuméfac. scrotum ; 1889, épididyme ; 1897, affec. actuelle. | Août 1898. Bon état général, fistule. |
| 21 | Baudet et Kendirdjy. 1" cas, *Gaz. des Hôpitaur*, 15 octobre 1898. | 17 | 25 juill. 1898 | Tub. test. épididyme, canal déférent, vés. sém. droite. | Ablat. unilatérale des v. génitales et prostatectomie, résect. partielle. | Six mois après noyaux tuberculeux dans l'autre épididyme. | 1 cas guérison avec fistulette. | » | » | Fistulette excisée fin 1899. 6 mois après opérat. noyau tuberc. dans l'autre épididyme. |
| 22 | *Id.* 2° cas, *Journ. méd. de Bordeaux*, 18 février 1900. | » | » | Tub. test. épididyme, canal déférent, vés. sémin. droite. | Ablat. unilatér. des v. génit. 1 côté ; ablat. la vésic. et de l'extr. corresp. du défér. de l'autre côté, bien qu'org. fuss. sains. | » | Guérison. | » | » | Aucune récidive depuis 2 ans. |

Tableau des opérations pratiquées pour tuberculose des vésicules séminales (*suite et fin*).

| NUMÉROS DES OBSERVATIONS | NOMS DES AUTEURS | AGE | DATE DES OPÉRATIONS | EXAMEN CLINIQUE | NATURE DE L'OPÉRATION | COMPLICATIONS | RÉSULTATS IMMÉDIATS | DATE DE SORTIE | AFFECTIONS ANTÉRIEURES AU DÉBUT | RÉSULTATS ÉLOIGNÉS |
|---|---|---|---|---|---|---|---|---|---|---|
| 23 | Chavannaz in Baudet, Trait. de tuberc. testic. par la castrat. précoce et par l'ablat. totale des v. génit. *Journ. de méd. de Bordeaux,* 18 févr. 1900. | » | » | » | Vésiculectomie par méthode de Baudet. | » | Plein succès. | » | » | » |
| 24 | Roux (Observation inédite). | j. h. | 1899 | » | « Castration totale » (ablat. testic., déf. vésic.). | Fistulette périnéale. | Bon. | » | Tub. épid. testic. (hernie inguinale. | » |
| 25 26 | Doyen (V. Opér. sur prostate). | » | » | » | » | » | » | » | » | » |
| 27 | Bolton (*Journ. of cut. and. g. v. dis.,* p. 551 et 579. | » | 1899 | » | Ablation de la vés. par v. sacrée. | » | Bon résultat. | » | » | » |
| 28 29 | M. Moulin (2 cas), *Edimbourg Medic. Society,* 8 janv. 1900. | » | » | » | Ablat. des 2 vés. sém. par inc. prérectale. | Persistance d'une fistule urin. pendant quelques mois dans un cas. | Guérison. | » | Tub. épid. testic. | » |
| 30 | Alb. Hogge (Obs. inédite). | 50 | Mai 1900 (six mois avant raclage de l'épididyme droit, guérison). | » | Raclage de la vésicule séminale droite caséeuse par la voie périnéale, sonde à demeure pendant 8 jours, drainage de la pl. périnéale. | Fistulette périnéale. | Grande amélioration au point de vue des douleurs et de l'état général, disparition de la rétention. | 1 mois après. | Cystite, tub. épid. testic., vésicule unilatérale, rétent. d'urine. Tub. pulmon. avancée. | Revu un mois après en bon état. |

lades, à un moindre degré peut-être, les vésicules séminales, la prostate, la vessie?

Certains le pensent, puisqu'il a été observé que les lésions cysto-vésiculo-prostatiques avaient rétrocédé à la suite d'opération radicale ou économique sur le testicule et son conduit excréteur. Il semble que Baudet a trouvé le mot juste quand il a écrit : « Ce n'est pas une raison parce que l'arbre génital est malade à ses deux bouts, qu'il faille l'abattre de suite et d'un seul coup..., mieux vaut tenter les traitements conservateurs et ne s'attaquer d'abord qu'aux lésions épididymo-testiculaires ». Pourtant, les faits encore peu nombreux, il est vrai, d'ablation totale des voies génitales pour tuberculose, semblent engager, par leurs résultats favorables, les chirurgiens à pratiquer plus souvent dans l'avenir ces tentatives hardies[1].

———

## VALEUR DE L'INTERVENTION CHIRURGICALE
## DANS LA TUBERCULOSE RÉNALE

RAPPORT

par M. le docteur Alfred POUSSON
de Bordeaux.

Les premières interventions pour tuberculose rénale semblent avoir été pratiquées par Bryant en 1870 (néphrotomie) et Peters en 1872 (néphrectomie). Résultant d'erreurs de diagnostic, elles demeurèrent longtemps isolées, et ce n'est qu'à partir de 1880, après les opérations intentionnelles d'Habershon et de Czerny, qu'on commence à trouver dans les recueils périodiques la relation de quelques faits. En 1886, Brodeur les analyse, mais malgré les résultats encourageants de sa statistique les chirurgiens montrent encore une certaine réserve vis-à-vis de cette nouvelle intervention. C'est à la suite d'une leçon de Guyon (1888), des statistiques de Newmann (1888), d'une communication de Herczel sur la pratique de Czerny à la *Réunion des médecins et naturalistes allemands* (1889), d'un travail de Morris à l'*Association médicale britannique* (1889), d'une discussion au sein du *Congrès des chirurgiens allemands* (1890), de la publication des mémoires de Küster et d'Israël dans le *Centrabl. f. chir.*, que l'intervention chirurgicale

1. La place limitée réservée à ce travail nous force à passer sous silence les indications bibliographiques qui lui sont relatives. — Voir ci-dessus les tableaux des opérations pratiquées pour tuberculose de la prostate et des vésicules séminales.

dans la tuberculose rénale est définitivement entrée dans la pratique.
Depuis lors les opérations se sont rapidement multipliées, qui ont
permis à Vigneron, Facklam, Palet de dresser des statisques impo-
santes, auxquelles nous avons ajouté, en vue de ce rapport, les faits
publiés dans ces huit dernières années.

I

### RÉSULTATS GÉNÉRAUX

1º Résultats immédiats. *a*) *Mortalité opératoire globale.* — Les statistiques impersonnelles, c'est-à-dire dressées avec les observations
éparses dans la littérature médicale, auxquelles nous joignons celle
que nous avons établie nous-même, montrent le peu de gravité de
cette intervention.

*Statistiques impersonnelles.*

| Statisticiens. | Interventions. | Décès. | Mortalité. |
|---|---|---|---|
| Brodeur. . . . . . . . . | 26 | 11 | 43,5  pour 100. |
| Vigneron . . . . . . . | 169 | 38 | 22,47  — |
| Palet . . . . . . . . . | 136 | 38 | 28,67  — |
| Facklam. . . . . . . . | 108 | 22 | 20,37  — |
| Pousson. . . . . . . . | 161 | 19 | 11,86  — |
| Ensemble . . . . . . | 600 | 128 | 21,35 pour 100. |

Si l'on songe à la gravité de la tuberculose rénale abandonnée à
elle-même, on ne pourra s'empêcher de trouver cette léthalité de
21,35 pour 100 relativement faible : pour être juste, il convient de la
réduire au pourcentage de la statistique que nous avons dressée en
recueillant 161 faits récents ayant bénéficié des progrès de la technique et par-dessus tout de la précision des indications opératoires.
Cette mortalité de 11,86 pour 100 s'abaisse encore, si on envisage les
statistiques personnelles de quelques chirurgiens rapportées dans ce
tableau.

*Statistiques personnelles.*

| Opérateurs. | Interventions. | Décès. | Mortalité. |
|---|---|---|---|
| Bardenheuer . . . . . | 7 | 0 | 0  pour 100. |
| Czerny . . . . . . . . . | 6 | 0 | 0  — |
| Israël. . . . . . . . . | 20 | 3 | 15  — |
| Küster . . . . . . . . | 11 | 2 | 18,18  — |
| Riss. . . . . . . . . . | 7 | 0 | 0  — |
| Tilden Brown. . . . . | 9 | 1 | 11,11  — |
| Albarran . . . . . . . | 35 | 2 | 5,71  — |
| Routier. . . . . . . . | 11 | 0 | 0  — |
| Tuffier . . . . . . . . | 16 | 2 | 12,5  — |
| Pousson . . . . . . . | 12 | 2 | 16,66  — |
| Ensemble . . . . . . | 134 | 12 | 8,95 pour 100. |

Une léthalité de 8,95 pour 100, voilà le bilan mortuaire actuel des opérations dirigées contre la tuberculose rénale.

*b) Mortalité opératoire respective de la néphrotomie et de la néphrectomie.* — Ces deux modes d'intervention se partagent inégalement la mortalité. Tandis que le bloc des statistiques impersonnelles indique une léthalité sensiblement égale pour la néphrotomie (20,8 0/0) et la néphrectomie (21,47 0/0), celui des statistiques personnelles aux opérateurs précités montre que l'incision simple du rein est autrement meurtrière que son extirpation (18,51 0/0 contre 6,54 0/0). Ce résultat, *a priori* inattendu, s'explique si l'on prend note qu'alors que l'ensemble des premières statistiques se compose de toutes les interventions publiées depuis vingt-cinq à trente ans, l'ensemble des secondes ne comprend que celles pratiquées depuis dix ans à peine. La mortalité de la néphrectomie en effet a diminué parallèlement aux progrès de la médecine opératoire secondée par l'antisepsie et au perfectionnement des moyens que nous avons d'apprécier la valeur fonctionnelle du rein opposé. Quant à la néphrotomie, sa gravité n'a pas sensiblement diminué (50 0/0 stat. de Brodeur, 27,5 0/0 stat. de Pousson) parce que tous les mauvais cas de nos jours lui demeurent réservés.

*c) Causes de la mort après la néphrotomie et la néphrectomie.* — Les 26 décès opératoires survenus à la suite des 125 néphrotomies réunies par Brodeur, Vigneron, Facklam et nous-même ont été déterminés par :

| | | | |
|---|---|---|---|
| L'anurie | 2 fois. | La septicémie | 4 fois. |
| L'insuffisance rénale. | 5 — | Des causes non détermi- | |
| Le shock | 5 — | nées | 12 — |

Les 102 décès opératoires consécutifs aux 475 néphrectomies des mêmes statisticiens et de Palet avec eux ont été imputés à :

| | | | |
|---|---|---|---|
| L'anurie | 9 fois. | La septicémie | 8 fois. |
| L'insuffisance rénale. | 37 — | La blessure de la veine | |
| La tuberculose généra- | | cave | 2 — |
| lisée | 13 — | Des causes non détermi- | |
| Le shock | 17 — | nées | 16 — |

On le voit, la suppression complète de la sécrétion urinaire et son insuffisance n'enregistrent à leur passif pas moins de 51 de ces 128 décès, c'est-à-dire près de la moitié. L'état anatomique et le mauvais fonctionnement physiologique du rein opposé sont les causes de ces accidents, naguère inéluctables, que les progrès réalisés dans le diagnostic des lésions rénales nous font espérer de conjurer désormais.

2° RÉSULTATS ÉLOIGNÉS. *a) Après la néphrotomie.* — Des 99 observations de néphrotomie suivie de succès opératoires, 65 sont suffisamment explicites pour juger les résultats éloignés. Sur ce nombre 39 malades succombèrent dans un délai variant de quelques mois à un an et parmi eux 22 furent emportés par les progrès de la tuberculose dans le rein opéré ou généralisation à l'appareil urinaire entier. En lisant les détails des observations de ces 22 malades, on ne peut s'empêcher de penser qu'un certain nombre sont morts par suite de l'insuffisance de la néphrotomie. Des 24 opérés, vivant encore au moment de la publication de l'observation, 6 étaient néphrotomisés depuis moins de un an, les autres depuis un à cinq ans (opéré de Guyon deux ans; Tuffier, Riss, trois ans, Thornton cinq ans).

Pour aucun de ces malades on ne peut affirmer que la guérison a été définitive, mais tous avaient l'apparence d'une santé excellente et leur état local s'était considérablement amélioré.

Ainsi la néphrotomie peut rendre des services de longue durée, mais la persistance d'une fistule est pour ainsi dire la règle après elle. Un seul sujet opéré par Küster semble en avoir été exempt; les observations de Haberson de Thornton, de Ris sont contestables; celles de Rafin et de Tuffier sont plus certaines; chez mes néphrotomisés personnels la fistule n'a jamais fait défaut.

*b). Après la néphrectomie.* — Sur les 575 observations de néphrectomie, 355 peuvent servir à l'appréciation de ces résultats. Sur ce bloc, 42 opérés succombèrent dans l'année suivante, dont 38 à la généralisation de la tuberculose à la vessie, à l'autre rein, aux poumons ou à quelques autres organes. Les 293 autres néphrectomisés vivaient encore lorsque leurs observations ont été publiées : 49 étaient opérés depuis moins de 1 an, 55 depuis plus de 1 an, 15 depuis 2 ans, 12 depuis 3 ans, 14 depuis 4 ans, 14 depuis 5 à 10 ans. Parmi ces derniers citons les opérés de Verneuil, de Verhoogen (5 malades), de Thornton, de Martin, de Bardenheuer, de Reynier, enfin d'Antona dont la malade néphrectomisée en 1882 vit encore et est bien portante.

La persistance d'une fistule si fréquente après la néphrotomie est exceptionnelle après la néphrectomie, car Palet ne l'a notée que 15 fois sur 85 opérations et encore ne fut-elle définitive que dans 5 cas; sur nos 105 faits nous l'avons relevée 7 fois et chez deux malade de Socin elle se ferma spontanément après quelques mois.

Fait des plus important, la survie après la suppression du rein est plus longue qu'après sa simple incision, car sur 63 néphrotomies nous notons 39 morts dans l'année suivante, soit 61,90 pour 100, tandis que sur 555 néphrectomies nous trouvons 42 morts seulement, soit 12,53 pour 100.

## II

### RÉSULTATS DANS LES DEUX PHASES DE L'ÉVOLUTION DE LA MALADIE
### ET SUIVANT LES DIVERSES CIRCONSTANCES CLINIQUES

*Indications et contre-indications opératoires.* — Il convient d'envisager ces résultats aux deux grandes phases de l'évolution de la maladie.

*a). Phase d'infection purement bacillaire.* — Cette phase, qui tend à prendre une place de plus en plus importante en pathologie rénale, ne s'observe vraisemblablement que dans la tuberculose descendante ou primitive. Les opérateurs, qui sont intervenus à cette période, y ont toujours été conduits par la nécessité de mettre un terme à quelques accidents (douleurs intenses, hémorragies profuses), mais aucun sauf Albarran n'a agi dans le seul but de supprimer un foyer bacillaire silencieux. Nous croyons avec Albarran que l'intervention dans ce cas est parfaitement légitime ; c'est alors qu'on a toutes les chances de guérir radicalement la tuberculose rénale par la néphrectomie. Sur 10 néphrectomies, commandées par l'existence de douleurs ou d'hémorragies, nous n'avons relevé aucun décès, et les malades ont pu être suivis longtemps conservant l'intégrité de leur appareil urinaire et voyant les lésions initiales de leur vessie, s'il en existait, s'améliorer. Citons parmi les résultats remarquables d'interventions pour douleurs ou hémorragies, les cas de Casper, de Schede, d'Israël, de Routier, de Loumeau.

*b) Phase d'infection mixte.* — Nous devons grouper en deux catégories les cas ressortissant à cette phase : les cas de tuberculose primitive dans lesquels l'infection peut être et demeurer limitée au rein, et les cas de tuberculose secondaire, dans lesquels la vessie, la prostate et les organes génitaux sont toujours pris conjointement. Malheureusement les auteurs ont rarement pris le soin d'indiquer à quelle variété ils ont eu affaire; après une lecture attentive des observations nous avons trouvé 49 interventions pour tuberculose primitive et 20 pour tuberculose secondaire.

1° *Tuberculose primitive.* — Les 49 interventions ont donné 8 morts rapides et 4 retardées. Chez les autres opérés, la survie, se prolongeant encore au moment de la publication de l'observation, était au-dessous de 1 an chez 13 malades, au-dessus de 1 an chez 5, de 2 ans chez 4, de 3 ans chez un opéré de Golberg, de 4 ans chez 1 de Czerny, de 6 ans chez 4 de Verhoogen, de 9 ans chez 1 de Doyen, de 10 ans chez

1 de Régnier. Tous ces malades, sauf 4 chez lesquels on pratiqua la néphrotomie avec 2 morts (une opératoire et une deux mois après), furent néphrectomisés.

2° *Tuberculose secondaire.* — Les 20 interventions ont donné 4 morts rapides et 5 retardées. Chez les autres opérés la survie existait depuis 2 mois 1/2 chez un malade de Carlier, 1 an 1/2 chez un Routier, 5 ans chez un de Poncet; temps inconnus chez X X. Sur ces 20 malades 6 furent néphrectomisés avec une seule mort opératoire (cas de Schuchardt), tous les autres furent néphrotomisés avec 5 morts opératoires (cas de Verhoogen, Tuffier, Socin).

c). *Comparaison des résultats des interventions dans la tuberculose primitive et secondaire.* — S'ils sont sensiblement les mêmes au point de vue des dangers immédiats (8 morts rapides sur 49 interventions pour tuberculose primitive et 4 morts rapides sur 20 interventions pour tuberculose secondaire), ils sont notablement meilleurs au point de vue des effets consécutifs dans la forme primitive. En effet dans cette forme nos 49 opérations n'ont donné lieu qu'à 4 morts retardées, tandis que nous en relevons 5 sur les 20 opérations dans la seconde forme.

d) *Circonstances cliniques.* 1° *Bilatéralité des lésions.* — Elle ne contre-indique pas formellement l'intervention, et il faut distinguer, au point de vue prohibitif, les cas où le rein opposé présente des lésions tuberculeuses à un certain degré de leur évolution, et ceux où il offre des lésions de néphrite bacillaire ou vulgaire peu avancée. Si dans les premiers on ne saurait raisonnablement pratiquer la néphrectomie, on peut tout au moins avoir recours à la néphrotomie palliative, de soulagement ou hémostatique; mais dans les seconds, alors que l'urine recueillie par le cathétérisme de l'uretère ne contient avec une légère diminution de l'urée et des sels qu'une faible proportion d'albumine, de rares cylindres et quelques micro-organismes, il est possible, sans grands risques et avec beaucoup de profit, de faire l'ablation du rein le premier et le plus profondément infecté. Vigneron signale cette « influence favorable de l'ouverture ou de l'ablation d'un rein tuberculeux sur les douleurs et la *fonction* du second rein » et nous-même avons démontré que sous l'influence d'une opération palliative, comme l'incision d'un rein pathologique, plus particulièrement d'un rein pyonéphrotique en rétention complète ou partielle, et encore mieux d'une néphrectomie, on voit les lésions initiales du rein adelphe rétrocéder.

2° *État de la vessie.* — Les phénomènes réflexes, tels que douleur, fréquence et caractère impérieux des mictions, cessant comme par enchantement après l'intervention, ne contre-indiquent pas l'opération, bien au contraire. A moins de lésions tuberculeuses très étendues et très profondes, aujourd'hui facilement appréciables par la cystoscopie, la cystite ne s'y oppose pas davantage. Même lorsque l'infection bacillaire de la vessie est antérieure à celle du rein, elle s'améliore toujours après l'opération et les différents topiques employés auparavant sans résultats peuvent en avoir raison. Quant aux infections banales, si fréquentes chez les tuberculeux rénaux (Albarran), la guérison est presque la règle après l'intervention sur le rein.

3° *État des autres organes et de la santé générale.* — Les indications et les contre-indications opératoires, qui en découlent, ne diffèrent pas de celles qu'on trouve à propos de toutes les interventions chirurgicales. Nous ne nous attarderons pas à les discuter.

4° *Sexe et âge.* — La tuberculose rénale plus fréquente chez la femme que chez l'homme a donné lieu à un nombre d'interventions 2 fois plus considérable dans le sexe féminin que dans le sexe masculin, et la léthalité opératoire a été un peu plus fréquente dans le premier que dans le second.

C'est à la période moyenne de l'âge adulte que la mortalité opératoire est le plus faible (21,55 0/0), dans l'enfance elle est notablement inférieure (35,35 0/0) à ce qu'elle est dans l'adolescence (47,56 0/0) où elle atteint son maximum; enfin dans la vieillesse, bien qu'elle soit considérable (42,85 0/0), elle est cependant moindre que dans l'adolescence et la première étape de l'âge adulte.


## III

### RÉSULTATS DES DIVERS MODES D'INTERVENTION

*(Choix de la méthode et du procédé opératoire.)*

*a) Néphrotomie.* — Elle ne saurait légitimement être employée dans la *tuberculose miliaire et nodulaire*, car même aidée du curettage et de la cautérisation elle ne pourrait atteindre tous les foyers disséminés dans le parenchyme. Dans la *forme massive*, Madelung et Duret y ont eu recours, le premier sans succès, le second avec un bon résultat; nous pensons que dans cette forme, le tissu rénal n'existant plus pour ainsi dire, mieux vaut pratiquer d'emblée l'extirpation de l'organe. C'est dans la *forme hydronéphrotique* avec conservation de la perméabilité de l'uretère que l'incision du rein donnerait vraisemblablement ses meilleurs résultats, mais nous ne croyons pas qu'elle ait jamais été pratiquée dans cette variété, tout à fait exceptionnelle

d'ailleurs. La néphrotomie jusqu'ici a été presque exclusivement pratiquée dans la *forme pyonéphrotique*, de beaucoup la plus fréquente. Or
si dans quelques cas rares, ressortissant plus probablement à l'infection mixte ascendante, le parenchyme entièrement détruit fait place à
une poche unique remplie d'un magma caséo-purulent, le plus souvent il existe une série de cavernes et de cavernules indépendantes les
unes des autres et du bassinet lui-même. L'incision du rein la mieux
combinée est ainsi incapable d'ouvrir tous les foyers, et après une
amélioration passagère, mais presque constante, il est juste de le reconnaître, on observe le retour offensif de tout le cortège de ces
symptômes graves, qui rendent la survie des néphrotomisés moins
longue que celle des néphrectomisés. La néphrotomie ne doit être en
définitive considérée que comme une opération de nécessité, que doit
compléter tôt ou tard une néphrectomie secondaire. En effet sur 86 néphrotomisés des statistiques de Brodeur, Vigneron et Pousson,
20 moururent d'accidents pour la plupart imputables à l'insuffisance
de l'intervention, et des 65 autres, 56 durent subir la néphrectomi
secondaire.

A l'exception d'un très petit nombre d'opérateurs qui ont eu recours à la voie transpéritonéale (Kuester), tous les autres ont ouvert
le rein par la voie lombaire ou paralombaire en dehors du péritoine.
C'est à cette méthode qu'on doit donner la préférence.

*b) Néphrectomie.* — C'est l'opération de choix, applicable à toutes
les phases de l'évolution de la tuberculose rénale.

1° *Mortalité comparée de la néphrectomie primitive et secondaire.* —
La mortalité de la néphrectomie en général étant de 21,47 pour 100,
voyons quelle est celle de l'exérèse pratiquée d'emblée et celle de
l'extirpation faite après une néphrotomie préalable. Pendant longtemps on a cru que la néphrectomie primitive était plus grave que
la secondaire. Les statistiques de Brodeur et de Palet viennent à
l'appui de cette opinion, celle de Vigneron et surtout la nôtre l'infir-
ment, et en additionnant les chiffres de ces quatre statistiques, on
voit qu'une grande supériorité revient à la néphrectomie primitive,
qui accuse 21,79 pour 100 de mortalité contre 50,76 pour 100, bilan
de la néphrectomie secondaire.

La néphrectomie secondaire pouvant rendre néanmoins de très
grands services, il importe de savoir à quelle époque il convient de la
pratiquer pour en retirer bénéfice. De la statistique que nous avons
dressée à ce sujet, le moment le plus propice pour la tenter est compris entre le deuxième et le quatrième mois après la néphrectomie.
Avant cette époque les chances de mort sont plus grandes parce que

l'état général des malades n'est pas encore suffisamment relevé ; après elles le sont, soit parce que l'opéré ayant fait de nouveaux foyers d'infection est redevenu cachectique, soit parce que les fusées purulentes et les adhérences inflammatoires exposent à des accidents opératoires.

2° *Gravité comparée de la néphrectomie extrapéritonéale et de la néphrectomie transpéritonéale.* — En groupant les faits de nos diverses statistiques, nous voyons combien plus meurtrière est la néphrectomie transpéritonéale, dont la léthalité est de 54,04 0/0 contre 21,21 0/0 que comporte l'extrapéritonéale. C'est donc à cette dernière qu'on doit donner la préférence.

En combinant judicieusement les incisions lombaires et paralombaires, on peut extirper par cette voie de très volumineuses tumeurs sans les rompre, condition des plus importantes pour éviter l'ensemencement de la loge lombaire. Le morcellement de Tuffier nous semble pour cette raison devoir être rejeté. Quant à la néphrectomie sous-capsulaire d'Ollier, c'est un procédé d'exception, ayant le grand inconvénient de laisser dans la gangue péri-rénale des follicules et nodules tuberculeux. La voie lombaire permet aussi, dans la majorité des cas, de bien former le pédicule, de lier les vaisseaux séparés du bassinet au catgut et non à la soie, qui s'infectant devient la source de suppuration intarissable, enfin de réséquer l'uretère dans la plus grande étendue possible.

*c) Néphrectomie partielle.* — Israël, Tuffier et quelques rares opérateurs, se trouvant en face de lésions tuberculeuses bien limitées, ont cru pouvoir faire la résection partielle d'une corne ou d'un coin du rein, et le premier de ces chirurgiens a pu suivre un sujet ayant subi une héminéphrectomie pendant dix-huit mois sans que le moindre accident se soit reproduit. Nous ne pensons pas que cette opération économique très exceptionnellement indiquée, par exemple dans le cas d'un tuberculome unique et bien circonscrit, ait jamais chance de passer dans la pratique. Selon nous, elle risquera toujours d'être insuffisante, car la portion du rein conservée, si elle n'est pas déjà envahie par l'infiltration tuberculeuse, est presque toujours atteinte de néphrite de voisinage.


## DISCUSSION

M. Carlier (de Lille). — Il me paraît indispensable d'envisager séparément la valeur de nos moyens d'action chirurgicale suivant qu'ils s'adressent à la tuberculose du rein ou à la tuberculose de la vessie.

Je partage les idées émises par M. Pousson dans son rapport sur la tuberculose rénale ; la néphrectomie me paraît l'opération de choix, la néphrotomie une opération de nécessité, un pis-aller. Les résultats immédiats et éloignés de la néphrectomie sont d'autant plus remarquables que l'opération est pratiquée à une époque plus rapprochée du début de la maladie, dans la *phase d'infection purement bacillaire* (Pousson).

Chirurgien et malade ont tout à gagner à ne pas temporiser longtemps; le premier opérera dans des conditions plus simples, le second n'en sera encore qu'à la période d'infection rénale avec une vessie non encore ou à peine infectée par le bacille de Koch.

Ce que nous savons de l'évolution habituelle de la tuberculose du rein et de l'unilatéralité fréquente de cette localisation du bacille de Koch nous engage à intervenir hâtivement, dès que le diagnostic est posé.

En effet, les lésions bacillaires du rein évoluent silencieusement plus souvent qu'on ne le pense, et l'on est parfois surpris, le rein une fois enlevé, d'y constater de grosses lésions dont on ne soupçonnait pas l'importance.

La néphrectomie n'est justifiée qu'autant que l'on a des renseignements précis sur la valeur fonctionnelle du rein supposé sain. Le cathétérisme des uretères, dont on peut être le partisan ou l'adversaire, nous donne évidemment ces renseignements indispensables. Je me suis pendant longtemps refusé à cathétériser l'uretère du côté supposé sain, mais je viens d'observer et d'opérer un malade dans des conditions qui m'ont rendu désormais méfiant à l'égard de l'épreuve du bleu : l'analyse chimique des urines m'avait permis de croire à l'intégrité du rein congénère. J'eus recours à la néphrectomie: or, mon malade est mort, et l'autopsie m'a permis de constater de très graves lésions dans le rein que j'avais laissé.

Je ne crois pas que la néphrectomie doive forcement être suivie de la résection de l'uretère. C'est en effet un second acte opératoire qui prolonge l'opération et dont le malade ne tire pas toujours grand profit. Je cherche même à ne pas trop diminuer la longueur de l'uretère, de façon à le fixer au fond de la plaie. Si l'uretère suppure consécutivement, j'ai de la sorte plus de facilité pour traiter le trajet fistuleux que si l'uretère avait été réséqué jusque dans le pelvis.

Je me déclare donc très partisan de l'intervention chirurgicale dans la tuberculose du rein. Par contre, je suis beaucoup plus réservé lorsqu'il s'agit d'une tuberculose de la vessie.

La tuberculose vésicale est secondaire à une tuberculose du rein ou à une tuberculose de la prostate ou des vésicules séminales; dans le premier cas, la néphrectomie pratiquée en temps opportun mettra la vessie à l'abri de toute atteinte bacillaire, et en cas d'infection déjà existante, elle restera le moyen le meilleur pour la combattre. Que de tuberculoses on eût évitées si l'on avait supprimé plus tôt la source de contamination, c'est-à-dire le rein !

Mais que faire à un malade dont la vessie s'est infectée consécutivement à une tuberculose de la prostate ou des vésicules? Il me paraît illogique d'intervenir du côté de la vessie sans supprimer d'abord la source de son infection. Les malades que j'ai opérés à une époque rapprochée du début de leur maladie en les soumettant à une taille hypogastrique suivie de curettage, de cautérisations ignées et d'excision des lésions, n'ont en général pas bénéficié de mon intervention et les douleurs réapparurent dès que je laissai se refermer la fistule vésico-hypogastrique. Je me suis bien mieux trouvé du traitement médical chez les malades dont les mictions sont surtout fréquentes et à peine douloureuses, et j'ai observé des cas où ce traitement a agi merveilleusement. Une fistulisation hypogastrique de la vessie n'eût pas mieux fait, et je n'avais pas créé une infirmité toujours très pénible. Si cependant l'examen bactériologique des urines me fait constater une association microbienne dont nous connaissons la gravité, j'interviens par des instillations appropriées, auxquelles je renonce vite d'ailleurs, si elles provoquent la moindre irritation.

Quand la cystite n'est influencée ni par le traitement médical, ni par les pansements intra-vésicaux, qu'elle épuise le malade par la fréquence et la douleur des mictions, j'interviens alors par la cystostomie que je préfère au drainage par le périnée. L'opération procure aux malades un soulagement réel qui peut en imposer parfois pour une guérison, mais je considère que ce drainage hypogastrique, une fois créé, sera souvent définitif.

M. Loumeau (de Bordeaux). — Comme dans toutes les tuberculoses chirurgicales, la suppression d'un foyer tuberculeux urinaire doit être aussi complète et aussi précoce que possible, qu'il s'agisse du rein ou de la vessie.

Pour le rein tuberculeux, une fois son congénère reconnu suffisant à assurer seul la dépuration urinaire, la néphrectomie s'impose et constitue la méthode de choix, la néphrotomie n'étant qu'une méthode de nécessité dont le chirurgien est obligé de se contenter en face d'un état général trop grave ou d'adhérences rendant trop périlleuse l'extirpation de l'organe ; en ce dernier cas, il faudra recourir le plus tôt possible à la néphrectomie secondaire.

J'ai opéré sept tuberculoses rénales, cinq par la néphrectomie primitive, deux par la néphrotomie, tous par la voie lombaire. Parmi les cinq premiers cas, il s'agissait une fois de tuberculose rénale à forme hématurique, et la malade, opérée à peu près exsangue et *in extremis*, se porte aujourd'hui très bien, quarante-cinq mois après mon intervention. Les quatre autres néphrectomies furent dirigées contre une pyonéphrose et trois néphro-tuberculoses caverneuses. Elles furent également suivies de guérison, et, dans deux cas, amenèrent la disparition d'une cystite concomitante. Ces guérisons datent aujourd'hui de six, neuf, onze et quatorze mois. Dans deux cas où la seule néphrotomie fut pratiquée, il s'agissait de pyonéphroses tuberculeuses adhérentes et de malades profondément affaiblis. L'un mourut quinze jours après l'opération de septicémie ; l'autre, du choc opératoire, quelques heures après une très laborieuse néphrectomie secondaire pratiquée un mois après l'incision et la fistulisation du foyer rénal. Chez ces sept opérés, l'examen cystoscopique, seul ou combiné avec le cathétérisme urétéral, dont je n'ai jamais eu qu'à me louer, m'avait préalablement démontré l'existence et la suffisante validité du rein opposé.

Contre la tuberculose vésicale, compliquée ou non de cystite et non imputable à l'inoculation d'un foyer rénal ou para-vésical, dont la suppression préalable s'imposerait tout d'abord, le traitement sanglant est commandé par l'inefficacité des autres moyens thérapeutiques.

L'ouverture sus-pubienne de la vessie permet le curettage, la thermo-cautérisation, au besoin l'abrasion de la muqueuse malade et la mise au repos longtemps prolongé du réservoir vésical par la cystostomie. J'ai opéré de cette manière douze malades, dont deux présentaient une tuber-culose commençante de la vessie sans cystite; neuf autres avaient une cystite tuberculeuse ancienne et le douzième une cystite chronique interstitielle, avec abolition de la capacité vésicale à la suite d'une instil-lation de nitrate d'argent pratiquée par erreur dans sa vessie tubercu-leuse. A part un seul de mes opérés, tuberculeux laryngé et pulmonaire en même temps que vésical, chez qui la cystostomie était dirigée contre les douleurs intolérables de la cystite et qui succomba d'infection tuber-culeuse généralisée deux mois après mon intervention, tous se sont par-faitement trouvés de l'opération. Elle a supprimé les troubles locaux, remonté l'état général et, dans trois cas, amené une guérison complète qui date actuellement de quatre, six et neuf mois, et a été obtenue après une fistulisation vésico-hypogastrique maintenue pendant trois, douze et dix-huit mois. Les huit autres cystostomisés conservent toujours leur méat sus-pubien, qui date de quatre mois à trois années, et que je lais-serai seulement oblitérer le jour où la tolérance de la vessie et l'indo-lence de la miction naturelle viendront, avec la disparition définitive des bacilles de Koch dans les urines, me démontrer la guérison complète. Seul le malade opéré pour sa cystite chronique interstitielle post-tuber-culeuse gardera vraisemblablement toute sa vie le méat contre nature qui a supprimé les besoins douloureux et incessants d'uriner, visés par mon intervention.

M. Albarran (de Paris). — Voici ma statistique personnelle dans la tuberculose rénale. J'ai pratiqué 29 néphrectomies dont 28 guéris et un mort, soit une mortalité de 5 1/2 pour 100. Sur 15 néphrostomies une mort opératoire.

Je suis heureux de voir M. Pousson accepter, contrairement à l'opinion de Tuffier, ce que j'ai toujours défendu, l'utilité des interventions pré-coces dans les lésions unilatérales : les succès immédiats sont beaucoup plus nombreux lorsqu'on opère de bonne heure, et on évite les redou-tables complications vésicales par voie descendante, dont la fréquence est grande dans la tuberculose. Je lis dans le rapport de M. Pousson que les opérateurs ont toujours été conduits par la nécessité de mettre un terme à des accidents (douleurs intenses, hémorragie), aucun n'a agi dans le seul but de supprimer le foyer bacillaire silencieux. Or, j'ai publié à la Société de Chirurgie, en octobre 1899, une observation où j'ai enlevé le rein sans aucun symptôme rénal; de même, mon dernier opéré, qui est encore dans nos salles, n'a jamais eu aucun symptôme rénal apparent.

Mais pour opérer lorsque les lésions ne se manifestent pas encore par les symptômes ordinaires, il faut diagnostiquer de bonne heure; or, ce diagnostic, que j'ai pu faire, le cathétérisme urétéral le permet. Par lui nous pouvons étudier comparativement dans les deux reins les qualités physiques et la composition chimique des urines, pratiquer leur analyse histologique et bactériologique, connaître enfin les modifications dans le pouvoir éliminateur des reins à l'égard du bleu de méthylène et de la fluoridzine. L'étude de l'urine globale ne peut, au contraire, pas nous renseigner sur les lésions légères ou même graves d'un seul rein. Voici des courbes de bleu de méthylène qui le démontrent.

Pour baser des indications opératoires précises il est nécessaire de connaître aussi exactement que possible l'état du rein qui doit rester en place. On peut se tromper en croyant les deux reins malades lorsqu'un seul est atteint; on peut, au contraire, penser que la lésion est unilatérale lorsque les deux reins sont gravement atteints. Vous pouvez voir en ce moment au n° 19, salle Laugier, une femme chez qui tout fait penser que seul le rein est malade : elle ne souffre que de ce côté; le rein gauche n'est pas augmenté de volume; l'urine a une composition ordinaire, le bleu de méthylène s'élimine bien; or, j'ai pratiqué le cathétérisme urétéral avant de l'opérer et j'ai trouvé des lésions graves doubles qui contre-indiquent toute intervention.

Comme l'a dit Pousson, on peut et on doit parfois extirper un rein lorsque l'autre est légèrement malade : mais il faut encore pouvoir dire avec certitude que cet autre rein suffira à la vie. J'ajoute que la néphrectomie ne sera alors indiquée que si le rein qu'on doit enlever cause une atteinte grave à la santé générale. Il est évident que si les lésions sont légères des deux côtés, il ne faut point intervenir.

J'entends souvent parler, comme dans le rapport, de deux phases dans la tuberculose rénale, une première d'infection bacillaire pure, avec lésions peu prononcées encore; une seconde d'infection mixte qui serait surtout caractérisée par la pyonéphrose. Or, on doit bien établir que la pyonéphrose tuberculeuse peut exister sans qu'il y ait d'infection mixte; les lésions sont souvent purement bacillaires comme le démontrent plusieurs observations personnelles avec cultures immédiates du pus.

Un dernier mot, enfin, au sujet de la résection de l'uretère. Dans mes premières opérations je la faisais; j'y ai renoncé aujourd'hui quand les lésions ne sont pas très limitées : 1° parce qu'on n'enlève jamais ou presque jamais toute la partie malade; 2° parce que cette extirpation urétérale aggrave l'acte opératoire; 3° parce que, chez plusieurs malades, j'ai constaté qu'ultérieurement l'uretère sectionné s'atrophie et parce que, chez aucun de mes opérés, je n'ai vu de fistule persistante.

Les succès opératoires seront plus nombreux, les survies plus longues lorsque nous ferons mieux le diagnostic précoce des lésions, déterminant avec exactitude l'état des deux reins. Ici encore le cathétérisme cystoscopique des uretères a réalisé déjà un progrès considérable.

# DEUX OBSERVATIONS D'INTERVENTION CHIRURGICALE DANS UN CAS DE TUBERCULOSE RÉNALE ET UN CAS DE TUBERCULOSE VÉSICALE

par M. le docteur HAMONIC,

de Paris.

Assez souvent j'ai été appelé à ouvrir la vessie pour la tuberculose chronique de cet organe.

Beaucoup plus rarement, j'ai eu à intervenir par la méthode sanglante pour la tuberculose rénale.

De ma série d'observations, je ne veux aujourd'hui en relater que deux dans lesquelles la guérison s'est produite dans des conditions inespérées. Les voici en quelques mots :

Il y a huit ans, je fus appelé auprès d'une hématurique qui avait un rein droit très volumineux et très douloureux. Aucun antécédent tuberculeux ni aucun signe de tuberculose pulmonaire. Tous les traitements médicaux ayant échoué, je proposai une intervention, mais on n'accepta en principe que la néphrotomie et en raison de la gravité du pronostic, on s'opposa à la néphrectomie.

J'isolai le rein avec d'assez grandes difficultés, et après incision suivant la technique habituelle, je trouvai dans le parenchyme une quantité assez considérable de tubercules miliaires désséminés. Après lavage au sublimé, je touchai la surface rénale avec de la solution au chlorure de zinc à 5 0/0, puis je suturai l'organe et le remis à sa place.

Après des péripéties diverses et au bout de 6 semaines environ, la guérison survint. Tous les symptômes disparurent peu à peu et ne se sont plus reproduits depuis 8 ans. Tout fait supposer que l'explosion rénale tuberculeuse est complètement effacée sous l'influence de modifications nutritives inflammatoires et traumatiques qui ont suiv la néphrotomie qui, dans le cas actuel, avait été bien plus une opéra tion exploratrice qu'une opération curative.

Dans une autre circonstance, en 1895, j'eus l'occasion chez un calculeux d'ouvrir la vessie pour retirer une pierre uratique très dure de 55 grammes.

Le réservoir une fois ouvert, je rencontrai une muqueuse parsemée de granulations miliaires tuberculeuses. Un lambeau de cette muqueuse excisée permit au microscope de confirmer le diagnostic.

Comme la vessie ne présentait pas d'ulcérations ni de fongosités, on ne pouvait songer à en pratiquer le curettage. Je me contentai donc de la suturer en partie en laissant pendant quelque temps un drainage hypogastrique et urétral.

Le malade a guéri très rapidement, et depuis son opération sa santé est toujours demeurée parfaite. A plusieurs reprises j'ai eu l'occasion de faire l'examen cystoscopique et je n'ai rien constaté d'anormal sur sa muqueuse.

Voilà encore un cas dans lequel l'action traumatique opératoire paraît avoir été suffisante pour enrayer et même guérir une tuberculose localisée à son début.

---

## DES INTERVENTIONS DANS LA TUBERCULOSE GÉNITO-URINAIRE

### par M. F. LEGUEU,

de Paris.

Les questions soulevées par les rapports que vous venez d'entendre sont des plus importantes, elles intéressent à la fois les chirurgiens et les spécialistes.

La tuberculose dans l'appareil génito-urinaire débute par deux points : elle commence par la prostate ou elle commence par le rein.

Elle commence par le rein, et de là descend vers la vessie et remonte vers le congénère.

Elle commence plus souvent par la prostate et les vésicules séminales et de ce point où elles ont pris naissance les lésions tuberculeuses évoluent vers le testicule par l'intermédiaire du canal déférent, et vers la vessie plus rarement.

La tuberculose génitale est donc toujours secondaire à une tuberculose profonde. Aussi suis-je opposé à toute tentative de castration dans la tuberculose testiculaire : je me contente d'enlever l'épididyme et de supprimer en même temps la plus grande étendue possible du canal déférent. Je n'aborde que rarement la prostate et les vésicules séminales ; en voici la raison. Je n'ai vu que très rarement ces lésions suppurer après infection secondaire : au contraire dans tous les cas que j'ai opérés ou vu opérer, la plaie est restée fistuleuse, et le malade a gardé une fistule. Je respecte donc ces lésions dont l'extension vers la vessie n'est heureusement pas fatale.

La tuberculose de la vessie m'apparaît comme presque toujours secondaire à une tuberculose rénale ou à une tuberculose vésico-prostatique. Jusqu'ici je n'ai pratiqué dans la tuberculose vésicale que des opérations tardives : leurs résultats ont été défectueux. Dans les tuberculoses vésicales au début, je n'ai fait jusqu'alors que le traitement médical conservateur, parce que je n'ai pas trouvé dans la littérature ni dans la pratique de mes collègues d'observations capables de plaider la cause des interventions précoces dans les tuberculoses vésicales.

En ce qui concerne la tuberculose rénale, je suis partisan de la néphrectomie primitive. Plus je vois de malades, et plus je suis convaincu du rôle prépondérant qui revient à la tuberculose rénale dans l'extension et la propagation de la tuberculose à l'appareil urinaire. La doctrine de la tuberculose descendante conduit naturellement à la pratique de la néphrectomie primitive. Je la pratique toutes les fois que les lésions vérifiées et reconnues unilatérales sont progressives et ne manifestent aucune tendance à l'amélioration sous l'influence du traitement général. J'ai vu des exemples anatomiques incontestables de tuberculoses rénales guéries avec oblitération de l'uretère. Ces cas dont je n'ai vu que trois exemples sont très rares, et en général la marche de la tuberculose est progressive. Aussi quand il y a des hémorragies, quand il y a des douleurs, ou seulement de la pyurie, mais à condition que les lésions soient unilatérales, je pratique la néphrectomie.

Pour la détermination de ces indications, j'ai recours au cathétérisme de l'uretère ; mais c'est surtout dans les cas douteux, alors qu'il y a doute sur la localisation, que le cathétérisme urétéral est utile et même nécessaire pour définir l'extension des lésions. Et chez un malade, que j'ai soigné il y a trois semaines, j'ai dû au seul cathétérisme de l'uretère de me montrer l'insuffisance fonctionnelle et l'altération commençante du congénère, et de m'éviter ainsi les accidents qui auraient inévitablement suivi la néphrectomie. Mais tout en reconnaissant les avantages et la nécessité de cette exploration dans certains cas, je dois reconnaître qu'il faut parfois s'en passer et qu'il est telle contre-indication du côté de la vessie ou de l'uretère qui la rendent impossible.

## QUELQUES REMARQUES SUR LA TUBERCULOSE URINAIRE

### par M. le docteur B. MOTZ,

de Pologne.

Depuis quelques années, messieurs, je poursuis des recherches sur l'évolution et les résultats éloignés du traitement de certaines lésions de l'appareil urinaire. Il y a un an, j'ai eu l'honneur de présenter à l'Association d'urologie les résultats éloignés de l'intervention chirurgicale dans les tumeurs de la vessie, où j'ai démontré que nous nous faisions beaucoup trop d'illusions sur ce sujet, c'est-à-dire que si les résultats immédiats sont excellents, les résultats éloignés sont absolument déplorables.

Je poursuis les mêmes recherches sur les tuberculoses urinaires. J'ai voulu voir ce que deviennent les malades atteints de la tuberculose urinaire qui arrivent en si grand nombre à la consultation et dans les salles de la clinique de mon maître, M. le professeur Guyon.

A mon grand regret, je ne suis pas en état de vous présenter des conclusions fermes sur ce sujet. Ce n'est pas le nombre de cas qui m'empêche de le faire, parce que, à ce moment, je possède dans mon dossier plus de 150 cas que je suis ; c'est la durée trop courte de la lésion tuberculeuse de la plupart des malades qui ne me permet pas de conclure.

J'ai fait des recherches pour retrouver les malades qui se sont présentés à la clinique il y a 6, 7, 8 ans, mais malheureusement le nombre de ceux que j'ai pu retrouver n'est pas assez grand, de telle façon que la plupart de mes malades ne sont atteints de la tuberculose que depuis 3 ou 4 ans.

Plusieurs années d'observations particulières des tuberculeux urinaires m'ont permis pourtant de faire quelques remarques qui sont en rapport intime avec le sujet que vous avez mis à l'ordre du jour de cette séance. Je me permets, par conséquent, de vous communiquer mes impressions personnelles et quelques faits qui se rattachent à la question de la guérison de la tuberculose urinaire.

Je m'arrêterai d'abord sur le point de départ et la localisation de la tuberculose urinaire.

Dans un rapport que vous avez devant vos yeux, le D^r Saxtorph, de Copenhague, affirme que la tuberculose urinaire « a comme origine

---

1. Motz. Les résultats éloignés de l'intervention chirurgicale dans les tumeurs de la vessie. Compte rendu de la quatrième session de l'Association d'Urologie, 1899.

toujours (ou presque toujours) un foyer tuberculeux pulmonaire plus ou moins ancien, souvent très ancien. « La confirmation de ce fait serait très importante parce qu'elle influencerait énormément la discussion du pronostic de la tuberculose urinaire. Heureusement l'histoire clinique des malades que nous avons examinés nous prouve que ce n'est qu'une simple hypothèse qui est, jusqu'à un certain point, en contradiction avec l'impression générale que produisent les tuberculeux urinaires ; dans la grande majorité des cas, il est tout à fait impossible de retrouver les traces de la tuberculose des autres organes chez nos tuberculeux urinaires.

La question du siège primitif de la tuberculose urinaire présente un intérêt capital. En examinant les malades à ce point de vue, j'ai constaté que sur 56 malades dont j'ai pu prendre personnellement les observations, la tuberculose a commencé dans les reins dans 41 cas. Dans 11 cas, elle m'a paru être d'origine vésicale et dans 4 cas, il m'a été impossible de déterminer le point de départ.

Ces 56 cas de la tuberculose urinaire ont été 22 fois précédés ou accompagnés de la tuberculose génitale.

Il n'est pas difficile, dans la grande majorité des cas, de déterminer le point de départ de la tuberculose urinaire. Nous n'avons qu'à interroger nos malades avec patience sur les premiers symptômes de leur maladie. Les uns vous diront que c'est déjà depuis longtemps qu'ils sont soignés pour une albuminurie, les autres qu'ils ont vu leur urine devenir trouble déjà depuis plusieurs mois avant l'apparition des symptômes qui les ont forcés de consulter le médecin. Chez les autres encore, vous serez frappé par la variabilité de la sensibilité vésicale. Ces malades, qui en apparence présentent les symptômes d'une inflammation vésicale qui se caractérise par la fréquence et la sensibilité anormale de leurs mictions, vous diront très souvent qu'il y a des moments où ils peuvent garder leurs urines 5, 6, 7 et quelquefois même 8 heures. La constatation de ce phénomène qui est extrêmement fréquent vous permettra d'affirmer que les symptômes que présente le malade ne sont pas dus à l'inflammation vésicale, mais que leur source est dans les reins, c'est-à-dire que vous êtes en présence de reflexes réno-vésicaux. Vous n'avez qu'à attendre l'accalmie dans l'état de votre malade et par l'examen cystoscopique vous confirmerez votre diagnostic.

Je vous signalerai encore un symptôme qui vous engagera très souvent à chercher du côté des reins chez les tuberculeux urinaires ; ce symptôme, c'est une douleur localisée au bout de la verge. Nous connaissons cette douleur chez certains malades atteints d'une lésion vésicale comme, par exemple, chez les calculeux, mais dans aucun maladie la localisation de la douleur au bout de la verge n'est aussi fréquente que dans la tuberculose rénale. Vous la trouverez au moins dans un tiers des cas.

Je passe maintenant à un chapitre de la tuberculose urinaire qui est peut-être le plus obscur. Je veux parler de la guérison spontanée de la tuberculose urinaire.

Je ne connais pas personnellement dans la littérature des observations bien prises. Il ne suffit pas de constater que les symptômes subjectifs aient disparu, il ne suffit pas que le malade se considère comme guéri, le microscope seul peut nous affirmer la guérison complète d'une inflammation urinaire.

En nous basant sur la pathologie générale, nous devons, *a priori*, jusqu'à un certain point, admettre que la guérison spontanée de la tuberculose urinaire doit exister. Nous connaissons, d'ailleurs, les résultats des autopsies de tuberculeux pulmonaires, où l'on a vu des cicatrices dans le tissu rénal, dues probablement à une lésion tuberculeuse guérie ; nous connaissons aussi une tendance à la guérison spontanée par la caséification complète du tissu rénal, mais il nous manque complètement jusqu'à présent, si je ne me trompe pas, des observations de la tuberculose rénale diagnostiquée cliniquement et complètement guérie sans aucune intervention chirurgicale.

Cette absence des observations de la guérison de la tuberculose urinaire est un signe certain de la gravité de la lésion. L'impression générale que produisent les tuberculeux urinaires est très mauvaise, le pronostic, par conséquent, est très défavorable ; il est, d'après moi, beaucoup plus défavorable que dans la tuberculose pulmonaire.

Parmi les malades que j'ai pu observer, je n'ai vu que 4 cas de la guérison complète de la tuberculose vésicale grave, dont j'ai communiqué 3 à la troisième session de la Société d'urologie. Dans un de ces cas, la malade a été soumise au curettage vésical ; dans les trois autres, les malades, en dehors du traitement général, ont suivi le traitement local par les instillations au sublimé (1/5000). L'examen histologique et bactériologique démontra l'absence de tous les éléments pathologiques.

Les malades qui ont été atteints de la tuberculose urinaire et qui se considèrent comme guéris sont au nombre de trois.

Un de ces malades, âgé de 35 ans, présenta, il y a 6 ans, les premiers symptômes de la tuberculose rénale. Au toucher rectal on a con-

1. Motz. Guérison complète de trois cas de tuberculose vésicale grave. C. R. de la 3ᵉ session de l'Association d'urologie, 1898.

staté la présence d'une prostatite tuberculeuse. L'examen bactériologique a démontré la présence de nombreux bacilles de Koch. Je l'ai
revu il y a quelques jours, en très bon état, se considérant comme
complètement guéri. Il n'urine qu'une fois la nuit et deux ou
trois fois le jour. Son urine est légèrement louche et contient encore
un certain nombre de leucocytes. L'examen bactériologique révéla la
présence des bactéries. Les recherches de bacilles de Koch ont donné
un résultat négatif.

Le deuxième malade, âgé de 44 ans, a été vu il y a 4 ans et on a
porté le diagnostic de la tuberculose génitale et rénale. Je l'ai revu au
mois de juillet de cette année en très bon état.

## DISCUSSION.

M. Lavaux (de Paris). — Je tiens à appuyer, au moins dans son
ensemble, l'excellent rapport de M. Saxtorph, surtout la première moitié
de ce rapport.

Il est évident que la question de la pathogénie de la tuberculose urinaire domine tout ce débat. Je vois avec plaisir que l'opinion que je
soutiens depuis plus de dix ans, après Conheim et Cayla, est aujourd'hui
à peu près unanimement admise. C'est bien par le rein que débute
l'infection tuberculeuse dans la grande majorité des cas.

Eh bien, ramenons la discussion, qui a trop souvent dévié, dans cette
séance, sur son véritable terrain. Tous les distingués orateurs que nous
venons d'entendre préconisent la néphrectomie *précoce* dans le traitement de la tuberculose rénale. Est-ce logique? Comment! Voilà des
malades prédisposés à l'infection tuberculeuse; on admet qu'il existe
chez eux préalablement, dans un point de l'organisme, un foyer tuberculeux primitif, et dès que la tuberculose a atteint l'un des reins, on vient
nous proposer d'admettre que la néphrectomie est immédiatement indiquée. Qui nous prouve que chez ces tuberculeux, qui conservent quelque
part un foyer de tuberculose et que la suppression d'un rein va mettre
dans un état d'infériorité physiologique manifeste, qui nous prouve, je
le répète, que l'infection tuberculeuse ne va pas envahir à son tour le
rein considéré jusque-là comme sain? Dans quelques semaines peut-être,
dans quelques mois, un an ou plus, ne constaterons-nous pas, chez ces
prédisposés, une nouvelle tuberculose urinaire?

Je m'attendais à voir une proposition aussi hardie appuyée sur de
nombreux faits cliniques probants, sur de nombreux cas de néphrectomies pratiquées dans ces conditions et suivies de guérisons constatées
cinq ans, dix ans, quinze ans après l'opération. Or, rien de semblable
n'a été apporté au Congrès.

Il y a une autre raison qui me fait rejeter la néphrectomie *précoce*.
C'est la puissance actuelle du traitement médical employé seul ou aidé
de la petite chirurgie lorsque la tuberculose vésicale s'ajoute à la tuberculose rénale.

M. Saxtorph rejette l'emploi du nitrate d'argent dans le traitement de la cystite tuberculeuse. Sur ce point, il faut préciser. S'il s'agit de solutions fortes, de solutions caustiques de nitrate d'argent, d'instillations par exemple, je suis de l'avis du distingué rapporteur : la contre-indication est formelle. Mais s'il s'agit de solutions faibles, au millième, ou même à 1/2000 et si l'on a soin de les injecter, *sans sonde*, après anesthésie directe de la muqueuse des voies urinaires inférieures, le nitrate d'argent peut donner dans certains cas d'excellents résultats. J'aurai du reste l'occasion, mardi prochain, de revenir sur cette intéressante question. J'ai publié un certain nombre d'observations qui prouvent combien sont rares aujourd'hui, aussi bien pour les reins que pour la vessie, les véritables indications des interventions sanglantes dans la tuberculose urinaire.

M. Casper (de Berlin). — Dans la tuberculose des reins il n'y a pas de meilleur moyen pour faire un diagnostic sûr et précoce que le cathétérisme des uretères. J'ai publié le premier cas dans lequel j'ai réussi à trouver le bacille de Koch dans l'urine prise d'un rein.

Pour faire un diagnostic précis, il faut comparer l'urine des deux côtés recueillie par le cathétérisme des uretères et examiner trois points : quantité des urines; concentration moléculaire, quantité de sucre éliminé après injection de fluoridzine. La concentration moléculaire est toujours diminuée du côté malade; diminuée aussi l'élimination du sucre. Je trouve que le bleu de méthylène ne donne pas de renseignements aussi sûrs que l'épreuve par la fluoridzine. Il y a entre les deux substances cette différence : que le bleu est éliminé par les reins comme beaucoup d'autres substances; mais le sucre est produit par le rein, et prouve ainsi la fonction du rein. La quantité de fluoridzine injectée étant de 5 milligrammes, il y a plus d'un gramme de sucre éliminé. Cet examen m'a permis d'éviter une néphrectomie qui aurait été fâcheuse chez une malade ayant une hématurie rénale droite, et chez qui je reconnus que le rein gauche était aussi malade.

M. Mankiewicz (de Berlin). — Je ne trouve pas que dans la tuberculose vésicale la douleur et la polliaturie sont améliorées et guéries par les lavages boriqués. Les lavages ne sont pas tolérés; ils produisent de la distension, de la douleur et des hémorragies. L'évacuation des résidus vésicaux serait utile, mais on doit introduire le moins possible d'instruments dans une vessie tuberculeuse. Le meilleur médicament est le sublimé en solution variant de 1/1000 à 1/10 000, en installation de 5 centimètres cubes, suivant la méthode de Guyon, de Casper.

M. Nicolich (de Trieste). — J'ai opéré six malades de tuberculose rénale, toutes par la néphrectomie, avec un décès et cinq guérisons. Je suis convaincu de l'utilité du cathétérisme urétéral que j'ai pratiqué dans tous les cas où il m'a été possible de le faire.

Il ne faut pas trop prolonger l'opération pour faire l'urétérotomie, même si le canal est tuberculeux; une malade opérée il y a dix-huit mois se porte très bien et n'a aucune fistule quoique j'aie été obligé de laisser en place l'uretère tuberculeux.

## QUATRIÈME SÉANCE

## SAMEDI 4 AOUT 1900

*à deux heures et demie.*

### Présidence de M. le professeur KÜMMEL,

de Hambourg.

*Communications diverses :*

## VESSIE

## DRAINAGE DE LA VESSIE PAR L'IRRIGATION CONTINUE APRÈS LA TAILLE SUS-PUBIENNE (CYSTOSTOMIE)

### par le docteur LE CLERC DANDOY

de Bruxelles.

Messieurs,

· J'ai l'honneur de vous exposer un système de drainage vésical après a taille hypogastrique, système que j'ai eu l'occasion d'appliquer quatre fois et qui m'a donné d'excellents résultats.

Permettez-moi d'abord de vous dire les motifs qui m'ont fait préfé-rer cette méthode au procédé généralement employé, c'est-à-dire le drainage au moyen du double syphon du professeur Guyon. Il est des cas, je pense, où cette dernière méthode ne suffit pas à remplir le but qu'on se propose, de plus elle expose parfois à des inconvénients que l'on peut résumer comme suit ;

Dans la grande majorité des cas, l'urine de l'opéré devient rapide-ment purulente ; en dépit des lavages antiseptiques répétés, son odeur est ammoniacale, fétide ; pour peu que le drainage ne marche pas régu-lièrement, le malade est souillé d'urine nauséabonde, les pansements sont fort désagréables à renouveler. De plus il peut se faire que le tube syphon cesse de fonctionner, soit pour un motif inexplicable, soit qu'un caillot bouche la lumière des drains, et la chose arrive facilement dans les tailles faites pour néoplasmes. L'urine, dès lors, se fait issue directement par la fistule, elle peut s'infiltrer entre les couches de tissus, et compromet la réunion immédiate des sutures posées au voisinage de la plaie.

D'autre part, toujours à cause de ses propiétés septiques, l'urine peut être cause d'abcès, d'infiltration, — fait assurément rare, mais signalé — ; une péritonite enfin pourrait, dans certains cas de taille difficile, être la conséquence d'une lésion de la séreuse exposée au contact dangereux de l'urine.

Un moyen fort simple parait tout indiqué pour prévenir ces complications : c'est de placer une sonde à demeure dans le canal de l'urètre et d'éviter de cette manière l'accumulation des urines dans la vessie.

Mais s'il est vrai que ce moyen réussit complétement dans les cas où la conformation anatomique de l'urètre prostatique est normale, il manque entièrement son but lorsqu'il s'adresse à des cas où les rapports sont changés (tumeur vésicale, hypertrophie de la prostate). La sonde a demeure est d'ailleurs une nouvelle cause d'infection si son séjour dans le canal doit se prolonger.

L'ennemi à craindre, dans l'opération de la taille sus-pubienne, est donc l'urine. Favoriser son élimination au fur et à mesure de son arrivée dans la vessie, l'empêcher de s'infecter, même d'une manière relative, en un mot soustraire les tissus, la plaie opératoire, le péritoine à son contact dangereux : tel doit être l'objectif du chirurgien.

Nous croyons l'avoir réalisé de manière fort simple en utilisant, pour assurer l'élimination de l'urine, un courant de sérum artificiel, pénétrant par le canal de l'urètre (au moyen d'une sonde de Nélaton) et ressortant de la vessie par les tubes de Guyon-Perrier. Le dispositif est le suivant : un grand injecteur d'Esmark (6 litres) est placé au pied du lit du patient à faible hauteur de celui-ci. Il est rempli d'eau salée (8°/₀₀) et stérilisée, que l'on maintient à une température tiède, grâce à un petit brûleur placé sous l'injecteur. Un robinet permet au sérum de s'écouler lentement.

L'injecteur est en rapport avec la vessie par sonde de Nélaton, ou mieux de Pezzer. Après avoir irrigué la vessie, le sérum s'échappe, comme nous le disions plus haut, par les drains de Guyon-Perrier, qui seront suffisamment longs pour remplir efficacement leur rôle de tubes-siphons.

Tel est le système de drainage que nous avons appliqué à deux premiers cas dont je vais résumer l'observation.

Obs. I. — D. Lambert, 60 ans, employé de chemin de fer. Hérédité : Père mort subitement à 50 ans. Mère morte à 85 ans. 6 frères morts. A eu 8 enfants dont 2 sont morts en bas-âge; les autres sont bien portants.

Depuis deux ans, le malade a uriné du sang à trois ou quatre reprises; ces hématuries ont été abondantes et le patient, à son entrée à l'hôpital — service de M. le professeur De Smet, — est dans un état d'affaissement très grand.

A l'examen de l'appareil urinaire, on constate que la vessie remonte jusqu'à 3 doigts sous l'ombilic; les mictions sont fréquentes, mais elles ne vident qu'incomplètement la vessie; les urines sont franchement sanglantes. Par l'examen cystoscopique, on constate l'existence d'une tumeur villeuse siégeant au pourtour du col vésical. On décide de faire la taille sus-pubienne.

Opération le 7 novembre 1899. Incision transversale de Trendelenbourg comprenant la peau, les muscles droits, la vessie. Le néoplasme est implanté largement sur le bas-fond vésical et au niveau du col, ce qui explique la rétention urinaire. Il est excessivement friable et on ne peut songer à l'enlever. Par arrachement, par curettage, on en extirpe la majeure partie. L'hémorragie abondante qui succède à cette manœuvre est arrêtée assez facilement par un tamponnement à la gaze iodoformée. Suture incomplète de la vessie, les tubes siphons de Guyon-Perrier ayant été fixés dans l'espace resté libre de la plaie. Puis suture des muscles droits au moyen d'un seul fil conduit de la manière suivante : il pénètre dans le bout inférieur de l'un des muscles sectionnés, ressort par le bout supérieur du même côté; puis il pénètre par le fragment supérieur du muscle opposé et ressort enfin par le fragment inférieur du même côté. Des petits fils complètent cette suture musculaire. La plaie cutanée est réunie à la soie.

Une sonde de Pezzer mise à demeure dans l'urètre, est reliée à un irrigateur d'Esmark contenant du sérum à 37 degrés; l'écoulement du liquide entraîne immédiatement le sang épanché dans la vessie.

Le lavage au sérum est continué sans arrêt pendant 8 jours. Les suites opératoires ne présentent rien de particulier. Pas de température. La réunion se fait *per primam* le long de la plaie cutanée; aucune suppuration au niveau du méat hypogastrique.

Au huitième jour, on supprime l'irrigation continue, les drains seuls sont conservés. La sonde à demeure avait été tolérée très facilement et n'avait provoqué aucune sécrétion.

L'état du malade, à partir de ce moment, va en s'améliorant; on remplace les drains par une sonde de Pezzer à pavillon plat autour duquel les téguments forment un anneau qui s'oppose complètement au suintement de l'urine. Celle-ci est recueillie dans un urinal fixé au membre inférieur.

L'analyse miscroscopique d'un fragment de la tumeur a démontré qu'il s'agissait d'un épithélioma.

Le malade a quitté l'hôpital le 17 février 1900. Sa santé s'est considérablement améliorée; il garde constamment à l'hypogastre la sonde de Pezzer qui constitue un moyen occlusif parfait. La miction n'a plus jamais été sanguinolente, sauf pendant un jour où l'on avait obturé la sonde et où le malade avait eu avec beaucoup de peine, quelques mictions volontaires.

L'aspect de la cicatrice est net; il n'existe aucune éventration. La méthode palliative de traitement semble avoir atteint parfaitement son but dans ce cas.

Obs. II. — Marie X..., ménagère, 52 ans. Rien dans l'hérédité, aucun antécédent personnel. Mariée depuis le mois de juin 1895; a toujours été bien réglée. Stigmates d'hytérie évidents. Souffre de la vessie depuis le mois de juin 1898; le début de l'affection fut marqué par les douleurs au commencement de la miction. Les urines étaient claires au dire de la malade. Plusieurs traitements furent essayés sans succès (lavages divers, instillations).

Au cystoscope, lorsque la malade vint nous consulter, on voyait une zone rouge, s'étendant sur le bas-fond de la vessie, à droite, en une bandelette longue de 2 à 5 centimètres. Par-ci par-là existaient quelques foyers de cystite bien circonscrits.

Pendant le courant de l'année 1899, nous pratiquâmes deux curettages vésicaux qui furent suivis, surtout le premier, de guérison complète, mais qui ne se maintint pas. Les douleurs reparurent plus intenses vers le mois de septembre 1899, elles se manifestaient sous la forme d'épreintes, de ténesme; le nombre des mictions s'accrut considérablement et les urines devinrent troubles. La malade réclama à toute force une intervention radicale, et, en présence des symptômes persistants de cystite douloureuse, la taille sus-pubienne fut pratiquée le 17 décembre 1899 dans l'espoir d'explorer aisément la vessie. Mais, l'organe n'ayant pu être distendu, il fallut, pour pouvoir l'inciser, se guider sur le bec d'un cathéter préalablement introduit par le canal de l'urètre. La vessie fut ouverte dans la profondeur, derrière la symphyse.

Malgré ces complications du manuel opératoire, les suites furent très simples, grâce au système de drainage établi comme dans l'observation I. Les douleurs disparurent immédiatement après l'opération et, chose curieuse, ne se montrèrent plus, tant que le courant de sérum artificiel fut maintenu; on irrigua ainsi la vessie pendant 5 semaines consécutives, tout arrêt du courant s'accompagnant des plus vives douleurs.

Actuellement, la situation de la malade, au point de vue douleur, est considérablement améliorée; il persiste une fistulette sus-pubienne; la patiente peut garder une sonde à demeure sans en éprouver la moindre gêne. Nous nous proposons de fermer la fistulette et avons bon espoir de pouvoir enlever d'ici peu la sonde à demeure.

Voici les avantages que nous avions reconnus à ce procédé :

1° Il n'existe absolument pas de fermentation urinaire ; l'odeur du patient est nulle ; aucun caillot ne peut se former dans la vessie ; le drainage est assuré (avantage incontestable dans les cystostomies pour néoplasmes ;

2° La sonde urétrale est parfaitement tolérée; aucune trace de pus n'est visible au méat après le quatrième ou cinquième jour si l'on a pris soin de stériliser la sonde à demeure avant son application et de laver convenablement l'urètre ;

5° Les dangers d'infection urineuse et d'infiltration sont écartés d'une manière complète ;

4° Les sutures au voisinage de la fistule se réunissent par première intention.

Le procédé que je viens de décrire a été modifié à propos d'une taille faite comme traitement palliatif d'une vaste tumeur ostéosarcomateuse de la prostate.

Le drainage vésical fut réalisé de la manière suivante :

Un réservoir métallique R contenant une dizaine de litres de sérum artificiel (chlorure de sodium à 8°/₀₀) chauffé à une température convenable, est disposé au pied du lit de l'opéré. Le liquide s'échappe par un tube en Y renversé, lequel est en rapport par une de ses branches avec l'un des tubes de Guyon-Perrier placés dans la vessie ; l'autre est relié à une trombe à eau, en verre (trombe de Geissler) (T) dont le tube d'appel est rattaché à l'autre drain vésical. Quelques robinets (r) permettent de régler le courant que l'on entretient pendant un temps variable (4-6 jours).

Voici l'observation résumée de la première application de ce système.

Obs. III. — D. Alphonse, 65 ans ; typographe. Syphilis à l'âge de 25 ans ; aurait souffert de trois atteintes de blennorragie il y a une vingtaine d'années ; le malade en aurait été bien guéri, mais les urines seraient restées troubles depuis lors.

Depuis plusieurs années, sa santé s'est altérée, il a présenté à différentes reprises des symptômes de prostatisme, de la rétention, des hématuries ; et depuis trois mois la miction volontaire a disparu d'une manière complète.

Il entre à l'hôpital Saint-Pierre, service de M. le professeur De Smet, le 22 février 1900.

A ce moment, nous relevons les symptômes suivants : Rétention complète, le cathétérisme évacue 500 centimètres cubes d'urine infecte dans laquelle le microscope décèle des globules rouges et blancs, tous les éléments du pus et quelques cylindres hyalins. Par le toucher rectal, on sent que la prostate a les dimensions d'une tête de fœtus à terme ; on ne peut atteindre les limites supérieures de la tumeur ; vers la droite, elle est intimement soudée au sacrum ; cet os et la prostate semblent ne faire qu'un tout avec lui.

La tumeur est cause non seulement de rétention urinaire, mais encore de constipation opiniâtre depuis deux mois. Le traitement consiste en cathétérisme régulier et lavages de la vessie à l'eau boriquée et au nitrate d'argent. Au bout d'un mois l'état vésical s'améliora quelque peu ; les hématuries disparurent presque complètement, mais les urines ne s'éclaircirent guère.

Le 28 mars, nous pratiquâmes une cystostomie sus-pubienne qui fut des plus simples ; on fixa la vessie par 6 points de suture à la paroi abdominale et le système de drainage décrit plus haut fut appliqué immédiatement après l'opération et permit de constater la rapidité de la cicatrisation, l'absence de toute odeur urineuse. Aucune élévation de température.

Le drainage fut continué pendant six jours ; on put alors enlever les fils, la cicatrisation était parfaite. Les suites n'ont rien présenté de particulier. Le malade a quitté l'hôpital le 15 mai, à sa demande, en proie aux progrès de la cachexie.

La dernière observation a trait à une cystite tuberculeuse ;

Obs. IV. — G. Joseph, 26 ans, ouvrier agricole. Entre à l'hôpital Saint Pierre, service de M. le professeur De Smet, le 10 mars 1900. Hérédité n'offre rien de particulier.

Le début de la maladie remonte au mois de septembre 1899, il fut marqué par la fréquence des mictions s'accompagnant d'hématurie terminale ; le malade à ce moment devait uriner toutes les demi-heures, mais les envies se rapprochèrent de plus en plus, et en mars, époque de l'entrée à l'hôpital, le patient urinait 190 à 250 fois par vingt-quatre heures. Les douleurs, le ténesme étaient constants, le sommeil faisait complètement défaut depuis quatre mois.

Le diagnostic de tuberculose vésicale s'imposait par exclusion ; il existait du reste des noyaux caractéristiques dans la prostate ; du côté de la poitrine principalement à gauche, on pouvait relever des symptômes manifestes de tuberculose. L'examen des urines ne décela pas de bacilles de Koch ; dans l'expectoration, au contraire, ils existaient en grand nombre.

En présence des douleurs intolérables éprouvées par le malade au niveau de la vessie et du canal de l'urètre, douleurs telles qu'il était impossible de pratiquer le cathétérisme, et que l'application des calmants locaux (iodoforme, gaïacol) n'était même pas tolérée, par suite de la faible capacité de la vessie, nous avons espéré soulager ce malade en lui faisant subir l'opération de la taille et en nous efforçant de traiter *directement* le réservoir urinaire, sans passer par le canal.

La taille hyppogastrique fut pratiquée le 6 avril ; elle présenta de très grandes difficultés, par suite de l'impossibilité absolue de distendre la vessie, malgré une narcose profonde. La vessie dut être incisée directement derrière le pubis, sur un catéther métallique introduit par l'urètre. Il ne fut pas possible d'attirer les lèvres de la plaie vésicale jusqu'au niveau de la peau et trois points de suture furent placés non sans peine (2 latéraux, 1 supérieur).

C'est dans ce cas que nous devions craindre les conséquences d'un drainage insuffisant, c'est-à-dire la péritonite et l'infiltration de l'urine dans le petit bassin. Le drainage avec aspiration nous mit certainement à l'abri de ces complications et les résultats immédiats de notre intervention furent excellents, c'est-à-dire que le malade cessa complètement de souffrir ; le double courant de sérum artificiel le soulagea à ce point qu'il demandait à ce qu'il fût entretenu d'une manière permanente ; de plus, ce mode de drainage, en écartant les dangers que je signalais plus haut, permit aux sutures de se consolider rapidement. Le courant fut entretenu pendant un mois et mit fin, pendant ce temps, aux douleurs.

L'aggravation des symptômes pulmonaires, l'amaigrissement progressif du malade, l'apparition de pus abondant dans les urines, nous empêchèrent de compléter le traitement vésical. Il semble du reste qui l'intervention ait donné un coup de fouet à la tuberculose. Le malade ne tarda pas à tomber dans un état de cachexie et mourut le 25 juillet.

On put, à l'autopsie, constater les lésions avancées de tuberculose dans les 2 poumons, et des lésions de néphrite tuberculeuse ascendante à droite. Quant à la vessie, elle présentait des ulcérations multiples et profondes, sa capacité ne dépassait pas 20 centimètres cubes.

Telles sont, messieurs, forcément résumées, les observations que j'avais à vous présenter.

Un point sur lequel je tiens encore à attirer votre attention, c'est que le drainage avec courant constant de sérum artificiel est extrêmement bien supporté par des vessies irritables, tuberculeuses, lesquelles, ainsi que vous le savez, tolérent difficilement le contact des drains ordinaires.

---

# LA SUTURE TOTALE DE LA VESSIE APRES LA TAILLE HYPOGASTRIQUE

## par M. V. CARLIER,

professeur agrégé à la Faculté de Médecine, à Lille.

Bien que la suture totale de la vessie après la taille hypogastrique constitue, à l'heure actuelle, un procédé chirurgical adopté par un grand nombre de chirurgiens, il m'a paru opportun de reprendre, devant le Congrès, l'étude de cette intéressante question.

Tous ceux qui ont assisté aux premiers essais de la suture totale se rappellent encore avec quelle hésitation on la pratiquait. On choisissait les cas pour l'appliquer, et on la déconseillait pour peu qu'on doutât de l'asepsie de la paroi vésicale et de son contenu.

Dans ces dix dernières années, la question s'est heureusement modifiée. La suture totale a bénéficié des grands progrès accomplis en chirurgie urinaire et beaucoup de chirurgiens ont à leur actif une série de cas heureux de fermeture complète de la vessie après la taille hypogastrique.

On se préoccupe moins de savoir si la paroi vésicale est saine ou non, si le milieu est aseptique ou septique, et les chirurgiens ont actuellement recours à la suture totale de la vessie chez des malades qui, il y a dix ans, ne leur eussent point paru justiciables de ce brillant procédé opératoire. Tellement il est vrai que la vessie, une fois ouverte, ne demande qu'à se fermer (Guyon).

Ce qui le prouve, c'est ce qui se passe chez l'enfant, où les plaies non suturées de la vessie aboutissent si rapidement à une entière et solide cicatrisation ; c'est encore ce qui se passe chez la femme, dont on a tant de peine à maintenir ouverte la plaie de la vessie après une taille vésico-vaginale. D'autre part, lorsqu'après une taille hypogastrique on suture partiellement la plaie vésicale en ne laissant que l'espace nécessaire pour la mise à demeure des tubes syphons, il est de règle de voir réussir ces sutures partielles, quel que soit le milieu dans lequel on opère.

En réalité, la seule condition indispensable pour le succès d'une suture totale, c'est d'assurer le bon drainage de la vessie. Or, avec l'emploi des sondes de Pezzer ou de Malécot, ce drainage s'effectue ordinairement d'une façon parfaite, du moins toutes les fois qu'on n'a pas à compter avec une hémorragie vésicale. C'est l'hémorragie qui compromet la suture, aussi une hémorragie abondante me paraît-elle être la seule contre-indication à l'emploi de la suture ; il y a longtemps d'ailleurs que M. Guyon a insisté sur ce point.

S'il est en effet possible, au moyen de petits lavages fréquemment répétés, d'empêcher l'obstruction de la sonde par des mucosités provenant d'une vessie infectée, par contre, il est plus malaisé de débarrasser la sonde et la vessie des caillots sanguins lorsque la vessie saigne, et malgré une étroite surveillance, le malade sera dès lors exposé aux douleurs et aux dangers de la rétention.

C'est ce qui se produisit chez un malade de 60 ans que j'ai opéré, il y a six mois, d'un néoplasme vésical. Malgré la persistance d'un léger écoulement sanguin que je croyais insignifiant, je terminai l'opération par une suture totale. Or, la vessie saigna pendant les deux jours suivants, et le malade nécessita une surveillance de tous les instants pour le bon fonctionnement de la sonde. Si ma suture ne lâcha pas, en revanche l'opéré ressentit de vives douleurs dont il eût été préservé si j'avais eu recours chez lui au drainage hypogastrique.

La suture réussit toujours chez l'enfant, elle réussit presque toujours chez la femme, elle réussit très souvent chez l'adulte.

La suture réussit toujours chez l'enfant pour les raisons suivantes : la vessie de l'enfant ne saigne pas, la suture est facile à exécuter chez lui, enfin, la paroi vésicale, ordinairement peu altérée, se prête admirablement à la réunion par première intention. Si l'on considère d'autre part toutes les difficultés inhérentes au drainage hypogastrique dans le jeune âge, on aboutit à cette conclusion qu'il faut toujours tenter la suture totale chez l'enfant. J'y ai eu recours plusieurs fois, et toujours avec un succès complet, chez des enfants calculeux dont la pierre était trop volumineuse pour pouvoir recourir à la lithotritie.

C'est sans doute à la brièveté de l'urètre de la femme qu'il faut attribuer la rapidité de la cicatrisation des plaies de la vessie dans le sexe féminin.

Les incisions sus-pubiennes résultant d'une taille hypogastrique se cicatrisent plus rapidement encore chez elle que les incisions vésico-vaginales, et c'est pour les cas de suture totale chez la femme que pourrait se discuter l'utilité de la sonde à demeure. Nous reviendrons dans un instant sur ce point.

J'ai dit que la suture totale est très souvent suivie de succès chez l'homme, si l'on a le soin de n'y pas recourir lorsqu'on a à craindre un saignement intra-vésical. Il faut encore excepter certains malades profondément infectés, soit par un calcul, soit par un néoplasme, et chez lesquels l'opération n'a de chances de succès que si elle est rapidement exécutée. Hormis en cas, il m'a paru que les malades ne pouvaient que bénéficier d'une occlusion complète et immédiate de la vessie.

J'ai toujours employé la suture à deux étages. Lors de mes premières opérations, je faisais un premier plan de sutures au catgut, et un second plan à la soie fine et à la Lembert. Depuis quelque temps je fais les deux plans de sutures au catgut, bien que l'emploi de la soie ne m'ait occasionné aucun ennui. Lorsque j'ai affaire à une vessie saine, je comprends dans la suture toute l'épaisseur de la paroi vésicale, y compris la muqueuse. Si la vessie est infectée, je fais la suture en en exceptant la muqueuse. Ainsi comprise, cette suture, qui est couramment employée à Necker, est remarquable par sa simplicité d'exécution, et je me suis souvent demandé pour quelles raisons MM. Jonnesco et Razimonsky ont cru devoir préconiser des sutures très compliquées, telles qu'ils les ont décrites dans des mémoires dont la lecture n'a pu entraîner ma conviction.

J'ai toujours pris soin, en suturant la paroi abdominale, de laisser un petit drain à l'angle inférieur de la plaie. Ce drain de sûreté doit être dirigé vers la cavité de Retzius, qu'il ne fait qu'effleurer. Sauf incident fâcheux, ce drain doit être enlevé le troisième ou quatrième jour après l'opération. Bien que je croie ce petit drainage inutile chez l'enfant, j'estime cependant qu'il donne une telle sécurité qu'il vaut mieux ne pas renoncer à son emploi.

Il me reste un dernier point à examiner, celui de la sonde à demeure après la suture totale de la vessie. Jusqu'ici j'ai toujours eu recours à la sonde à demeure ; je crois cependant qu'elle n'est pas toujours nécessaire. Je suis décidé à ne plus l'employer chez les enfants, qui la supportent parfois assez mal, ainsi que chez la femme. En tout cas, il m'a paru que le séjour de la sonde à demeure pouvait être considérablement réduit.

Son emploi, pour être utile et surtout pour n'être pas nuisible, nécessite une grande surveillance. J'ai opéré en janvier 1900, pour un minuscule polype de la vessie, un malade de trente-cinq ans. J'avais mis à demeure une sonde de Pezzer. Dans la seconde nuit qui suivit l'opération, par suite des mouvements du malade qui déplacèrent la bouteille-urinal, la sonde s'infléchit sur elle-même et fit un obstacle absolu à l'écoulement des urines. La vessie se remplit au point que le malade dut faire de grands efforts pour uriner et réussit à uriner entre la sonde et l'urètre. Bien que ces efforts se soient renouvelés plusieurs fois dans la nuit, la suture de la vessie n'en avait point souffert. Il est bien évident que ce malade eût couru moins de risques s'il n'avait pas eu de sonde à demeure.

Le même fait s'est produit chez une jeune fille de 26 ans que j'ai opérée en 1897 pour une tuberculose de la vessie. Pendant la nuit, la sonde mal fixée sortit de la vessie et son extrémité resta dans l'urètre en y formant bouchon. A la visite du lendemain, je trouvai la vessie très distendue par l'urine, mais la suture n'avait pas lâché et le pansement n'était nullement souillé.

Ces deux cas prouvent tout simplement qu'on peut se passer de la sonde à demeure chez une certaine catégorie de malades, mais il ne faut pas se dissimuler que ces malades-là doivent être choisis avec un grand discernement. Quoi qu'il en soit, lorsque je ne mettrai pas de sonde à demeure, je sonderai mes opérés toutes les trois ou quatre heures, de façon à éviter la distension de la vessie.

---

## DE LA CYSTORRHAPHIE TOTALE

### par M. DELAGRAMMATICA,

de Constantinople.

Messieurs,

La cystorrhaphie totale qui a fait de la taille hypogastrique une des plus belles opérations de la chirurgie urinaire n'est pas encore entrée dans le domaine de la chirurgie courante. Malgré son innocuité démontrée par l'expérimentation et constatée cliniquement depuis longtemps déjà, nombre de confrères hésitent ou ils négligent d'en faire profiter leurs malades. Mais si le drainage hypogastrique de la vessie offre une sécurité incontestable, il importe cependant à plusieurs points de vue de tenir compte de l'avantage capital que présente la fermeture immédiate de la vessie, à savoir que par son fait la guérison arrive plus vite et le séjour du malade à l'hôpital est notablement abrégé.

Je ne vais pas passer en revue tous les procédés techniques préconisés jusqu'à nos jours. Je crois du reste que la question de leur choix est d'un intérêt secondaire, que le succès de la suture vésicale dépend principalement d'un bon drainage du réservoir urinaire par l'urètre et que c'est la défectuosité de ce drainage jointe à une suture mal faite qui ont peut-être fait naître les procédés en question. En tout cas, le plus simple parmi eux, c'est-à-dire la suture des lèvres opératoires sur un seul plan, a donné à bien d'autres comme à moi-même de bons résultats, aussi bons que les autres procédés plus compliqués. Pourvu que l'on évite l'adossement de deux muqueuses autant qu'on peut le faire, surtout chez l'enfant, et qu'on ferme soigneusement la vessie; et cette suture réussira non seulement lorsque les urines seront aseptiques, mais aussi lorsqu'il y aura cystite. Ainsi dans deux cas de calculs vésicaux que j'ai dû extraire par la taille hypogastrique, dans lesquels j'ai pratiqué la fermeture immédiate et complète de la vessie sur un seul plan, celle-ci malgré la cystite existante et un état général mauvais chez mes malades, réussit dans tous les deux. Il importe même de noter qu'un de ces malades a eu le jour de l'opération une congestion pulmonaire, laquelle avec des étapes successives a évolué pendant dix jours et envahi la totalité presque de ses poumons, ce qui nous a inspiré de sérieuses craintes pour sa vie.

Un second plan de suture constituerait en cas de cystite un surcroît de précaution, mais il ne sera, il me semble, indispensable, que lorsque la vessie, par le fait d'une inflammation chronique et intense ou d'une sclérose sénile, sera profondément altérée et sa vitalité bien compromise. Mais dans ce cas une autre question, celle d'opportunité même de la suture totale de la vessie, doit être examinée pour ne pas aller ainsi au-devant d'un échec certain. Quant aux espèces microbiennes causes de la cystite, elles constitueraient *a priori* un facteur important à cet égard, et il serait intéressant par exemple de savoir si une anaérobie, ou une aérobie décomposant rapidement l'urée, comme le proteus, font échouer plus fréquemment que les microbes ordinaires la suture totale de la vessie; mais il me semble qu'en pratique on peut ne pas en tenir compte, car la présence de ces microbes constatée, une sonde à demeure, ou bien un traitement plus simple de la cystite, modifieront rapidement le milieu vésical dans lequel on va agir.

Dans la question spéciale de la cystorrhaphie totale, la septicité donc de l'urine, prise isolément, ne joue pas le rôle prépondérant que l'on serait porté, par des considérations théoriques, à lui assigner, et de ce fait à première vue paradoxal, mais qui trouve son explication dans l'extraordinaire vitalité de la vessie, devaient être frappés ceux surtout qui drainent systématiquement la vessie par l'hypogastre, car la suture partielle de la vessie que nécessite ce drainage n'échoue jamais comme on le sait. On aurait pu concilier la théorie et la clinique en admettant que dans ce cas la vessie drainée par les tubes-siphons resterait constamment vide dans l'hypothèse que cet instrument aspire l'urine de la vessie, comme il aspire la solution boriquée pendant les lavages, à mesure que les uretères l'y déversent. S'il en était ainsi la plaie vésicale suturée serait restée à l'abri d'un contact immédiat avec l'urine septique. Mais il évident que la vessie drainée par ces tubes, tout en étant rétractée, reste pleine d'une certaine quantité d'urine; car ces tubes en dehors des lavages se comportent comme des simples drains, et car leur jeu de siphon ne pourrait continuer qu'à la condition que les uretères débitassent autant d'urine qu'il en peut sortir par ces tubes.

Il est donc hors de doute que ce ne sera pas l'infection vésicale qui empêchera à elle seule le succès de la suture totale de la vessie, dans un cas donné, mais bien sa mise en tension, et c'est celle-ci qu'il faut tâcher toujours de prévenir par l'emploi d'une sonde d'un calibre suffisant, que l'on tiendra perméable, par des petits lavages vésicaux plus ou moins fréquents suivant l'abondance du pus sécrété par la vessie.

Mais s'il est vrai que la vessie oppose une résistance vraiment extraordinaire contre la plupart des micro-organismes pathogènes, je ne néglige pas cependant de mettre la plaie vésicale dans des conditions d'une asepsie rigoureuse, en écartant toutes les causes possibles d'une contamination de la cavité prévésicale presque fatale en cas de cystite. Pour atteindre ce but, en dehors des moyens d'asepsie usuels, je prends soin de vider par la sonde préalablement la vessie enflammée avant de l'inciser; car il est douteux que le liquide qui garnit la vessie, et qui, à son ouverture, viendrait inonder, sans cette précaution, le champ opératoire, puisse être, malgré les lavages réitérés, absolument aseptique. Pour ce faire je saisis la vessie avec une pince à griffes et je dis à l'aide d'ouvrir alors le robinet de la sonde en place. Lorsque la vessie a été totalement vidée, je la soulève avec ma pince et pendant que l'aide en déprime le fond au moyen de la sonde métallique laissée en place à cet effet, j'y plonge mon bistouri sans crainte et je prolonge mon incision sur la longueur voulue. De cette façon je n'ai plus de liquide à éponger à l'ouverture de la vessie et celle-ci étant à sec je suis en mesure en écartant les lèvres de l'incision d'inspecter sa cavité et d'y intervenir de suite s'il y a lieu.

La garniture de la vessie avec de l'air stérilisé présente, elle aussi, les mêmes avantages, mais je préfère son évacuation pure et simple comme plus expéditive et décongestionnant simultanément l'organe. C'est ainsi que j'agirai môm si j'ai affaire à une vessie rétractée, car une vessie vide doit *a priori* se laisser attirer en longueur pour être incisée plus facilement qu'une vessie pleine.

Plus que la cystite, la cautérisation de la vessie est regardée par beaucoup d'auteurs comme une contre-indication formelle à la fermeture complète de la vessie.

S'il est vrai que la plupart des cystites rebelles contre lesquelles on est finalement obligé d'intervenir chirurgicalement et de cautériser les lésions, causes de leur ténacité, demandent un long repos et exigent par conséquent le drainage hypogastrique, nous savons cependant qu'il en est d'autres, à lésions peu profondes et circonscrites, ou consistant en une simple hyperémie diffuse, lesquelles après une première intervention guérissent bien et définitivement dans 15 ou 20 jours. Comme ces cystites s'observent surtout chez les femmes, la sonde à demeure même prolongée, n'aura pas d'inconvénients et elle sera bien tolérée si les lésions ne siègent pas au voisinage immédiat du col. Il en est de même de la cautérisation du point d'implantation d'un néoplasme de la vessie, lorsque celui-ci n'infiltre pas toutefois largement la paroi vésicale, car dans ce dernier cas, comme dans l'abrasion au fer rouge du lobe médian de la prostate, des hémorragies secondaires sont à redouter et c'est cette dernière éventualité qui impose alors le drainage hypogastrique de la vessie. Hormis ces deux circonstances : nécessité pour la vessie enflammée d'un repos prolongé et crainte d'hématurie secondaire, je ne vois pas d'inconvénient si l'on fait bénéficier des avantages de la cystorrhaphie totale les malades opérés pour une cystite ou un néoplasme de la vessie et chez lesquels on s'est servi du cautère. La formation des escarres résultant d'une cautérisation étendue et énergique, qui pourraient obstruer la sonde, sont loin d'être la règle. Toutefois mon expérience personnelle ne me permet pas d'avoir une opinion nette à cet égard; je signale seulement que je ne les ai pas vues dans les cas de deux néoplasmes de la vessie, où j'avais tout lieu de m'y attendre, parce que j'avais pratiqué une cautérisation large et énergique de leur point d'implantation. De mémoire, je ne connais qu'un malade opéré par M. le Prof. Albert de Vienne, malade qui expulsa deux mois après l'opération une escarre large de plusieurs centimètres carrés et déjà chargée de dépôts calcaires. Du reste ces lambeaux de tissus nécrosés, résultat de l'inflammation circonscrite d'élimination, commencent à se détacher généralement à partir du sixième jour, mais ils ne tombent le plus souvent qu'au douzième ou quinzième jour après l'opération et à cette date s'ils venaient obstruer, soit la sonde à demeure, soit l'urètre, et provoquer un ischurie momentanée et la distension de la vessie, la suture vésicale sera déjà assez consolidée pour résister et le malade pourra sans inconvénient attendre l'intervention du médecin pour vider sa vessie.

Ce que j'ai dit pour la cautérisation ignée s'applique à plus forte raison à la cautérisation chimique de la vessie. Je n'insiste donc pas.

Ces réserves faites, je ne vois d'autres contre-indications à la cystorrhaphie totale que celles qui découlent des six circonstances suivantes :

1° Impossibilité de placer une sonde à demeure, intolérance de cette sonde et accidents infectieux devant fatalement survenir à cause d'un très mauvais état du canal urétral, compliqué ou non d'une infection péri-urétrale, ou à cause d'une inflammation aiguë ou subaiguë du reste de l'appareil génital : prostatite, épididymite, etc.

2° Nécessité pour la vessie d'un repos prolongé, simple ou combiné avec des attouchements de la muqueuse dans les cas des cystites tuberculeuses, douloureuses ou présentant simplement des altérations pathologiques profondes, dont la régression complète demande beaucoup de temps ;

3° Participation des voies urinaires supérieures à l'inflammation de la vessie avec ou sans fièvre ;

4° Troubles dyspeptiques ou autres dénotant une intoxication urinaire avancée et faisant présumer un mauvais état anatomique de l'appareil urinaire et en particulier des reins et une résistance moindre de l'organisme à l'infection;

5° Possibilité d'hémorragies secondaires dans les cas d'extirpation partielle de la prostate, d'abrasion au fer rouge des tumeurs volumineuses de la vessie ;

6° Taille hypogastrique pour remédier à une rétention d'urine chez les prostatiques.

En somme, je crois que si le drainage hypogastrique de a vessie offre une sécurité certaine, la cystorrhaphie totale est elle aussi exempte de tout danger. Les accidents du côté de l'urètre, etc., peuvent être prévenus ou arrêtés dans leur évolution, ils sont du reste exceptionnels avec l'asepsie des sondes et du canal urétral que nous pratiquons aujourd'hui ; l'infiltration d'urine par l'hypogastre, possible en cas de cystite, est sûrement conjurée par le drainage préventif de la cavité de Retzius, et la péritonite étant la conséquence de la blessure de la séreuse, cet accident, loin de contre-indiquer la cystorrhaphie totale, la demande au contraire impérieusement. Tout en reconnaissant donc qu'on ne saurait jamais être trop prudent en chirurgie urinaire, je crois qu'il y a lieu d'élargir un peu le cadre des indications de la fermeture complète de la vessie, car en tentant cette opération qui complète si heureusement la taille hypogastrique, on ne risque rien, je le répète, tandis que sans elle la guérison et la sortie du malade de l'hôpital est retardée, et si l'ouverture sus-pubienne de la vessie se fistulise, il est exposé par ce fait à subir une seconde intervention pour l'oblitération de sa fistule.

---

## NOTE SUR LA RÉPARATION SPONTANÉE DES PLAIES INTRA-PÉRITONÉALES DE LA VESSIE

par le docteur LÉON IMBERT,

professeur agrégé à la Faculté de Montpellier.

J'ai communiqué l'année dernière à la Société de chirurgie une observation dont l'interprétation présentait quelques difficultés ; il s'agissait d'une rupture traumatique de la vésicule biliaire, survenue à la suite d'une contusion et spontanément cicatrisée sous le couvert d'une péritonite localisée. Ce fait curieux m'a engagé à rechercher dans quelles conditions se faisait la réparation spontanée des viscères creux. Ce sujet a du reste été déjà abordé : Schwartz a publié dans la *Riforma medica* une étude de ce genre ; je n'ai pu malheureusement me la procurer. D'autre part, Cornil et Carnot ont publié l'année dernière une série de recherches à ce sujet ; mais ils se sont placés surtout au point de vue histologique et expérimental et n'ont guère envisagé les conséquences pratiques de leurs travaux. Il me semble cependant que l'expérimentation peut fournir quelques données intéressantes pour la détermination chirurgicale dans le cas de rupture vésicale ; et c'est à ce dernier point de vue que j'ai repris la question. Je me suis adressé de préférence à la vessie, organe plus facile à aborder chez le lapin, que la vésicule biliaire ; cependant j'ai fait une expérience sur ce dernier organe ; j'en rapporterai les résultats à la fin de cette note. Il y aurait lieu assurément de répéter ces recherches sur les diverses cavités aseptiques de l'économie et principalement sur celles qui sont le siège d'une circulation assez active, comme l'uretère.

Les expériences de Cornil et Carnot sont fort intéressantes : mais elles s'éloignent des conditions cliniques en ce sens que la plaie n'est pratiquée que lorsque une ligature a préalablement interrompu le cours de l'urine : ces auteurs lient en effet la vessie et l'uretère, puis ouvrent le segment ainsi isolé. Ils ont constaté non seulement la cicatrisation des lèvres de la plaie, mais encore la reconstitution du conduit urinaire et enfin la résorption de la ligature et le rétablissement de la circulation des urines. L'épithélium reconstitue un revêtement continu par greffe, glissement et multiplication.

L'année dernière, de Rouville a communiqué à la Société de biologie les résultats de ses recherches sur les fonctions de la vessie et montré comment l'organe reformait immédiatement sa cavité lorsqu'il n'était pas malade.

Les expériences que j'ai entreprises dérivent des précédentes ; elles ont été conçues de la façon suivante : une vessie étant ouverte dans le péritoine, purement et simplement, sans aucune ligature protectrice, se cicatrisera-t-elle et comment? Ces recherches ont porté à la fois sur le côté clinique et le côté histologique. Au point de vue clinique, elles montrent en effet qu'une plaie vésicale peut, dans certaines circonstances, se cicatriser par les seules ressources de la nature. Au point de vue histologique, nous avons vu la formation d'une cicatrice mince, mais assez résistante pour rétablir la continuité parfaite de la vessie, même sous tension.

Voici comment j'ai procédé d'une façon générale : sur un lapin bien portant, je commençais par faire soigneusement disparaître les poils dans la région sus-pubienne. Puis, avec les précautions d'asepsie habituelle, je pratiquais sur la ligne médiane une laparotomie : arrivé sur la vessie, je la faisais saillir hors de l'abdomen et pratiquais alors sur elle soit une incision, plus ou moins large, soit une résection. L'organe était alors réintégré dans l'abdomen sans autre ligature que celle qui pouvait être nécessitée par la section de quelque artériole : section que j'évitais du reste d'habitude aisément. Enfin la paroi abdominale était refermée.

Mes expériences ont porté sur 17 lapins que j'ai opérés de la façon
uivante :

Sur 15 d'entre eux, j'ai pratiqué une incision vésicale, aux ciseaux,
de courte étendue, un à deux centimètres en moyenne. Sur ce nombre
1 seul est mort, de péritonite septique; un autre a été tué alors que
la péritonite était déjà déclarée, il doit donc être rangé dans la catégorie des morts opératoires. Il y a donc eu 2 morts sur 15 animaux
opérés. Cette mortalité est très faible assurément, mais je ferai
remarquer qu'elle doit être encore considérée comme trop forte. En
effet les deux morts sont dues à la péritonite : elles relèvent évidemment
d'une infection opératoire; il n'est pas toujours facile, en effet,
d'opérer aseptiquement sur un champ opératoire aussi réduit qu'un
abdomen de lapin. Il est probable en définitive que si l'opération
avait été bien aseptique, ces lapins eussent guéri comme les autres.

Par contre, il faut tenir compte de ce fait que sur les 15 lapins
opérés par incision, 5 ont été sacrifiés, l'un au bout de vingt-quatre
heures, l'autre après quarante-huit heures, le dernier après soixante-
douze heures; il n'est donc pas démontré en somme qu'ils eussent
guéri, surtout le dernier dont la vessie n'était pas encore complètement fermée et dont le péritoine renfermait encore beaucoup d'urine.

En résumé, on voit que, dans la grande majorité des cas, une incision
vésicale courte se cicatrise facilement et spontanément chez le lapin.

Sur un seul animal, j'ai pratiqué une large incision, divisant le
réservoir urinaire en deux valves antérieure et postérieure. Cet animal
est mort un peu plus de vingt-quatre heures après l'opération, il ne
présentait par de lésions de péritonite et son péritoine était plein
d'urine. On ne peut guère admettre que la mort soit due à la résorption
urineuse, car les lapins opérés par une incision courte ne se cicatrisent
pas en moins de vingt-quatre heures, comme je le dirai plus loin.
Peut être cet animal a-t-il succombé à une infection à marche très rapide
et n'ayant pas déterminé de lésions appréciables.

Trois autres lapins ont subi une résection de la vessie. Chez l'un
d'eux la résection a été de faible étendue : un centimètre environ; il
a parfaitement guéri. Chez un autre, j'ai réséqué la moitié supérieure
du globe vésical; il est mort soixante heures environ après l'opération. Le péritoine était plein d'urine; il n'y avait pas trace de péritonite; il a dû succomber à la résorption urineuse. Enfin le troisième
animal a subi une résection des parois latérales, de trois centimètres de
long environ sur un centimètre de large. Il a parfaitement guéri,
mais est mort un mois après; l'autopsie n'a pu en être faite pour
diverses raisons; mais en considération de sa longue survie, je suis

porté à croire qu'il a dû succomber à une épidémie qui atteignit à cette époque plusieurs lapins non opérés.

Il faut donc conclure de tout cela, au point de vue clinique, que :

Les plaies de la vessie guérissent spontanément chez le lapin lorsqu'elles sont de peu d'étendue; leur danger augmente donc avec leurs dimensions.

Les résections de la vessie guérissent aussi spontanément lorsque le fragment réséqué n'est pas trop considérable.

Telles sont les conclusions cliniques que l'on peut tirer de ces recherches. Mais il est intéressant de savoir comment les choses se passent macroscopiquement et microscopiquement.

Voici d'abord les phénomènes que l'on constate aisément à l'œil nu :
*Incision de la vessie.*

Dès que la vessie est ouverte, toute l'urine qu'elle contenait s'en écoule et l'organe perd de son volume et devient une poche flaccide dont les parois sont accolées. Quelques heures après, on constate le début de phénomènes des réparations qui ont une double origine : d'une part, on voit que les lèvres de la plaie vésicale se sont accolées en même temps que la muqueuse s'est renversée en dehors, et s'est mise en ectopie; mais la fermeture n'est pas effectuée et la vessie est toujours vide, bien que contenant parfois quelques gouttes d'urine; d'autre part, le péritoine lui-même renferme une quantité d'urine plus ou moins considérable, le liquide est absolument clair et mélangé sans doute à la sérosité péritonéale; mais en outre il s'est produit un exsudat péritonéal plastique qui a déjà créé des adhérences, très faibles du reste, entre les bords de la plaie et les organes abdominaux, ou la paroi abdominale elle-même.

Ce n'est qu'au bout de quarante-huit heures que la vessie est fermée; elle renferme une certaine quantité d'urine et son étanchéité est désormais assurée; mais la moindre traction déchire la jeune cicatrice. En outre, on voit bien que la fermeture paraît être consolidée soit par la paroi abdominale, soit par un organe quelconque (intestin grêle ou gros intestin) dont la surface péritonéale est venue s'accoler à la plaie et en facilite l'occlusion. Le simple fait de décoller cet organe suffit à rouvrir la vessie.

A partir de ce moment la cicatrice se consolide progressivement et au bout de trois semaines, on la trouve forte et résistante. A ce moment les adhérences qui unissent l'intestin à la vessie peuvent être rompues sans difficulté; l'organe demeure étanche; la cicatrisation est parfaite; la cicatrice, vue du côté vésical, présente un enfoncement relativement profond, pouvant loger une tête d'épingle, punctiforme bien que l'incision ait été longitudinale; en outre les environs sont gaufrés et soulevés par des plis qui convergent en rayonnant vers le point central. J'ai dit que de toutes les vessies incisées, une seule avait paru ne point se cicatriser : elle appartenait à un lapin que j'ai sacrifié au bout de trois jours dans l'intention d'étudier histologiquement les lésions à cette époque; mais dans d'autres expériences, la vessie était complètement fermée dans ce délai.

*Résection de la vessie.* — Pour les résections de peu d'étendue, la marche de la cicatrisation est absolument identique, et cela se comprend facilement : une fois ouverte en effet, la vessie vide devient une simple membrane molle dont les deux feuillets s'accolent l'un à l'autre : l'abrasion d'une petite partie de cette membrane n'en saurait gêner la cicatrisation. Au contraire lorsque la résection est étendue la réunion est beaucoup plus difficile car, d'une part la capacité du réservoir à reconstituer est notablement diminuée et il sera par conséquent soumis à des pressions plus fortes et, d'autre part les dimensions de la plaie étant plus grandes, la réparation nécessitera plus de temps. Cela explique que, chez le lapin auquel j'ai réséqué environ la moitié du réservoir urinaire, la plaie ne s'est pas cicatrisée; l'animal est mort en soixante heures environ. A l'autopsie j'ai trouvé la vessie ouverte; cependant le travail de réparation était déjà commencé : la plaie était comme rétrécie en anneau.

Enfin, j'ai fait, au point de vue histologique, les constatations suivantes :

Le phénomène le plus important et le plus net est le renversement de la muqueuse qui s'ectropionne pour recouvrir en quelque sorte la surface de section. Ce fait est constant : il m'a paru résulter de plusieurs facteurs.

D'une part, le derme de la muqueuse vésicale augmente considérablement d'épaisseur au niveau des bords de la plaie : il s'infiltre de liquide suivant une zone très limitée et, trouvant libre expansion du côté de la plaie, il s'y développe, entraînant avec lui et ectropionnant la muqueuse; ces détails se voient sur toutes les coupes avec une parfaite netteté. Le bourrelet rétrécit la plaie; il est cependant peu favorable à sa cicatrisation, car il rejette en dehors les surfaces avivées qui se trouvent de la sorte sur le même plan que la surface externe de la vessie, et ne peuvent pas s'adosser à elles-mêmes : les lèvres de la plaie sont donc tapissées d'une muqueuse qui doit évidemment nuire à la cicatrisation; le rebroussement de la muqueuse m'a paru expliquer la forte dépression que présente la cicatrice constituée; d'autre part, elle permet de comprendre que la surface de section ainsi repoussée en dehors prenne adhérence sur les organes voisins qui vont former ainsi comme une valve de fermeture.

Pendant que le derme de la muqueuse s'ectropionne ainsi, l'épithélium suit le mouvement, il recouvre donc intégralement le bord de la solution de continuité et même la lèvre externe sur une certaine étendue. Seulement il est obligé de s'aplatir considérablement et de diminuer sa hauteur de moitié environ. Se produit-il ici les phénomènes de greffe, glissement et multiplication dont parlent Cornil et Carnot? C'est probable, mais je n'ai pu vérifier ce point.

Tels sont les phénomènes qui se passent dans la première journée.

Un peu plus tard, la surface de section prend un point d'appui sur un viscère environnant, et cela malgré la continuité de la sécrétion urinaire. La surface avivée, qui a pris une forme circulaire s'accole à l'intestin grêle ou au gros intestin : à partir de ce moment, la cicatrisation fait de rapides progrès; l'épithélium vésical qui recouvre le bourrelet ectropionné prolifère rapidement et bientôt il va recouvrir l'organe qui est venu s'accoler à la vessie; à partir de ce moment, l'étanchéité, bien que fragile encore, est assurée : il n'est plus besoin que de renforcer la cicatrice qui se double d'une couche de tissu conjonctif.

Enfin, au bout de trois semaines ou un mois, on voit que l'épithélium, entièrement reconstitué, recouvre toute la vessie; au-dessous une cicatrice indique le lieu de la section : elle est fortement déprimée et, au microscope, on voit que les faisceaux musculaires qui l'environnent sont plus épais que sur d'autres points : ils semblent s'être repliés sur eux-mêmes à la façon de fils élastiques coupés pendant leur extension. La cicatrice est d'habitude entièrement fibreuse; j'y ai trouvé cependant des fibres musculaires, ce qui semblerait indiquer que la tunique musculaire peut, au bout de quelque temps, retrouver sa parfaite continuité.

On voit donc, en somme, que les plaies vésicales peuvent se cicatriser parfaitement par leurs propres moyens à la condition qu'elles soient peu étendues et aseptiques.

J'ai répété ces expériences sur la vésicule biliaire d'un lapin qui survécut et ne fut sacrifié que plus de deux mois après. L'animal a commencé par maigrir durant quelques semaines; au moment où je l'ai sacrifié il avait repris une bonne santé. La vésicule biliaire avait été incisée sur une étendue de 1 centimètre environ. A l'autopsie, j'ai trouvé des adhérences très nombreuses, très épaisses, unissant l'intestin, le foie et l'estomac; ce dernier était le siège d'une dilatation considérable, due probablement aux adhérences. Quant à la vésicule, il m'a été impossible de la trouver : elle était probablement ratatinée et perdue dans les adhérences unissant l'intestin au foie.

### Principales expériences.

I. — Lapin n° 9. *Incision courte de la vessie*. Tué 15 heures après une incision courte de la vessie. Péritoine plein d'une sérosité limpide. Vessie ouverte, mais renfermant quelques gouttes de liquide; quelques adhérences larges et minces entre la vessie et la paroi abdominale. Au niveau de la plaie, la muqueuse est fortement éversée en dehors, si bien que la surface de section très petite paraît être sur le prolongement de la face extérieure de la vessie.

Il s'est produit là un bourrelet considérable, recouvert de muqueuse sur presque toute son étendue et constitué principalement par le derme de la muqueuse épaissi et infiltré de sérosité, mais sans abondance notable de leucocytes. Quelques hémorragies au niveau de la surface de section. Tout le bourrelet muqueux est entièrement dépourvu de fibres musculaires. Celles-ci sont comme rétractées un peu en deçà de la section.

Un fort grossissement montre la confirmation des détails précédents; mais on note que l'épithélium, au lieu d'être cylindrique comme au niveau de la muqueuse vésicale normale, est très aplati, et son épaisseur totale paraît diminuée au moins de moitié. Cela résulte vraisemblablement, conformément aux conclusions de Cornil et Carnot, à la fois de l'étalement et de la multiplication des cellules.

II. — Lapin n° 10. *Incision courte de la vessie*. Tué 40 heures après une incision courte de la vessie, Vessie complètement fermée mais peu distendue. Pas de liquide dans l'abdomen. Cicatrice vésicale légèrement adhérente au gros intestin. A la coupe, on voit bien que l'orifice, bordé entièrement de muqueuse est oblitéré par le gros intestin comme par une soupape. Le bourrelet signalé dans la précédente préparation existe, mais il est notablement réduit dans ses dimensions. Par contre, l'épithélium a complètement envahi sa face externe; il s'étend sur celle-ci sur une assez grande longueur pour que l'on puisse admettre qu'il a mis obstacle à la cicatrisation. L'intestin ne devient donc adhérent qu'en couronne et sur un point où une masse de fibrilles l'unit à la vessie. L'épithélium possède à peu près sa hauteur normale. Les fibres musculaires vésicales présentent les mêmes caractères que plus haut.

III. — Lapin n° 1. *Incision courte de la vessie*. Autopsie trois semaines après l'opération. La vessie adhère légèrement à la abdominale et au gros intestin. Elle est complètement fermée.

La paroi est pleinement reconstituée en tissu conjonctif avec une cicatrice déprimée et gaufrée Les fibres musculaires demeurent éloignées de l'ancienne solution de continuité. L'épithélium tapisse tout l'entonnoir. Il est un peu diminué de hauteur.

IV. — Lapin n° 3 *Résection peu étendue du sommet de la vessie*. Tué 7 jours après l'opération. Vessie complètement fermée, légèrement adhérente à la cicatrice abdominale et à une anse intestinale qui s'en détache facilement. La cicatrice est profondément déprimée et gaufrée. A un faible grossissement, on voit que la paroi vésicale possède une épaisseur bien moindre au point qui a été blessé. A ce niveau existe une profonde dépression, tandis que les bords de la cicatrice paraissent au contraire surélevés par rapport aux régions vésicales environnantes.

L'épithélium descend sans aucune discontinuité dans toute cette fosse et remonte sur la berge opposée; la muqueuse y présente les replis qui existent sur le reste de la surface. L'épaisseur de l'épithélium paraît être sensiblement la même que dans les autres points. Tout au plus, le derme paraît-il davantage infiltré de cellules rondes.

C'est surtout la couche musculaire dont l'épaisseur est diminuée. Au lieu de présenter une grande épaisseur de faisceaux orientés en divers sens elle montre seulement 2 ou 3 assises, dirigées toutes parallèlement à la muqueuse et dans un même plan. Dans les environs de la cicatrice, les fibres musculaires paraissent comme retroussées et semblent avoir ainsi accru l'épaisseur des bords de la cicatrice vésicale. Un gros vaisseau se voit sur la couche profonde, vis-à-vis de la cicatrice.

A un très fort grossissement, on voit que l'épithélium se présente sur la cicatrice avec les caractères qu'il possède ailleurs; il est seulement un peu moins épais. Au-dessous se voit un derme dont l'épaisseur est variable et augmente du fond de la cicatrice à sa surface. Enfin et profondément se voient de minces et rares faisceaux de fibres musculaires lisses.

V. — Lapin n° 5. *Résection de la moitié de la vessie.* Mort spontanément 60 heures après l'opération. Vessie petite ; mais la plaie est retrécie comme une bourse. Pas de péritonite

Les bords de l'incision paraissent épaissis. A un faible grossissement on voit cette éversion déjà signalée de la muqueuse. L'épithélium continue en apparence jusque sur la face extérieure de la vessie, mais son épaisseur y diminue progressivement et il disparaît bientôt. Les plis de cette dernière partie sont moins nombreux et moins profonds que sur la muqueuse vésicale normale. Au-dessous de l'épithélium se trouve un derme assez épais, mais qui diminue progressivement d'épaisseur avec l'épithélium et disparaît avec lui Au-dessous vient la couche musculaire épaissie et comme rétractée sur elle-même. Les deux dernières couches dermiques et musculaires sont infiltrées de foyers hémorragiques, ainsi que la sous-muqueuse.

Tous ces détails se voient plus nettement à un fort grossissement. On voit bien que l'épithélium éversé diminue d'épaisseur : cela résulte d'un nombre moindre d'assises de cellules et aussi d'un abaissement de la hauteur des éléments cellulaires en général. Toutefois, la couche épithéliale conserve une certaine hauteur dans le fond des sillons. Au reste, il faut se souvenir qu'il s'agit d'une pièce d'autopsie qui a pu être plus ou moins altérée.

## DISCUSSION

M. Nicolich (Trieste). — Il n'y a pas longtemps que le professeur Albert, de Vienne, écrivait que la suture totale de la vessie est une utopie, mais cela ne veut pas dire qu'en Allemagne et en Autriche on ne fait pas la suture de la vessie; au contraire, on la fait très souvent.

Quand l'urine est aseptique et quand il n'y a pas de probabilité d'hémor-

ragie secondaire comme c'est le cas chez les prostatiques, je fais toujours
la suture totale de la vessie, ainsi que des parois abdominales, et je
ne laisse qu'un petit drain dans la cavité de Retzius. Dans les cas où
la suture complète est indiquée, je ne laisse pas même la sonde à demeure
comme M. Bassini le fait depuis longtemps, et je suis très content de ce
procédé qui, surtout chez les enfants, est d'une grande utilité. La suture
que j'emploie est celle qu'on utilise à Necker, et je ne peux pas comprendre l'utilité des sutures compliquées comme celles de Razimonsky et
Jonnesco.

Je préfère toujours le catgut, vu que j'ai dû une fois faire une lithotritie à
un malade pour une pierre qui s'était formée sur un fil de soie qui était
tombé dans la vessie après une section faite pour une plaie de cet
organe.

M. Preindlsberger (Sarajevo). — Je suis presque tout à fait de l'avis
de M. Nicolich. Comme élève du professeur Albert, j'ai pratiqué la suture
de la vessie après l'intervention chirurgicale dans la lithiase.

Au point de vue du drainage, je ferai remarquer l'impossibilité du
drainage chez les enfants de 2 à 4 ans, surtout à cause de l'urétrite qui
en est la conséquence.

M. F. Legueu (Paris). — J'ai eu le regret de ne pouvoir assister au début
de la séance, et je n'ai pu entendre toutes les communications de nos
confrères relatives à la suture de la vessie.

Cependant je viens d'entendre adresser à la sonde à demeure, après la
taille, des reproches que je ne puis accepter et contre lesquels je veux
tout au contraire protester : si j'ai bien compris, notre distingué confrère
M. le D<sup>r</sup> Nicolich vient de nous dire que la sonde à demeure était dangereuse après la suture de la vessie.

Qu'on puisse obtenir la réunion par la première intention d'une
suture de vessie sans sonde à demeure je le conçois parfaitement. Mais
de là à dire que la sonde est dangereuse, il y a loin ; la sonde, au contraire, me paraît une garantie dont on ne saurait se passer toutes les fois
qu'il y a menace d'hémorhagie, comme il arrive si souvent chez l'adulte.

Je fais en général la suture à un seul plan, toujours au catgut.

Chez l'enfant, la suture réussit toujours. Chez l'adulte, elle réussit beaucoup plus rarement ; on voit vers le septième jour une petite fistule qui
se ferme avant le vingtième jour.

## NOUVEAUX CAS DE FISTULES VÉSICO-VAGINALES
## TRAITÉES PAR LE PROCÉDÉ DE DÉDOUBLEMENT

### par le docteur LOUMEAU,

de Bordeaux.

J'apporte cinq nouveaux succès à l'actif du procédé de dédoublement dans le traitement des fistules vésico-vaginales, procédé que j'avais déjà utilisé trois fois chez des malades. (Association française d'Urologie, 1897). Cette opération consiste à dédoubler tout le pourtour de la fistule par un avivement de 1 à 2 centimètres et affronter ensuite par leurs faces cruentées : d'une part, au catgut, les deux lèvres vésicales refoulées vers la vessie, et, d'autre part, au fil d'argent, les deux lèvres vaginales dont les bords libres forment un relief saillant dans le vagin.

Sur mes cinq dernières opérées, deux avaient subi pour cystite douloureuse une cystostomie vaginale maintenue pendant plus d'un an fistuleuse et offraient une fistule peu étendue qui fut très rapidement oblitérée. Les trois autres fistules étaient beaucoup plus graves en raison de leur siège élevé, n'intéressant pourtant pas le col utérin ; de leurs dimensions, variant entre celle d'une pièce de 1 franc et d'une pièce de 2 francs, et de plusieurs échecs opératoires antérieurs. L'une d'elles était d'origine obstétricale ; la seconde avait succédé à l'ablation d'un épithélioma vésical dont j'avais dû poursuivre profondément l'implantation dans l'épaisseur de la paroi vésico-vaginale : la troisième avait eu pour point de départ, chez une femme de 75 ans, l'ulcération d'une vieille cystocèle vaginale habitée par un énorme calcul phosphétique. Chez toutes mes malades, l'opération réussit à la première tentative, secondée par le tamponnement aseptique du vagin et la mise à demeure dans la vessie, par l'urètre, d'une sonde de Malécot constamment ouverte, et maintenue jusqu'à l'ablation des fils métalliques, réalisée du huitième au douzième jour.

### DISCUSSION

M. LEGUEU. — Je considère que le procédé du dédoublement dans le traitement des fistules vésico-vaginales est le procédé de choix. Son efficacité maintes fois éprouvée le met bien au-dessus du procédé américain et de la suture transvésicale ; pour ma part, je lui dois plusieurs succès complets et immédiats dans des cas où le procédé américain avait complètement échoué.

Dans un cas entre autres, il s'agissait d'une double fistule à la fois recto et vésico-vaginale, consécutive à une hystérectomie difficile. A l'aide d'une seule et même incision, je pus dédoubler la muqueuse du vagin des muqueuses vésicale et rectale, et combler dans la même séance les deux brèches de ces conduits. Pendant quelque temps, grâce à une désunion profonde, les gaz passèrent dans la vessie, mais la guérison se compléta rapidement.

Dans un autre cas, que j'ai opéré très récemment, toute la face inférieure de la vessie faisait presque défaut, à la suite d'un accouchement pénible et laborieux. La face antérieure du col utérin faisait partie de la fistule ; j'ai pu dans ce cas isoler la muqueuse vésicale de la paroi antérieure de l'utérus, et combler dans une seule séance la brèche qui était énorme. Une petite désunion, il est vrai, se produisit au niveau d'un des angles de la plaie; mais la fistule insignifiante qui persiste actuellement, sera guérie d'emblée et facilement dans une seconde séance.

En somme, à mon avis, ni l'étendue, ni l'élévation de la fistule ne la mettent en dehors des indications du procédé du dédoublement, et ce procédé est de beaucoup préférable, dans les cas difficiles, à la suture transvésicale.

J'ai l'habitude de suturer isolément au catgut l'orifice vésical et au fil d'argent l'orifice vaginal. Les sutures isolées de chaque orifice sont disposées dans un sens réciproquement perpendiculaire, et j'ai soin, autant que possible, de solidariser les deux plans de manière à éviter la désunion entre les deux.

---

## CHRONIC CYSTITIS DUE TO THE BACILLUS TYPHOSUS
## REPORT OF A CASE OF SEVEN YEARS DURATION

by Hugh H. YOUNG, Md. D.,

Head of the department of Urinary Surgery, Johns Hopkins hospital dispensary (Abstract of Remarks Reported in full in vol. VIII Johns Hopkins hospital reports.

The case here reported has been under the writer's care since March 1898, and has been referred to previously in articles by Gwyn, and also by Richardson.

History. T. C. male, aet. 59 years, single.

Complaint. Bladder trouble. Family history unimportant.

Past history. Indefinite history of prostatorrhoea beginning fifteen years ago. No previous history of gonorrhoea or bladder trouble.

Present illness. Dates back to an attack of typhoid fever, for which he was admitted to the hospital under Prof. Osler's care in August 28th, 1895. For several weeks before admission the patient had been suffering with headaches, pain in the limbs, and in the region of the right kidney, with fever.

On admission he complained of pain in the back and pain on urination, which was much more frequent than normal. He was very constipated but complained of no abdominal pain.

On last admission to the hospital in January. 1900, he had a slight gleety discharge. Urine still cloudy, but voided only every four to six hours and without pain, in amounts varying from 400 to 600 c.c. Urine (freshly voided) dark grey turbidity, with soft cheesy masses which sink at once to the bottom. Sp. Gr. 1014, reaction : slightly acid, albumin 0,25 per cent. No sugar. Microscopically pus cells and bacilli. General health of the patient fairly good. Cultures made on numerous occasions from urine taken from the bladder with aseptic precautions still showed the bacillus typhosus in pure cultures. Widal tests again positive.

*Cystoscopic Examination.* Mucosa generally red in color, individual vessels not visible. Numerous small ulcers covered with fibrin present. Ureteral orifices deep red in color, and surrounded by swollen mucous membrane. Examination considerably interfered with by the impossibility of obtaining a clear fluid in the bladder (owing to the great amount of pus and fibrin present). Diagnosis : general chronic cystitis with small ulcerations.

*Clinical course of the Disease.* General condition. The patient constantly complained of slight malaise, nausea, chronic constipation, and pain in the back, but was never acutely sick.

Pyrexia. Often slight evening elevation of the temperature to about 99°.

Urinary symptoms. Practically free from subjective symptoms. No increased frequency, no pain, stream forcible. No blood. Urine always very cloudy, reaction generally slightly acid, though sometimes neutral, or even slightly alkaline, albumin averaging 0.05 per cent. Microscopically, pus cells, few epithelial cells, bacilli, motile, and proved by cultures to be the bacillus typhosus present in large quantity.

*Note* : After cystoscopic examination an acute exacerbation of the gonorrhoea occurred, followed by an invasion of the bladder with the gonococcus, at first only a few diplococci appearing in the last urine, but finally great numbers, fully as many as the bacilli, intracellular, decolorizing by Gram, growing with typical colonies on hydrocele-agar, and refusing to grow on ordinary media. The cultures were obtained from the bladder by suprapubic aspiration.

It is interesting to note that this invasion of the bladder occurred and persisted despite the constant usage of urotropin, and bichloride irrigations of the bladder (1 to 50000). And when last seen, four months after the infection of the bladder with the gonococcus occured, typhoid bacilli and gonococci were both present in considerable numbers and both intracellular. The urine had not changed in appearance, and was still slightly acid. Cystocopic examination still showed a chronic ulcerative cystitis.

*Cases in the Literature.* While reports of cases of typhoid fever accompanied by acute cystitis have of late become considerable only two cases of chronic cystitis due to the typhoid bacillus are to be found, viz : by Rovsing, and by Houston. Rovsing's case had had typhoid fever eighteen months before, followed by very painful and frequent micturition. Vesical tenesmus became so severe that the patient begged for operation. Urine was acid, of very milky color. Culture obtained with a sterile catheter, gave a pure growth of the bacillus typhosus. At operation (sectio alta) the bladder was found much contracted, the mucous membrane dark red, and with numerous ulcerations simulating tuberculosis. Both kidneys were enlarged, and at autopsy (one month later) double pyonephrsis, with a stone in the right kidney was found.

Houston's case was a young woman of 35 years of age, who had never had typhoid fever, but who had, three years previously, nursed a child with presumably typhoid, and had soon begin to have frequent and painful micturition. On admission she had a chronic cystitis. The urine was turbid, strongly acid, contained a small amount of albumen, epithelium, leucocytes and bacilli, which proved to be typhoid bacilli. The blood gave the Widal test. Houston thought the bacillus had gained entry through the mamma and localized in the bladder without producing an attack of typhoid fever. In this respect his case is entirely different from the other two. Unfortunately no cystoscopic examination was made in Houston's case, and no note made as to the size of the bladder, an important point since Rovsing's case showed contracture of that viscus, while mine did not, though both were ulcerated. The peculiar milky appearance of the urine was present in all the cases, though the reaction was strongly acid in Houston's, while neutral in mine. The difference in the severity of symptoms in the three cases is remarkable, requiring operative interference in Rovsing's and causing no inconvenience in mine.

The accidental contamination of the bladder in the case here reported with the gonococcus, and its persistence after four months of treatment, adds fresh interest to the case, and furnishes another case of chronic cystitis, infected with the gonococcus to the one previously reported by the writer in vol. IX, *Johns Hospkins Hospital Reports*.

On examination the liver and spleen were both enlarged, abdomen sunken, neither kidney palpable, No rose-spots found. No urethral discharge. Urine : neutral, cloudy, albumen abundant; sediment composed of pus cells. No diazo. Blood negative. Temperature 103.8°, but after four days it became normal, and remained nearly so for ten days when the patient suffered a relapse, which lasted about eleven days. Prof. Osler considered it a definite case of typhoid fever. On October 21ˢᵗ 1895, the patient was discharged and soon returned to work, but still noticed the pus in his urine.

In July 1897 the patient had gonorrhoea, which was soon cured, but his urine remained purulent, as before.

In March 1898 when first seen by the writer his urine was very cloudy, of a peculiar thick grey opacity, due to pus cells, and small thin bacilli which decolorized by Gram. No other bacteria present.

A culture taken from the bladder with a searcher after thorough cleansing of the penis and urethra, showed on plate cultures a pure culture of the bacillus, which decolorized by Gram. Inoculation into various media resulted as follows : Glucose agar : no gas. Bouillon : cloudy; actively motile bacilli. Milk : slightly acidified, but not coagulated. Potato : no visible growth. Gelatine : flat nail head growth, no liquefaction. Dunham no indol. Flagella present, shown by Loeffler's method. Cultures taken from various other colonies also proved to be the same organism.

In order to eliminate the possibility of urethral contamination a specimen of urine was obtained by suprapubic aspiration of the bladder, but cultures again showed the same organism identical with the bacillus typhosus.

Widal tests : Patient's blood-serum with a known bacillus typhosus; reaction positive. Bacillus from the bladder with the blood-serum of a known typhoid fever patient ; reaction positive. Patient's blood-serum with bacillus from his bladder, reaction positive.

Diagnosis Chronic Cystitis with pure culture of the bacillus typhosus.

The patient remained in the hospital 18 days. Urinations about normal in frequency, and a large amount of urine each time. No bladder irritation. On discharge from hospital the condition of the urine was about as bad as at entrance.   He soon went to work, and suffered no great inconvenience.

In September 1899 the patient again acquired gonorrhoea, and has never gotten entirely free from it.

---

## LEUCOPLASIE VÉSICALE PRIMITIVE HÉMORRHAGIQUE,

TAILLE HYPOGASTRIQUE, ESCHARIFICATION IGNÉE DES LÉSIONS, AMÉLIORATION [1].

### par M. J. ESCAT,

de Marseille.

A côté des leucoplasies secondaires de la muqueuse urinaire, existe-t-il une leucoplasie primitive ; indépendante des lésions inflammatoires connues et capable de constituer un type clinique distinct?

Je suis porté à répondre par l'affirmative en ce qui concerne la vessie.

Les deux observations qui font l'objet de cette communication ne répondent en aucune façon au type clinique connu sous le nom de cystite leucoplasique ou de cystite verruqueuse tel qu'il est admis. Dans ces deux cas, de la plaque leucoplasique ou de la nappe verruqueuse, on passe sans transition à la muqueuse saine. Quant aux signes cliniques, ils ne rappellent en rien les affections inflammatoires de la vessie, mais plutôt les néoplasies ou les ulcérations simples de cet organe.

Chez deux jeunes gens de vingt-deux et vingt et un ans, de constitution très vigoureuse sans lésions et sans antécédents inflammatoires urinaires, j'avais porté le diagnostic de papillomasie vésicale dans les conditions suivantes : l'un avait des hématuries vésicales spontanées depuis quatre ans avec alternatives d'urines limpides, la capacité vésicale cependant ne dépassait pas 80 grammes et la cystoscopie pleine de difficultés resta sans résultat positif, la réplétion vésicale était impossible sous le chloroforme malgré l'absence de cystite ; l'autre malade, de race égyptienne, exempt de Bilharzia urinait du sang depuis huit ans, mais, depuis un an seulement, l'hématurie est abondante avec caillots, il y a des alternatives d'urines non purulentes

1. Mes deux malades ont été opérés dans les hôpitaux de Marseille, grâce à l'extrême obligeance de mon collègue Delanglade et de M. le professeur Combalat. Je suis heureux de les remercier de m'avoir ainsi ouvert leurs services.

mais bactériuriques fétides, et d'urine sanglante. La capacité vésicale était normale, la cystoscopie très facile montra des masses papillaires mamelonnées sessiles avec reflets nacrés et resplendissants comme dans la cystite leucoplasique, une ulcération siégeait autour de l'uretère gauche, la partie de la vessie non dégénérée avait un aspect sain, sans cystite. Dans ce dernier cas, je crus à des masses papillaires néoplasiques non villeuses non pédiculée. L'état général des deux malades était excellent. La taille suspubienne démontra chez le premier une dégénérescence verruqueuse de la moitié gauche de la muqueuse vésicale, le bas fond et le col sont pris, le doigt a la sensation d'un semis de grains de plomb sur un derme fibreux et comme cicatriciel. Au niveau du col petites masses masses épithéliales friables où l'examen microscopique pratiqué par M. le professeur Nepveu de Marseille ne décèle pas l'organisation du papillome; la moitié droite de la vessie est saine et extensible, la vessie est petite, la portion atteinte ayant perdu son extensibilité.

Chez l'Égyptien l'ouverture de la vessie montra un semis de granulations leucoplasiques sur toute la surface vésicale à côté de grandes plaques leucoplasiques nacrées. L'une siège à la partie supérieure de la vessie, l'autre au niveau de l'uretère gauche grande plaque exulcérée, fissurée et saignante avec derme fibreux. En dehors et à droite une petite végétation jaune, très friable non saignante repose sur noyau dermique, dur fibreux. Entre ces lésions, muqueuse saine, la moitié droite du trigone l'est également, la paroi est souple, la vessie est très vaste, il n'y a pas de sclérose envahissante comme chez le premier malade. L'absence de toute lésion inflammatoire primitive et de toute affection organique autre que la leucoplasie prouve que cette dernière a été la lésion primitive et unique. Elle a évolué ici sans cystite. Le terme de cystite verruqueuse comme celui de cystite leucoplasique doit être rejeté pour ces deux cas. Il semble qu'à côté des leucoplasies urinaires secondaires à une inflammation quelconque de la vessie, leucoplasies dont Hallé a fait une étude désormais classique, et dont il a montré l'évolution vers le globe épidermique et l'épithélioma, il existe une dégénérescence leucoplasique de la muqueuse vésicale primitive dont l'étiologie reste obscure, qui produit la plaque leucoplasique, les granulations verruqueuses. l'infiltration dermique, les végétations friables la fissuration ulcérative et les hémorrhagies. Quant à la dégénérescence cancroïdale elle est plus que probable si les

---

1. Les limites imposées à cette publication ne me permettent pas de reproduire les observations *in extenso*.

malades ne succombent pas avant aux complications urinaires possibles.

Dans les cystites leucoplasiques le traitement de choix est la taille hypogastrique suivie de drainage et le curettage énergique de la muqueuse qui doit être profondément cruentée. J'ai publié en 1897, plusieurs observations de cystite rebelles recueillies dans le service de M. Guyon et de M. Albarran et je me suis attaché à mettre en relief les bons effets de ce traitement.

Chez mes deux malades l'usage de la curette était impossible, je n'ai pu entamer ces lésions dures, cornées : il faudrait ici une curette à dents de scie ou dont la face convexe fût munie de pointes de lime une sorte de râpe. J'ai eu donc recours à l'escharification ignée, très profonde, par le thermocautère, usant tantôt de la pointe tantôt du gros cautère. Mes deux malades opérés depuis peu vont bien, l'Égyptien a encore la vessie fistulisée. Mais je n'espère pas le résultat complet obtenu ordinairement dans les cystites devenues leucoplasiques. Quant à l'épithélioma il reste toujours possible.

Au moment d'imprimer ces lignes je puis ajouter que mes deux malades ayant la vessie fermée depuis deux mois vont bien, mais tous les deux reviennent uriner un peu de sang à la fin de la miction. Je crains donc que l'amélioration, considérable actuellement, ne soit éphémère.

---

## DES ULCÉRATIONS VÉSICALES ET DE L'ULCÉRE SIMPLE DE LA VESSIE

par M. RENÉ LE FUR,

de Paris,

Ancien interne des hôpitaux de Paris, Chirurgien à l'hôpital Péan.

Le chapitre des ulcérations simples de la vessie est encore peu connu, et tout entier à refaire sur bien des points.

Ces ulcérations peuvent revêtir deux types cliniques : soit le type de l'*ulcère simple chronique et solitaire*, bien décrit par Fenwick en 1896 ; soit le type de l'*ulcération aiguë, perforante d'emblée*.

La *pathogénie* de ces ulcérations simples de la vessie est très variable. Toutes les explications données à propos des ulcérations gastriques peuvent être invoquées ici ; mais nous devons surtout en retenir trois.

Je voudrais montrer qu'il existe dans la vessie, comme dans l'estomac, comme dans l'intestin, des ulcérations simples, non symptomatiques d'une lésion vésicale primitive. Ulcérations dont la symptomatologie est souvent obscure, dont le diagnostic, impossible autrefois, peut être fait aujourd'hui grâce aux perfectionnements apportés à la cystoscopie ; et dont l'évolution peut reproduire toutes les modalités des ulcérations de l'estomac : soit le type aigu, perforant d'emblée, accompagné d'hémorrhagies abondantes et de perforation rapide — soit le type chronique, à évolution lente, accompagnée de lésions inflammatoires, d'abord au niveau de la lésion (ulcère à bords indurés et épaissis), diffusant ensuite dans toute la vessie, en donnant de la cystite et de la péricystite, et jusqu'au niveau des reins, créant ainsi les lésions ascendantes de pyélonéphrite auxquelles finit par succomber le malade.

La pathogénie de ces ulcérations est encore loin d'être éclaircie : j'essaierai de donner une interprétation pathogénique basée à la fois sur la clinique, l'anatomie pathologique, et sur un certain nombre d'expériences de laboratoire que j'ai entreprises sur les animaux.

Quant au traitement, il importe de ne pas le négliger car une intervention appropriée, faite en temps opportun peut très bien sauver le malade qui court les plus grands dangers si l'affection est méconnue et abandonnée à elle-même.

Il est nécessaire dès le début, de distinguer *deux grands groupes* d'ulcérations vésicales :

1º Les ulcérations qu'on peut appeler *symptomatiques* d'une lésion vésicale primitive et qu'on peut observer par exemple à la suite de néoplasme, tuberculose, calculs, corps étrangers, cystites chroniques, cystites aiguës, etc. — Je ne m'occuperai pas ici de ces ulcérations qui sont les plus connues et dont les caractères ont été bien étudiés, surtout depuis la période cystoscopique. — Je me contenterai seulement de faire remarquer combien on a de tendance à agrandir aujourd'hui le cadre de ces ulcérations symptomatiques, notamment des ulcérations tuberculeuses, au détriment des ulcérations simples, et à y renfermer toutes les ulcérations douteuses, ou de cause inconnue.

2º Les ulcérations *simples* qu'on pourrait encore appeler primitives, essentielles, pour les opposer aux premières et qui ne sont dues ni à une lésion primitive de la paroi, ni à une cystite antérieure : à ce groupe appartient notamment l'ulcère simple de la vessie ce sont les plus intéressantes ; les moins connues ; ce sont les seules dont je m'occuperai ici.

3º En dehors de Mercier et d'Oliver qui ont décrit des ulcères simples de la vessie avec quelques erreurs d'interprétation, on rencontre éparses dans la littérature médicale, un certain nombre d'observations de ce genre. Moi-même j'ai retrouvé trois pièces très intéressantes d'ulcère simple de la vessie dans le musée de mon maître M. le professeur Guyon, et dans son service de l'hôpital Necker, j'ai eu l'occasion dernièrement encore d'en observer un cas.

Parmi les auteurs actuels, trois seulement ont nettement pris parti dans la question, affirmant la fréquence de l'ulcération simple de la vessie, et en étudiant les caractères cliniques, anatomo-pathologiques, et la pathogénie.

*Fenwick*, par ses multiples publications, par ses nombreuses cysto-scopies (il a observé au moins dix cas d'ulcération simple à lui seul) a fourni des documents très importants pour l'étude de cette question : « Huit années de cystoscopie soignée et persévérée, écrivait-il déjà en 1896, m'ont montré que le chapitre des ulcérations non malignes de la vessie était à refaire. — Je suis arrivé à la conviction qu'il existe plusieurs formes simples d'ulcération diagnostiquées à tort comme tuberculeuses et considérées aussi à tort comme incurables. — Une des variétés les plus fréquentes et les plus intéressantes, comme aussi la plus simple, parmi les ulcérations chroniques de la vessie, est l'ulcère simple isolé ou solitaire de la vessie. »

J'ai écrit dernièrement à Fenwick pour savoir si sa conviction s'était encore fortifiée depuis lors en faveur de la fréquence de l'ulcération simple; il m'a répondu affirmativement, me disant qu'il en avait observé plusieurs autres depuis.

*Castaigne* a publié en mars 1899, dans les *Bulletins de la Société anatomique*, une observation excessivement intéressante d'ulcère simple de la vessie, accompagné d'hématuries très abondantes et de perforation vésicale; c'est l'observation la plus complète que nous possédions, car l'histoire clinique, la description de l'ulcération, les examens histologiques et bactériologiques y sont relatés avec de minu-tieux détails.

Enfin *Gandy*, dans sa thèse remarquable de doctorat : *l'Ulcère simple et la névrose hémorragique des toxémies*, a réuni quelques cas d'ulcération simple de la vessie et leur attribue la même patho-génie qu'aux ulcérations gastriques.

Parmi ces ulcérations simples de la vessie, il en existe deux types bien différents au point de vue des symptômes, de l'évolution, et de l'anatomie pathologique; et qu'on peut superposer aux variétés cor-respondantes d'ulcération gastriques : l'un *chronique*, l'autre *aigu perforant*.

Le premier groupe comprend toutes les ulcérations qui évoluent lentement et sont habituellement superficielles, ne dépassant ordinairement pas la muqueuse. Dans ce groupe, *l'ulcère chronique solitaire de la vessie*, déjà cité et décrit par Fenwick est un des plus intéressants. — Il apparaît ordinairement chez les jeunes gens de vingt à vingt-cinq ans, sans aucun antécédent vésical, ni même vénérien. On peut le retrouver dans les deux sexes. Le début en est soudain, caractérisé par une légère fréquence des mictions, accompagnée ordinairement d'hématuries intermittentes. — Un symptôme de première importance et sur lequel Fenwick insiste beaucoup est une douleur violente et constante en un point de l'urèthre pénien.

Lorsqu'on soumet ces malades à la *cystoscopie*, on constate ordinairement une ulcération le plus souvent unique, exceptionnellement multiple, dans la région du trigone, en dedans et en arrière d'un des orifices urétéraux. Ses dimensions peuvent être variables, ordinairement de 2 à 5 centimètres de diamètre. Au début, ses bords sont à pic, gélatineux ; son fond paraît bourbeux et sanguinolent. Mais peu à peu, l'ulcère se recouvre d'incrustations calcaires, de pseudo-membranes qui le dissimulent et qu'il faut enlever si on veut le voir nettement. — Quelquefois, il se forme sur la paroi opposée de la vessie, juste en face du premier, un second ulcère qu'on peut appeler *ulcère par contact*.

L'*évolution* de ces ulcères est très caractéristique. On peut la diviser en trois périodes : dans la première, l'ulcération est simple, sans complications de voisinage ; il n'y a aucune cystite, ce qui permet d'affirmer qu'on a affaire à une ulcération simple ; c'est le moment d'intervenir par un curettage énergique de la lésion. La deuxième période est caractérisée par l'apparition de la cystite, d'où une tendance marquée à l'incrustation calcaire. La croûte phosphatique s'accumule rapidement ; de temps en temps, des morceaux s'en séparent et des fragments calcaires sont expulsés par l'urèthre, ainsi que des débris de pseudo-membranes, au prix de douleurs plus ou moins violentes. Quelquefois, ces fragments calcaires sont retenus dans la vessie et forment des calculs nécessitant la lithotritie. — La vessie s'enflamme de plus en plus ; les exsudats inflammatoires traversent les couches musculaires (cystite interstitielle), entravant d'abord la distension de la vessie, et finissant par réduire de plus en plus la capacité du viscère. Enfin, dans une troisième et dernière période, la vessie est transformée en une poche non élastique pouvant contenir à peine quelques grammes d'urine. — Mais on a rarement l'occasion de constater cette dernière période, car la pyélo-néphrite ascendante emporte généralement le malade dès la fin de la seconde période.

Les *ulcérations aiguës* de la vessie sont rares en dehors de l'*ulcère simple perforant*. Ce dernier offre des caractères bien spéciaux. *Cliniquement*, il est le plus souvent latent, pendant une période plus ou moins longue, et s'annonce alors brusquement par une des deux complications suivantes : hématurie ou perforation. L'hématurie peut être très abondante et anémier rapidement le malade au point de faire croire, par son intensité et sa spontanéité, à une hématarie d'origine rénale (cas de Castaigne). La perforation semble être la règle au cours de ces ulcérations de la face postérieure et survient ordinairement du quatrième au huitième jour ; elle peut être parfois révélée par une douleur intense, d'emblée excessive ; mais le plus souvent elle se produit sans grand bruit et peut facilement passer inaperçue ; la réaction péritonéale est en effet très peu marquée, ce qui tient à l'asepsie normale du contenu vésical, comme l'a d'ailleurs montré Castaigne ; on sait en effet que l'ulcération aiguë perforante évolue ordinairement dans des vessies non atteintes de cystite. Dans presque tous les cas, on constate une rétention complète ou incomplète, et les urines recueillies par la sonde sont ordinairement sanguinolentes. — Latence, hématurie, perforation, telle est, pourrait-on dire, la triade symptomatique caractérisant l'ulcère aigu perforant de la vessie.

*Au point de vue anatomo-pathologique*, certains détails sont à retenir : la forme souvent ovalaire de la perforation, à grand axe d'ordinaire transversal ; sa délimitation nette, à pic l'unicité habituelle. Le *siège* aussi paraît constant : ces ulcères se produisent presque toujours au niveau de la paroi postérieure sous-péritonéale de la vessie, près du sommet. Il est même intéressant d'opposer ce siège élevé de l'ulcère aigu perforant à celui de l'ulcère chronique, solitaire, situé ordinairement plus bas, dans la région du trigone.

Certaines ulcérations aiguës de la vessie présentent des bords rouges, vascularisés, offrant même parfois la trace d'un cercle éliminatoire ; si on examine avec soin le reste de la muqueuse vésicale, on retrouve souvent des plaques de congestion, des ecchymoses qui semblent indiquer une diffusion des lésions plus grande qu'on ne l'avait pensé au premier abord.

Quelle est la *pathogénie* de ces ulcérations aiguës de la vessie ou ulcères simples perforants de la vessie ?

Toutes les explications données à propos des ulcérations gastriques peuvent être invoquées ici ; mais nous devons surtout en retenir trois : l'influence des *lésions vasculaires*, des *lésions infectieuses* et des *lésions trophiques*. Quant à l'acidité du milieu, si elle peut être invoquée au niveau de l'estomac, elle ne pourrait l'être au même titre au niveau de la vessie, car l'acidité normale, d'ailleurs très faible, de l'urine, fait bientôt place à l'alcalinité, dans le cas de vessie enflammée.

*L'embolie et la thrombose artérielle* sont invoquées par quelques auteurs; et Castaigne, dans sa dernière observation, note expressément qu'une artère vésicale était oblitérée près de l'ulcère. — Mais on peut se demander si toutes ces lésions vasculaires ne sont pas d'ordre secondaire. J'ai tenté sur des chiens quelques expériences de ligature des artères se rendant à la vessie; je n'ai jamais obtenu aucune lésion de la muqueuse vésicale. Sans donc rejeter absolument cette explication, nous devons être plus près de la vérité en accordant une grande importance aux *lésions infectieuses d'ordre général.*

Nous n'avons d'ailleurs qu'à nous reporter aux examens histologiques pratiqués dans le cas d'ulcère aigu perforant et mentionnés notamment dans la thèse remarquable de Gandy, Paris 1899.

Voici ce que nous y voyons souvent constaté :

Vaso-dilatation générale excessive des vésicules de la sous-muqueuse et des capillaires de la muqueuse; nécrose spéciale frappant tous les éléments en bloc; infiltration hémorrhagique abondante, à la fois de la sous-muqueuse et de la muqueuse; quelquefois thrombose spéciale hyaline des petits vaisseaux de voisinage. Enfin, à la périphérie, infiltration inflammatoire d'éléments embryonnaires jeunes, sous forme de liséré périnécrotique, de traînées périvasculaires s'étendant plus ou moins loin. Œdème de la sous-muqueuse.

A quoi attribuer ces lésions, sinon à un principe infectieux (ordinairement toxine, rarement bactérie), transmis par la voie vasculaire sanguine et qui est venu se déposer pour ainsi dire au niveau des capillaires de la muqueuse et de la sous-muqueuse, réalisant alors le processus histologique de la nécrose hémorrhagique aiguë, et arrivant à produire successivement toutes les lésions suivantes : infarctus hémorrhagique — escarre — érosion hémorrhagique — exulcération de la muqueuse — enfin ulcération profonde à fond encore hémorrhagique ou escarrifié.

Cette hypothèse rationnelle, déjà confirmée par l'histologie, je vais essayer maintenant de la démontrer par des faits *d'ordre clinique et expérimental.*

D'abord on a parfois retrouvé les lésions décrites précédemment : ecchymoses, infiltrations sanguines, érosions hémorrhagiques, exulcérations, ulcérations constituées — non seulement dans l'estomac et

---

1. GANDY. *L'ulcère simple et la nécrose blennorrhagique des toxémies.* Th. Paris 1899.

l'intestin, mais encore au niveau de la muqueuse vésicale, au cours de diverses infections (érysipèle, septicémies post-opératoires, pyohémies — infection puerpérale — scarlatine — variole — diphtérie — fièvre typhoïde — dysenterie — étranglement herniaire — tuberculose pulmonaire); et même dans quelques affections septiques locales (phlegmon diffus ou gangréneux). On peut les constater aussi dans les intoxications : soit étrangères à l'organisme (par les sels de mercure par exemple, surtout le sublimé) soit autochtones (comme dans l'urémie, le cancer, et en général toutes les cachexies). — Mais il est deux cas où on les retrouve peut-être encore plus fréquemment : à la suite de brûlures étendues de la surface cutanée qui s'accompagnent, comme on le sait, d'une intoxication profonde, et dans cette affection que Parrot désignait sous le nom d'œdème des nouveau-nés : sous l'influence des modifications profondes que subit l'organisme à la naissance de la vie extra-utérine, amenant sans doute une brusque fabrication de toxines, surviennent des ulcérations aiguës de l'estomac, de l'intestin, ou même de la vessie, accompagnées d'hémorrhagies abondantes et de perforation.

Si dans toutes ces affections les diverses lésions vésicales énumérées précédemment ne sont pas plus souvent mentionnées, c'est qu'on néglige souvent d'observer l'état de la muqueuse vésicale.

Mais dans un grand nombre d'autopsies que j'ai faites à l'hôpital Necker, portant sur des affections fort diverses d'ailleurs, et où j'examinais systématiquement la muqueuse vésicale, j'ai été surpris de retrouver parfois ces lésions que je n'aurais pas même eu l'idée de rechercher.

Enfin je voudrais exposer rapidement en terminant une autre série de faits qui me portent à considérer comme vraie dans un certain nombre de cas cette pathogénie des ulcérations vésicales adoptée par Gandy dans sa thèse : La nécrose hémorragique au cours d'une toxémie.

Sur un grand nombre de chiens, lapins, cobayes, j'ai injecté par la voie sanguine des cultures de différents microbes (coli-bacille, b. pyocyanique — b. lactique, etc.). — Je procédais ordinairement de trois façons : ou bien j'injectais la culture dans la circulation veineuse générale, et je produisais alors un traumatisme au niveau de la muqueuse vésicale — ou même une simple rétention d'urine momentanée; ou bien, après avoir découvert une artériole se rendant à la vessie, j'y introduisais un ou deux centimètres cubes de culture virulente; ou bien j'injectais directement dans la paroi vésicale, sous la muqueuse, une ou deux gouttes de culture.

Un certain nombre de mes expériences sont restées négatives : parmi les autres, certaines n'ont donné qu'un résultat incomplet (plaques d'injection, ecchymoses). — Huit sont très concluantes : J'ai obtenu deux fois avec du coli-bacille, deux fois avec du pyocyanique, des nécroses hémorrhagiques frappant en bloc tout un îlot de muqueuse vésicale ; ou des ulcérations constituées, depuis la simple exulcération jusqu'à l'ulcération profonde atteignant la musculeuse et même jusqu'à l'ulcération perforante. — Dans un cas même, j'ai pu suivre la transition d'une lésion à l'autre : il existait deux gros îlots de nécrose hémorrhagique reliés par un pont et soulevant la muqueuse qui présentait une coloration noire à ce niveau ; on aurait dit deux gros hématomes, mais l'on voyait sur l'un des îlots un sillon ou cercle éliminatoire qui avait déjà soulevé le bloc nécrotique et le séparait nettement des portions voisines de la muqueuse vésicale saine. Si j'avais sacrifié l'animal un jour plus tard, j'aurais eu sans doute l'occasion de constater la chute de cet îlot nécrotique intéressant toute la paroi et il s'en serait suivi une perforation. Dans deux cas, j'ai obtenu une ulcération taillée à l'emporte-pièce et ayant perforé toute l'épaisseur des parois vésicales.

Il faut aussi, croyons-nous, faire une part assez importante aux *lésions trophiques* dans la pathogénie de ces ulcérations vésicales, comme pour toutes les autres ulcérations. — Spillmann, Herting, Blocq, Tuffier ont beaucoup insisté sur la fréquence de ces ulcérations chez les paraplégiques, les tabétiques, les aliénés paralytiques, en un mot chez tous ceux qui présentent des troubles trophiques prononcés. Il se peut qu'on décrive un jour un mal perforant vésical comme on a décrit un mal perforant buccal après le mal perforant plantaire.

Deux points restent encore obscurs dans l'histoire des ulcérations vésicales :

1° La bactériurie peut-elle suffire à créer de toutes pièces une ulcération vésicale ?

2° Une ulcération aiguë de la vessie peut-elle s'indurer comme au niveau de l'estomac, et se transformer en ulcère chronique à bords épaissis ?

Je ne saurais répondre absolument à ces deux questions. Mais je crois que la bactériurie ne peut que favoriser l'apparition d'une ulcération, si les autres conditions pathogéniques se trouvent réunies. Quant à la transformation d'une ulcération aiguë en ulcère chronique, je crois qu'elle est possible. Oliver l'admettait, et sans être fréquente au niveau de la vessie, elle doit cependant exister.

Voici, pour terminer, mes conclusions :

En dehors des ulcérations vésicales symptomatiques d'une lésion primitive de la paroi, il existe des ulcérations simples, essentielles, qu'on doit opposer aux premières. Ces ulcérations peuvent, comme dans l'estomac, revêtir deux types — soit le type chronique de l'ulcère simple, solitaire, de la vessie, bien décrit par Fenwick, et souvent confondu avec la tuberculose, bien à tort, car il est curable — soit le type aigu : ces ulcérations aiguës dont le type est l'ulcère simple, perforant, peuvent avoir une pathogénie variable; il faut savoir être éclectique, et tout en admettant les lésions vasculaires (embolie et thrombose), d'ailleurs rarement constatées, savoir faire une place beaucoup plus grande aux lésions trophiques et surtout aux lésions infectieuses de nécrose hémorrhagique, prouvées à la fois par la clinique, l'histologie, l'expérimentation.

---

## PROPAGATIONS GANGLIONNAIRES DANS LES NÉOPLASMES VÉSICAUX

### par M. O. PASTEAU,

de Paris.

Il était encore classique il y a quelques années de dire que les néoplasmes vésicaux ne s'accompagnaient pas de propagations ganglionnaires. Ces conclusions étaient basées sur des idées théoriques et des constatations cliniques. En effet, ne pouvant arriver à injecter les lymphatiques de la vessie, on en était arrivé à dire que ceux-ci n'existent pas; d'autre part, chez les malades on ne trouve pour ainsi dire jamais de propagations ganglionnaires.

A la suite de travaux de Teichmann, Sappey, Albarran et Lluria, j'ai repris l'étude des lymphatiques vésicaux, en même temps que Gerota les étudiait à Berlin au point de vue purement anatomique.

En 1898, j'avais déjà réuni à Necker, chez M. le professeur Guyon, 89 observations, dont 49 personnelles avec 62 cas de propagations ganglionnaires. Les 25 cas de tumeurs que j'ai observés depuis n'ont pas changé mes conclusions.

L'étude de la *nature* et du *siège des tumeurs* n'amenant aucun résultat au point de vue de l'étiologie de ces propagations, j'ai cherché ce qu'on trouverait en étudiant le *mode d'implantation* de ces néoplasmes. Sur 71 cas où l'implantation est nettement indiquée on trouve :

25 pour 100 de propagations ganglionnaires dans les tumeurs pédiculées;

44 pour 100 de propagations ganglionnaires dans les tumeurs sessiles;

35 pour 100 de propagations ganglionnaires dans les tumeurs infiltrées.

Si cliniquement on ne trouve rien, c'est que :

Dans 79 pour 100 des cas il y a dégénérescence des ganglions iliaques;

Dans 24 pour 100 des cas il y a dégénérescence des ganglions lombaires, et ces ganglions sont trop profonds pour être perçus.

Cependant comme il est possible par la cystoscopie et surtout par le palper abdominal combiné au toucher rectal ou vaginal de sentir si la tumeur est infiltrée, *on peut pour ainsi dire toujours faire indirectement le diagnostic de l'existence des propagations ganglionnaires dans les tumeurs vésicales.*

Ces lésions ne sont donc pas rares; d'autre part, elles sont possibles à diagnostiquer. Aussi, lorsqu'on ne peut intervenir de bonne heure, même si on fait une large opération, on ne doit pas compter sur une guérison définitive et on peut prévoir que les lésions continueront à évoluer au loin, si elles n'évoluent pas sur place.

---

## CURETTAGE DE LA VESSIE POUR LITHIASE CHEZ UNE FEMME

### par le docteur EDGARD CHEVALIER,

Chirurgien des Hôpitaux de Paris.

La malade dont je relate ici l'observation est une femme de 44 ans que j'ai opérée en septembre 1899 à l'hôpital Necker.

Elle est entrée le 14 août 1899 salle Fouché et nous raconte ainsi son histoire pathologique.

Il y a quinze mois, sans cause appréciable, elle remarqua quelques hématuries peu abondantes, qui durèrent environ trois mois.

Les mictions peu fréquentes, peu douloureuses donnaient des urines troubles avec dépôt gluant.

Survinrent quelques douleurs rénales sans coliques néphrétiques proprement dites.

Cet état subsista sans grandes modifications jusque six mois avant l'entrée à l'hôpital. A ce moment survinrent les phénomènes de cystite :

Fréquence de la miction qui se répète toutes les heures ou demi-heures le jour, et 5 à 6 fois la nuit;

Douleur dans la miction, non exagérée par la marche et non calmée par le repos, urines glaireuses, puis plus simplement troubles.

Rien de particulier aux règles.

A l'examen de la malade on ne constate rien de particulier du côté de la santé générale, ni du côté de l'appareil génital. Tout se concentre sur son appareil urinaire :

Reins et uretères : rien de spécial.

Vessie : l'exploration de la vessie avec l'explorateur à boule est un peu douloureuse et ne donne pas de sensation de corps étranger vrai (calcul), mais l'exploration avec l'explorateur métallique montre que toute la paroi de la vessie est tapissée d'une couche pseudo-calcaire qui donne un son étouffé; nulle part on ne perçoit de calcul libre.

Capacité vésicale — environ 60 grammes — au delà de ce chiffre vives douleurs.

Urines troubles avec dépôt phosphatique.

Urèthre : rien de spécial.

Diagnostic : Lithiase vésicale.

Je fais endormir la malade et à l'aide d'un lithotriteur introduit dans la vessie je fais des tentatives infructueuses pour saisir des portions de cette boue calcaire.

Devant l'impossibilité d'opérer avec cet instrument, je prends une curette de Wolkmann ordinaire, je l'introduis par l'urèthre dans la vessie, et je pratique le curettage complet de cet organe comme je l'ai déjà fait un certain nombre de fois pour des cystites simples ou rebelles chez des femmes. Grâce à ce procédé je débarrasse complètement la vessie d'une boue phosphato-calcaire qui incrustait toute la muqueuse.

Je termine par un grand lavage à la solution de nitrate d'argent à un 1000° et place une sonde à demeure.

Les suites furent des plus simples, les urines devinrent claires, les douleurs disparurent, les mictions redevinrent normales, et la malade sortit du service guérie de ses accidents.

Telle est l'observation de ma malade. Je crois que l'on peut dire qu'elle n'avait pas encore eu le temps d'agglomérer en un calcul unique les sels terreux qui précipités dans ses urines troubles s'étaient fixés sur la muqueuse enduite d'un vernis glaireux. Je crois plutôt à cette hypothèse qu'à celle d'une fragmentation spontanée de son calcul.

# DE LA BOUTONNIÉRE PÉRINÉALE AVEC DILATATION IMMÉDIATE PROGRESSIVE DE L'URETHRE POSTÉRIEUR

COMME VOIE D'EXTRACTION DES PETITS CALCULS SURTOUT CHEZ LES ENFANTS,
AVEC TROIS OBSERVATIONS DE LITHOTRITIE CHEZ L'ENFANT

## par MAURICE HACHE,

professeur de chirurgie à la Faculté française de médecine de Beyrouth.

Pour les enfants comme pour les adultes, la lithotritie a mainte nant gagné sa cause en France ; les travaux du professeur Guyon et de son École ont démontré que c'est l'opération de choix des calculs et que la taille ne doit bénéficier que de ses contre-indications

La plus fréquente de ses contre-indications chez l'enfant résulte du petit calibre de l'urèthre antérieur et de l'impossibilité de lui faire admettre même après incision du méat, un lithotriteur assez puissant pour broyer le calcul ou même à mors assez longs pour le saisir solidement, s'il est arrondi, la longueur des mors étant pour des questions de résistance, étroitement liée au calibre de la tige de l'instrument.

A ces cas où la lithotritie est matériellement impossible je crois qu'il faut ajouter ceux dans lesquels le lithotriteur passe très juste ; dans ces cas, en effet, l'instrument peut déchirer l'urèthre au retour pour peu qu'il soit engravé.

Cet accident m'est arrivé chez un enfant de 4 ans porteur d'un calcul phosphatique de 1 centimètre de diamètre écrasé en 6 minutes. Le lithotriteur nº 0 à mors plein de Collin avait difficilement franchi le bulbe à l'aller, son retrait fut très laborieux. Suites simples, sans fièvre, mais deux mois et demi après l'enfant me revenait avec un rétrécissement naissant de l'angle pénien admettant le béniqué 29. Il avait en outre un calcul enchatonné d'urates méconnu la première fois et que j'ai dû enlever par la taille hypogastrique après une boutonnière exploratrice : je reviendrai plus loin sur cette partie de son observation.

J'y ajoute la fréquence de l'enchatonnement ou des adhérences du calcul à la paroi vésicale que j'ai rencontrées 4 fois, sur une vingtaine de cas de calculs de l'enfance.

Il y a donc chez les enfants un certain nombre de petits calculs qui échappent à la lithotritie ; c'est pour eux que la boutonnière périnéale me paraît l'opération de choix, ainsi que pour les petits corps étrangers non broyables de la vessie de l'adulte.

La boutonnière périnéale est en effet beaucoup plus simple comme opération et comme suites que la taille hypogastrique, et elle est exempte des dangers qui ont fait rejeter avec raison les tailles périnéales, section d'un ou des deux canaux déférents et incontinence d'urine persistante. Je ne parle pas des hémorragies qui sont exceptionnelles chez l'enfant.

Si l'on n'utilise pas souvent dans ce but cette opération si simple et si anciennement connue c'est certainement parce que l'attention n'a pas été suffisamment attirée sur la largeur de la voie qu'elle peut donner, et c'est à ce point de vue que les observations que j'apporte pourront être de quelque utilité.

J'ai pratiqué 6 fois la boutonnière périnéale chez l'enfant. Une fois sur l'enfant de 4 ans cité plus haut chez lequel j'ai pu reconnaître ainsi l'enchatonnement du calcul, ultérieurement enlevé par la taille hypogastrique; une seconde fois chez un enfant de 6 ans auquel j'ai fait la lithotritie périnéale, et un troisième chez un enfant de 5 ans et demi auquel j'ai enlevé quelques graviers phosphatiques développés après une taille hypogastrique faite trois mois auparavant.

Je passe rapidement sur ces 3 cas qui ne font que confirmer l'innocuité bien connue de la boutonnière, pour insister seulement sur les trois derniers.

Obs. IV. — Enfant de 15 ans, Aziz Abou H. de Chypre, porteur d'un calcul de la région prostatique à côté duquel passait facilement l'explorateur métallique sans le révéler, mais qui donnait avec la boule d'un explorateur souple une sensation de frottement caractéristique. Les symptômes fonctionnels datant de 7 ans étaient d'ailleurs anormaux : envies impérieuses, mictions pénibles à la fin, non influencées par la marche, plus fréquentes et plus douloureuses la nuit que le jour. Je choisis la boutonnière périnéale à cause du siège du calcul et je la pratique le 5 avril dernier.

Après incision en arrière du bulbe sur le conducteur cannelé, j'introduis dans l'urèthre postérieur les dilatateurs de Hégar n° 7, 8, 10, 12 et 15, ce dernier correspondant au 59 filière Charrière (15 millimètres de diamètre), je peux alors très facilement introduire le petit doigt dans la vessie et sentir le calcul que les dilatateurs y ont refoulé, une tenette courbe n° 2 d'Aubry mesurant un centimètre et demi de diamètre et un centimètre d'épaisseur y pénètre très facilement et ramène le calcul qui s'est logé dans sa concavité sans augmenter l'écartement des mors.

C'est un petit calcul mûriforme d'oxalate de chaux ayant la forme d'un triangle à bords arrondis et mesurant environ un centimètre sur chaque bord et un demi centimètre d'épaisseur.

Tamponnement iodoformé de la plaie, sonde à demeure retirée au bout de 24 heures. Léger accès de fièvre le soir de l'ablation. Aussitôt la sonde enlevée les mictions se sont faites toutes les trois heures.

L'urine commence à passer par la verge le 5e jour, et le 11e jour moins de la moitié passait par la fistule. L'enfant est retourné chez lui en cet état et je n'en ai plus eu de nouvelles.

Obs. V. — Enfant de 10 ans, Georges Yousef d'Aïn Terez, ayant depuis un an et demi des douleurs à la miction qui était difficile et douloureuse; mais ces douleurs n'étaient pas constantes, et certaines mictions étaient tout à fait normales. L'explorateur de Guyon fait sentir un calcul d'un centimètre et demi.

Le 6 juin 1900 tentative de lithotritie avec le lithotriteur n° 1 de Collin; ce n'est qu'après 14 minutes que j'arrive à saisir le calcul, l'instrument dérape sur une première prise de 15 millimètres et en fait une seconde solide de 2 centimètres. Mais le calcul résiste absolument au broiement. Je procède immédiatement à la boutonnière périnéale.

Même manuel opératoire, mandrins de Hégar jusqu'au n° 14 (14 millimètres de diamètre). Prise facile du calcul avec la tenette n° 1 d'Aubry mais la pierre déborde latéralement les bords de l'instrument et s'oppose à l'extraction; ne pouvant faire de prise correcte malgré plusieurs essais, je dois introduire le petit doigt par la plaie en même temps que la tenette pour redresser le calcul dans ses mors, l'extraction peut alors être faite avec une force modérée. Le calcul mesure 25 millimètres de long sur 15 millimètres de large et 2 millimètres d'épaisseur. Une de ses faces présente des aspérités d'un millimètre de hauteur environ où adhèrent encore des débris épithéliaux.

Grand lavage boriqué de la vessie et de l'urèthre, pas de sonde à demeure, pansement à plat.

Dans la journée mictions pénibles qui surprennent l'enfant et se font par la plaie : impossible de lui faire préciser leur fréquence. Boissons abondantes, aucune réaction locale ni générale. Le lendemain 4 à 5 mictions encore brûlantes pour lesquelles il demande le vase; pour une seule d'entre elles, il ne peut attendre qu'on le lui apporte. Ces mictions se font moitié par la verge et moitié par la plaie. Dès le 5e jour elles se font exclusivement par la verge et sans douleur.

Il sort de l'hôpital le 9e jour, avec une plaie périnéale granuleuse ne donnant plus issue à l'urine, avec 4 à 5 mictions en 24 heures encore un peu impérieuses.

Obs. VI. — Marcel A... 2 ans et demi, demeurant à Malacca-Zachlé, gêne de la miction observée depuis une huitaine de jours, crise de rétention complète depuis deux jours. Le cathétérisme montre un calcul engagé à l'entrée de la prostate et très facilement repoussé dans la vessie.

Opération le 26 mai 1900. Même manuel opératoire, dilatateurs de Hégar 5 à 9 (9 millimètres de diamètre). Un petit calcul est aussitôt pris et broyé avec une pince à pansement utérin. Croyant à une pierre plus volumineuse, je prolonge mes recherches, et ne trouvant rien, j'introduis péniblement le bout du petit doigt jusqu'au bord de la vessie, dont j'amène toute la surface à son contact par la palpation hypogastrique. La dilatation ainsi imposée au col correspond au 35 Charrière, comme je l'ai vérifié.

Lavage boriqué de la vessie et de l'urèthre, pas de sonde à demeure pansement à plat à la gaze boriquée.

Mictions fréquentes par la plaie le premier jour et la nuit, mais pas d'incontinence. Le lendemain, légère tuméfaction des bourses, 58°6; le surlendemain, cette tuméfaction a disparu, la miction est presque indolente, il commence à passer de l'urine par le canal qui était oblitéré par un petit caillot sanguin.

Atténuée par la quinine, la fièvre persiste cependant deux jours encore, mais elle disparaît immédiatement quand l'enfant est ramené à la montagne le 29 mai. La plaie périnéale reste fistuleuse 12 jours, elle est complètement cicatrisée le 15°. A cette date, l'enfant urine sans douleur 5 à 6 fois en 24 heures, et résiste facilement au besoin d'uriner.

J'ai donc pu, sans provoquer d'incontinence, enlever sur un enfant de 10 ans un calcul de 16 millimètres de diamètre minimum et chose plus intéressante dilater l'urèthre postérieur et le col d'un enfant de 2 ans et demi jusqu'à y introduire l'extrémité de mon petit doigt, c'est-à-dire jusqu'à permettre le passage d'un calcul de 1 centimètre de diamètre environ, en tenant compte de l'épaisseur des mors de la ténette.

L'inconvénient de cette voie est de ne pas permettre une grande précision dans les manœuvres intra-vésicales, surtout chez les très petits sujets où la pince ne peut être ouverte qu'avec effort, ses branches étant serrées dans le canal. M. Collin veut bien me construire pour ces cas une petite ténette sur le modèle de sa pince à corps étrangers de l'urèthre. Le toucher rectal et mieux encore le toucher vésical sont d'un grand secours pour aider les manœuvres et contrôler le résultat.

Le manuel opératoire est des plus simples; le cathéter cannelé sur lequel on ouvre l'urèthre est un conducteur très suffisant pour introduire les dilatateurs de Hegar dans l'urèthre postérieur, en ayant soin de le retirer jusqu'à ce que son extrémité boutonnée affleure le bord antérieur de l'incision uréthrale.

Je joins à ces faits le résumé des trois opérations de lithotritie que j'ai eu l'occasion de pratiquer chez des enfants de 3, 4 et 5 ans.

Obs. VII. — Yousef Seman, âgé de 5 ans, entre dans mon service le 11 mars 1898 pour un calcul vésical. Il y avait déjà passé huit jours au mois d'octobre précédent pour une rupture de l'urèthre par engagement d'un petit calcul. Lithotritie le 11 mars avec le n° 0 de Collin qui passe facilement : calcul de un centimètre de diamètre, 14 prises en 4 minutes Aspiration de 4 minutes donnant la poussière café au lait des calculs uriques.
Suites simples.

Obs. VIII. — Ouieh Nammoum, âgé de 4 ans, entre le 11 décembre 1897 avec un calcul léger, ne donnant aucune sensation avec l'explorateur métallique, reconnaissable seulement par l'explorateur à boule et le toucher bimanuel. Lithotritie le 15 décembre avec le n° 0 de Collin qui passe difficilement au niveau du bulbe. Presque immédiatement, prise d'un centimètre d'un calcul qui s'écrase, puis trois petites prises en 6 minutes. Le retrait du lithotriteur est très laborieux à cause de l'engravement des mors par la bouillie phosphatique. Lavages. Sonde à demeure, qui est arrachée au bout de quelques minutes.

Suites simples, sort le 5° jour avec des mictions douloureuses, mais commençant à s'espacer.

Deux mois et demi après l'enfant m'est ramené avec un rétrécissement de l'angle pénien qui est dilaté jusqu'au n° 34 Beniqué; je reconnais un calcul enchatonné qui est extrait le 24 mars par la taille hypogastrique. C'était un calcul urique de 5 grammes qui avait été méconnu pendant la lithotritie. L'enfant a quitté l'hôpital, guéri, le 19 avril.

Obs. IX. — Yousef Abdallah 5 ans entre le 10 décembre 1893 pour une rétention d'urine avec miction par regorgement due à un calcul. Lithotritie le 18 décembre avec le n° 0 de Collin, 24 prises en 9 minutes; calcul de un centimètre et demi à broiement un peu laborieux composé d'oxalate de chaux, mais beaucoup moins foncé que ne le sont en général les calculs mûraux. La sonde à demeure mise après l'opération n'est pas tolérée et la miction par regorgement continue jusqu'au 31 décembre, époque où elle cède à l'application pendant trois jours d'une sonde de Pezzer. Il sort guéri le 4 janvier.

---

# FRAGMENTATION SPONTANÉE DES CALCULS URINAIRES DANS LA VESSIE

## par M. le professeur SEVEREANU,

de Bucarest.

Le 5 décembre de l'année écoulée, il nous est amené dans notre service, par son père, le jeune *Marin Tziganila*, âgé de 18 ans, roumain, de la commune rurale Ghimpatzi, district de Vlashca, qui souffrait, depuis plusieurs semaines, des voies urinaires.

Voici l'historique du malade tel qu'il nous est donné par son père : L'enfant, dès sa naissance, était bien constitué, suffisamment fort; à l'âge de 2 à 3 ans il a commencé à ressentir des douleurs très violentes pendant les mictions, qui étaient très fréquentes sans que jamais l'urine fût mélangée de sang. Ces douleurs ont persisté jusqu'à ce que l'enfant ait atteint l'âge de 9 ans, époque à laquelle elles ont complètement cessé, sans traitement et sans autre cause connue, et l'enfant a pu vaquer aux travaux habituels des paysans sans être incommodé.

Cet état satisfaisant a duré 9 ans, et les parents avaient complètement oublié les souffrances de leur garçon dans son enfance; il vaquait à ses travaux journaliers, courait, montait à cheval, se transportait en chariots non suspendus, etc., sans ressentir la moindre douleur.

Au mois de septembre 1897, conduisant la nuit un troupeau de moutons en pleine obscurité, il tombe dans un trou et ressent immédiatement une violente douleur dans le bas de l'abdomen. A partir de ce moment, les mictions sont devenues très fréquentes, et surtout la nuit, très pressées, toujours accompagnées de douleurs violentes; l'émission de l'urine, s'interrompant brusquement pendant la miction, ne reprenait son cours qu'après que le patient faisait mouvoir le bassin dans différentes directions. Les douleurs ne s'irradiaient dans aucune autre partie du corps, elles restaient limitées à la verge, et surtout à son extrémité. Jamais l'urine n'a contenu de sang. Quand le malade était à cheval ou en chariot, il ressentait des douleurs dans la vessie, douleurs qui disparaissaient aussitôt qu'il restait au repos.

L'urine a toujours été limpide et jamais ni sable ni gravier n'ont été émis par l'urèthre, le malade n'a jamais eu d'affection de nature génitale. Quand il entra dans notre service, il se trouvait dans l'état suivant : Bien constitué, suffisamment fort, par rapport à son âge, n'avait aucun vice organique, se plaignait de douleurs violentes pendant les mictions; celles-ci étaient fréquentes et rapides. Urine normale et en quantité ordinaire (1200—1500 gr.). Le pénis ne présentait pas d'état anormal, le prépuce, même, n'était pas allongé comme il l'est ordinairement chez les calculeux. On ne trouvait aucune tumeur dans la région hypogastrique, le périnée se trouvait de même dans l'état normal.

Par le rectum, avec le doigt, on trouvait la prostate augmentée de volume, et dans la vessie on sentait une tumeur; par la pression avec la partie charnue de l'index on pouvait remarquer qu'il existait un corps étranger dans la vessie, et même la sensation du doigt semblait indiquer l'existence de plusieurs corps étrangers, qui glissaient les uns sur les autres, exactement comme si l'on avait senti la présence de plusieurs corps durs dans une vessie inerte.

De ces indications, nous avons pu déduire la présomption de la présence d'un calcul dans la vessie et même, pour nous, il était à peu près certain que le calcul n'était pas unique.

*Examen de l'urèthre et de la vessie.* — Après avoir fait le lavage de l'urèthre à l'eau boriquée à 5 pour 100, nous sommes entré dans la vessie avec une sonde métallique n° 18, et, aussitôt dépassé le col de la vessie, nous avons rencontré un corps solide, mais la vessie ne contenant pas d'urine, nous n'avons pu faire l'examen complet. Au moyen de notre sonde, nous avons introduit 200 grammes d'eau boriquée et nous avons pu alors examiner la vessie dans tous ses détails; nous avons trouvé dans le cul-de-sac inférieur un corps étranger dont le diamètre nous a paru dépasser 3—4 centimètres, présentant une grande résonance, ce qui nous a fait supposer que le calcul était ou uratique ou oxalatique, et surtout nous supposions une composition d'oxalates, parce que la sonde nous indiquait la présence d'aspérités sur sa surface, aspérités qui ne se trouvent que dans les calculs oxalatiques. Toujours avec la sonde, nous avons supposé la présence de plusieurs calculs. De ces quelques caractères que nous avions pu constater, nous avons cru avoir affaire à plusieurs calculs que nous supposions être de composition oxalatique.

Les quelques jours qu'il a fallu pour préparer le malade à l'opération, ont suffi à l'effrayer; soit de ce qu'il voyait autour de lui et les souffrances qu'il endurait au moment des lavages, soit que d'autres personnes l'aient effrayé, il refuse absolument de se laisser opérer. Le père nous priait d'autre part d'opérer son enfant à tout prix, quel qu'en soit le résultat, car les souffrances rendaient la vie difficile non seulement à l'enfant, mais à toute sa famille.

Ayant l'autorisation du père, nous avons chloroformisé le malade malgré lui et nous l'avons opéré par la taille transversale sus-pubienne. Après avoir ouvert la vessie et fixé les bords de l'ouverture au moyen de pinces, nous avons introduit l'index gauche et nous avons constaté la présence de deux calculs occupant la partie basse de la vessie et qui étaient indépendants l'un de l'autre. Nous avons fait glisser une tenette droite le long du doigt et nous avons extrait les deux calculs l'un après l'autre. Nous avons ensuite lavé la vessie à l'eau boriquée; nous avons de plus constaté que la muqueuse était très injectée, sans ulcérations. Comme nous ne faisons souvent la suture de la vessie, et pour que ses parois ne se retirent pas au fond, laissant ainsi un vide entre elles et celles de l'abdomen, dans lequel s'introduirait l'urine, ainsi que pour arrêter le sang, nous avons cru qu'il serait plus avantageux d'appliquer quatre points de suture en croix entre les bords de la plaie vésicale et les chairs voisines, sous la peau. Ces sutures ont été faites avec du catgut n° 1.

Nous avons introduit un drain de gaze iodoformée, la plaie et les environs ont été enduits de vaseline iodoformée, et par dessus le tout un pansement contentif.

*Examen du calcul.* — Les deux calculs extraits sont les deux moitiés d'un seul et même calcul.

Réunis, ils forment un calcul elliptique, aplati sur deux faces, long de 57 millimètres, d'une grosseur de 40 millimètres sur un des diamètres transversaux et de 25 millimètres sur l'autre. Le poids total est de 30 grammes. Une des moitiés pèse 20,6 grammes, l'autre 9,4 grammes. La surface est nette, luisante, la consistance est forte, la résonance très prononcée. Les deux surfaces de réunion sont irrégulières, présentant, sur chacune des moitiés, des convexités et des concavités qui s'adaptent exactement les unes sur les autres; sur l'une des surfaces de rupture, il existe les noyaux de cristallisation qui s'adaptent exactement à l'excavation qui se trouve sur la surface articulaire de l'autre moitié.

Des caractères des surfaces de rupture, il ressort d'une façon certaine et indiscutable que les deux calculs sont les moitiés d'un seul et même calcul qui s'est rompu dans la vessie d'une façon qu'il nous est difficile d'expliquer.

Tout ce que nous pouvons admettre dans le cas présent serait une contraction violente de la vessie au moment de la chute dans le fossé, en pleine nuit.

Du poli des surfaces de rupture, on peut aussi déduire que le temps qui s'est écoulé depuis la fragmentation correspond à celui écoulé depuis la chute et le moment où le malade a commencé à ressentir ces douleurs violentes dans le bas de l'abdomen.

Nous ne pouvons admettre comme cause de cette rupture que la contraction violente de la vessie, produite au moment où le malade est tombé dans un trou en faisant un faux pas, pendant la nuit.

L'usure et le poli des surfaces nous incitent à reconnaître que la rupture s'est produite plusieurs semaines, ou même plusieurs mois avant, c'est-à-dire vers l'époque où le malade, au moment de la chute, a ressenti des douleurs très fortes dans le bas de l'abdomen.

## VINGT-HUIT CAS DE LITHIASE VÉSICALE CHEZ L'ENFANT, TRAITÉS PAR LA TAILLE HYPOGASTRIQUE ET LA SUTURE TOTALE DE LA VESSIE

### *RAPPORT*

### par M. le docteur DIMITRI MICHAILOWSKY,

ex-chirurgien en chef de l'hôpital de Philippopoli.

Messieurs, j'ai eu l'occasion de pratiquer la taille hypogastrique avec suture totale de la vessie chez 28 sujets atteints de calculs, j'ai employé chez eux deux procédés de suture de la vessie. Dans 20 cas j'ai eu recours à la suture de la vessie à un seul plan selon le procédé de « Halsted's plain guilt suture », dans huit cas j'ai eu recours à la suture à deux plans, un profond et un superficiel (suture Lembert).

Mon intention ici n'est pas d'établir un parallèle entre la taille hypogastrique et la lithotritie. La supériorité de cette dernière est aujourd'hui pleinement reconnue ; et elle est devenue la méthode de choix depuis les perfectionnements que lui a fait subir en France mon très vénéré maître, M. le professeur Guyon. Je n'ai pu malheureusement la pratiquer, les instruments me faisant défaut. Je ne veux pas vous présenter une analyse complète de mes observations, je désire seulement attirer votre attention sur quelques points de technique et de clinique.

Sur mes 28 opérés il y a 22 enfants de deux à seize ans et 6 adultes.

Deux de mes opérés ont succombé : le premier est mort cinq jours après l'opération d'une péritonite circonscrite sans élévation de température (37°,1) et malgré un état général très bon. Le second succomba le matin du deuxième jour de l'opération avec des symptômes d'anurie.

Ces deux morts ne sauraient être attribuées à l'opération, elles ne sont pas dues non plus à une intoxication par des agents antiseptiques, ceux-ci n'ayant été employés qu'à très faible dose. (Acide borique 20 pour 1000 ou nitrate d'argent 1 pour 1000.)

Sur les 28 opérés guéris la suture a été hermétique dans 25 cas, 4 fois les sutures de la vessie ont cédé et il s'est produit une légère infiltration d'urine de la cavité de Retzius, vers le cinquième jour de l'opération, mais la guérison s'est toujours effectuée sans autre incident, au bout de vingt à trente jours.

Une seule fois j'ai été obligé de rouvrir la vessie, c'est chez un petit hémophile qui quatre jours après la première opération, fut pris d'hématurie assez grave pour mettre sa vie en danger.

Je fais toujours l'incision vésicale assez haut de façon à éviter de manœuvrer l'aiguille au voisinage du col de la vessie. Les fils suspenseurs mis en place et la vessie ouverte, j'explore la cavité avec l'index droit pour me rendre compte de la forme, du volume et du nombre de calculs. J'ai fait vingt fois la suture de la vessie suivant le procédé d'Halsted à un seul plan, huit fois suivant le procédé classique à deux plans. J'emploie pour la suture vésicale des fils de soie n° 2 ; et pour la suture de la paroi abdominale deux plans de sutures à la soie n° 4. Je place chez presque tous les opérés une petite mèche de gaze iodoformée dans la cavité de Retzius et je l'enlève vingt-quatre heures après.

Je mets toujours une sonde à demeure que je laisse en place un temps variable, suivant la tolérance du canal, le bon ou le mauvais fonctionnement de la sonde ; en même temps surtout chez les enfants je fais lier les pieds et les bras au lit. Sur un urètre tolérant, chez un petit malade laissé une dizaine de jours dans le décubitus dorsal, la sonde à demeure bien surveillée est un important facteur pour le succès de l'opération et donne une grande sécurité au chirurgien. Je lave la vessie du malade pendant les dix jours qui précèdent l'opération et les quelques jours suivants avec de l'acide borique et du nitrate d'argent.

Au point de vue étiologique et pathogénique les calculs de mes opérés étaient tous primitifs, les sujets étaient tous de sexe masculin et appartenaient à la classe pauvre. Au point de vue chimique la plupart des calculs étaient uriques ; quelques-uns d'oxalates de chaux. Leur poids variait entre 10 grammes et 150 grammes.

J'arrive maintenant aux remarques classiques : vous savez Messieurs que le diagnostic positif chez les enfants calculeux ne peut être fait que par l'emploi de l'explorateur du professeur Guyon ou de la sonde en argent, mais vous savez aussi quelles difficultés rencontre chez ces petits êtres l'examen de la vessie ; quelle résistance il faut vaincre, combien de paroles inutiles il faut prononcer, bref nous sommes obligés de recourir le plus souvent au chloroforme.

Il existe malheureusement encore chez nous des services chirurgicaux où le manque de personnel médical et quelquefois une surcharge de travail empêchent le chirurgien de recourir toujours à la chloroformisation : dans ce cas j'ai recours au toucher rectal bimanuel. Les enfants se prêtent aisément à cet examen, qui est facile et sûr pour le diagnostic, d'autre part, le toucher est inoffensif et donne des renseignements précis sur le nombre, la forme et le volume des calculs.

Je ne me sers pas du ballon de Petersen chez les enfants, il n'a pas de raison d'être vu la situation anatomique de leur vessie.

Je me permets d'informer le Congrès que toutes mes opérations aseptiques sont faites dans une salle d'opération étroite, petite, près de quatre water-closets et je peux dire que mes opérés sont traités plutôt antiseptiquement qu'aseptiquement.

Tels sont, Messieurs, les quelques détails que j'ai tenu à vous soumettre, je me bornerai, en terminant, à relever les quelques particularités, qui me paraissent les plus intéressantes dans ma communication.

1° En présence d'un calcul de la vessie chez l'enfant on ne doit songer qu'à deux méthodes de traitement : la lithotritie ou la taille hypogastrique avec suture totale de la vessie à un seul plan (Halsted's suture) ou à deux plans. Je dirai comme bien d'autres, que la lithotritie a le seul tort d'exiger une main très exercée et un outillage spécial.

2° Pour le dignostic des calculs vésicaux chez les enfants, on peut recourir à l'explorateur du professeur Guvon, à la sonde en argent ou encore au toucher rectal combiné.

---

## LES CALCULS URINAIRES EN ÉGYPTE

### par le docteur TREKAKI,

Médecin de l'hôpital hellène, d'Alexandrie.

Les calculs urinaires sont très fréquents en Égypte. Si cette fréquence est relativement très grande dans certaines régions de l'Europe, en Égypte elle est immensément supérieure.

Un relevé des statistiques des hôpitaux d'Égypte convaincra le lecteur mieux que tout autre commentaire.

### HOPITAUX DU CAIRE.

*Hôpital de l'État* (Kasr-el-Aïn) :

Année 1899. Sur 1582 malades indigènes il y a eu : 150 calculs urinaires.

### *Hôpital Allemand*

Sur 71 calculs vésicaux il y a eu 68 indigènes et 5 Européens seulement dans un hôpital où la majeure partie de la population est composée d'Européens.

## HOPITAUX D'ALEXANDRIE.

### *Hôpital Allemand.*

**Année 1894.** — Sur une population de 1285, dont 770 indigènes, il y a eu 101 calculeux vésicaux.

**Année 1895.** — Sur 1112 malades dont 598 indigènes, il y a eu 68 calculeux.

**Année 1896.** — Sur 1110 malades traités, dont 611 indigènes, on a compté 58 calculeux. Ce qui fait pour les 5 années réunies, le 7 pour 100 de calculeux vésicaux sur le chiffre total des malades traités, et de 16 pour 100 environ de calculeux, sur le nombre total des indigènes soignés à l'hôpital allemand.

Quant au rapport qu'il y a entre les malades indigènes porteurs des calculs urinaires, et ceux de diverses autres nationalités reçus à l'hôpital, voici les chiffres :

.  Année 1895. — Sur 68 calculeux il y a eu 67 indigènes et un Syrien.

Année 1896. — Sur 58 calculeux, on compte 55 indigènes et 3 Syriens.

### *Hôpital européen.*

**Année 1898.** — Sur 1294 malades dont 245 indigènes, il y a eu 15 calculeux urinaires.

**Année 1899.** — Sur 1555 malades, dont 295 indigènes, il y a eu 10 calculeux.

### *Hôpital Hellène.*

(Clientèle presque exclusivement européenne.)

Année 1899. — 5 calculeux, dont 3 indigènes et deux Grecs.

Le relevé donc de cinq hôpitaux d'Égypte donne la proportion de 448 calculeux urinaires sur 4167 indigènes, ce qui fait le 17 pour 100 de lithiasiques sur le nombre total d'Égyptiens hospitalisés.

Si donc certaines contrées européennes tiennent une prépondérance au point de vue de cette fréquence, cela est dû à des causes inhérentes à l'individu. Le genre de vie du Français, de l'Italien, de l'Anglais, prédispose à la formation de la lithiase urinaire, à l'essence même de la précipitation des substances chimiques de l'économie qui serviront à former le calcul, à cette biochimie enfin qui sera le point de départ de la genèse d'un corps étranger dans le sein de l'organisme.

Dans la vallée du Nil, il est nécessaire, au contraire, de viser plus haut et s'adresser à d'autres éléments pour avoir une explication pathogénique plus nettement démonstrative.

Le genre de vie en effet du fellah diffère quelque peu de celui de l'Européen. Mais cette différence n'est pas suffisante par elle-même pour nous arrêter, ne fut-ce qu'un instant, sur le mode d'explication d'un fait de ce genre. Si l'Arabe est la plupart du temps végétarien, si le fellah des campagnes préfère l'alimentation végétarienne à l'alimentation carnée, si, en d'autres termes, le paysan arabe se nourrit d'aliments hydrocarbonés et rejette l'alimentation azotée, cela est dû moins à ses goûts qu'à son genre particulier de vie. Mais cela est surtout dû à sa tempérance et plus particulièrement aux ressources naturelles du sol de l'Égypte et à la richesse de la vallée du Nil.

Tout est là en effet. Le Nil avec ses eaux bienfaisantes tant de fois chantées par les anciens Égyptiens, charrie avec lui des éléments nécessaires mais néfastes à l'alimentation du paysan égyptien.

L'eau du Nil, par elle-même, peut être considérée innocente de tous les méfaits dont on l'accuse.

C'est « un air liquéfié » disaient les historiographes égyptiens pour mieux démontrer sa nature, et mieux établir l'essence de sa constitution chimique.

La vérité de cet adage nous est démontrée par un grand nombre de phénomènes qu'on observe journellement chez les fellahs et l'Européen de l'Égypte. Il nous démontre que l'eau du Nil, claire, limpide, débarrassée de toutes les souillures qu'elle charrie dans son sein, est éminemment innocente. Il nous démontre, d'autre part, que l'Européen qui consomme de l'eau claire et filtrée peut se mettre à l'abri d'une foule de circonstances capables d'entraver le fonctionnement de son organisme; témoins en effet de la fréquence relativement minime des calculs vésicaux chez l'Européen habitant ces contrées.

Le fellah au contraire qui fait de l'eau du Nil une de ses principales ressources de nourriture se contente bien souvent d'une alimentation simple dans laquelle entre pour une grande part l'eau du Nil chargée de limon. Son instinct le pousse à l'usage presque exclusif d'une eau boueuse comme portant avec elle le plus d'éléments nutritifs possibles. C'est un héritage séculaire que lui ont légué ses ancêtres.

Le fellah de l'Égypte ne boit donc que de l'eau du Nil chargée de limon. Toute autre eau lui répugne comme contraire et insuffisante à l'alimentation journalière.

Ainsi donc il avale des éléments chimiques et des éléments organiques qui doivent avoir une influence néfaste sur l'urination. Leur abondance surtout met le fonctionnement de l'arbre urinaire dans des conditions particulièrement déplorables. L'eau du Nil, en effet, exempte de toute souillure, et complètement filtrée, telle qu'elle sert dans l'alimentation de l'Européen qui habite l'Égypte, est une eau dont la teneur en éléments minéraux est extrêmement faible. Toutes les analyses témoignent de ce fait. Ceci est d'ailleurs facile à comprendre, car le sol Égyptien et le lit du Nil en particulier sont privés d'éléments capables d'être dissous dans la masse aqueuse qui les charrie. C'est un sol éminemment favorable à ce point de vue.

Mais l'Arabe, nous l'avons déjà dit, fait usage de l'eau non filtrée, et qui plus est, de l'eau boueuse où le limon, qui est partie intégrante de l'eau du Nil, entre pour une très grande part dans la boisson. Or ce limon offre des substances chimiques capables de produire des dégâts considérables. Une analyse complète nous en procurera les éléments intéressants à l'étude que nous avons entreprise.

Voici donc la composition d'un échantillon de limon en n'importe quel mois de l'année.

100 parties de limon sec contiennent : [1]

| Silice | 50,40 | Alumine | 19,80 |
|---|---|---|---|
| Potasse | 1,10 | Sesquioxyde de fer | 11,70 |
| Soude | 1,20 | Acide carbonique | 0,91 |
| Chaux | 4,70 | Acide phosphorique | 0,08 |
| Magnésie | 3,20 | Eau combinée | 8,20 |

Voyons maintenant la composition moyenne du limon du Nil, d'après les analyses du Professeur Letheby du « London Hospital » exécutées sur des échantillons prélevés dans le fleuve, chaque mois, pendant une année entière, par ordre du khédive et d'après celles du Muséum d'histoire naturelle de Paris.

| | PENDANT LA CRUE | PENDANT L'ÉTIAGE | MUSEUM SANS INDICATION DE PROVENANCE |
|---|---|---|---|
| Acide phosphorique | 1,78 | 0.57 | 0,24 |
| Chaux | 2,06 | 3,18 | 2,65 |
| Magnésie | 1,12 | 0,99 | 3,42 |
| Potasse | 1,82 | 1,06 | 0,91 |
| Soude | 0,91 | 0,62 | 2,52 |
| Alumine | » | » | 21,90 |
| Oxyde de fer | 20,92 | 25,55 | 4,72 |
| Silice | 55,09 | 58,22 | 50,57 |
| Matières organiques et humidité | 15,09 | 10,57 | 11,52 |
| Acide carbonique | 1,28 | 1,44 | 0,11 |
| Pertes | » | » | » |
| TOTAL | 100,00 | 100,00 | 100,00 |

1. SCHLŒSING de l'Institut de France (*Bull. Inst. Égyp.*, 1890).

D'autre part, voici une analyse de l'eau du Nil en septembre (en pleine crue).

Sur 10000 parties de substances totales contenues, Muntz trouve[1] :

|  | En dissolution. | En suspension. |
|---|---|---|
| Azote. | 1 gr. 07 | 5 grammes. |
| Acide phosphorique. . | 0 gr. 40 | 4 gr. 10. |
| Potasse. | 5 gr. 66 | 150 grammes. |
| Chaux | 48 grammes. | 70 gr. 50. |

La chaux serait sous la forme de carbonate de chaux.

Poursuivons nos investigations. Un litre d'eau du Nil prise par Figari au confluent de deux Nils au nord de Khartoum, le 30 juillet, a déposé au bout de quarante-huit heures, 5 millimètres et demi de limon, qui, reçu sur un filtre séché au soleil, puis chauffé à l'étuve pesa 1 gramme. La même expérience répétée, au Caire en août de la même année, donna cette fois un précipité de 4 millimètres qui, desséché comme précédemment se réduisit à 1 gr. 8 centig.

D'après tous les auteurs, c'est vers la fin de juillet (crue) que la quantité de limon en suspension est la plus grande, et cette quantité augmente au fur et à mesure que l'on avance vers le nord de l'Égypte mais diminue beaucoup vers la fin de la crue, bien que l'eau soit encore assez trouble.

Quel enseignement doit-on tirer de toutes ces analyses? Il nous semble qu'on doit se faire cette opinion :

Si on suppose que l'habitant des villages consomme deux litres d'eau non filtrée par jour, on doit en conclure qu'il absorbe ainsi *deux grammes seize centigrammes* de limon dans les vingt-quatre heures. Or savez-vous ce que contiennent ces deux grammes seize centigrammes de limon, et ce que par conséquent le fellah avale des substances minérales par vingt-quatre heures?

Le tableau suivant nous le dira :

| | | |
|---|---|---|
| Silice. | 1 gramme. | |
| Potasse. | 5 centigrammes. | |
| Soude | 5 | — |
| Chaux | 10 | — |
| Magnésie. | 7 | — |
| Acide phosphorique | 16 milligrammes. | |
| Acide carbonique. | 2 centigrammes. | |

Donc l'Arabe absorbe avec l'eau, 1 gramme et demi à 2 grammes environ de matières minérales par jour ! Chiffre exhorbitant comme on le voit.

1. Compte rendu de l'Académie des Sciences de Paris, séance du 11 mars 1889.

Que doit-on conclure de tous ces faits? La première idée qui vient à l'esprit de l'observateur, c'est qu'une telle quantité de substances minérales absorbées journellement par l'Égyptien, doit nécessairement porter une perturbation dans le fonctionnement de l'appareil de l'urination.

Voilà un premier fait qui reste acquis, et qui semble avoir une influence considérable sur la genèse des calculs urinaires dans les contrées de la vallée du Nil.

Mais à côté de cette cause étiologique de la lithiase en Égypte, il y a à en considérer une autre non moins importante, celle qui reconnaît la présence dans l'arbre urinaire du ver trématode connu sous le nom de *Bilharzia Hématobia* qui par son habitat presque exclusif dans l'appareil urinaire et par les multiples altérations qu'il produit, est, lui aussi, un élément sérieux dans la genèse des calculs. Ce ver, en effet, par les myriades d'œufs qu'il dépose dans la vessie et sur la paroi de ce réservoir produit la précipitation des sels de l'urine qui, comme nous l'avons dit plus haut, s'en trouve sursaturée.

De fait de nombreuses analyses démontrent les œufs de Bilharzia comme noyau primitif de certains calculs vésicaux.

Donc pour terminer et en matière de conclusion générale, il découle de toutes ces notions, que l'eau du Nil par son limon qui est partie intégrante de l'alimentation du fellah expose celui-ci à la sursaturation de l'urine par les nombreux sels qu'il avale quotidiennement; et en second lieu la présence chez plusieurs d'entre eux des œufs de la Bilharzia aide puissamment dans la formation des calculs urinaires en Égypte.

---

# LA LITHIASE EN BOSNIE CONSIDÉRÉE AU POINT DE VUE DE SES RAPPORTS AVEC LES CONDITIONS GÉOLOGIQUES ET HYDROLOGIQUES DU PAYS

par M. J. PREINDLSBERGER[1],

de Sarajevo.

C'est une contribution à l'étude encore obscure de cette étiologie, fondée sur 176 cas observés depuis cinq ans et demi presque exclusivement en Bosnie et en Herzégovine. Les recherches géologiques ont été contrôlées par M. J. Grimmer, les analyses chimiques par M. M. Teich.

L'auteur a présenté un mémoire, *Essay, thèse,* sur le sujet en titre. au *Congrès.*

*Géographie.* — L'étude de la répartition géologique présente encore des lacunes ; la lithiase répandue sur toute la terre est plus fréquente en certains pays. En Bosnie, où elle est quatre à cinq fois plus fréquente qu'en Bohême, on a relevé ainsi qu'en Herzégovine, 176 cas depuis quinze ans. La fréquence va en augmentant depuis 1894, depuis la disparition des empiriques.

*Géologie et eau.* — L'eau potable, surtout contenant des éléments calcaires et magnésiens aurait de l'influence : or, sa teneur minérale dépend de la constitution géologique du sol. La lithiase serait donc plus fréquente dans les terrains crétacés, le jurassique et les autres formations calcaires plus récentes. En Bosnie et en Herzégovine, la lithiase prédomine, en effet, dans une zone coupant transversalement le pays, suivant la haute chaîne la plus orientale des Alpes dinariques et constituée surtout par du calcaire triasique. Contrairement à la théorie de Stamm, on trouve, sur 26 cas de calculs, 24 non composés de phosphates, bien que provenant de localités pourvues d'eau également calcaires.

*Age.* — La fréquence serait grande surtout dans l'enfance et au début de la vieillesse. Le maximum, d'après les observations, porte sur des gens de moins de 20 ans.

*Sexe.* — Le calcul vésical est rare chez la femme.

*Race.* — Il est plus fréquent dans la population chrétienne que dans la population mahométane.

*Climat.* — Semble peu important, bien qu'on ne relève que 14 cas provenant d'Herzégovine, dont le climat diffère de celui de Bosnie.

*Genre de vie.* — Surtout chez les enfants pauvres. Le chrétien est moins riche que le mahométan et est soumis à des jeûnes rigoureux : il est presque végétarien.

*Connexions avec d'autres maladies.* — En Bosnie, les infections intestinales des enfants ne sont pas plus fréquentes que dans les autres pays. Il n'y a guère de cas de goutte. Dans les observations, on n'a pas de corps étrangers à incriminer.

A signaler dans les causes favorisantes les infections uriques des tubes urinifères des nouveau-nés.

## LES CALCULS DE LA VESSIE EN GRÈCE

### par M. le docteur E. KALLIONZIS,

Professeur de Médecine opératoire et d'Anatomie topographique à l'université d'Athènes.
Délégué de Grèce.

Messieurs,

C'est depuis 1881 que l'affection de calculs de la vessie en Grèce me préoccupe, vu sa fréquence relative, que j'eus l'occasion de constater pour la première fois pendant mon internat à la clinique chirurgicale de la Faculté de médecine de l'Université d'Athènes, sous le feu professeur Aretaéos (1881-1882) et j'ai cru devoir en rechercher les causes pathogéniques ; je les ai étudiées pendant une dizaine d'années (1890-1900) et c'est le résultat de cette étude que j'ai l'honneur de vous communiquer.

L'époque est déjà loin où Civiale dans son Traité de l'affection calculeuse (Paris, 1858, p. 567) écrivait que c'est dans les Iles Ioniennes de Grèce qu'on a constaté depuis 1820-1850 quelques cas de calculs de la vessie. Je viens vous prouver qu'aucune province de Grèce n'est pas exempte de la maladie, et de plus que la Grèce est un pays où les calculs de la vessie se rencontrent en fréquence relative.

C'est à tort que les traités classiques, même les plus récents, ne mentionnent même pas la Grèce parmi les pays où s'observent les calculs de la vessie.

La péninsule hellénique, la plus orientale des péninsules de l'Europe méridionale, présente des calculeux de la vessie à toutes les classes et à tous les âges.

Si j'examine ma statistique personnelle de treize ans (1887-1900), je trouve 79 cas opérés par moi (les 4 cas provenant de la Turquie d'Europe exceptés) tant en ville dans la clientèle privée, qu'à la clinique chirurgicale de la Faculté de médecine de l'Université d'Athènes de mon éminent maître et déjà collègue à la Faculté, M. le professeur J. Galvani, dont j'ai eu l'honneur d'être chef de clinique pendant six ans et son suppléant pendant les vacances. Tous ces opérés (75) provenaient de Grèce, excepté 4 cas de Turquie d'Europe.

Dans la clinique chirurgicale universitaire du professeur Galvani (d'Athènes) où chaque année sont traités 300, 400 malades de la chirurgie générale et gynécologique, sans exception ou prédilection, les calculs de la vessie prédominent relativement ; sur 2 015 malades traités du 1er septembre 1893 au 1er septembre 1899, 72 étaient des calculeux dont 8 provenaient de la Turquie d'Europe et les autres, 64 de Grèce.

La même proportion relative s'observe à peu près dans l'autre clinique chirurgicale universitaire d'Athènes, de chirurgie générale et gynécologique de mon maître et déjà collègue à la Faculté, M. le professeur Magginas, qui a opéré, pendant ce même laps de temps, 69 calculeux, dont 62 de Grèce et 7 de Turquie d'Europe.

M. le professeur Galvani (d'Athènes), dans sa belle et riche clinique chirurgicale de chirurgie générale et gynécologique à l'hôpital de l'Annonciation (d'Athènes), a opéré pendant ces dernières années (1884-1900) 178 calculeux de la vessie provenant d'Athènes et des différentes provinces de la Grèce, non compris ceux qui venaient de la Turquie (50 autres cas).

M. le professeur Magginas (d'Athènes), dans l'autre clinique chirurgicale de chirurgie générale et gynécologique de l'hôpital Arétaéios (d'Athènes) qu'il dirige depuis le 1er mai 1899, a opéré, parmi 262 malades entrés pendant une seule année (1er mai 1899-1er mai 1900), 14 calculeux, dont 10 de Grèce et 4 de Turquie. Frappé lui aussi depuis longtemps de la fréquence relative de la maladie en question en Grèce, il a fait une très intéressante communication [1] au deuxième Congrès des médecins grecs tenu à Athènes en 1887 sous le titre « Essai sur la classification géographique de calculs de vessie en Grèce » et il relate 406 cas de calculeux bien observés tant par lui que par différents confrères de provinces, dont 304 provenaient de toute la Grèce et 102 de Turquie ; il y promet de faire ultérieurement la classification de calculeux de Grèce par pays de provenance.

Aussi le feu professeur Arétaéios (d'Athènes) a communiqué au même Congrès des médecins grecs (1887) sa statistique personnelle des 215 calculeux qu'il a opérés à Athènes pendant sa longue carrière chirurgicale (et il en a opéré bien d'autres depuis 1887 jusqu'à sa mort en 1895) de provenance de toute la Grèce, y compris les quelques cas de Turquie ; il se proposait, lui aussi [2], de faire la classification géographique des calculs de la vessie en Grèce, vu la fréquence relative de la maladie, comme il l'a annoncé au dit Congrès et comme je le lui ai entendu dire bien des fois dans ses leçons de clinique chirurgicale de l'Université d'Athènes pendant mon internat, mais sa mort survenue en 1895 a interrompue son œuvre.

Cet état de choses m'a amené à examiner la maladie en question de plus près, au point de vue de sa fréquence relative par département,

1. Compte rendu du 2e Congrès de Médecins grecs, tenu à Athènes en 1887. Athènes, 1888, p. 101.
2. Compte rendu du 2e Congrès de Médecins grecs, tenu à Athènes en 1887. Athènes, 1888, p. 875.

provinces et communes et voici les renseignement fournis pour les quinze dernières années (1885-1900) par des confrères exerçant depuis des années aux chefs-lieux de départements dans les provinces, villes et villages de Grèce, y compris les données de ma propre observation.

*D'après les derniers résultats, statistiques du recensement de la population du Royaume de Grèce de 1896 (Ministère de l'intérieur. Total des habitants : 2 453 806).*

A) Département d'Attique et Boétie (515 069 habitants) :

| | | | |
|---|---|---|---|
| α) | Province d'Attique (224 125 hab.). | 81 | cas de calculs. |
| ε) | — d'Egine (8 944 hab.). . . | 4 | — |
| γ) | — de Mégaris (22 911 hab.). | 12 | — |
| δ) | — de Thèbes (29 750 hab.). | 24 | — |
| ε) | — de Levadie (27 561 hab.). | 6 | — |
| | Total. . . . . . | 127 | cas de calculs. |

B) Département de Phtiotis et Phocis (147 297 habitants) :

| | | | |
|---|---|---|---|
| α) | Province de Phtiotis (59 086 hab.). . . . . . | 24 | cas. |
| ε) | — de Parnassis (34 261 hab.) . . . . . | 6 | — |
| γ) | — de Locris (27 759 hab ). . . . . . . | 9 | — |
| δ) | — de Doris (26 211 hab.) . . . . . . . | 4 | — |
| | Total. . . . . . . . . . . | 43 | cas. |

Γ) Département d'Aetolie et Acarnanie (170 565 habitants) :

| | | | |
|---|---|---|---|
| α) | Province de Missolonghi (27 912 hab.) . . . . | 8 | cas. |
| ε) | — de Valtos (17 569 hab.). . . . . . . | 5 | — |
| γ) | — de Trichonia (23 776 hab.) . . . . . | 5 | — |
| δ) | — d'Euritanie (45 667 hab.). . . . . . | 4 | — |
| ε) | — de Naupactie (30 258 hab.) . . . . . | 6 | — |
| ζ) | — de Vonitsa et Zéromero (27 585 hab.). | 4 | — |
| | Total . . . . . . . . . . . . | 52 | cas. |

Δ) Département d'Arta (39 144 habitants) :

| | | | |
|---|---|---|---|
| α) | Province d'Arta (39 144 hab.) . . . . . . . . . | 2 | cas. |
| | Total . . . . . . . . . . . | 2 | cas. |

E) Département de Larissa (181 542 habitants) :

| | | | |
|---|---|---|---|
| α) | Province de Larissa (40 470 hab.). . . . . . . | 9 | cas. |
| ε) | — de Tyrnavos (19 866 hab.) . . . . . | 8 | — |
| γ) | — d'Agya (15 796 hab.) . . . . . . . . | 2 | — |
| δ) | — de Volo (70 709 hab.). . . . . . . . | 7 | — |
| ε) | — d'Almyro (12 381 hab.). . . . . . . . | 3 | — |
| ζ) | — de Pharsala (10 381 hab.). . . . . . | 2 | — |
| η) | — de Domoco (11 959 hab.) . . . . . . | 2 | — |
| | Total . . . . . . . . . . . | 33 | cas. |

Z) Département de Tricalla (Thessalie) (176775 habitants) :

α) Province de Tricala (67454 hab.). . . . . . . . 10 cas.
ϐ)    —    de Kalambaca (28556 hab.). . . . .   2  —
γ)    —    de Karditsa (80766 hab.) . . . . . . .   5  —
                    Total . . . . . . . . . .  15 cas.

H) Département d'Eubée (115515 habitants) :

α) Province de Chalcis (41721 hab.). . . . . . . .   8 cas.
ϐ)    —    de Xerochori (15828 hab.). . . . .   4  —
γ)    —    de Karystie (49228 hab.). .  . . . .  10  —
δ)    —    de Scopelo (8758 hab.) . . . . . . .   5  —
                    Total . . . . . . . . . .  25 cas.

Θ) Département de Cyclades (134747 habitants) :

α) Province de Syra (32177 hab.). . . . . . . . .  10 cas.
ϐ)    —    de Kéa (15325 hab.). . . . . . . . .   5  —
γ)    —    d'Andros (18809 hab.). . . . . . . .   5  —
δ)    —    de Ténos (12500 hab.). . . . . . . .   4  —
ε)    —    de Naxos (25944 hab.). . . . . . . .   4  —
ζ)    —    de Théra (4454 hab.) . . . . . . . .   2  —
η)    —    de Mélos (12722 hab.). . . . . . . .   4  —
                    Total . . . . . . . . . .  34 cas.

I) Département de Corfou (Ile Ionienne) (124578 habitants) :

α) Province de Corfou (90872 hab.). . . . . . . .   9 cas.
ϐ)    —    de Paxo (5814 hab.) . . . . . . . . .   1  —
γ)    —    de Leucas (29892 hab.) . . . . . . .   2  —
                    Total . . . . . . . . . .  12 cas.

K) Département de Kephalonie (85565 habitants (ile Ionienne) :

α) Province de Kranéa (53044 hab.) )
ϐ)    —    de Palle (18928 hab.) ' . . . . .  17 cas.
γ)    —    de Same (17708 hab.) )
δ)    — ·  d'Ithaque (ile Ion.) (15286 hab.) . .   2  —
                    Total . . . . . . . . . .  19 cas.

A) Département de Zante (45052 hab.) (ile Ionienne) :

α) Province de Zante (45052 hab.) . . . . . . .  10 cas.
                    Total . . . . . . . . . .  10 cas.

M) Département d'Argolis et Corinthie (157578 hab.) :

α) Province de Nauplie (18697 hab.). . . . . . .  15 cas.
ϐ)    —    d'Argos (27657 hab.). . . . . . . .  10  —
γ)    —    de Corinthie (64577 hab.). . . . . .  54  —
δ)    —    de Spetzia et Hermionis (17075 hab.)  12  —
ε)    —    d'Hydra (7177 hab.) . . . . . . . .   7  —
ζ)    —    de Trézène (10111 hab.) . . . . . .   8  —
η)    —    de Cythères (ile Ion.) (12306 hab.) .   6  —
                    Total . . . . . . . . . .  90 cas.

N) Département d'Arcadie (167 092 habitants) :

    α) Province de Mantinée (58 469 hab.). . . . . . .  26 cas.
    ϐ)     —     de Kynourie (55 599 hab.). . . . . . .   9 —
    γ)     —     de Gortynie (51 960 hab.). . . . . .  22 —
    ᵟ)     —     de Mégalopolis (25 264 hab.) . . . .  14 —
                 Total . . . . . . . . . . .  71 cas.

Ξ) Département d'Achaïa et Élis (256 251 habitants) :

    α) Province de Patras (78 443 hab.) . . . . . . .  20 cas.
    ϐ)     —     d'Aegialie (21 544 hab.). . . . . . .  11 —
    γ)     —     de Kalavryta (44 859 hab.). . . . . .   9 —
    ᵟ)     —     d'Élie (91 425 hab.). . . . . . . . .  24 —
                 Total . . . . . . . . . . .  64 cas.

O) Département de Laconie (155 462 habitants) :

    α) Province de Lacédemon (58 205 hab.). . . . .  18 cas.
    ϐ)     —     de Gythion (18 841 hab.) . . . . . .   9 —
    γ)     —     d'Oetylos (51 692 hab.) . . . . . . .  25 —
    ᵟ)     —     d'Epidaure-Limira (26 726 hab.). . .  16 —
                 Total . . . . . . . . . . .  66 cas.

Π) Département de Messénie (205 798 habitants) :

    α) Province de Kalamata (59 872 hab.). . . . . .  22 cas.
    ϐ)     —     de Messénie (44 280 hab.). . . . . .  17 —
    γ)     —     de Triphylie (50 386 hab.). . . . . .  16 —
    ᵟ)     —     de Pylie (55 175 hab.). . . . . . . .  15 —
    ε)     —     d'Olympie (56 085 hab.). . . . . . .  12 —
                 Total . . . . . . . : . . . .  80 cas.

Si incomplets que soient les tableaux ci-dessus — parce qu'il y a évidemment bien d'autres cas dont je n'ai pas eu connaissance — ils suffisent, je crois, pour pouver qu'aucune province des différents départements du royaume hellénique n'est exempte de la maladie et constater sa fréquence relative dans quelques-unes. Je crois même, sur les assertions de vieux confrères de province, que cette fréquence relative existait toujours ; et si dans les dix dernières années, elle est devenue plus évidente, on pourrait peut-être l'attribuer, à mon avis, tant à l'augmentation de la population qu'au changement de la diète, mais surtout à ce que les moyens de diagnostic et de traitement ont été perfectionnés et que les malades eux-mêmes vont réclamer le secours du chirurgien à Athènes, aussi bien que dans les provinces, où l'on trouve aujourd'hui d'excellents opérateurs, avec beaucoup plus de confiance qu'auparavant où l'on mourait par crainte d'être opéré.

De tout temps, les médecins grecs ont recherché les causes de cette fréquence relative. On a incriminé l'eau potable du pays — parce que le climat de Grèce fait des habitants de grands buveurs d'eau pendant l'été — ainsi que la manière dont se nourrit la population hellénique.

Dans la plupart des départements de la Grèce, ce sont les sources qui fournissent l'eau potable directement sans intermédiaire d'aqueducs ; mais dans plusieurs petites îles de la Grèce (surtout à Hydra, Spetzia, Théra, Syra, Paxos, ainsi que dans la partie méridionnale du Taygète (Peloponèse) l'usage de l'eau pluviale prédomine. Dans bon nombre d'îles, on fait aussi un grand usage de l'eau de puits, mais cet usage est beaucoup plus faible dans le Peloponèse et dans la Grèce continentale.

L'analyse de l'eau du réservoir d'Athènes, dont toute Athènes fait usage, due à M. A. Dambergis, professeur de chimie de l'Université d'Athènes, a prouvé :

Dans 1 litre au 1000<sup>e</sup> centimètre cube :

| | | |
|---|---|---|
| 1) | Substances fixes . . . . . . . . . . . . . . | 0,5962 |
| 2) | Calcium . . . . . . . . . . . . . . . . . . | 0,1406 |
| 3) | Magnésie . . . . . . . . . . . . . . . | 0,0511 |
| 4) | Acide sulfurique . . . . . . . . . . . . . | 0,0175 |
| 5) | Chlorium . . . . . . . . . . . . . . . . | 0,0622 |
| 6) | Matières organiques non azotées . . . . . . | 0,0080 |
| 7) | — — azotées . . . . . . . . | 0 |
| 8) | Acide azotique . . . . . . . . . . . . . . | Traces. |
| 9) | — azoteux . . . . . . . . . . . . . | 0 |
| 10) | Ammoniaque . . . . . . . . . . . . . . | 0 |
| 11) | Degrés hydrotimétriques (Fr.) . . . . . . . | 37°,8 |
| 12) | Température . . . . . . . . . . . . . . . | 16°,6 |

Je laisse de côté l'eau des autres chefs-lieux de départements et de provinces dont fait usage la population et dont l'analyse n'est pas encore faite pour toutes les sources, et je vais examiner — ce qui est très important pour la maladie en question — la manière dont se nourrit la population hellénique et surtout la basse classe qui fournit le plus fort contingent de calculeux.

Le pain forme la partie fondamentale de l'alimentation des paysans, des ouvriers et des basses classes en Grèce. A part le pain, la nourriture du paysan se compose ordinairement de légumes verts ou secs, le plus ordinairement en soupe, d'olives et d'herbages assaisonnés avec de l'huile ; la tomate fraiche, comme mets, pendant l'été et l'automne, prédomine ; on en abuse même. Parmi les éléments azoteux, ceux dont on use le plus sont le fromage et les poissons salés et plus rarement des poissons frais.

Dans la plupart des contrées helléniques, l'usage de la viande, chez les paysans, est très limité ; le paysan mange de la viande une seule fois par semaine, mais il y a des provinces où celà n'arrive que très rarement dans l'année, c'est-à-dire seulement pendant les grandes fêtes religieuses (Noël, Pàques, Carnaval). L'usage de laitages n'est fréquent que chez les gens les plus aisés, sauf dans les districts pastoraux.

Dans les chesf-lieux des départements et à Athènes même, la nourriture des basses classes ne diffère pas beaucoup de celle des paysans, mais on y mange généralement moins d'herbages et de poissons salés, tandis qu'on fait un plus grand usage de viande, des poissons frais, surtout dans les villes maritimes ou peu distantes de la mer, et de toutes sortes de nourriture chaude. Chez la bourgeoisie, on mange de la viande deux ou trois fois par semaine, rarement tous les jours, ce qui est le cas dans les classes aisées. C'est du veau et du mouton qu'on consomme le plus.

Comme vin, c'est le vin résiné, blanc ou rouge, du pays dont usent les paysans, les ouvriers et les basses classes. La bourgeoisie fait usage de vins du pays non résinés et sur la table des classes aisées, on voit aussi des vins étrangers.

Après ce qui précède, je crois que la cause de la fréquence relative de la maladie en question en Grèce est à rechercher, pas tant dans l'usage des eaux qu'on boit, mais surtout dans la nourriture non azotée des basses classes, qui fournissent le plus grand nombre de calculeux ; la diète *exclusivement végétale* dont on *abuse* et surtout *l'abus* de la *tomate fraîche*, en est, à mon avis, la cause prédominante, d'autant plus que le D_r Arapidès (d'Athènes), ex-préparateur au laboratoire de chimie biologique de l'Université d'Athènes, a trouvé que le noyau de calcul vésicaux qu'il a analysé, était toujours formé par d'oxalates.

Les graveleux sont très fréquents en Grèce et s'ils ne deviennent pas tous des calculeux, c'est que la crainte de le devenir, surtout après une colique néphrétique, qui les a fait souffrir le martyre, les pousse à se faire soigner à temps.

L'hérédité même de la maladie se voit très fréquemment en Grèce, surtout chez de petits garçons de pères ou mères graveleux. Du reste la population grecque use en grande échelle et abuse même quelquefois contre la gravelle, des eaux minérales abondantes du pays, lesquelles, combinées à une diète appropriée, empêchent la gravelle de tourner en calcul de la vessie.

Nous avons en Grèce les eaux minérales de *Loutraki*, tout près de l'isthme de Corinthe, vers son côté nord. Ces eaux jaillissent par de nombreuses fentes tout près du bord de la mer, de dessous de la roche

*Gerania*, de constitution calcaire et forment trois différents groupes.

D'après le professeur Dambergis (d'Athènes), voici l'analyse chimique de ces trois groupes :

| Le groupe A donne : | Le groupe B donne : | Le groupe C donne |
|---|---|---|
| 25 litres d'eau à 1″. | 80 litres d'eau à 1″. | La même du B. |
| 1500 — — à 1′. | 4000 — — à 1′. | — |
| 90 cc. à l'heure. | 288 cc. à l'heure. | — |
| 2160 — en 24 heures. | 6912 — en 24 heures. | — |
| Température : 30°,9 C. | Temp. 31°, 30°,6, 36°,0 C. | Temp. 29°,8 C. |
| (Temp. de l'air : 18°,8 C. | (Temp. de l'air : 18°,8 C. | -- |
| — de la mer : 22°,8 C.) | — de la mer : 22°,8 C.) | — |
| 1) Chlor. de sodium. 0,949 | 0,996 | 0,988 |
| 2) — de potass. 0,055 | 0,053 | 0,076 |
| 3) — de magnés. 0,099 | 0,121 | 0,080 |
| 4) Sulf. de calcium. . 0,045 | 0,049 | 0,048 |
| 5) -- de magnés. . 0,088 | 0,079 | 0,078 |
| 6) Bicarb. de calcium 0,511 | 0,291 | 0,294 |
| 7) — de magnés. 0,211 | 0,203 | 0,180 |
| 8) — de sodium. 0,095 | 0,106 | 0,084 |
| 9) Ox. de fer et d'alum. 0,001 | 0,001 | 0,001 |
| 10) Acide pyritique. . 0,014 | 0,013 | 0,015 |
| 11) Mat. organ. azot. Traces. | Traces. | Traces. |
| 12) Ammoniaque . . . — | — | — |
| 13) Acide phosphoriq. -- | — | — |
| 14) — azotique . . — | — | — |
| 15) Manganium. . . . — | — | — |
| 16) Bromium. . . . . — | — | . . |
| 17) Iode . . . . . . — | — | . . |
| 18) Lithium. . . . . . — | -- | — |
| Total de mat. fixes. 1,866 gr. | 1,912 gr. | 1,844 gr. |

Ces eaux sont très limpides, inodores, et ne laissent en coulant aucun résidu ; elles sont de goût au commencement doux et agréable et peu après très légèrement salin.

D'après l'analyse du professeur Dambergis, ces sources sont classées dans les thermes alcaliques, légèrement muriatiques et ressemblent aux eaux de Bourbon-Lancy, Bourbon-Archambault, Vittel et Contrexéville (France), de Drivurg et Marienbad (source Rodolphe, d'Autriche), de Bath (d'Angleterre), Jinselbad et Leuck (Suisse).

Il y a aussi en Grèce une autre source dans l'île d'Andros (Cyclades) ; c'est l'eau minérale d'*Apikia*, source *Sariza* qui a été découverte par hasard par les paysans qui voyaient que chaque année le fond du bassin où l'eau coulait était percé.

Cette eau est incolore, très limpide et inodore ; elle a le goût agréable et la température moyenne ; l'analyse chimique faite par le professeur Dambergis (d'Athènes) a donné le résultat suivant et ressemble au contenu de l'eau minérale d'Evian (Savoie).

Poids spécifique : 1 gr. 0001525 (14° C.).
Réaction faiblement alcaline.
Sur 10 000 centimètres cubes contiennent :

| | | |
|---|---|---|
| 1) Carbonate de soude | 0 gr. | 12066 |
| 2) — de chaux | 0 gr. | 83000 |
| 5) — de magnésie | 0 gr. | 25140 |
| 4) Sulfate de chaux | 0 gr. | 24010 |
| 5) Chorure de sodium | 1 gr. | 11996 |
| 6) — de potassium | 0 gr. | 09586 |
| 7) — de magnésium | 0 gr. | 018192 |
| 8) Alumine | 0 gr. | 0600 |
| 9) Silice | 0 gr. | 144000 |
| Somme de substances fixes | 3 gr. | 04570 |
| Acide carbonique de bicarbonate | 0 gr. | 54680 |
| — — libre | 0 gr. | 15640 |
| Total | 3 gr. | 74690 |

Carbonate de fer
Ammoniaque
Acide azotique } . . . . . . . . . . En traces.
— phosphorique
Substances organiques

L'emploi de cette eau est renommée en Grèce pour ses excellents résultats sur la gravelle ; et au premier congrès des médecins grecs tenu à Athènes en 1882, le D[r] Papalexopoulos (de Syra-Cyclades) a même communiqué la guérison d'un calcul de la vessie par l'emploi de cette eau. Il s'agissait d'un garçon de 14 ans qui portait un calcul de la vessie de volume d'une noisette, comme l'a prouvé l'examen de la vessie par la sonde métallique fait par M. le D[r] Papalexopoulos[1], assisté d'un autre confrère. L'opération de la taille n'ayant pas été acceptée, le malade a été soumis à l'emploi de l'eau d'Andros, source *Saritza*, pendant cinq mois (deux litres par jour). L'examen ultérieur fait après ce laps de temps au moyen de la sonde métallique et par le même docteur, a prouvé la disparition de la pierre et de tous les autres symptômes concomitants ; le malade s'est porté bien depuis, sans plus de détails.

Encouragé de ce résultat, notre confrère a employé la même eau sur un autre calculeux de la vessie de 55 ans, qui portait un gros calcul du volume d'une noix. Le malade en question n'a pas accepté

1. Compte rendu du 1[er] Congrès de Medecins grecs, tenu à Athènes, en 1882. Athènes, 1883, p. 157.

l'opération et a été soumis pendant de longs mois à l'eau d'Andros et se portait si bien qu'il ne se souciait plus de sa maladie.

La communication de ce distingué confrère m'a vivement intéressé et depuis je n'ai pas cessé de soumettre les calculeux que je voyais, à l'emploi de cette eau et surtout ceux qui ne voulaient accepter aucune opération. Malheureusement, je n'ai pas observé les mêmes résultats et tôt ou tard, je les opérais. Cependant ce qui est plus que certain, c'est que l'emploi de cette eau de l'île d'Andros dans la gravelle donne des résultats excellents et peut très efficacement remplacer l'eau d'Evian et de Contrexéville.

Quant aux eaux alcalines d'Hermione (Peloponèse) qui suintaient des parois d'un puits dans le couvent des Saint-Anargyres non loin du village auquel elles doivent leur nom, je viens d'apprendre qu'elles sont taries. Ces eaux, très limpides, incolores et inodores étaient d'une saveur franchement alcaline et renommées en Grèce pour leurs bons résultats contre la gravelle. Dans l'antiquité, selon toute probabilité, s'élevait près de leur source, le fameux temple d'Esculape d'Halyké.

De ce qui précède, il résulte :

1) Que les calculs de la vessie en Grèce sont une maladie relativement fréquente.

2) Qu'aucune province de Grèce n'est exempte de la maladie en question.

3) Que très probablement, c'est la *diète végétale exclusive* et l'*abus* de la *tomate fraîche*, qui en est la cause prédominante.

4) Que les basses classes fournissent le plus grand nombre de calculeux.

5) Qu'en Grèce aussi de tous les âges, c'est l'enfance surtout qui, de l'avis de tous les confrères de Grèce qui se sont occupés de la maladie et de ce que j'ai vu, présente la plus grande fréquence absolue.

6) Que les eaux minérales de Loutraki et d'Andros peuvent très efficacement remplacer le Contrexéville et l'Evian.

## DISCUSSION

M. Delagrammatica — M. Kallionzis vient de soutenir que le genre d'alimentation et spécialement l'abus des tomates fraîches est la cause de la fréquence de la lithiase en Grèce. Cela est en désaccord avec les nouvelles théories d'après lesquelles la formation des calculs est la conséquence des troubles dyspeptiques, d'une préparation insuffisante des éléments d'assimilation et d'une désassimilation, d'une combustion imparfaite. Cependant si cela est vrai pour la généralité des cas, il ne faut pas, je crois, pour cela, renier toute influence aux *ingesta*. L'ancienne théorie donc de l'action lithogène de l'ingestion d'eau ou des substances trop chargées en matières terreuses et en particulier d'acide oxalique, ne doit donc être complètement abandonnée, surtout lorsque des statistiques si importantes viennent à son appui.

M. Preindlsberger. — Je ne me flatte pas d'avoir trouvé l'étiologie de la lithiase, je ne me flatte non plus de vous avoir dit du nouveau. Tout ce que j'ai pu vous offrir, ce sont des recherches exactes sur les rapports de la lithiase avec les conditions géologiques et hydrologiques des pays, car nous avons recherché la situation géologique de chaque petit village d'où venait un malade atteint de lithiase.   .

## VOLUMINOSO CALCOLO VESCICALE INTORNO AD UNA FORCINA DA CAPELLI IN UNA DONNA

par M. le docteur MICHELE PAVONE,

da Palermo.

Nel mese di aprile scorso fui gentilmente invitato dal D$^r$ Michele Noto ad operare una donna G. P. di anni 23, nubile affetta da voluminoso calcolo vescicale per il quale soffriva da 4 anni.

La paziente é di statura media, sviluppo scheletrico regolare, colorito della pelle bianco pallido, mucose apparenti pallide, pannicolo adiposo scarso. Ella é molto isterica.

L'urina appena emessa é di reazione neutra ma lasciata un poco in riposo diventa di reazione nettamente alcalina e di odore ammoniacale. All' analisi chimica si riscontrano traccie d'albumina e molto muco-pus. All' osservazione microscopica, oltre a numerosi corpuscoli di muco-pus, abbondanti cristalli di triplo fosfato, qualche corpuscolo sanguigno e qualche cellula epiteliale della vescica ma nessun cilindro nè alcuno elemento renale.

Osservando gli organi genitali esterni, si nota il meato urinario un pó edematoso ed iperemico. Introducendo un exploratore metallico, si riscontra subito un grosso calcolo in vescica.

Tenuto conto del volume del calcolo e dell' iperestesia della paziente, dipendente sia dalla cistite sia dal suo carattere eminentemente isterico, preferisco operare sotto la cloroformizazione.

Dopo aver ben lavato l'uretra e la vescica con dell' acqua borata tiépida al 1 0/0; introduco un frangipietra e frantumo buona porzione di calcolo; ad un certo punto pero avverto una sensazione diversa da quella fornita dal calcolo non solo ma percepisco che una porzione di calcolo é aderente alla vescica in guisa da non poterla assolutamente staccare col frangipietra. Allora estraggo la porzione di calcolo già ridotto in frantumi ed invito il collega a cloroformizzare più profondamente l'ammalata; quindi pratico la dilatazione rapida dell' uretra mediante l'introduzione graduale e successiva delle sonde Hégar e immediatamente introduco l'indice della mano destra, sfiancando completamente l'uretra ed il collo vescicale. In tal modo constato un calcolo molto allungato, disposto trasversalmente ed immobilizzato per le suedue estremità, specialmente in alto e a destra ove una delle sue estremità é completamente aderente alla vescica.

Col dito comincio a staccarte una del l'estremita quando, poco dopo avverto una punta metallica; proseguendo, percepisco, a breve distanza, un altra punta metallica e continuando a staccare da esse delle concrezioni e seguendo il loro tragitto, mi formo la convinzione che si trattasse di una lunga forcina da capelli. Denudo come meglio posso, la detta forcina dalle concrezioni calcolose e provo ad estrarla dalla parte curva ma non riesco, essendo appunto questa parte completamente saldata colla vescica. Allora sono òbligato a tentare di estrarla dalla parte delle due punte; ciò che riesco a fare con manovre delicatissime e pazienti onde evitare di pungere e forare la vescica e l'uretra.

Infine, colla guida dell' indice della mano destra in vescica e colla mano sinistra sulla regione ipogastrica, riesco con movimenti combinati e dolci ad immettere le due punte nell' uretra, a tenerle vicine fraloro ed a stringerle insieme mercè un laccio a nodo scorsoio fattomi passare lungo il mio indice dal collega. Allora, colla mano sinistra faccio delle trazioni delicate sulla forcina e, coll indice della mano destra, riesco finalmente astaccare completamente l'altra porzione della forcina, che sembrava addirittura saldata alla vescica. In questo momento avvenne una leggiera emorragia. Col dito continuo a staccare dalla vescica qualche altra porzione di calcolo aderente e quindi lavo abbondantemente l'uretra e la vescica con dell' acqua borata tiepida al 4 0/0.

La forcina estratta è lunga circa 10 centimetri. L'operata in breve tempo si rimise completamente in salute.

Se l'inferma mi avesse informato della manovra che ella avea fatto colla forcina e della penetrazione di questa in vescica avrei compreso subito che la formazione del calcolo vescicale era dovuta al depositarsi dei sali dell' urina attorno alla forcina da capelli e, dato il volume del calcolo, avrei preferito eseguire la cistotomia ipogastrica ed estrarre ad un tempo il grosso calcolo col suo nucleo cioè colla forcina. L'inferma peró non accenno mai a nulla di tuttoccio ma fortunatamente io potei, in unica seduta, frangere la pietra, praticare la dilatazione rapida dell' uretra e del collo vescicale ed estrarre la forcina da capelli con felice esito.

Da questo caso sono a dedurre le seguenti considerazioni cliniche :

1º Allorché in tutte le esplorazioni della vescica si riscontra un calcolo che mantiene sempre una posizione anormale bisogna sospettare un corpo estraneo nonostante che il paziente neghi assolutamente ció poiché queste cose si fanno manon si confessano.

2º In questi casi é preferibile la cistotomia ipogastrica.

---

# UN CAS DE CORPS ÉTRANGERS DE LA VESSIE APRÈS UNE LAPAROTOMIE

## par M. SEPP

d'Amsterdam.

Si les corps étrangers qui sont venus dans la vessie par l'urètre ne sont pas rares, ceux au contraire qui y ont pénétré par un processus inflammatoire sont moins fréquents. Le Dʳ Héresco, dans un mémoire paru dans les *Annales* de 1898, n'en a pu trouver que 14, recueillis par le Dʳ Gayet. M. Héresco y a ajouté deux observations de notre maître, M. Guyon, dans lesquelles des calculs s'étaient formés autour des fils de soie.

Dans tous les ouvrages traitant de chirurgie urinaire on trouve mentionné des corps étrangers les plus variés et les plus étonnants. Je ne citerai que le cas décrit par le Dʳ Lohnstein de Berlin : un jeune marié, un peu trop craintif et trop pressé, se trompe d'étage et introduit la nuit de nóces dans la vessie de sa femme un pessaire occlusif, qui ne tarde pas à la faire souffrir.

Les corps étrangers dont je désire parler devant vous ont pénétré dans la vessie de ma malade d'une manière plus chaste.

Il s'agit d'une dame de 46 ans, mariée, nullipare, qui avait été ovariotomisée par un de mes confrères d'Amsterdam. Elle avait un kyste multiloculaire de l'ovaire droit : la tumeur était très grande et elle avait un pédicule très large qui avait été lié du côté de l'utérus avec six ou sept fils de soie, tandis que la partie périphérique fut liée avec une sonde de Nélaton. Pas le moindre accident pendant l'opération, pas de blessure de la vessie. Seulement, sept semaines après, cette malade, qui n'avait auparavant aucune plainte de la part de ses voies urinaires, commençait à se plaindre d'une fréquence très augmentée et de douleurs très fortes pendant et après la miction. De temps en temps quelques gouttes de sang à la fin de la miction. Les urines parfaitement normales auparavant devenaient alcalines et contenaient un dépôt considérable de pus et de phosphates. Les difficultés augmentaient au jour le jour, et il survint même une rétention d'urine qui nécessitait un sondage. En retirant la sonde, les yeux de cet instrument étaient bouchés par une fausse membrane. Quelques jours après, élimination spontanée d'une autre fausse membrane, large comme la paume de la main, et dont l'examen microscopique ne révélait rien de particulier : c'était du tissu nécrotique. Bientôt après émission spontanée d'un petit concrément phosphatique. La malade n'a jamais eu de fièvre. On m'appela en consultation et je constatai à l'aide du cystoscope qu'il y avait une grande quantité de concréments de grandeur très variable, et des incrustations surtout du côté droit. Par-ci par-là des fils blanchâtres auxquels pendaient des concréments.

Je résolus d'enlever autant que possible de ce que j'avais vu et, en quelques séances, j'ai pu débarrasser cette vessie par un lithotriteur à mors plats de plus de trente grammes de pierre et de six fils de soie que je pouvais arracher très facilement. La malade allait beaucoup mieux, mais elle avait encore souvent de fortes douleurs. J'introduisis de rechef un cystoscope et je trouvai à mon grand étonnement la sonde de Nélaton, qui avait été mise comme ligature autour du pédicule de la tumeur abdominale : elle se trouvait comme un anneau autour du col vésical. Je pus la retirer assez facilement. Après quelques lavages ma malade est complètement guérie, et elle se trouve aujourd'hui aussi bien que possible.

---

## DEUX CAS INTÉRESSANTS DE LITHIASE VÉSICALE

### par M. Suarez de MENDOZA-

de Madrid

Dans le premier cas, il s'agit d'une vessie biloculaire ou du moins paraissant telle, formée de deux loges communiquant à la partie supérieure par un orifice de la dimension d'une pièce de un franc.

Chaque loge contenait une pierre ; celle de la loge antérieure mesure 4 centim. 1/2 de longueur, 5 de largeur et 2 1/2 de hauteur ; tandis que pour l'autre, ces mesures se réduisent à 4, 2 1/2 et 2 centimètres respectivement. Le septum qui séparait les deux loges avait l'aspect d'une véritable paroi et non d'une bride. Le malade fut débarrassé de ces calculs au moyen de la taille hypogastrique.

Le second cas a trait à un calcul enkysté, présentant un prolongement intra-vésical en forme de champignon, chez un prostatique à la troisième période avec infection antérieure. La partie enkystée fusiforme mesure 5 centimètres de long sur 2 de large. Il fallut pratiquer une section de 4 centimètres dans la paroi vésicale pour extirper de sa loge la partie enkystée. La taille hypogastrique permit de mener à bien cette délicate opération.

## DISCUSSION

M. O. PASTEAU (de Paris). — A propos de la communication précédente sur la présence des calculs dans les vessies biloculaires, je ferai remarquer qu'il y a lieu de distinguer plusieurs genres de ces vessies.

Les unes sont bilobées à proprement parler et j'ai vu un cas de gros calcul en sablier dont chaque moitié dilatée était située dans une des deux loges vésicales.

Les autres sont des vessies d'apparence normale qui présentent un ou deux diverticules. Ceux-ci sont presque toujours latéraux, et s'ouvrent juste en dehors des orifices uretéraux ; s'il y a deux diverticules, ils sont le plus souvent symétriques ; ils peuvent aussi bien exister chez l'homme que chez la femme et j'en ai vu plusieurs exemples. Dans un cas, il existait chez une jeune fille de 18 ans un gros calcul vésical urique réuni par un mince pédicule avec le calcul arrondi qui remplissait le diverticule latéral droit et dont le diamètre était de 5 centimètres et demi.

---

## EXTRACTION, A L'AIDE DE LA CYSTOSCOPIE, DES CORPS ÉTRANGERS DE LA VESSIE, CHEZ LA FEMME

par M. le docteur HENRY REYNÈS,
de Marseille.
Ex-chef de Clinique chirurgicale à la Faculté de Médecine de Montpellier.

Les cas d'extraction cystoscopique des corps étrangers de la vessie, chez la femme, n'étant pas très communs, je crois pouvoir rapporter l'observation suivante.

OBSERVATION. — Il s'agit d'une jeune fille de 18 ans, internée à l'asile des aliénés de Saint-Pierre, à Marseille, qui s'introduisit dans l'urètre et dans la vessie un crochet à cheveux. On s'aperçut du fait cinq jours après.

Les médecins de l'asile, les D<sup>rs</sup> Boubila, médecin-chef, et Cossa, médecin-adjoint, pratiquèrent le cathétérisme, sentirent le corps étranger, mais ne purent l'extraire. Ils firent alors appel à M. le professeur Roux, de Brignoles, chirurgien des hôpitaux de Marseille, dont les tentatives d'extraction furent également infructueuses.

Devant cette impossibilité, le D<sup>r</sup> Roux, d'accord avec ses confrères de l'asile, était disposé à pratiquer une taille hypogastrique ; mais auparavant on voulut bien me faire appeler pour pratiquer la cystoscopie et essayer l'extraction.

Cette intervention eut lieu le neuvième jour après l'introduction de l'épingle à cheveux, en présence de MM. les D<sup>rs</sup> Boubila, Cossa, Roux de Brignoles, et de MM. les internes Jourdan et Aglot.

Comme générateur d'électricité, je me servis d'accumulateurs transportables, d'un modèle léger et très pratique construit chez Gaiffe.

La vessie fut lavée et soigneusement désinfectée, puis remplie d'eau.

La malade étant agitée, et souffrant, elle fut chloroformée.

Le cystoscope, introduit dans la vessie, me montra immédiatement le crochet à cheveux, et me permit, avec une grande netteté, d'en repérer la situation et d'en apprécier les dimensions : les médecins présents purent également se convaincre de la perfection de cet examen cystoscopique.

Nous essayâmes alors, sous le contrôle de l'examen cystoscopique, d'extraire le crochet.

J'introduisis la longue et mince pince de Collin dans l'urètre, le long et à coté du tube cystoscopique : je confiai cette pince à M. le D<sup>r</sup> Roux en le priant de la manœuvrer suivant mes indications, pendant que, l'œil au cystoscope, je m'efforcerai de lui faire prendre avec la pince le crochet par la partie courbe.

Nous eûmes quelques tâtonnements inévitables à cause de l'inversion des images, et parce qu'il fallait combiner nos mouvements : une même personne ne pouvant pas commodément et, en même temps, avoir l'œil au cystoscope et manœuvrer la pince.

Cependant dans le champ optique je voyais nettement la pince et la partie courbe du crochet, si bien qu'à un moment, jugeant la prise bonne et solide, je retirai le cystoscope, et priai M. Roux de retirer prudemment sa pince.

Effectivement le crochet sortit.

Un lavage vésical compléta cette intervention qui n'eut aucune suite, et évita ainsi à la malade une importante opération tranchante.


L'idée d'appliquer la cystoscopie à la connaissance des corps étrangers de la vessie, surtout depuis que de grands perfectionnements ont été apportés aux instruments en Allemagne par Nitze et Casper, en

France par Boisseau du Rocher et Albarran, est venue tout naturellement à l'esprit des chirurgiens,

L'endoscopie vésicale permet en effet de connaître la nature, les
dimensions, et la situation des corps étrangers ; comme le dit Casper[1],
« cet examen est en général facile, et un simple coup d'œil suffit souvent pour reconnaître un bout de sonde, une épingle, un crochet à
cheveux, repérer sa situation, apprécier sa mobilité ou sa fixité, et sa
grandeur ». Pousson[2], Goizet[3], signalent également l'utilité de la
cystoscopie en ce qui concerne le diagnostic des corps étrangers de
la vessie.

Cependant si on peut citer d'assez nombreuses observations d'examens endoscopiques pratiqués pour reconnaître des corps étrangers
intra-vésicaux, qu'on a ensuite enlevés avec des crochets spéciaux,
des lithotriteurs ou par la taille vésicale, par contre les cas sont moins
nombrenx où la prise et l'extraction du corps étranger ont été faites
sous le contrôle cystoscopique. Albarran[4] signale ce procédé; Casper[5]
en agissant de la même façon a pu, chez une femme qui lui était
adressée par le professeur Dührssen, faire pénétrer à la fois dans la
vessie le cystoscope et une pince avec laquelle il put extraire un fil à
ligature en soie. Chevalier[6] a également extrait par ce moyen une
canule à lavement, et Pousson[7] un crochet à cheveux.

Tous les chirurgiens cependant ne sont pas assez pénétrés du secours
que la cystoscopie peut fournir en pareil cas.

J'en veux pour preuve la discussion qui a eu lieu dans une séance
récente de la Société de chirurgie[8].

M. Rochard, pour extraire un crochet à cheveux de la vessie d'une
femme, fut amené à pratiquer la taille vaginale, après avoir, dit-il,
épuisé tous les moyens connus : mais il n'indique pas si parmi ces
moyens il a essayé la cystoscopie, ce que je ne crois pas.

M. Picqué naguère encore, parlant des crochets à cheveux, disait
qu'il fallait délaisser tous les procédés d'extraction par les voies naturelles, et qu'il se ralliait délibérément à la pratique de la taille. Il est
aujourd'hui moins absolu dans sa formule depuis qu'il a signalé à la

1. CASPER. *Handbuch der Cystoskopie.* Leipzig, 1898, p. 120 : Fremdkorper in der
Blase.
2. POUSSON. Précis des maladies des voies urinaires.
3. GOIZET. Cystocopie et cystoscopes. Thèse de Paris, 1898-1899.
4. ALBARRAN. In Leçons clin. sur les maladies des voies urinaires, par Guyon;
3e édit., 1897; t. III, p. 241.
5. CASPER. *Loc. cit.*, p. 124.
6. CHEVALIER. Congrès d'Urologie, 4e session, 1899.
7. POUSSON. Congrès d'Urologie, 4e session, 1899.
8. Soc. de Chirurgie. *Bulletin.* Séance du 10 janvier 1900, p. 20.

Société de chirurgie deux faits d'extraction de crochets par les voies naturelles. Dans ces deux faits, dus à MM. Mougeot (de Chaumont) et Guillet (de Caen), l'extraction se fit simplement avec un doigt introduit dans la vessie après dilatation extemporanée de l'urèthre; il s'agissait d'épingles à cheveux; M. Guillet s'aida en même temps d'un doigt introduit dans le vagin.

On voit par ces exemples qu'il ne faut point se hâter de recourir à des interventions sanglantes, à des tailles, alors qu'on peut presque toujours arriver à extraire le corps étranger par les voies naturelles. On voit aussi toute l'importance de la cystoscopie dans ces cas là, et qu'on doit toujours avoir recours à ses lumières, c'est le cas de le dire, avant d'en arriver à de plus graves procédés.

CINQUIÈME SÉANCE

## MARDI 7 AOUT

*à 9 heures du matin.*

Présidence de M. SEVEREANU,

de Bucarest.

---

*Troisième question mise à l'ordre du jour :*

# RÉSULTATS ÉLOIGNÉS DES TRAITEMENTS OPÉRATOIRES
# DE L'HYPERTROPHIE PROSTATIQUE

*Rapporteurs :* Von Frisch (Vienne) et Legueu (Paris).

---

## RÉSULTATS ÉLOIGNÉS DES TRAITEMENTS OPÉRATOIRES
## DANS L'HYPERTROPHIE DE LA PROSTATE

*CONCLUSIONS DU RAPPORT*

de M. le professeur A. VON FRISCH,

de Vienne.

Parmi les différentes opérations radicales de l'hypertrophie prostatique, ce n'est que celles qui tendent à écarter directement l'obstacle prostatique s'opposant au libre écoulement de l'urine, qui puissent promettre un succès durable. On peut regarder comme telles la prostatectomie sus-pubienne et périnéale, la prostatectomie latérale et l'incision galvanocaustique d'après Bottini.

Les anciens procédés de Mercier et d'autres sont actuellement abandonnés comme en étant trop dangereux.

L'effet durable d'une pareille opération est d'autant plus sûr, que plus l'élimination de l'obstacle a mieux réussi, et plus le conduit est resté libre après la cicatrisation.

Il est évident qu'un procédé contrôlé par l'œil, comme les différentes prostatectomies, satisferait le mieux à ces conditions ; mais ces opérations doivent être regardées comme graves et trop dangereuses, vu que l'âge avancé et la faiblesse si fréquente de ces malades ne sont pas des conditions favorables. L'opération de Bottini paraît être moins dangereuse, pourtant elle n'est pas si inoffensive que le croient certains auteurs.

Les prostatectomies, de même que l'incision galvanocaustique, fournissent parfois des résultats irréprochables et très satisfaisants au point de vue de la durée. Même lorsque la vessie est distendue et que sa paroi musculaire paraît avoir perdu sa contractilité, le résultat définitif peut encore être parfait, lorsque l'obstacle a été complètement enlevé.

Cependant, il n'existe pas à ce jour une ligne de conduite précise, qui puisse nous assurer un succès durable par l'opération. Même si nous tâchons d'enlever les parties de la prostate, qui font l'obstacle, aussi complètement que possible par les prostatectomies, les conditions mécaniques, qui donnent lieu à l'obstruction, sont tellement variables dans les différents cas, qu'aucun des procédés en usage ne nous permet de les découvrir toujours dans leur totalité. Il en est de même de l'opération de Bottini, dans laquelle nous opérons dans l'obscurité et où, malgré l'emploi du cystoscope, nous ne pouvons souvent pas trouver la vraie cause de la rétention de l'urine. C'est là la cause de l'échec de ces opérations dans un certain nombre de cas.

L'effet durable de toutes ces opérations peut devenir illusoire plus tard par la formation de cicatrices dures et hypertrophiques, qui constituent un nouvel obstacle, ou bien par le progrès de l'hypertrophie de la glande et par la formation de nouveaux bourrelets et proéminences.

---

## RÉSULTATS ÉLOIGNÉS DES TRAITEMENTS OPÉRATOIRES
## DE L'HYPERTROPHIE PROSTATIQUE

---

### RAPPORT

**par M. FÉLIX LEGUEU,**

Chirurgien des hôpitaux, professeur agrégé à la Faculté de Médecine de Paris.

Les éléments dont se compose la maladie constituée par l'hypertrophie de la prostate sont multiples. Leurs rapports n'ont pas été compris de la même façon, et, suivant les théories en cours, des opérations très différentes ont été proposées et pratiquées pour traiter la même affection. Je ne m'arrêterai pas à signaler et à étudier des tentatives louables peut-être, mais qui, défectueuses dès le principe, n'ont eu qu'une fortune éphémère. Au contraire, me plaçant à un point de vue plus élevé, je ne suivrai que les grandes lignes, j'étudierai les méthodes plus que les procédés opératoires, et je chercherai à dégager des résultats éloignés qu'elles ont donnés une orientation pour l'avenir.

Les opérations qui s'adressent à l'hypertrophie prostatique sont de trois ordres : 1° celles qui ont pour but la dérivation des urines ou le drainage vésical; 2° celles qui se proposent de modifier la prostate en agissant sur les testicules; 3° celles qui cherchent à modifier directement la prostate par la section ou la suppression de l'obstacle.

### I. — *Drainage vésical. Cystostomie.*

En présence d'un obstacle prostatique reconnu ou supposé inattaquable, on a pratiqué et on pratique encore la déviation des urines ou le drainage vésical.

Cette opération s'exécute par la voie *périnéale* ou par la voie *hypogastrique*.

· *Par la voie périnéale*, on aborde la vessie dans sa partie déclive; mais qu'on fasse ici la *boutonnière périnéale* de Thompson, la *prostatomie périnéale* de Harisson, c'est un drainage temporaire qui est établi; son efficacité est à peu près toujours limitée à la période d'application, et il n'y a pas à envisager les résultats éloignés de ces opérations, malgré les bons résultats transitoires qu'elles ont donnés.

Par la *voie hypogastrique*, on peut aussi créer une voie de dérivation des urines; dans ce but on fait l'abouchement de la muqueuse vésicale à la peau, et la fistule a des chances de durer. Ce n'est plus une cystotomie, c'est la cystostomie telle que Mac Guire et que Poncet nous l'ont apprise.

*a.* Pratiquée contre des *accidents généraux d'infection urinaire*, cette opération ne soulève que peu d'objections : elle constitue dans les *formes suraiguës* et *aiguës*, une ressource précieuse, malgré la gravité des circonstances. Dans les *formes chroniques*, elle intervient encore et très heureusement, mais seulement après l'échec de la sonde à demeure : et celle-ci réussit si souvent à Paris, que nous n'avons que de rares occasions de recourir à la cystostomie dans ces conditions.

*b.* Mais la cystostomie est proposée et pratiquée par Poncet pour remédier *aux accidents locaux de l'hypertrophie prostatique*, elle est faite pour parer aux difficultés et aux nécessités du cathétérisme, pour substituer à la vie de sondage un état plus compatible avec les exigences sociales ou professionnelles, elle est faite enfin, quoique accessoirement, pour amener la diminution du volume de la prostate.

Jusqu'où et dans quelle proportion la cystostomie a-t-elle rempli son programme?

J'emprunte aux observations de Poncet lui-même les observations qui vont me servir; 55 malades cystostomisés par Poncet ou par ses élèves ont été suivis au moins six mois et au maximum neuf ans. Ces cystostomisés se répartissent en trois groupes :

1º *Il y en a 14 qui sont absolument incontinents*, il perdent continuellement leurs urines par leur méat sus-pubien et doivent porter un appareil.

2º *Il y en a 7 qui sont des demi-continents*, c'est-à-dire que tantôt ils retiennent leurs urines et tantôt ils les perdent involontairement. D'autres urinent toutes les dix minutes par leur méat et cet état équivaut bien à l'incontinence.

5º *Enfin il y en a 14 qui sont continents*, c'est-à-dire, que chez eux, la miction ne s'effectue qu'à certains intervalles réguliers, toutes les trois ou quatre heures par exemple. Elle se fait ou par la fistule seule, ou à la fois par la fistule et par l'urètre. Mais il est aussi des malades chez lesquels la miction ne se fait ni par le méat, ni par l'urètre, ils sont obligés de se sonder par la fistule à chaque besoin.

Et en somme, après comme avant, le cystostomisé est un infirme : l'opération a substitué une infirmité à une autre. La seconde vaut-elle mieux que la première?

Lorsque la continence est parfaite, lorsque la miction par la fistule se fait volontairement, l'infirmité est atténuée, mais cette continence, on ne peut l'obtenir à volonté. Car si nous connaissons bien quelques-unes des conditions qui l'assurent, il n'est aucun procédé qui puisse se vanter de la réaliser. Au contraire, pour les malades incontinents, l'infirmité s'accroît d'un orifice anormal, toujours souillé, mal protégé par un appareil délicat à appliquer et difficile à entretenir. Par ailleurs la vessie se vide mal, il y a stagnation permanente, des calculs se forment. Je comprends dès lors que tous ces malades, qui pouvaient avant la cystostomie se sonder facilement, regrettent leur état antérieur et réclament avec insistance la fermeture de leur fistule.

Et quant à ceux qui étaient, avant la cystostomie, condamnés à des sondages difficiles, quelquefois impossibles, parfois hémorragiques, je ne suis pas persuadé que la sonde à demeure n'aurait pas, chez quelques-uns au moins, assoupli le canal, régularisé le trajet et décongestionné le prostate.

C'est dire que pour nous la cystostomie reste une ressource ultime et toujours palliative.

## II. — *Opérations testiculaires.*

La castration chez l'animal détermine l'atrophie de la prostate : le fait est indiscutable, les expériences de White, de Kirbey, de Legueu, de Bazy et d'Albarran l'ont établi.

Mais cette influence atrophique s'exerce-t-elle dans les mêmes proportions sur la prostate malade et hypertrophiée?

White, Griffith, Keloy, Mansell Moullin, Watson, de Rouville, Albarran et Motz ont examiné à ce point de vue la prostate de malades qui étaient morts quelque temps après la castration, et n'y ont vu aucune trace d'atrophie. Mais la période de temps qui s'était écoulée entre l'opération et l'autopsie n'était que de quelques semaines; il n'est pas étonnant que l'atrophie n'ait pu se produire. Bryson cependant a examiné une prostate quatorze mois après la castration et n'y a rien vu qui ressemble à de l'atrophie. Durant ce laps de temps, la prostate pouvait au moins commencer sa régression. Mais c'est là un fait unique, on ne saurait généraliser : mieux vaut reconnaître que les faits anatomiques ne sont pas suffisants pour juger la question, et contentons-nous des documents cliniques.

Pour apprécier sur le terrain clinique l'influence de la castration sur l'hypertrophie prostatique, il y a avantage à étudier successivement les modifications qui se passent du côté de la prostate, et les résultats thérapeutiques.

1° *Action sur la prostate.*

Tous les faits sont d'accord pour signaler une modification réelle et précoce dans le volume de la prostate après la castration. Immédiatement après l'opération, la prostate diminue de volume; cette diminution, le toucher rectal, l'exploration avec la sonde permettent de la constater dans les quelques jours ou dans les quelques semaines qui suivent l'opération. Elle est cependant trop précoce pour relever d'une atrophie vraie, histologique : elles résultent exclusivement de la décongestion. Elles s'observent en effet surtout sur les prostates molles et vasculaires, on les voit surtout chez les malades opérés au cours de la première attaque de rétention. Au contraire, ce premier bénéfice fait même défaut ou reste inappréciable sur les prostates scléreuses et fermes, ou chez les malades opérés en dehors de toute phase aiguë.

Que devient la prostate dans les années qui suivent la castration? L'atrophie vraie, réelle, complète de la prostate est exceptionnelle; ce qu'on observe habituellement, c'est une diminution de volume, ou une modification dans la consistance qui devient plus molle, moins ferme. Sur 68 prostates examinées cliniquement de huit mois à quatre ans après l'opération, je trouve en effet :

Atrophie évidente. . . . . . . . . . . . . . . . . . .   4 cas.
Diminution de volume. . . . . . . . . . . . . .  41  —
État stationnaire ou augmentation . . . . . . .  23  —
                         Total. . . . . . . . . . .  68 cas.

L'atrophie s'observe surtout sur les prostates à hypertrophies glan dulaires : au contraire, celles dans lesquelles domine le tissu fibreux ne subissent que de faibles modifications. L'action atrophique de la castration, quoique incontestable dans certains cas, est donc incons- tante et incertaine.

Cependant le bénéfice thérapeutique n'est pas nécessairement pro- portionnel à l'atrophie de la prostate : le rapport entre le facteur prostate et l'élément vésical n'est pas fixe, et l'étude des résultats thé- rapeutiques va nous montrer des améliorations sérieuses malgré que la glande ait conservé à peu près son volume primitif d'hypertrophie.

2º *Action sur la vessie. Résultat thérapeutique.*

Il est facile d'apprécier les *résultats immédiats* de l'opération : les observations sont nombreuses, les documents sont précis. Et on peut dire sans exagération que dans la grande majorité des cas, il se pro- duit dans les quelques jours ou les quelques semaines qui suivent l'opération une amélioration très appréciable. Cette amélioration rapide se manifeste chez les rétentionnistes complets, comme chez ceux qui n'ont encore que de la rétention incomplète; il est pourtant des degrés dans cette amélioration.

*Chez ces rétentions chroniques incomplètes*, on voit le résidu dimi- nuer, la contractilité vésicale reparaître; comme conséquence, les sondages sont moins fréquents ou deviennent inutiles. La cystite s'améliore ou disparaît.

Dans ces *rétentions chroniques complètes*, les résultats immédiats sont souvent aussi favorables. La contractilité vésicale reparaît, alors qu'elle était perdue depuis des années; la miction spontanée devient possible, la vessie se vide quelquefois complètement, plus souvent la rétention devient incomplète et les sondages peuvent être réduits à deux ou trois dans les vingt-quatre heures.

Mais ce ne sont là que des résultats immédiats et il est plus difficile d'apprécier exactement *les résultats éloignés de la castration*. On ne trouve pour les établir qu'un nombre de faits très inférieur. La plu- part des observations sont publiées dans les quelques semaines, tout au plus dans les deux ou trois premiers mois qui font suite à l'opération, et le chirurgien, sous l'impression de résultats immédiats toujours favorables, a une tendance naturelle à parler de guérison.

Au contraire, si on ne tient compte que des malades longuement suivis et pour lesquels la période d'observation a été au minimum de *huit mois*, on voit que les résultats éloignés ne sont pas toujours aussi favorables que les résultats immédiats. Les malades alors se comportent de l'une ou de l'autre des trois façons que voici.

1º Les uns (et ce sont les plus nombreux, 60 pour 100) continuent à bénéficier de l'amélioration primitive qu'ils ont ressentie à la suite de l'opération ; ce sont des rétentionnistes complets, qui ont passé à la rétention incomplète avec des résidus très diminués, avec, comme conséquence des sondages rares, une prostate qui reste grosse ; ce sont encore des rétentions incomplètes dont le résidu a diminué sans disparaître.

Pour eux, le bénéfice quoique minime se maintient : *ils restent améliorés*.

2º Les autres (30 pour 100) perdent au bout d'un certain temps le bénéfice primitivement obtenu, ou continuent à s'aggraver, si l'opération n'avait rien donné immédiatement. Chez eux, la contractilité vésicale, qui avait reparu, diminue à nouveau : les sondages deviennent plus fréquents, la prostate reste stationnaire ou augmente et les complications se surajoutent les unes aux autres. *Il n'y a aucun bénéfice*.

3º Enfin reste une troisième catégorie de malades, ceux qui marchent vers la guérison (10 pour 100). Chez eux le bénéfice immédiat s'accentue progressivement, en même temps que la prostate diminue ; la contractilité redevient parfaite, et les sondages deviennent inutiles. Il est permis en somme de parler de *guérison*.

Malheureusement les malades qui composent cette dernière catégorie sont très rares : les rétentionnistes complets ou incomplets ne figurent dans cette catégorie que par quelques unités, et les seuls malades chez lesquels on observe cette vraie guérison, ce sont ceux qui ont subi la castration à la phase des troubles prémonitoires, c'est-à-dire soit à la période de dysurie, soit à l'occasion d'une première rétention aiguë. Chez eux, la miction reparaît spontanée, le soir ou le lendemain de l'opération ; la vessie se vide et continue à se vider, la prostate diminue et s'atrophie et ces malades sont mis à l'abri des accidents qui se seraient fatalement réalisés dans la suite.

Comment interpréter ces résultats?

La rapidité de l'amélioration dans tous les cas, l'indépendance qui existe à ce moment et se maintient plus tard entre l'amélioration fonctionnelle et le volume de la prostate permet de penser que l'influence de la castration s'exerce d'abord sur l'élément vasculaire. L'action décongestive de la castration est immédiate et reste définitive, elle met le malade à l'abri des crises de congestion, qui jouent un si grand rôle dans l'évolution du prostatisme.

Puis, en seconde ligne, intervient l'action de la castration sur l'élément glandulaire; mais cette influence, quoique incontestable, est tardive, aléatoire et quelquefois nulle.

La castration agit encore, et le fait n'est pas douteux, sur la contractilité vésicale : comment et pourquoi? est-ce une action directe? Je ne le saurais dire : trop d'éléments sont en cause, dont beaucoup sont mal connus, pour qu'il me soit permis de trancher ces hypothèses.

Les *indications* de la castration sont déjà et deviendront très restreintes.

Au début, à la phase première des rétentions aiguës, la castration a une valeur réellement préventive et curative. Mais quels sont, à cette période, les malades qui consentiront à ce sacrifice excessif?

Ce serait cependant le meilleur moyen de permettre à la castration de donner tout ce qu'elle peut : car, plus tard, elle n'est plus qu'une ressource palliative pour prévenir les orchites à répétition, pour prévenir et traiter les attaques de congestion avec hémorragie et pour améliorer quelquefois l'état vésico-prostatique.

En parlant de la castration, je n'ai en vue que la castration double, la seule dont l'efficacité est établie : la *castration unilatérale* étant très inférieure.

Quant à l'*angioneurectomie* du cordon, qui fut mise en parallèle avec la castration, les observations ne me semblent pas encore suffisantes pour qu'il soit permis de dire qu'elle est bien supérieure.

La *résection des déférents*, la *vasectomie* a eu un moment une certaine vogue, et des observations longuement suivies nous permettent très facilement de juger de sa valeur. La résection des déférents vient loin derrière la castration, sa valeur est presque nulle. Je suis d'autant moins suspect de partialité en formulant cette appréciation, que j'ai été un des premiers ici à étudier cette question au point de vue expérimental et à appliquer sur l'homme cette opération.

En ce qui concerne l'influence de la vasectomie sur la prostate hypertrophiée, il n'est pas une observation, en effet, dans laquelle on ait noté une atrophie nette et évidente de la glande. On voit souvent la prostate diminuer de volume le lendemain ou dans les jours qui suivent l'opération, et cela surtout chez les malades opérés en pleine attaque de congestion avec rétention. Mais, plus tard, à distance, on voit la glande reprendre son volume et continuer à s'hypertrophier.

En ce qui concerne les résultats vraiment thérapeutiques de la vasectomie, ils ne sont favorables que chez les congestifs; chez eux, on voit, comme après la castration, mais moins qu'après la castration, reparaître la contractilité vésicale et s'effectuer les mictions spontanées. Mais chez les rétentionnistes incomplets et surtout complets, suivis au delà de huit mois, le bénéfice n'existe plus s'il a jamais existé, et le bilan de l'opération se résume à un insuccès absolu, augmentation de volume de la prostate, difficultés de sondage, rétention, cystite, calcul, etc.

Le seul bénéfice réel de la vasectomie, et c'est aussi la seule indication qui lui reste, c'est de supprimer les orchites répétées dont souffrent si souvent les prostatiques qui se sondent.

Nées d'une assimilation défectueuse et erronée, portées très haut par une faveur exagérée, les opérations testiculaires, malgré les améliorations qu'elles ont causées, verront peu à peu leurs applications se restreindre au profit des opérations d'exérèse directes jusqu'au jour prochain où elles iront rejoindre dans l'histoire la méthode de Battey, la castration ovarienne appliquée au traitement des fibromes utérins.

### III. — *Opérations prostatiques.*

A. *Prostatotomie.* — Avec la prostatotomie j'aborde les opérations qui s'adressent directement à la prostate, et se proposent de sectionner ou de supprimer l'obstacle.

La prostatotomie se fait surtout par la voie périnéale; elle consiste suivant la technique de Harrisson à dilater à l'aide du doigt l'urètre prostatique et à sectionner au bistouri l'obstacle dont le doigt constate la présence. Ensuite on draine par la mise à demeure d'une sonde de fort calibre, et la brèche est ainsi maintenue longtemps ouverte. C'est peut-être à ce drainage surtout que sont dues les améliorations observées à la suite de cette opération. Mais la brèche se referme, l'obstacle se reproduit, et l'amélioration primitive disparaît au bout de peu de temps.

Au lieu de passer par le périnée, Bottini reprenant, en la modifiant, l'idée de Mercier, fait la section de l'obstacle prostatique au galvano-cautère. Il incise le tissu prostatique en arrière, en avant, à

droite et à gauche, suivant les cas. La brèche est profonde : elle
porte sur l'obstacle ou sur les saillies dont la situation a été préalablement établie.

Les résultats s'annoncent immédiatement comme très brillants : le
jour même de l'opération, le soir, le lendemain au plus tard le réten-
tionniste évacue sa vessie, le résidu diminue ou disparaît, des malades
qui depuis des années vivaient de la sonde peuvent uriner seuls. Et
la proportion de ces succès est véritablement considérable. Freudenberg communiquait dernièrement au 29e Congrès de la Société allemande de chirurgie à Berlin une statistique de 685 cas opérés par
cette méthode avec 17 décès. Les résultats ont été contrôlés dans
666 cas : dans 42 cas, il n'y a eu aucun résultat; chez 624 malades,
on a constaté soit la guérison, soit une amélioration; le nombre des
guérisons serait à peu près le double du nombre des cas de simple
amélioration.

Tout en attachant à ces chiffres la signification incontestable qu'ils
comportent, il est impossible de ne pas faire remarquer qu'il s'agit ici
surtout de résultats immédiats. Les résultats immédiats de l'opération
de Bottini sont presque toujours favorables, je dirai même plus favorables qu'aucune autre méthode ne saurait les donner si simplement.
La rapidité avec laquelle on obtient un bénéfice thérapeutique très
réel, engage à publier l'observation de bonne heure et sans suivre le
malade. C'est ainsi, par exemple, que sur les 70 opérations que rapporte Cuellar dans sa thèse, il en est près de 40, c'est-à-dire les deux
tiers, pour lesquelles la période d'observation a été inférieure à 3 mois,
et a été souvent réduite à 2 ou 3 septénaires.

Les résultats éloignés de l'opération de Bottini sont ainsi plus difficiles à établir, et le nombre des faits qui sert à l'apprécier est beaucoup plus restreint. A distance, 4, 5 mois après, il n'est pas
exceptionnel de voir la récidive survenir, la brèche s'est fermée, la
prostate continue à augmenter. Bottini refait une nouvelle opération,
et la simplicité avec laquelle elle se pratique sans anesthésie, la fait
accepter facilement des malades.

Quelques inconvénients en sont cependant la conséquence, c'est
parfois l'incontinence d'urine pendant les premiers jours, ce sont
d'autres fois des accidents infectieux généraux ou locaux, cystite,
phlébite, épididymite. La mort survient dans environ 3 pour 100
des cas.

Mais, en regard de ces accidents qui survenaient, il faut l'observer,
chez des individus profondément infectés, remarquons que l'opération
de Bottini a donné de vraies guérisons, et cela chez des malades que

la castration avait à peine modifiés; elle donne des améliorations très réelles qui se caractérisent par le retour de la contractilité vésicale, la diminution ou la disparition des résidus, elle donne enfin la facilité du sondage pour ceux qui sont encore obligés de recourir à la sonde. La méthode de Bottini, surtout dans les cas où il existe un obstacle localisé, constitue une opération palliative simple, expéditive, bénigne et efficace.

### B. *Prostatectomie.*

Au lieu de sectionner l'obstacle, on a cherché à le supprimer : de là est venue la prostatectomie. Celle-ci on l'a faite jusqu'ici par la voie sus-pubienne, on commence à la faire par le périnée, et à côté des exérèses partielles, qui jusqu'alors ont été seules tentées on commence à envisager la perspective et la possibilité d'une prostatectomie totale.

La *prostatectomie sus-pubienne* inaugurée à l'étranger par Mac Gill, Dittel, Schmidt, Kümmel, défendue en France par Desnos, recherche la suppression à travers la vessie ouverte de l'obstacle pédiculé ou non. Suivant la forme et la nature de cet obstacle, il doit y avoir et il y a en effet entre toutes les opérations des différences très sensibles, et une cause avérée d'inégalité. Depuis la section d'une barre transversale jusqu'à l'excision d'un gros lobe médian pédiculé, ou à l'évidement d'un lobe latéral sessile, il y a bien des intermédiaires.

Sans tenir compte de ces différences, prenons en bloc les observations et voyons ce qu'elles donnent.

En laissant de côté les morts, qui suivant les statistiques s'élevaient de 5 à 15 pour 100, en négligeant toutes les observations, celles-là très nombreuses, qui sont trop récentes, je reste en présence de 242 observations de prostatectomies sus-pubiennes. Elles ont donné 140 guérisons ou améliorations, et 102 résultats nuls.

Les bons résultats ne sont pas tous comparables; il y a de vraies guérisons, des guérisons complètes et absolues, et cela même chez des malades opérés très tardivement. Tels ces opérés de Browne et de Füller, qui rétentionnistes depuis des années ont retrouvé une contractilité vésicale perdue et n'ont plus eu à faire usage du cathéter.

Plus souvent le résultat est moins brillant; il ne se traduit que par une amélioration, mais par une amélioration très réelle. C'est la contractilité vésicale qui reparaît partiellement, c'est le résidu qui diminue, c'est la cystite qui s'atténue. Certains malades cessent de se servir de la sonde, ou ne s'en servent plus que par intermittence, et le cathétérisme s'effectue facilement chez ceux qui avaient avant les plus grandes peines à passer leur sonde.

Sans doute les facteurs de cette amélioration sont multiples et ne relèvent peut-être pas tous de la prostatectomie. On a ouvert la vessie, celle-ci est restée quelque temps fistuleuse et drainée, on a supprimé quelques calculs qui causaient de la douleur. Et déjà il y a de quoi améliorer une prostatique.

Mais aussi remarquez que les seuls résultats dont je tiens compte sont les résultats vraiment éloignés, et lorsque l'amélioration se maintient des mois et des années, je crois qu'on peut sans conteste la rattacher à la prostatectomie elle-même. Et le bénéfice de l'opération dans ces circonstances est d'autant plus remarquable que ces malades ont presque toujours été opérés tardivement, en désespoir de cause ; souvent même la prostatectomie ne fut décidée qu'au cours d'une taille, tentée pour enlever un calcul ou drainer une vessie. On opérait pour une cystite, et trouvant une saillie prostatique accessible, le chirurgien se décidait à l'enlever et à accorder à son malade le bénéfice imprévu d'une prostatectomie partielle.

Et cependant la prostatectomie compte aussi des revers, des échecs absolus : après une amélioration transitoire, le bénéfice a été perdu, l'état s'aggrave à nouveau, la prostate continue à croître et on voit peu à peu le malade revenir à son état primitif.

On arrive ainsi à penser que chez les malades le bénéfice aurait été beaucoup plus appréciable ou plus durable si l'opération avait été plus précoce et aussi l'exérèse plus large.

C'est en effet le reproche qu'on peut faire à la prostatectomie sus-pubienne de ne permettre qu'une ablation minime et partielle. Sans doute, je le sais, on a enlevé à travers la vessie des lobes latéraux hypertrophiés, on a réalisé une sorte d'énucléation transvésicale. Mais l'attaque des lobes latéraux est très difficile par cette voie, et l'exérèse une fois réalisée laisse à sa suite une brèche ouverte, et le chirurgien n'a rien pour la combler.

Aussi la prostatectomie haute ne s'adresse qu'à l'obstacle saillant du côté de la vessie ; or tous les obstacles que constitue la vessie ne se développent pas de ce côté, et sur 333 observations d'hypertrophie prostatique que j'ai réunies, je trouve à ce point de vue les résultats que voici :

<pre>
Hypertrophies localisées au lobe médian ou aux
    glandes cervicales. . . . . . . . . . . . . . .  121
Hypertrophies portant à la fois sur les lobes laté-
    raux et le lobe médian. . . . . . . . . . . . .  156
Hypertrophie des lobes latéraux seuls . . . . . . .   56
</pre>

Ainsi donc la prostatectomie sus-pubienne n'a sa raison d'être que dans 121 cas sur 555, soit dans un tiers des cas seulement : et dans les autres, elle reste insuffisante et inefficace à moins de s'attaquer aux lobes latéraux en même temps, ce qui me paraît difficile et surtout dangereux de ce côté.

Il faut alors si l'on veut recourir à une opération s'adresser à une autre voie, quelle sera-t-elle?

La *voie périnéale* permet au contraire d'enlever largement à l'aide d'une incision prérectale une étendue considérable des lobes latéraux sans ouvrir ni l'urètre ni la vessie. C'est l'opération de Nicole, substituée comme plus compréhensive à la prostatectomie très restreinte telle que la faisait Dittel. Déjà Macewen, Alexander, Hochkis, Albarran ont fait cette extirpation sous-capsulaire de la prostate. Mais ces opérations sont récentes, elles ont donné avec une mortalité relativement minime des résultats immédiats très bons; mais on ne peut encore envisager leurs résultats éloignés.

L'avenir dira ce qu'ils sont; mais déjà nous pouvons espérer que les meilleurs résultats appartiendront aux opérations d'exérèse *précoces* et *très larges*.

Actuellement en effet, l'hypertrophie prostatique nous apparaît de plus en plus comme une maladie primitive, et n'agissant que secondairement sur une vessie dont elle trouble et altère mécaniquement le fonctionnement. Quelle que soit la nature intime et la cause de l'adénome prostatique, quelles que soient les influences congestives qui s'associent à elle et modifient le cycle régulier de son évolution, la prostate fait obstacle sur le trajet de l'urine et la rétention puis l'infection en est la suite. Dès lors la faveur doit revenir aux opérations qui suppriment cet obstacle.

Le bénéfice sera d'autant plus appréciable que l'opération aura été pratiquée plus tôt, avant que la vessie troublée n'ait déjà perdu sa contractilité, avant que l'infection n'ait ajouté ses lésions difficilement réparables.

Il faudra aussi que l'exérèse soit large, c'est-à-dire qu'elle porte sur toutes les parties hypertrophiées ou susceptibles de le devenir. La prostatectomie sus-pubienne est suffisante pour les obstacles limités; mais pour les lobes latéraux la voie périnéale offrira une voie plus large, sinon plus facile. Elle a le tort de ne pas permettre d'enlever en même temps les saillies intravésicales. Dans ces conditions, faudra-t-il combiner deux opérations successives, la taille hypogastrique pour enlever un lobe saillant, la voie périnéale pour enlever les lobes latéraux?

Ce sont là questions tout entières à résoudre. Je pense pour ma part, que prochainement la prostatectomie totale dont je vois les premières ébauches, et dont j'entrevois la prochaine réalisation, viendra trancher et simplifier ces hésitations. La chirurgie a déjà résolu des problèmes plus difficiles et elle s'en est toujours tirée avec honneur.

## TRAITEMENT DE L'HYPERTROPHIE PROSTATIQUE

### *COMMUNICATION RÉSUMÉE*

### par M. POUSSON
de Bordeaux.

Je m'associe sans réserve aux conclusions du remarquable rapport de notre collègue Leguen, et avec lui je considère que les opérations indirectes n'ont d'autres résultats que de prévenir les poussées congestives, origine d'accidents et de complications fréquentes chez les prostatiques, il est vrai, mais que l'emploi méthodique de la sonde à demeure prévient également et à moins de frais.

Parmi ces opérations indirectes, les unes (vasectomie, angionévrectomie) présentent peu de danger pour l'avenir des vieillards qui les subissent ; les autres (orchidectomie simple ou double) en supprimant la sécrétion interne diminuent incontestablement leur résistance organique. N'ayant qu'une foi médiocre dans les arguments des chirurgiens qui ont préconisé la castration, je n'ai jamais fait cette opération, mais j'ai fait un assez grand nombre de fois les opérations sur le cordon pour me convaincre que leurs résultats ne sont jamais curatifs et ne sont pas supérieurs à ceux que fournit la sonde à demeure.

La cystostomie sus-pubienne, à mon avis, est une opération bien rarement — sinon jamais — indiquée chez les prostatiques. Tout d'abord, elle ne combat pas mieux les phénomènes d'infection aiguë que la sonde à demeure, je crois même que quelque rapidité et quelque habileté qu'on mette à exécuter l'ouverture de la vessie, on fait courir de grandes chances de mort à ces malades en les opérant. Quant aux accidents d'infection chronique, résultant du croupissement des urines dans le bas-fond, la disposition de la fistule sus-pubienne ne permet ni de mettre ce bas-fond à sec ni de le nettoyer et de l'aseptiser.

C'est l'existence de ce bas-fond et sa disposition par rapport à l'embouchure de l'urètre à la vessie qui, pour moi, doivent commander les indications opératoires chez les prostatiques. Il existe évidemment chez tous, mais tandis que chez les uns l'absence de saillie prostatique sur la lèvre inférieure du col permet à l'urine, moyennant certains artifices, de sortir en totalité par la sonde et aux liquides modificateurs et antiseptiques de bien déterger cette partie du réservoir, chez d'autres, la saillie des lobes de la prostate crée un sinus au-dessous du col, que les sondages ne peuvent jamais complètement évacuer, que les lavages sont impuissants à atteindre efficacement et dans lequel croupissent et s'altèrent les urines précisément au point où s'ouvrent les uretères. Dans le premier cas, de beaucoup le plus fréquent, la sonde suffit à l'exclusion de toutes les autres opérations; dans le second, la prostatectomie seule est capable d'assurer la désinfection de ce cloaque. La vessie ouverte par-dessus le pubis et le col bien éclairé à l'aide de l'écarteur à lampe électrique dont je me sers habituellement, le ou les lobes prostatiques sont sectionnés, suivant les circonstances, à l'aide du bistouri, des ciseaux ou de la pince coupante sans crainte d'hémorragie. Dans les premiers temps, je drainais toujours par l'hypogastre, aujourd'hui je ferme le plus souvent la vessie après avoir placé une sonde de Pezzer dans l'urètre.

Sur 20 interventions, j'ai eu 5 morts chez des malades très âgés et profondément infectés. Des 15 survivants, 6 ont recouvré le pouvoir de vider complètement leur vessie; chez un 7ᵉ ce résultat a été temporaire, chez un 8ᵉ il a été partiel; mais tous ces malades étaient relativement jeunes, la dysurie n'était pas très ancienne et la vessie n'était pas trop altérée par l'infection. Chez tous les autres, j'ai obtenu la cessation de la cystite et des accidents infectieux.

---

# RÉSULTATS ÉLOIGNÉS DE QUELQUES CAS D'HYPERTROPHIE PROSTATIQUE TRAITÉS PAR LA VASECTOMIE, LA CASTRATION ET LA CYSTOSTOMIE

par M. le docteur P. HAMONIC,

de Paris.

J'ai déjà eu l'occasion de communiquer à la Société un certain nombre de cas d'hypertrophie prostatique traités par ces différentes méthodes.

Parmi les malades dont j'ai rapporté les observations, quelques-uns ont été perdus de vue.

Par contre, il m'est donné d'en suivre d'autres dont je désire dire quelques mots.

Deux prostatiques que j'ai opérés, en 1897, par la *castration double* et qui ont vu rapidement leurs accidents décroître et disparaître sont toujours dans une situation très satisfaisante.

L'extirpation des testicules a agi nettement sur l'élément prostatique et a amené une atténuation telle qu'elle équivaut à la guérison. Celle-ci se maintient depuis trois ans.

La *vasectomie* a donné des résultats éloignés beaucoup moins brillants.

Je continue à donner mes soins à cinq de mes opérés chez lesquels la section double des canaux déférents avait paru exercer une action décongestivante immédiate sur la glande prostate hypertrophiée.

Chez ces cinq sujets, après une période de temps variant de 8 à 24 mois, le prostatisme s'est reproduit comme au début. Deux des malades sont même devenus complètement rétentionnistes, ce qui a nécessité l'emploi de la sonde.

Je vois souvent trois malades à qui j'ai fait la *cystostomie*, l'un depuis cinq ans, les deux autres depuis trois ans pour prostate énormément hypertrophiée. Ces sujets, sauf l'ennui de leur infirmité, se portent bien. Deux retiennent même leur urine pendant plusieurs heures.

De ce petit nombre d'observations, nous pouvons déduire les conclusions suivantes :

La *castration double* est une opération dont l'effet ne saurait être récusé en doute dans l'hypertrophie prostatique.

L'amélioration qu'elle produit sur la glande hypertrophiée est durable. C'est donc une intervention utile qu'on doit conseiller et qu'on peut pratiquer avec la certitude de donner au sujet une amélioration notable. On lui fait perdre des organes qui ont, dans l'espèce, peu d'importance, étant donné l'âge habituel des malades chez lesquels on la pratique.

La *cystostomie*, quoique étant une opération palliative, est bonne en ce sens qu'elle permet une survie parfois considérable. Mais elle a l'inconvénient de créer une infirmité définitive autrement pénible que la castration double.

Quant à la *vasectomie*, malgré les espérances qu'elle avait données au début, elle me paraît constituer une opération insuffisante, et ne donnant, dans les cas où elle semble réussir, que des résultats transitoires. Elle me paraît s'appliquer surtout aux cas de congestion prostatique, car son action s'exerce principalement sur l'élément vasculaire. Elle n'a pas d'action sur l'hypertrophie glandulaire et à plus forte raison sur l'hypertrophie scléreuse de la prostate. Somme toute, c'est la *castration double* qui me paraît devoir être l'opération à préconiser chez les prostatiques réfractaires aux moyens thérapeutiques ordinaires.

## PROSTATIC HYPERTROPHY

### par M. HARRISON,

de Londres.

During the past seven years I have practised a large number of operations on the prostate when it has become so enlarged as to seriously obstruct the function of micturition.

I shall, however, confine myself to day to some remarks on the operation of vasectomy or obliteration of the vasa deferentia either by section or torsion which, I believe, I was the first to practice. I was led to do this mainly in consequence of D^r White's observations on castration, which appeared to me to throw considerable light on the pathology and treatment of prostatic hypertrophy. From the observations I have made during the past seven years on cases where the continuity of the vasa deferentia has been destroyed either by accident as in operations for the radical cure of varicocele, or by design, I am led to the belief that in vasectomy we have a means of preventing prostatic overgrowth taking place which is likely to prove of much service when the sexual as well as the urinary function are both threatened with serious damage.

Before proceeding further, I should like to ask you what are the usual effects of permanent obliteration of the seminal ducts by section, ligature or torsion in a healthy man, we will say, of 40 years of age whose sexual and urinary functions are both normal? I believe these to be inability to procreate, in the first place by mechanical occlusion of these ducts, and later on from atrophy of the secreting portion of the testes, processes which are not necessarily attended with loss of sexual appetite or power of indulging it, as follows in the case of castration. Coincidentally with this the prostate shrinks. What applies under these circumstances to the man of 40 years of age applies equaltrye to the man of 65 years of age, both in respect to the structure and function of these parts.

In a recent article in *The Lancet* (vol. ij 1900), I have published the particulars of some cases which would come under the latter category where both the sexual and urinary powers of the individuals referred to were threatened with extinction by the rapid development of prostatic hypertrophy, and where it was obvious that whatever became of the sexual function the prospect of substituting an artificial or aided micturition for a natural one was imminent.

This brings me to the main point of my observations today and to
traise the question before this distinguished assembly, can anything
further be done with reasonable safely to life and intellect, to prevent
the incidence of catheter life or dependence?

In the instances referred to in y paper in *The Lancet* where I
obliterated both trasa in the manner I have described, he process of
micturition has continued to remain normal and tunaided for long
periods whilst as far as I am aware, the sexual function has not
abnormally suffered.

It may be argued with fairness that there was no positive proof
that though the symptoms in these people just referred to appeared
to indicate they were all on the verge of catheter life or dependence, the latter may not have really happened. On the other
hand, judging from a fairly large and long exprience of cases of
prostatic retention of urine I hardly think I can have been entirely
wrong in my anticipations in all the instances and in concluding
that unless vascular or structural shrinkage of the prostate could
be quickly induced, the process of normal micturition would completely break down.

In contra-distinction to thesee cases where I believe the permanent
use of the catheter was averted by the early adoption of vasectomy
and the artificial induction of prostatic shrinkage, let me take the
class of cases in which this operation has been the most extensively
employed. In my own practice this would include something over
100 persons upwards of 60 years of age, where this operation was
practised. I refer to the cases where persons had been more or less
dependent on the catheter for long periods of time previously, and
where complications had arisen either by reason of catheterism
being difficult, painful or frequent or from some other cause of a
like nature it appeared necessary, to induce shrinkage of the prostate artificially. In this class of cases, from the observations of
persons so operated upon, for some years subsequently, the results
of vasectomy have been variable. In some apparently but little has
been gained, through in by far the great majority relief usually
followed and continued. Putting aside cases of fibrotic degeneration
of the prostate which are best treated by suprapubie prostatectomy
or by perineal prostatotomy these variable results are largely dependent upon the permanent effects produced upon the bladder by that
long continued obstruction and back pressure of the urine which
usually accompany all cases of progressive prostatic hypertrophy.

Though the prostate may shrink after vasectomy as I have seen to

small dimensions and become atrophied the bladder may be so
permanently damaged by pouching, trabeculation, and sacculation
as to never be likely to regain its power of voluntarily holding and
expelling urine even if it were possible to get rid of the prostate
altogether. On President Professor Guyon has well expressed it
that we must not look to the condition of the prostate alore as
explaining the entire series of morbid effects on urination with which
it is so frequently associated.

Vasectomy is an operation when performed as I have ventured to
describe which is free from risk to life and intellect. I have had
good opportunities of arriving at this conclusion as I have already
performed the operation considerably over 100 times. In this respect
it differs materially from castration which I cannot support under
these circumstances except when one or both testis happens to be
the seat of disease and requires removal. My contention to day is
to the purport that obliteration of the vasa should in many instances
preceed the adoption of catheter life, and that of this course were more
frequently taken persons might preserve their natural function of
micturition indefinitely or until their existence was terminated in
less painful ways than are frequently associated with this process.

## L'OPÉRATION DE BOTTINI DANS LE TRAITEMENT
## DE L'HYPERTROPHIE PROSTATIQUE

### par M. le docteur G. NICOLICH.

A la troisième session de l'association française d'urologie, en 1898,
j'avais fait connaître les résultats de cinq opérations de Bottini; dans
cette occasion j'ai démontré l'instrument de Bottini, modifié par
Freudenberg, et l'accumulateur de Kiss. Depuis cette époque, un peu
partout, mais surtout en Allemagne et en Amérique, l'opération de
Bottini a été pratiquée en proportions toujours croissantes. Freudenberg, W. Meyer, Gujtéras et tant d'autres ont publié les résultats de
cette opération. Bottini, dans un mémoire tout récent (*L'iscuria prostatica, Biblioteca della clinica moderna, Firenze* 1900), après avoir fait
l'histoire de son opération et des difficultés qu'il a dû vaincre pour
arriver à obtenir un bon instrument et une source électrique suffisante
pour rougir le couteau de l'inciseur, fait connaître les résultats de sa

pratique qui, naturellement, est la plus étendue de tous les autres chirurgiens.

Ma première opération de Bottini date du mois d'août 1898. Depuis cette époque j'ai pratiqué 29 fois cette opération; les résultats ont été très satisfaisants et ils m'encouragent à faire une relation pour mieux faire connaître l'utilité de cette opération. Il ne suffit pas de faire une statistique sommaire des cas opérés et donner tout simplement le chiffre des guéris et des morts, quand il s'agit d'une maladie multiforme comme l'hypertrophie de la prostate et quand il y a encore un grand nombre de praticiens qui, faute d'avoir jamais vu cette opération ou influencés par les enseignements de quelque grand maître, ne croient pas à l'opération que Bottini, depuis un quart de siècle, s'efforce de faire connaître. Dans notre art, on voit bien souvent de ces anomalies, et, sans aller trop loin de notre champ, il me suffit de rappeler ce qui se passe à présent en Autriche vis-à-vis de l'urétrotomie interne. A Vienne, à Graz, et partout où il y a des chirurgiens qui ont étudié à l'école de Dittel ou de ses élèves, on considère cette innocente opération comme meurtrière, et il faut voir la trépidation craintive des jeunes médecins, qui suivent mon service, quand ils assistent pour la première fois à une urétrotomie interne, qu'ils craignent tellement dangereuse, qu'ils ne peuvent pas se persuader que sur 344 urétrotomies internes, je n'ai eu qu'un cas de mort.

J'ai opéré avec la méthode de Bottini 29 prostatiques; je considère comme deux cas un malade qui a été opéré une deuxième fois un an et demi après la première. De ces malades, quatre étaient à leur première attaque de rétention complète et sont tous guéris; quatorze souffraient de rétention chronique incomplète qui, à intervalles variables devenait complète; de ceux-ci, dix sont guéris, un n'a eu aucune amélioration et trois sont morts; onze malades étaient en rétention complète, huit sont guéris, un n'est pas guéri, et deux sont morts. Ainsi, sur 29 opérés, j'ai eu 22 guéris, 2 non guéris, 5 morts.

Selon l'âge, mes opérés étaient :

De 51 à 60 ans. . . . . . . . . . . . . . . . . . . . .   1 cas.
De 61 à 70  — . . . . . . . . . . . . . . . . . . . . .  16  —
De 71 à 80  — . . . . . . . . . . . . . . . . . . . . .  11  —
De 81 à 90  — . . . . . . . . . . . . . . . . . . . . .   1  —

Le plus jeune avait 55 ans, le plus âgé 86 ans. Sur 29 malades, j'ai pratiqué 33 opérations, parce que j'ai dû dans quatre cas faire une deuxième opération, la première n'ayant pas atteint son but.

J'ai toujours fait usage comme source électrique de l'accumulateur Kiss avec l'ampèremètre; je me suis servi de l'inciseur de Bottini trois

fois seulement, parce que je trouve plus pratique et simple l'inciseur
modifié par Freudenberg. Une seule fois il m'est arrivé que le couteau
ne pouvait plus entrer dans sa niche; heureusement cet accident n'a
eu aucune mauvaise suite. J'ai presque toujours opéré à vessie vide,
seulement dans les derniers cas j'ai rempli la vessie d'air. Autrefois,
je chauffais le couteau à rouge, maintenant je le chauffe à blanc sans
avoir observé aucun inconvénient. Pour anesthésier la vessie et l'urètre
je me suis servi de la solution de cocaïne à 2 pour 100, qui n'a pas
eu toujours le pouvoir d'empêcher complètement les douleurs. La
sonde à demeure, sauf quelques cas, a toujours été le traitement post-
opératoire de choix; cinq ou six jours ont suffi, quelquefois j'ai dû
prolonger la demeure de la sonde à cause de la fièvre, très rarement
à cause de l'hémorragie.

L'examen cystoscopique des malades est à mon avis indispensable;
je l'ai pratiqué presque toujours, sauf dans quelques cas à urètre et
vessie intolérantes; cet examen m'a fait découvrir deux fois l'existence
d'un calcul caché derrière la protubérance du lobe moyen et, dans un
cas, cet examen m'a encouragé à faire une deuxième incision sur une
petite saillie du lobe moyen que le toucher rectal ne pouvait pas déce-
ler; cette deuxième incision a guéri le malade.

Parmi les malades guéris, j'ai observé les complications suivantes :

```
Fièvre . . . . .  2 fois très légère pendant 1 ou 2 jours.
  —    . . . . . .  2   —        —         —   1 semaine.
  —    . . . . . .  1   —        —         —   1 mois.

Hémorragie. .  1 fois le 1er et 12e jour après l'opération.
  —      . .  1  —  le  4e jour après l'opération.
  —      . .  1  —  le  5e   —            —
  —      . .  1  —  le  8e   —            —
  —      . .  1  —  le 12e   —            —

Incrustations phosphatiques sur l'escarre déta-
    chée. . . . . . . . . . . . . . . . . . . . . . . . . 1 fois.
Abcès péri-urétrale. . . . . . . . . . . . . . . . . 1  —
Incontinence d'urine. . . . . . . . . . . . . . . . 1  —
```

Trois malades avaient été déjà opérés de vasectomie plusieurs mois
auparavant.

Les malades en rétention complète étaient dans cet état depuis un
mois jusqu'à dix-huit mois.

J'ai pu constater que mes malades se portaient bien

| | | | | |
|---|---|---|---|---|
| 1 | fois | 25 | mois après | l'opération. |
| 1 | — | 22 | — | — |
| 1 | — | 18 | — | — |
| 1 | — | 17 | — | — |
| 2 | — | 15 | — | — |
| 1 | — | 15 | — | — |
| 1 | — | 8 | — | — |
| 1 | — | 6 | — | — |
| 1 | — | 5 | — | — |
| 1 | — | 2 | — | — |

Causes du décès :

Une fois : pyélonéphrite avec formation d'abcès dans la substance corticale du rein, vingt jours après l'opération.

Une fois : pyélonéphrite dans l'unique rein fonctionnant ; l'autre était atrophié et rempli de calculs, trois mois après l'opération.

Une fois : embolie de l'artère pulmonaire, quinze jours après l'opération.

Une fois : suppuration périprostatique et vésicale, et perforation de la paroi postérieure de la vessie, vingt-deux jours après l'opération.

Une fois : nécrose des os pubiens, quatre mois après l'opération.

L'enthousiasme avec lequel il n'y a pas longtemps beaucoup de chirurgiens accueillirent les opérations testiculaires contre l'hypertrophie de la prostate s'est vite baissé et maintenant tout laisse croire que les opérations testiculaires finiront par être oubliées. A vrai dire, il ne pourrait en être autrement, parce qu'aucune de ces opérations n'a des indications nettes et nous ne savons pas d'avance quels sont les cas qui pourront être traités avec succès. Mon expérience, basée sur l'observation prolongée et attentive de plusieurs prostatiques opérés de vasectomie, m'autorise à ne pas ôter toute valeur à cette opération, mais d'autre part l'opération de Bottini m'a donné de si bons résultats que je dois la préférer, même avec ses dangers. Défaut des indications d'un côté, bons résultats de l'autre, il n'y a pas de doute qu'on doive choisir ce dernier.

Quand doit-on pratiquer l'opération de Bottini? Le professeur de Pavie donne à son ouvrage le titre de traitement de l'iscurie prostatique. Ce titre donne selon moi les indications pour l'opération ; « *iscuria* » veut dire rétention complète, et quand un prostatique a eu une attaque de rétention complète, il en aura presque toujours d'autres à échéances plus ou moins prolongées, et la sonde lui sera indispensable. Quand un prostatique arrive à devoir vivre avec la sonde, il a bien des chances de s'infecter et dans ce cas l'opération est indiquée. Je ne veux pas affirmer qu'on doit pratiquer cette opération dans tous les cas. Dans la pratique il faut faire une distinction entre malades et malades. Je ne crois pas indiqué d'opérer un malade, qui est à sa première attaque de rétention, dont il peut guérir et rester plusieurs mois et même des années sans avoir plus besoin de la sonde. Il faut aussi prendre en considération le fait qu'il y a des malades en rétention complète depuis longtemps qui, grâce aux précautions antiseptiques, peuvent conserver l'urine claire et n'ont besoin de se sonder que trois ou quatre fois dans la journée. Dans ces cas, selon moi, l'opération n'est pas indiquée; mais dans la grande majorité des cas, et particulièrement chez les prostatiques qui vivent loin de la ville et qui ne peuvent pas observer une rigoureuse antisepsie, l'opération est indiquée. Ce n'est pas toujours avec la sonde que les prostatiques s'infectent; nombre de cas présentent des phénomènes d'infection même très grave sans jamais avoir été sondés. L'existence de l'infection n'est pas une contre-indication pour l'opération; j'ai opéré des malades infectés avec cystite et pyélite, et le résultat a été des plus satisfaisants, quelquefois même splendide. On a dit que l'affaiblissement de la contractilité vésicale contre-indique l'opération, mais rien n'est plus difficile de juger d'avance de l'état de cette contractilité; j'ai vu des malades dont la vessie présentait tous les signes de l'atonie, pouvoir très bien uriner une fois ôté l'obstacle à l'émission de l'urine. Le muscle vésical, avec le temps et l'exercice, devient toujours plus actif; plusieurs de mes opérés m'ont assuré un an et plus après l'opération de pouvoir uriner mieux que dans le premier temps après avoir été opérés.

Il paraît incroyable qu'une opération qui avait donné des bons résultats ait tant tardé à entrer dans la pratique courante. On peut expliquer peut-être ce fait par les défauts des instruments, par la difficulté qu'on avait de se procurer une source électrique suffisante et facile à être maniée, et peut-être aussi par l'opposition que les meilleures idées trouvent très souvent à faire leur chemin. Si plusieurs des adversaires de cette opération, au lieu de répéter ce que les autres ont dit, l'avaient eux-mêmes mise en pratique en observant les règles données par Bottini, je suis sûr qu'ils auraient changé d'avis. M. Legueu, dans son dernier rapport sur les résultats éloignés des traitements opératoires de l'hypertrophie prostatique, n'est pas bien informé quand il dit que l'opération de Bottini est une prostatomie électrolytique et quand il affirme qu'elle ne peut être jugée dans ses résultats éloignés faute de documents suffisants. Dans la presse médicale américaine, allemande et italienne, on trouve dans ces dernières années très souvent publiées des observations qui maintes fois sont de vrais documents, sans parler des publications de Bottini, qui sont pour moi de la plus grande valeur. Les adversaires de cette opération ont très souvent l'air de mettre en doute ce que Bottini affirme ; j'avoue que je ne peux pas comprendre cette manière de discuter. Il y en a quelques-uns qui trouvent très curieux que Bottini n'a pas eu de cas de mort ; il y en a d'autres qui trouvent très drôle que Bottini n'a pas observé des récidives ou des échecs. Tout ça n'est pas vrai. Bottini a eu aussi des morts et des récidives, comme je le dirai plus tard, quand je m'occuperai de la mortalité de cette opération. Si Bottini a eu de meilleurs résultats, cela se comprend très facilement si l'on considère sa longue expérience et son habileté.

Je suis persuadé que nombre de chirurgiens ont eu de mauvais résultats de l'opération de Bottini ou parce qu'ils ne disposaient pas de bons instruments et d'une bonne source électrique ou parce qu'ils n'ont pas observé une bonne technique, ou parce qu'ils ont mal choisi leurs cas.

A propos de la technique il est très important de savoir d'avance la direction et la profondeur des incisions qu'on doit pratiquer sur la prostate, et si l'on doit opérer à vessie vide ou remplie. W. Meyer (*Medical Record New-York*, 28 avril 1900), croit qu'il est très difficile de déterminer d'avance la longueur de l'incision ; si la prostate est dure, le toucher rectal fait en même temps que l'inciseur accroche la prostate, pourra donner la mesure de l'incision ; si l'extrémité de l'index touche la pointe de l'instrument, on calcule la distance de l'extrémité de l'index au bord de l'anus, on ôte de cette mesure la distance entre le bord inférieur de la prostate et l'anus, et on aura la longueur de l'incision ; l'expérience a démontré qu'il faut que l'incision soit au moins un centimètre plus grande. Dans les cas à prostate molle, on ne peut pas procéder de cette manière, parce que l'organe se laisse comprimer par l'instrument et l'on pourrait faire une incision trop longue. Meyer est d'avis de faire des incisions même de huit centimètres dans les prostates dures et très grosses, mais seulement de un à deux dans les prostates molles.

Freudenberg (*Deutsche Medizinische Zeitung*, janvier 1900) est d'avis que dans certains cas il peut être nécessaire de faire une incision même de six centimètres; il n'a pourtant jamais atteint cette longueur; trois centimètres et demi lui ont toujours suffi, et plusieurs fois encore moins.

Bottini (*l'Iscuria prostatica*, Firenze, 1900) ne donne à présent aucune importance à la longueur de l'incision ; il fait toujours une ou plusieurs incisions, mais toujours de la même longueur. Autrefois, il dirigeait l'incision sur le sommet de la protubérance prostatique et les résultats étaient souvent faibles ; maintenant qu'il suit une voie tout à fait différente, il obtient des effets plus prompts et sûrs. Il ne fait pas l'incision sur le lobe prostatique hypertrophié, mais sur l'entonnoir placé à la base de ce lobe et sur un point vis-à-vis de ce dernier sur la section antérieure du col de la vessie. De cette manière, l'incision tombe sur le sphincter vésical et l'on obtient une ouverture suffisante au passage de l'urine. *A priori*, on jugerait comme peu rationnel ce procédé qui ne touche pas le lobe hypertrophié et attaque la partie saine, mais on le trouve rationnel, dit Bottini, quand on pense que du côté sain on arrive immédiatement sur l'anneau fibreux qui, comme un sphincter, ferme le méat urinaire interne.

Freudenberg (*loc. cit.*) croit aussi que quelquefois il est plus indiqué dé diriger l'incision dans le sillon, entre deux saillies prostatiques.

A. v. Frisch (*Die Krankheiten der Prostata*, Wien, 1899) est d'avis que l'incision complète du sphincter vésical interne soit nécessaire au bon succès de l'opération.

Doit-on opérer à vessie vide ou remplie ?

Freudenberg, Meyer, préfèrent opérer à vessie remplie d'une solution stérile d'acide borique pour éviter le cas qui est arrivé une fois à Freudenberg qui, pendant une opération à vessie vide, accrocha un pli de la vessie. Autrefois j'opérais à vessie vide, maintenant je remplis la vessie d'air, parce que je ne peux admettre qu'il est dangereux d'injecter l'air dans la vessie, comme le croit Lewis. Selon cet auteur, l'absorption de l'air par les veines rénales pourrait tuer le malade.

Bottini opère toujours à vessie vide parce qu'il craint que le liquide injecté s'infiltrant entre les branches de l'instrument puisse diminuer l'intensité de la chaleur du couteau, et alors il peut arriver qu'au lieu de faire un sillon thermique on en fasse un mécanique, sans dire que le couteau refroidi peut se plier.

Mortalité :

Bottini partage ses opérés en deux séries ; dans la première sont groupés tous les cas traités avec des instruments imparfaits, sans appareil réfrigératif, et chauffés par des batteries électriques primitives ; dans la deuxième, les opérés avec des instruments perfectionnés.

Bottini (série I) . . . . . 200 cas, 14 décès, mortalité  7     pour 100.
    — (série II) . . . . . 255  —  3  —     —    1.27    —
W. Meyer[1] . . . . . . . . 24  —  6  —     —    25      —

1. *Loc. cit.*

A. v. Frisch[1] . . . . . . . .    10 cas,    1 décès,    mortalité,    10      pour 100.
Freudenberg[2] . . . . . .    51    —    6    —        —        11.76    —
Nicolich . . . . . . . . . .    29    —    5    —        —        17.24    —

Il est très difficile de bien juger de la valeur de ces chiffres, comme du reste il arrive trop souvent dans les statistiques médicales. Il y a des auteurs qui ne considèrent les décès comme causés par l'opération si l'opéré meurt quelques semaines plus tard, en conséquence de l'affection rénale qui, très souvent, existait aussi avant l'opération.

Je ne crois pas juste cette manière de voir, parce qu'il est certain que l'affection rénale préexistante peut être aggravée par l'opération et devenir mortelle à cause de celle-ci. Si j'avais aussi suivi cette manière de faire la statistique, j'aurais pu très bien ne pas compter parmi les décès deux de mes opérés qui sont morts, le premier trois mois après l'opération de pyélonéphrite calculeuse et le deuxième de nécrose des os pubiens quatre mois après. Parmi les causes qui ont déterminé la mort des opérés, on cite les suppurations prostatiques, périprostatiques et périvésicales, l'embolie de l'artère pulmonaire, suite de la thrombose des veines prostatiques, la perforation de la vessie, l'hémorragie et la pyélonéphrite.

La mortalité après l'opération a été assez forte pour tous excepté pour Bottini, mais il faut penser que l'on opère des malades presque toujours dans de très mauvaises conditions. Sur 220 prostatiques dont l'état était assez grave pour les faire entrer à l'hôpital, M. Motz[3] a trouvé 31 cas de mort, c'est-à-dire 14 pour 100. Si nous prenons en considération que la majorité de ces opérations ont été pratiquées chez les prostatiques les plus graves, la mortalité de l'opération de Bottini ne doit pas nous étonner.

Récidives après l'opération :

On dit que les récidives multiples signalées dans quelques cas témoignent de la rapidité avec laquelle doit se fermer la brèche que crée le galvanocautère. A ce propos, il faut faire une distinction entre récidive et succès incomplet de la première opération ; et je crois d'autant nécessaire de la faire que je vois quelques auteurs affirmer qu'il y a eu récidive dans les cas où on doit faire une deuxième opération à bref délai de la première. Ce n'est pas juste de parler de récidive quand il s'agit tout bonnement d'insuffisance de la première opération et on ne peut considérer récidivé un malade qui est encore en traitement. Il est arrivé presque à tous les opérateurs

1. *Wiener Klinische Wochenschrift.* Dezember 1898.
2. *Loc. cit.*
3. Compte rendu de l'Association Française d'urologie, 1897.

de devoir faire une deuxième et même une troisième incision pour vaincre l'obstacle et guérir leurs malades, mais dans ces cas il ne s'agissait pas de récidive, et ces deuxième et troisième opérations n'auraient pas été nécessaires si la première incision avait été suffisante.

Il y a récidive si après un délai plus ou moins long le malade qu'on considérait guéri souffre de nouveau dans l'émission de l'urine, comme il est arrivé chez un de mes opérés qui, après 18 mois de parfaite santé, a eu une nouvelle attaque de rétention. Ce malade guérit parfaitement après une deuxième opération

Si les récidives sont possibles, cela n'est pas une raison pour condamner l'opération, comme on ne condamne pas la cystotomie ou la lithotritie si une autre pierre se forme après l'opération. Les adversaires de la prostatotomie galvanique se servent pour la combattre des insuccès qui quelquefois suivent l'opération. On ne peut pas nier qu'il y a des cas où l'opération n'a eu aucun résultat; Bottini même, sur les 255 dernières opérations, a eu 4 insuccès; mais quelle est l'opération qui réussit toujours chez les prostatiques? Jusqu'à présent elle n'est pas encore trouvée.

Je crois qu'il ne faut pas toujours juger comme insuccès les cas cités comme tels; je suis persuadé que plusieurs fois ou le chirurgien n'a pas osé faire une deuxième ou une troisième opération, ou le patient n'a pas voulu s'y soumettre; et ces cas qui seraient guéris en répétant l'opération sont considérés comme insuccès. A ce propos, je dois mentionner un cas très instructif observé par Freudenberg qui, seulement après la troisième opération, guérit un malade de la rétention complète dont il souffrait depuis 5 ans. J'aurais aussi eu trois insuccès de plus si je n'avais pas pratiqué une deuxième incision à trois malades qui n'avaient obtenu aucun résultat de la première opération.

Dans les publications qui ont été faites ces dernières années, on trouve cités des cas de guérison d'ischurie prostatique avec l'opération de Bottini, qui démontrent, s'il était encore nécessaire, la grande utilité de l'incision galvanique de la prostate. A. v. Frisch[1] fait l'histoire d'un malade que l'on avait opéré en 1894 de prostatectomie latérale, en 1895 de taille médiane avec extirpation d'une grande partie du lobe moyen; en 1897 de taille hypogastrique et prostatectomie. Après toutes ces opérations, le malade était toujours en rétention complète quand Frisch, en 1898, lui pratiqua l'opération de Bottini; neuf jours après, le malade vidait sa vessie.

1. *Loc. cit.*

L'étude de ce qu'on a écrit sur l'opération de Bottini, mais surtout les faits de mon observation m'encouragent à la préférer à toutes les autres comme la plus sûre, la plus prompte et la moins dangereuse.

## DISCUSSION

M. Carlier (de Lille). — Dans mon rapport de 1896 sur le traitement de l'hypertrophie de la prostate par les opérations sur le cordon et le testicule, je me montrais très réservé sur l'avenir de la castration et j'exprimais des doutes sur la valeur de la vasectomie. Mes résultats personnels d'alors et ceux que j'obtins par la suite ne m'ont pas fait changer d'avis, la section des déférents ne m'a pas paru agir sur l'hypertrophie prostatique, elle décongestionne simplement un peu les congestifs.

Quant à la castration, je l'ai peu employée, ce moyen chirurgical qui répugne au malade et au chirurgien ne me paraît devoir donner des résultats que chez les prostatiques jeunes et au début de leur maladie; or, ce sont surtout ces malades qui accepteront le plus difficilement la castration.

J'ai pratiqué l'angioneurectomie, j'ai même eu recours dans six cas à la section complète de tous les éléments du cordon, artères, veines, nerfs et canal déférent. Dans aucun de ces cas je n'ai eu de gangrène du testicule, cet organe n'a pas toujours subi l'atrophie à laquelle je m'attendais. Quant à l'influence exercée sur les troubles urinaires, elle n'a été manifeste que chez deux malades de 48 et de 50 ans, c'est-à-dire chez des malades jeunes et qui étaient au début de leur maladie.

Chez trois malades, la cystostomie avec drainage permanent a fait cesser des accidents de fièvre et de dépérissement contre lesquels j'avais lutté en vain avec la sonde à demeure.

Il me paraît donc que les opérations pratiquées sur le testicule et le cordon ne sont que des moyens d'arrêt et non de guérison de la maladie, grâce à ces moyens la maladie marque le pas. Et c'est pourquoi leur action est très recommandable et surtout favorable si l'on a affaire à des sujets qui sont au début de leur hypertrophie de la prostate.

Restent donc les moyens chirurgicaux s'adressant directement à la prostate. Je n'ai pas d'expérience de l'opération de Bottini, cette section galvanocaustique de l'obstacle prostatique, dans un milieu souvent septique, m'inspire les craintes les plus vives, et la statistique de M. Nicolich n'est pas faite pour me rassurer.

Quant à la prostatectomie, son emploi est trop récent pour qu'on puisse s'appuyer sur les résultats qu'elle donne. Il m'apparaît bien cependant que c'est là l'opération de l'avenir pour l'hypertrophie de la prostate, mais il en sera de la prostatectomie comme des autres modes de traitement de l'hypertrophie de la prostate, il faudra la pratiquer très tôt pour qu'elle ne soit pas une opération septique et qu'elle ne soit ni trop meurtrière ni incertaine comme résultats. Or, il sera toujours très difficile au chirurgien de faire accepter une opération de cette nature à un malade parfois jeune encore, et chez lequel la maladie, prise au début, peut rester longtemps très supportable par une bonne hygiène, l'emploi judicieux de la sonde et la mise en pratique des opérations sur le cordon et sur le testicule, opérations non curatrices, il est vrai, mais au moins inoffensives.

M. D. GIORDANO (de Venise). — Je n'ai opéré que les prostatiques chez lesquels les cathétérismes patiemment répétés, la sonde à demeure amorcée par un siphon, ne donnèrent point de résultats.

J'ai pratiqué deux prostatectomies périnéales avec un résultat nul et une amélioration, et une prostatectomie hypogastrique, avec guérison. Il me semble cependant que ces opérations cruentes sont trop graves, ne donnant pas des résultats proportionnés au mal auquel elles s'adressent.

L'ignipuncture au paquelin de lobes latéraux, à travers le rectum, selon Negretto de Lodi, m'a donné deux résultats nuls, un médiocre, un bon. La simple cautérisation avec le cautérisateur galvanique de Bottini m'a donné un résultat bon et un nul.

La division avec le diviseur galvanique du même Bottini m'a donné 5 améliorations, 5 résultats nuls et 9 guérisons, qui ont duré de 7 mois à 2 ans. Après des mois, quelques-uns des guéris, à la suite de libations trop copieuses, ont dû se représenter avec de la rétention, qui a cédé en général au cathétérisme répété. Chez deux de ces récidivés, j'ai fini par répéter la division galvanique, en obtenant à nouveau qu'ils puissent vider spontanément leur vessie.

D'après ces quelques observations, il me paraît que le meilleur traitement opératoire de l'hypertrophie de la prostate, avec rétention, soit en ce moment la division avec l'appareil de Bottini. Les résultats immédiats sont bons en général, mais il faut s'attendre après un an en moyenne à de nouvelles attaques de rétention, qui doivent être traitées selon les méthodes courantes et sont susceptibles d'une nouvelle intervention au galvano-cautère.

M. CHEVALIER (de Paris). — Je reste convaincu que les opérations dites radicales de l'hypertrophie prostatique ne sont que des opérations d'exception, et que le traitement par le cathétérisme raisonné reste le traitement de choix. Je tiens, comme résultat éloigné, à donner des nouvelles du malade que j'ai opéré en avril 1896, par la castration double, et qui, ainsi que je l'ai déjà communiqué aux congrès de l'Association d'urologie 1896-97-98-99 avait subi antérieurement la vasectomie, la cystostomie, etc. Ce malade avait quitté Necker parfaitement guéri. Sa guérison s'est maintenue complète, ainsi que les nouvelles qu'il me donne régulièrement en témoignent.

M. LOUMEAU (de Bordeaux). — Voici les résultats de ma pratique relativement aux opérations pratiquées chez des prostatiques :

J'ai opéré par la *castration totale* cinq prostatiques atteints de rétention chronique complète et dont la prostate, très dure, rendait le cathétérisme laborieux, sinon impossible. Trois fois la rétention a complètement disparu, deux fois elle a été transformée en rétention partielle avec résidu, variable de 60 à 80 grammes, facile à évacuer par la sonde. Quant à la prostate, elle a dans quatre cas diminué de volume et de consistance. Chez mon cinquième opéré, elle est devenue, deux mois après la castration, le siège d'un cancer à marche rapide auquel le malade succombait trois mois plus tard, dans d'horribles souffrances à peine atténuées par une cystostomie sus-pubienne destinée à assurer le drainage vésical, devenu impraticable par le canal.

La *résection bilatérale des canaux déférents*, que j'ai pratiquée cinquante-six fois, ne m'a jamais paru modifier ni l'état de la prostate, ni la rétention chronique dont étaient précédemment atteints mes opérés. Le seul résultat acquis depuis a été de prémunir le patient contre les orchites du cathétérisme et c'est là, à mon sens, le seul bénéfice incontestable que l'on puisse attendre de cette opération.

La *cystostomie sus-pubienne*, que je crois exceptionnellement indiquée contre les difficultés mictionnelles du prostatisme auxquelles satisfait d'ordinaire l'emploi de la sonde, n'a été pratiquée qu'une seule fois par moi, dans l'hypertrophie de la prostate non compliquée d'infection vésicale. Il s'agissait d'un vieux médecin, à prostate très grosse, ligneuse, peut-être même néoplasique, provoquant une rétention complète et ne permettant pas l'introduction de la plus petite sonde. Le malade aima mieux subir et garder jusqu'à sa mort, survenue au bout de quatre mois de broncho-pneumonie, une fistule vésico-hypogastrique que d'être privé de ses testicules.

Quant à la *prostatectomie*, je ne l'ai pratiquée que trois fois pour une saillie prépondérante du lobe médian de la prostate, gênant la miction et finalement le cathétérisme devenu, par elle, douloureux, hémorragipare ou impossible. Par la voie sus-pubienne, j'excisai le lobe prostatique dont je cautérisai au fer rouge le point d'implantation. En même temps, chez mes deux derniers opérés, je lardai profondément au thermocautère toute la portion de la glande bombant vers la cavité vésicale. Ces trois prostatectomies partielles, effectuées sans aucun incident, datent de 7, 9 et 15 mois : mes opérés en ont retiré une facilité beaucoup plus grande du cathétérisme au moment des crises de rétention, devenues d'ailleurs moins fréquentes, et une puissance bien supérieure du jet urinaire. Chez les deux malades auxquels j'ai en même temps pratiqué l'ignipuncture de la prostate, l'organe a subi une très notable diminution de volume, appréciable par le toucher rectal et le palper bimanuel. Cette cautérisation interstitielle me paraît un heureux auxiliaire de la prostatectomie partielle dirigée contre l'hypertrophie sénile de la prostate.

## STATUS OF THE TREATMENT OF PROSTATIC HYPERTROPHY
## IN THE UNITED STATES

par M. RAMON GUITERAS,
de New-York.

The operative methods that have been used are : Ligation of the internal iliac arteries ;

Castration;

Vasectomy;

Prostatectomy;

Bottini operation.

Of these the first three have been practically discarded, the ligation of the internal iliacs was long ago abandonned and is now never heard of except in the history of the treatment of such cases.

Castration, an operation devised by one of our best surgeons, was discarded some years ago, as it was found that the mortality was over 20 per 100 and that of those living some became maniacal, some melancholic, while others developed nervous disorders or lost [their mental equilibrium.

Vasectomy was also an operation of but little popularity with us, and although some still perform it or angioneurectomy the vast majority of surgeons do not. The only argument in its favor is that it is not called dangerous, which is not the case, however, as numbers of deaths have been reported as following it.

We then come to the two operations most in vogue, prostatectomy and the Bottini operation. The advocate of both these methods argue strongly in their favor and the followers of one are wont to condemn the other operation. The supporters of prostatectomy claim that the Bottini operation is a blind one and that the surgeon cannot see what he is doing while the advocates of the Bottini operation claim that enucleation is extremely dangerous both at the time of the operation and afterwards.

Both are right, but luckily most of us do not confine ourselves to one operation, and are willing to try the procedure that is indicated in each case.

The Bottini operation is a blind one, but so is litholopaxy; in the one case we determine the size of the prostate and the required length of the cut by the rectal touch and by means of a searcher passed into the bladder, the end of which in that sac can be felt through the anterior wall of the rectum and so its position determined, while in litholopaxy we must always rely on the touch of the instrument itself.

Prostatectomy is a bloody and dangerous operation it is true and it is also blind, for we can see but little while at work, as in both the suprapubic and the perineal operation the hand is so large that the work of the enucleating finger is hidden and it is practically the touch alone that guides over in these operations.

What are then the indications that would help us in deciding which operation to perform?

Age is important, as the older is the patient the lower is his resisting power and the more liable he is to die from shock or asthenia. Therefore in a very old man if the prostate is of the right variety a Bottini should be performed and patients over 90 years of age have been operated upon by this means successfully. Old age, however, is not a contre-indication to prostatectomy as men over 80 years of age with sound kidneys and non-infected urine are clearly cases for enucleation,

The *size and shape* of the prostate indicate the operation in this way. The large prostate feeling like an apple or an orange on rectal examination indicate an enucleation. The smaller ones, not showing much enlargement by rectal touch, but where there is a distinct impediment in the prostatic urethra in introducing a sound together with quite a quantity of residual urine are better for the Bottini.

A general practitioner might ask how we can tell the size of the prostate, as it may not seem particularly large on rectal examination, when there may be a middle lobe projecting to a marked extent into the bladder. In answer to such a question I would say that one can never tell exactly what the size of a prostate is, but the trained genito-urinary finger can tell it a great deal by feeling the gland, and when added to this in note at urethral examination an impediment in the prostatic portion, an increased length of the canal and the presence of a considerable amount of residual urine, we can form a fair idea of the prostate we are dealing with. Beside this cystoscopy tells us something of the shape of the base of the gland.

The *condition of the bladder and kidneys* is very important. In the case of the former, however, not so much importance should be attached as in the latter, in governing the question of an operation; because it does not make any difference how badly bladder is involved; much can be done for it by internal and local treatment.

Diseased Kidneys, however, whether medically or surgically involved, are always a contre-indication to surgical interference in prostatic cases, as any operation on the urinary tract may be followed by an exacerbation of the condition, uræmia and death.

But if, when the Kidneys are involved, an operation is necessary the Bottini should be the case of choice. It must not be thought however that this operation is not dangerous as a most alarming reaction often follows it.

The indications then for the operations are as follows.

For a Bottini a prostate not markedly enlarged per rectum but presenting an impediment in the deep urethra giving rise to a considerable amount of residual urine in a man fairly well preserved.

For a prostatectomy a prostate of very large size per rectum, the larger the better, in a patient with healthy kidneys and good urine.

A Bottini may, however be performed in almost any case in which the instrument can enter the bladder and may be of benefit even in marked cases of hypertrophy when an enucleation is indicated; whereas in many cases of small sclerosed prostate with middle lobe impediment and considerable residual urine an enucleation could not possibly be made.

The method of performing the Bottini operation to day is the same everywhere, following Freudenberg.

In doing prostatectomy two methods are now in vogue with us, one is called the suprapubic and the other the perineal.

The both cases a suprapubic cystotomy is performed which enable us to see and to feel the tumor distinctly from the interior of the bladder.

If a large middle lobe is found called by some an intravesical tumor then the enucleation of the gland should be by the suprapubic route, but if it is found that the enlargement is principally of the lateral lobes then it is perhaps better to remove it through the perineum.

The *suprapubic operations* are practised by us as follows.

After opening the bladder suprapubically cut down through the tissues covering the gland antero-posteriorly with the scissors or knife, insert the end of the finger into this incision and procede to enucleate while pressure is made against the perineum from without.

Personally I make counter pressure in this 'operation by means of the finger of the other hand inserted into the rectum. In this way the bulk of the prostate gland can often be shelled out in three large pieces, while at other times it must be removed piecemeal.

Enucleation cannot always be performed by this means and the surgeon sometimes has to be content with the removal of the piece forming the barrier. A boutonniere operation is then performed and suprapubic and perineal drainage established.

In the perineal operation, after the suprapubic cystotomy is performed, a perineal incision is made on an urethral guide down to the apex of the prostate after which the capsule of the gland is cut through and the finger inserted and enucleation begun, counter pressure being made by the fingers of the other hand in the bladder. After the lateral lobes have been enucleated the middle one is pushed down and removed. The drainage is the same as in the other operations.

As by this last method the principal roll played by the suprapubic cystotomy was to allow pressure to be made upon the prostate from above, a very ingenious device has been made to obviate the necessity of this. It consists of a hard rubber tube with a soft rubber balloon at the end. This can be inserted with the balloon collapsed through the perineal opening into the bladder and is inflated. This can then be pulled down against the base of the prostate during enucleation thus keeping us constant direct pressure.

In conclusion I will say that it seems to be the tendency among us to enucleate all the troublesome prostates that in think we can remove safely, judging from the size, shape, the age of the patient and the condition of the kidneys and bladder, and to operate on the remainder by the Bottini operation.

## DISCUSSION

M. Frank (de Berlin). — Je m'associe, quant aux opérations mutilantes (vasectomie et castration), aux idées de Legueu. J'ai fait l'opération de Bottini, et de Nicolich 7 fois, 1 fois sans résultat, 6 avec résultat, c'est-à-dire le malade n'avait plus besoin de la sonde, l'urine résiduelle était presque ou complètement disparue; la musculature vésicale récupéra sa contractilité, l'urine qui était auparavant purulente devint claire.

Quant à la technique, il faut établir par le toucher rectal et l'examen cystoscopique le nombre et la profondeur des sections à faire. On doit opérer, à couteau blanc et très lentement, afin que l'opération soit galvanocaustique et non coupante. — Ainsi on évite des hémorragies. On ne doit pas faire l'opération, quand on se trouve en présence de reins très malades et quand il s'agit d'une infection des voies urinaires par des microbes qui décomposent l'urine.

Quant à dire qu'il s'agit ici d'une opération aveugle, on pourrait en dire autant de la lithotritie. Et il faut de plus remarquer que, si on fait la cystoscopie avant la lithrotripsie, les conditions changent pendant l'opération, tandis que dans l'hypertrophie de la prostate on a affaire à des conditions anatomiques qui restent toujours les mêmes.

L'auteur a traité son dernier cas avec un instrument qui a été construit par son assistant le D<sup>r</sup> Bierhoff avec M. Freudenberg et qui permet un contrôle cystoscopique pendant l'opération. On arrive en effet, avec l'instrument, à voir les endroits sur lesquels on incisera ; et on peut voir après l'opération si la profondeur des incisions est suffisante ; la longueur échappe naturellement au contrôle.

M. Frank a pu constater avec le cystoscope dans un des cas qu'il avait opéré auparavant que ses 4 incisions qu'il avait faites étaient complètement conservées dans leurs profondeurs ; le drainage fait par l'opération était encore suffisant pour l'évacuation de la vessie.

M. le D<sup>r</sup> A. Hogge (de Liège). — J'ai fait trois castrations doubles pour prostatisme. Dans le premier cas, je n'ai pu suivre mon malade que trois semaines après l'opération qui ne produisit aucun résultat en ce laps de temps.

Mon deuxième cas était un homme de 62 ans, prostate plutôt petite, très dure. Rétention complète depuis 5 mois, et incomplète depuis très longtemps. Le rétablissement a été immédiat mais partiel des fonctions vésicales, nécessitant deux ou trois sondages par jour. L'amélioration était progressive quand le malade mourut d'affection intercurrente 6 mois après l'intervention.

Mon troisième cas était celui d'un homme de 75 ans, prostatique à la seconde période, laissant après miction un résidu moyen de 90 grammes. Mictions impérieuses et fréquentes sans cystite (bactériurie récidivante). Castration double en février 1898 — immédiatement après, résidu moyen de 30 grammes et mictions nocturnes tombées de 10 ou 12 à 4 ou 5. L'amélioration continue, et actuellement le malade ne doit plus jamais recourir à la sonde. Il n'urine jamais plus involontairement, ce qui lui arrivait quelquefois avant la castration ; son état physique et psychique est excellent.

Le quatrième cas est dû à la pratique du professeur Von Winiwarter, de Liège : homme de 68 ans, passant très souvent de la rétention incomplète à la rétention complète nécessitant la ponction de la vessie. La dysurie remontait à des années. Castration double en 1896. Depuis cette époque, plus aucun accident dysurique. État général et local excellent. Le volume de la prostate semble avoir diminué. Il n'y a jamais eu de cystite ni avant ni après la castration.

Enfin, j'ai fait trois fois la vasectomie double pour hypertrophie de la prostate, et cette opération ne m'a jamais donné que des résultats passagers dus à la décongestion de l'organe en cause.

---

## INDICATIONS DE LA PROSTATECTOMIE
### par M. E. DESNOS,
de Paris.

La cure radicale de l'hypertrophie de la prostate, que vise la prostatectomie, est-elle possible chez tous les prostatiques, ou tout au moins peut-elle être envisagée comme méthode générale de traitement chez ces malades ? Je crois qu'aujourd'hui il faut répondre hardiment par la négative : si la prostatectomie donne dans des cas particuliers de bons résultats, ses indications sont exceptionnelles et ce sont elles que je désire tout d'abord préciser.

La grande majorité des prostatiques trouve un soulagement réel, et si prononcé que pour certains d'entre eux on pourrait dire guérison, dans l'ensemble des soins généraux et locaux devenus classiques aujourd'hui. Ce traitement a été formulé d'une manière si précise et si lumineuse par le professeur Guyon qu'aujourd'hui encore, après plus de vingt années, on n'a trouvé presque aucune modification à lui faire subir. Je n'ai même pas à en retracer ici les principales lignes et je considérerai comme admis par tous les chirurgiens que lorsque le cathétérisme ne présente pas de danger et ne rencontre aucun obstacle, lorsqu'il procure un soulagement complet au malade, il ne saurait être question pour ce dernier d'une opération qui pourrait lui faire courir quelques risques.

Mais il est loin d'en être toujours ainsi : quand l'amélioration apportée par le cathétérisme est insuffisante et de courte durée, on est en droit de songer à un traitement radical et, à ce titre, les opérations portant sur la prostate hypertrophiée sont légitimes.

Celles-ci réclament la réunion de conditions toutes spéciales dont les deux principales sont la présence d'un lobe prostatique plus ou moins bien isolé, saillant dans la vessie, d'une part, et d'autre part la conservation de la contractilité vésicale. Un diagnostic précis est indispensable. La conservation de la contractilité vésicale est facile à déterminer; il importe pour cela d'examiner la force de projection du jet d'urine expulsé par une sonde, le malade étant dans le décubitus dorsal. Toutefois une première et unique constatation ne suffit pas; il arrive souvent qu'une vessie forcée par une rétention datant de longtemps a perdu momentanément sa contractilité; mais si on la soumet à un cathétérisme régulier, on voit après quelques jours la pression vésicale augmenter au point de produire un jet d'urine assez puissant; ce n'est donc qu'après une observation prolongée qu'on est en droit d'affirmer l'atonie définitive du muscle vésical. Lorsque celle-ci est bien réelle, la prostatectomie doit être rejetée, car elle ne donnerait aucune amélioration.

Plus difficile est la détermination de la forme d'hypertrophie à laquelle on a affaire. Seule, une exploration intra-urétrale donne des renseignements, car l'intensité de la dysurie n'est pas en rapport absolu avec le volume de la prostate, et le toucher rectal ne fournit ici que des indications imparfaites; on ne peut conclure du développement de la masse totale de la prostate ou de sa face rectale, aux dispositions que cette glande affecte du côté de la vessie. Toutefois en combinant le palper hypogastrique et le toucher rectal on arrive à constater la présence d'une tumeur intra-vésicale, mais encore faut-il que cette dernière soit d'un volume important.

Déjà le cathétérisme renseigne mieux, et à l'aide d'une exploration en gomme on perçoit les saillies et les irrégularités du canal prostatique et du col vésical ; de même, un explorateur métallique à courte courbure permettra de contourner le col vésical et d'y reconnaître les saillies prostatiques.

Mais ces renseignements ne sont qu'approximatifs et ne permettraient pas d'asseoir un diagnostic topographique suffisant et assez précis pour faire décider une opération. C'est au cystoscope qu'il faut recourir ; on se rend de cette façon un compte absolument exact des dispositions des tumeurs prostatiques et de la prise qu'elles offrent à l'action chirurgicale.

La présence d'un lobe moyen bien saillant dans la vessie, formant une sorte de luette vésicale constitue la disposition la plus avantageuse, elle est aussi la plus rare ; la disposition en éventail, en barre, est également favorable ; en troisième ligne viennent les saillies des lobes latéraux dont l'excision, ainsi que nous le verrons, donne des résultats moins bons que dans d'autres formes. Enfin il est des cas, fort nombreux, dans lesquels aucune saillie n'apparaît autour du col. Ailleurs on voit seulement une sorte de bourrelet circulaire qui circonscrit tout le col. Dans ces cas, c'est à d'autres méthodes qu'il faut s'adresser pour tenter une cure radicale, car l'excision ne donnerait aucune amélioration, et je reste persuadé que beaucoup d'opérations de prostatectomie suivies d'échec ont été pratiquées dans des cas de ce genre.

Ainsi donc, on le voit, la réunion de ces deux conditions est nécessaire : fibre musculaire vésicale bien contractile, d'une part ; saillie prostatique faisant manifestement obstacle à la miction, d'autre part. Un tel obstacle joue un rôle évident dans le mécanisme de la dysurie, et les malades de ce genre peuvent être assimilés à des rétrécis urétraux ; chez ces derniers la vessie, fatiguée par une lutte prolongée, finit cependant par céder et plus d'un malade ayant conservé longtemps un rétrécissement de l'urètre très serré, voit s'établir l'incontinence par regorgement ; que l'obstacle soit levé, presque toujours la miction normale se rétablira et la rétention cessera ; il en est de même du prostatique dans les conditions que je viens de déterminer.

C'est dire que l'âge a une importance très grande. La conservation de la contractilité des fibres musculaires est d'autant plus probable que l'opéré sera plus jeune ; après une prostatectomie, la vessie, n'ayant plus à lutter contre un obstacle permanent se vide, se contracte normalement et son bas-fond ne se distend pas, si la puissance musculaire de la vessie est encore peu atteinte ; si au contraire le muscle est sclérosé ou si les fibres en sont déjà divisées et ne produisent plus que des contractions partielles sans synergie musculaire, la distension aura lieu de nouveau au bout de quelque temps, et ces malades, malgré l'excision prostatique, deviendront semblables à ces prostatiques, sans saillies prostatiques, à vessie primitivement sclérosée qui se distend parce que ces parois ont faibli et non parce qu'elle a rencontré un obstacle au-devant d'elle.

L'infection des voies urinaires crée-t-elle une contre-indication ? Non, si elle est limitée aux voies inférieures ; une opération dans laquelle on incise largement la vessie et qui ouvre une large issue aux produits infectés paraît même trouver ici une indication particulière, et l'on sait combien nombreux sont les cas où M. Poncet et l'École de Lyon conseillent d'intervenir ainsi. Quant aux manœuvres opératoires qui intéressent la prostate elle-même, après ouverture de la vessie, il est à souhaiter que celles-ci soient faites dans un organe non infecté, mais les suites ne sont pas dangereuses si on prend la précaution de ne pas chercher la réunion immédiate de la vessie.

Par contre, on se montrera très réservé quand les voies supérieures sont infectées ; il sera bon de tenir le malade en observation pendant un temps prolongé et de soumettre sa vessie à une évacuation régulière soit au moyen de cathétérismes répétés, ou de la sonde à demeure, soit par une cystostomie ; si les signes d'infection rénale disparaissent, on pourra réséquer les lobes saillants de la prostate ; on s'abstiendra en cas contraire.

Je ne dirai que deux mots du manuel opératoire ; c'est presque toujours la voie sus-pubienne que j'ai suivie, car elle donne plus de jour et permet mieux que toute autre de régler les manœuvres et de les suivre par la vue et le toucher. La prostatotomie peut suffire, dans certaines formes d'hypertrophie en barre. Quelquefois, à mesure que le bistouri intéresse cette saillie, on voit les lèvres de l'incision s'écarter comme s'il s'agissait de la section d'un muscle strié ; il se produit alors une excavation qui permet le libre écoulement de l'urine et le résultat est aussi bon et aussi complet que lorsque la résection est effective. C'est là une exception : presque toujours il est nécessaire de pratiquer une excision, une exérèse du tissu prostatique. Celle-ci varie suivant les formes d'hypertrophie. Quand il s'agit d'une véritable luette, d'une tumeur pédiculée, une incision transversale au niveau du col vésical suffit encore quelquefois ; mais le plus ordinairement je pratique une incision cunéiforme ; le sommet du V pénétrant plus ou moins profondément dans la glande et permettant d'enlever un segment assez important de la prostate. Cette manœuvre s'applique aussi bien au lobe moyen qu'aux lobes latéraux.

J'ai tenté assez souvent la réunion des lèvres de la plaie prostatique ; j'ai échoué ordinairement, le tissu glandulaire se déchirant sous la traction des fils ; dans les cas où j'ai réussi je n'ai pas remarqué que la guérison fût plus rapide, aussi ai-je renoncé à la réunion depuis longtemps déjà. Je ne crois pas d'ailleurs qu'il faille faire des délabrements considérables, il suffit d'aplanir le pourtour de l'orifice cervical, en creusant une sorte de gouttière qui se prolonge dans le canal prostatique pour obtenir le résultat cherché.

C'est dire qu'il s'est agit dans toutes mes opérations de prostatectomie partielle. Je n'ai jamais cherché l'ablation totale de l'organe, comme l'ont fait encore récemment M. Proust et M. Gosset, qui ont décrit une opération radicale sur les résultats de laquelle il est impossible de porter un jugement aujourd'hui. J'estime d'ailleurs que dans la grande majorité des cas, une résection partielle est suffisante.

J'ai pratiqué 29 opérations portant sur les saillies prostatiques, prostatotomie et prostatectomie, sur lesquelles j'ai eu 5 morts à déplorer ; un seul de ces décès paraît dépendre directement de l'opération le malade ayant succombé dans le collapsus au troisième jour ; un malade est mort subitement en faisant un effort pour se relever au huitième jour ; enfin, un troisième malade a succombé pendant la deuxième semaine avec des frissons et des phénomènes de néphrite aiguë, les dix premiers jours ayant été apyrétiques.

Dans 2 cas il y eut une dégénérescence secondaire de la prostate ; l'un d'eux fut opéré deux fois, et les examens histologiques pratiqués firent constater un tissu normal après la première opération, épithéliomateux après la seconde. Dans 7 cas l'opération ne donna pas de résultats immédiats, et chez l'un de ces malades, dont l'hypertrophie était d'ailleurs peu considérable, la rétention parut même augmenter, mais chez les 6 autres, si l'amélioration ne se produisit pas, au moins chez 4 d'entre eux, suivis régulièrement, l'affection paraît s'être arrêtée dans sa marche, la rétention et les symptômes restant les mêmes.

Dans 17 cas l'amélioration a été des plus remarquables ; d'abord les difficultés de cathétérisme, réelles chez plusieurs d'entre eux avant l'opération, ont complètement et immédiatement disparu ; chez tous également la rétention a diminué et disparu même complètement chez 5 d'entre eux. Enfin le point sur lequel j'attirerai surtout l'attention en terminant est la persistance de la guérison et de l'amélioration : sur 6 malades opérés à des époques déjà éloignées de cinq à dix années vivant encore et conservant sans modification les bénéfices de leur opération.

Dans cette communication j'ai entendu me borner à relater des faits personnels, sans établir de comparaison entre les diverses opérations qui visent la cure radicale de l'hypertrophie prostatique. D'après ces cas, on reconnaîtra que la résection partielle de la prostate, appliquée avec discernement et après une étude attentive et prolongée des indications, est peu meurtrière et assure un bon et surtout un durable résultat fonctionnel.

---

## CONTRIBUTION A L'ÉTUDE DU PROSTATISME

### par M. le docteur B. MOTZ,

de Paris.

Messieurs, je viens de passer devant vos yeux les projections des lésions prostatiques observées chez les « prostatiques sans prostate », c'est-à-dire chez les personnes avec la prostate petite et dont les troubles urinaires ressemblent absolument à ceux qu'on observe dans l'hypertrophie de la prostate.

Un des chapitres des plus obscurs de la pathologie urinaire, c'est justement celui des « prostatiques sans prostate ».

Quand vous avez devant vous les malades avec la prostate grosse plus ou moins molle ou avec la prostate dure, bosselée, irrégulière, vous vous expliquez jusqu'à un certain point la cause des troubles dont ces malades sont atteints. On sait maintenant, depuis les travaux qui ont été faits à la clinique de Necker, que le point de départ de ces troubles urinaires est la prolifération épithéliale anormale de la prostate ; on sait que dans les hypertrophies simples, on est en présence d'une prolifération bénigne, adénomateuse, tandis que dans le cancer la même prolifération épithéliale se caractérise par une tendance à l'envahissement ganglionnaire et par la production des toxines qui tuent le malade. Mais si vous êtes devant un malade dont la prostate au toucher rectal ne présente rien d'anormal, vous ne serez pas capables d'expliquer les phénomènes cliniques qu'il présente. Le nombre de ces malades est pourtant très considérable. En faisant mes recherches sur l'hypertrophie de la prostate, j'ai constaté que sur 120 sujets atteints de prostatisme, chez 55, c'est-à-dire chez un quart, la prostate n'était pas augmentée. Vous voyez donc, messieurs, que ce ne sont pas des cas rares. L'étude de ces cas s'imposait après celle des prostates hypertrophiées.

J'ai eu l'occasion d'étudier l'appareil urinaire de 16 cas de « prostatiques » sans prostate et je vous ai fait voir les projections des coupes de prostate de 15 de ces malades.

Au point de vue du diagnostic histologique, ces prostates peuvent être divisées en 4 catégories :

1° Prostates avec adénomes. . . . . . . . . . . . . 6 cas
2°      —      avec adéno-épithélioma . . . . . . 5 —
3°      —      avec cancers au début . . . . . . . 2 —
4°      —      sans aucune lésion. . . . . . . . . . 5 —

En résumé, sur 16 prostates, j'ai trouvé dans 15 cas une prolifération épithéliale anormale, c'est-à-dire *la même lésion histologique que vous trouverez dans les cancers et dans l'hypertrophie de la prostate.*

Les adénomes et les adéno-épithélioma de la prostate sont à présent bien connus (8 cas), mais nous connaissons moins bien les proliférations épithéliales à cellules claires (5 cas). Leur point de départ est nettement glandulaire. Si on suit leur évolution, on voit autour des culs-de-sac glandulaires tapissés très souvent d'épithélium bien conservé, l'apparition d'un stroma fibrillaire formant des mailles remplies par des cellules épithéliales à protoplasma clair. A une étude plus avancée, on observe la disparition du revêtement épithélial des culs-de-sac glandulaires et leur remplacement par l'épithélium de nouvelle formation. On peut observer encore là, en dehors de cette variété lacunaire, une forme en plaques composées de cellules polygonales tassées les unes contre les autres.

Les vessies des malades avec cette prolifération épithéliale anormale ne *présentent rien de particulier* : la plupart ressemblent aux vessies de nos prostatiques ordinaires.

Je viens de dire que dans 5 cas la prostate ne présentait rien de particulier. Je dois cependant vous prévenir que dans ces cas mon examen n'a pas été complet parce que je n'ai pas pu faire un nombre suffisant de coupes de la prostate.

Pas plus dans ces cas que dans les autres, nous ne pouvons nous expliquer l'insuffisance vésicale, le prostatisme par l'artério-sclérose vésicale.

L'examen histologique m'a fait voir qu'il n'y a qu'une de ces vessies qui est véritablement sclérosée et dont les vaisseaux sont atteints d'une endo et péri-artérite. La coïncidence d'une inflammation chronique ne nous permet pas de décider si cette sclérose a été primitive ou secondaire.

Les deux autres vessies présentaient les vaisseaux normaux. L'une d'elles produisait l'impression d'une vessie tout à fait normale, et c'est seulement avec un examen minutieux que j'ai pu constater qu'il y avait une légère sclérose de certains faisceaux musculaires. L'autre, au contraire, avait une notable hypertrophie musculaire avec le commencement d'atrophie; elle présentait, par conséquent, l'aspect des vessies si bien décrites par mon ami et compatriote Bohdakowicz.

Vous êtes probablement frappés, messieurs, de la contradiction qui existe entre l'évolution clinique et l'état néoplasique des prostates de ces malades. Cette contradiction n'est qu'apparente. Depuis la publication du remarquable mémoire de MM. Albarran et Hallé, le doute sur la possibilité de cette variété de dégénérescence néoplasique de la prostate est inadmissible.

En étudiant 100 prostates, prises en bloc, des malades qui sont morts avec l'hypertrophie de la prostate à la clinique de Necker, MM. Albarran et Hallé ont constaté que dans 14 cas il y avait une dégénérescence épithéliomateuse typique. Cette constatation a été faite presque toujours seulement à l'examen histologique : ni l'examen clinique, ni l'examen macroscopique à la table d'autopsie n'avaient fait penser à la dégénérescence maligne de ces prostates. Le grand mérite de ce travail, c'est de nous faire voir pour la première fois qu'il existe dans la prostate des tumeurs à une évolution tout à fait distincte de celle de tumeurs connues, à une évolution lente qui peut probablement durer de très longues années sans aucune infiltration ganglionnaire, sans aucun symptôme de néoplasie.

La possibilité d'une pareille lésion est tout à fait compréhensible si nous nous plaçons au point de vue de l'anatomie pathologique générale. Vous tous, messieurs, connaissez bien une variété de tumeurs épithéliales qui peuvent traîner de longues années et qui ont une tendance à la guérison spontanée. Je parle de ces tumeurs de la mamelle, de ces squirrhes qu'on observe dans les hospices de vieilles femmes et qui peuvent évoluer des dizaines d'années.

Le nombre de cas que j'ai observés n'est pas suffisant pour pouvoir faire des conclusions définitives. Je ne doute pas que vous poursuiviez l'étude de cette intéressante question et que peut-être, dans une de nos prochaines réunions, nous la discuterons définitivement en nous basant sur un grand nombre de cas observés. Pour le moment, je ne veux que souligner ce fait que sur 146 malades qui sont morts à la clinique de Necker avec les symptômes du prostatisme et qui ont été étudiés par MM. Albarran, Hallé et par moi-même, dans 145 cas, le point de départ de ces symptômes a été *une prolifération anormale bénigne ou maligne du tissu épithélial de la prostate.*

## RESULTATE DER BOTTINI'SCHEN OPERATION BEI PROSTATAHYPERTROPHIE
## DEMONSTRATION EINES GEMEINSAM MIT DR. BIERHOFF CONSTRUIRTEN
## KYSTOSKOPISCHEN PROSTATA-INCISOR'S

par M. le docteur ALBERT FREUDENBERG,

in Berlin.

Meine Herren,

*a)* Da die Behandlung der Prostatahypertrophie auf der Tagesordnung steht, gestatte ich mir, Ihnen über die Resultate, welche mir die Behandlung dieses Leidens mit der galvanokaustischen Incision respective Cauterisation nach Bottini im Laufe einer nahezu vierjährigen Erfahrung ergeben hat, zu berichten, und Ihnen ferner eine Statistik vorzulegen, welche die gesammten nach sorgfältiger Durchforschung der Literatur zu meiner Kenntniss gelangten Fälle mit umfasst.

Ich selbst habe die Bottini'sche Operation nunmehr 86 mal bei 69 Patienten ausgeführt, 78 mal mit dem „Incisor", 8 mal mit dem „Cauterisator". Darunter befinden sich 4 Todesfälle in Folge der Operation, wovon aber bei zweien der eine sicher, der andere mit hoher Wahrscheinlichkeit der Unvollkommenheit der damals noch üblichen Technik zur Last zu legen ist.

2 weitere Fälle (beides 78 jährige Patienten) habe ich 24 Tage resp. 49 Tage nach der Operation an bereits lange vor derselben bestehender chronischer Pyelonephritis verloren. Sie sind meiner Ansicht nach nicht *infolge*, sondern *trotz* der Operation gestorben.

Uebrigens bestand auch bei den 4 erst erwähnten Todesfällen bereits vor der Operation chronische Pyelitis resp. Nephritis. Fälle, deren Nieren noch intact waren, habe ich überhaupt nicht verloren.

Rechnet man jene beiden Fälle ab, so habe ich also 4 Todesfälle auf 69 Patienten = 5,8 0/0 Mortalität; rechnet man sie hinzu, — was ich nicht für berechtigt halte —, so ergeben sich 6 Todesfälle auf 69 Patienten = 8,7 0/0 Mortalität.

Unter den 86 Operationen bei 69 Patienten, die ich im Ganzen ausgeführt, finden sich 8 Operationen (7 mit dem „Cauterisator", 1 mit dem „Incisor") bei 8 Patienten, bei welchen ich die Operation nicht wegen Prostatahypertrophie, sondern aus andrer Indication, meist chronische Prostatitis mit sexueller Neurasthenie, ausgeführt habe.

Lassen wir diese 8 Fälle, unter denen sich kein Todesfall durch die Operation findet, ausser Betracht, beschränken wir uns also auch für die Frage der Mortalität auf die Fälle, in welcher wirkliche Prostatahypertrophie die Indication zum Eingriff abgegeben, so bleiben 4 resp. 6 Todesfälle auf 61 Patienten (mit 78 Operationen) = 6,56 resp. 9,85 0/0 Mortalität.

Was die *Erfolge* der Operation bei Prostatahypertrophie betrifft, so sind von meinen 61 operirten Prostatikern 51 = 50,82 0/0 als geheilt, 16 = 26,25 0/0 als wesentlich gebessert zu bezeichnen, das sind zusammen 47 = 77,05 0/0 „gute Resultate".

Ich bemerke dazu, dass ich unter „geheilt" verstehe, dass die betreffenden Patienten den Katheter zum Zwecke der Urinentleerung gar nicht mehr gebrauchen, dass sie mit einer sie absolut nicht belästigenden Häufigkeit in freiem Strahle ohne jede Beschwerde uriniren, und dass der Residualurin ganz verschwunden oder auf ein bedeutungloses geringes Quantum — sagen wir höchstens 40 bis 50 Ccm. — herabgesunken ist. Unter „wesentlich gebessert" verstehe ich, dass, neben einer beträchtlichen Hebung des Allgemeinbefindens, Körpergewichts, u. s. w. Patienten mit completer Retention zu ausgiebiger Spontanmiction gelangt sind, solche mit incompleter Retention eine wesentliche Verminderung des Residualurins und damit der Mictionshäufigkeit resp. des Kathetergebrauchs erzielt haben. Von dieser Begriffsbestimmung bin ich in meiner Statistik bezüglich „Heilung" niemals, bezüglich „Besserung" nur in einem einzigen Falle abgewichen, der trotz ausbleibender mechanischer Wirkung nach der Operation, bei sonst vollständig gleichbleibenden äusseren Verhältnissen, eine solche eclatante Besserung des Allgemeinbefindens, mit Gewichtszunahme von 28 bis 31 Pfund aufwies, dass man ihn unmöglich als ungebessert bezeichnen konnte[1].

Als „ohne Erfolg" operirt habe ich 8 Fälle zu verzeichnen = 13,10/0.

---

1. Der betreffende Fall findet sich in meiner in der *Deutschen Medizinalzeitung*. Nr. 1-6, 1900, mitgetheilten Casuistik unter Nr. 12 ausführlich berichtet.

In dreien dieser Fälle habe ich zwei Sitzungen vorgenommen. Einen der 8 Fälle will ich noch einer zweiten Sitzung unterziehen, die hoffentlich Erfolg bringen wird; aber auch unter den übrigen 7 Fällen sind mindestens 5, die meiner Ansicht nach noch auf einen Erfolg rechnen können, wenn sie sich zu einer Wiederholung der Operation entschliessen würden.

Ebenso befinden sich übrigens unter den als „gebessert" Rubricirten noch mehrere, von denen ich annehme, dass sie durch Wiederholung der Operation zu einer vollständigen Heilung gelangen könnten.

Was die *Dauerhaftigkeit* meiner Erfolge betrifft, so habe ich bisher — in allerdings nur vierjähriger Erfahrung — nur *ein* wirkliches Recidiv erlebt. Die Neigung zu solchen scheint im Ganzen sehr gering zu sein; sei ist um so geringer, je vollständiger der Erfolg war. Ich habe eine ganze Reihe von Fällen Jahre lang verfolgt und immer von Zeit zu Zeit wieder ihren Residualurin controlirt, ohne dass irgend eine Veränderung zum Schlechteren zu bemerken war. Besonders eclatant waren, wie in Bezug auf den Erfolg selbst, auch in Bezug auf die Dauerhaftigkeit dieses Erfolges 2 Fälle, die ich vor 2 3/4 resp. 5 1/4 Jahren operirt habe, nachdem sie vorher 5 resp. 5 1/2 Jahre complete Retention gehabt, der eine auch ohne jeden Erfolg castrirt worden war. Beide uriniren seit der Operation in ausgezeichneter Weise, ohne jede Schwierigkeit, ohne jede Beschwerde, sie haben nie wieder den Katheter nöthig gehabt, haben beide einen absolut klaren Urin bekommen, ihr von Zeit zu Zeit geprüfter Residualurin schwankt zwischen 15 und 41 resp. 24 und 58 Ccm. — und, wie gesagt, das Resultat ist jetzt 2 3/4 resp. 5 1/4 Jahre absolut constant geblieben. Ich habe die beiden Fälle auf dem letzten Congress der Deutschen Gesellschaft für Chirurgie vorgestellt. — Vielleicht wird Ihnen diese geringe Neigung zu Recidiven nach der Bottini'schen Operation weniger merkwürdig erscheinen, wenn Sie diese Abbildung eines über 15 Monate nach erfolgreicher Bottini'scher Operation gewonnenen Praeparates — der Patient starb an einer intercurrenten Krankheit — betrachten und sehen, welch ein mächtiger Trichter für den Urinabfluss am Blaseneingang durch den Eingriff erzeugt worden ist[1].

Was nun die *Gesammtstatistik* der Bottini'schen Operation betrifft[2], so habe ich für die Frage der Mortalität zusammenstellen können 755 Fälle mit 44 Todesfällen, das wäre eine Mortalität von 5,84 0/0.

---

1. *Archiv. f. klin. Chirurgie*, 1900, Heft 4, p. 950, Fig. 5.
2. Die Einzelzahlen, aus welchen sich die folgende Gesammtstatistik der Bottinischen Operation zusammensetzt, sindinzwischen in dem Centralbl. f. d. Krankheiten der Harn- und Sexualorgane, 1900. p. 515, genau publicirt worden.

Unter den 44 Todesfällen finden sich aber mindestens 12 Fälle, bei denen es fraglich sein muss, ob sie wirklich der Operation zur Last fallen. Ziehen wir diese ab, so bleiben 32 Todesfälle = 4,25 0/0.

Für die Frage „Erfolg oder Misserfolg" lassen sich verwerthen 718 Fälle mit 55 Misserfolgen = 7,66 0/0 und mit 622 „guten Resultaten", das heisst Heilungen  Besserungen = 86,65 0/0. Von den guten Resultaten sind etwa 61,5 0/0 als Heilungen und 58,7 0/0 als Besserungen zu bezeichnen.

Wie man sieht ist diese Gesammtstatistik noch besser als die meinige. Es dürfte dies der bekannten Thatsache entsprechen, dass Statistiken eines Einzeloperateurs fast immer ungünstiger ausfallen, als aus der Literatur zusammengestellte und vielfach aus Einzelfällen sich zusammensetzende Gesammtstatistiken, — eine Thatsache, die sich aus der Neigung der menschlichen Natur erklärt, über günstige Resultate lieber und schneller zu berichten, als über ungünstige. Ausserdem kommt vielleicht in Betracht, dass ich gerade die leichtesten Fälle im Anfangsstadium nicht operire, hingegen selbst im vorgerücktesten Stadium und bei ausgesprochener Pyelitis den Patienten bisher die Operation nicht verweigern zu dürfen geglaubt habe.

Jedenfalls ist sowohl meine, wie die Gesammtstatistik der Bottini'schen Operation eine sehr günstige. Und dabei können wir hoffen, dass die Erfolge der Operation noch wesentlich bessere sein werden, wenn wir einerseits die Fälle in Zukunft rechtzeitiger zur Operation bekommen, namentlich bevor secundäre Nierenbecken — und Nierenaffectionen irreparable Veränderungen gesetzt und gleichzeitig die Gefährlichkeit der Operation bedeutend gesteigert haben, und wenn andererseits die Erfahrungen der einzelnen Operateure grössere und die Vervollkommungen der Operationstechnik immer mehr Gemeingut ge worden. Nicht nur mir, sondern auch anderen Operateuren ist es ja so gegangen, dass sie im Anfange ihrer Erfahrungen Todesfälle und Misserfolge zu beklagen hatten, die der noch unvollkommenen Technik zur Last zu legen waren, und dass die Resultate erst mit der Zeit immer bessere wurden. Ich darf als Beweis dafür für mich vielleicht hervorheben, dass ich unter meinen letzten 12 Fällen (mit 14 Operationen) keinen Todesfall zu verzeichnen hatte, hingegen 10 vollkommene Heilungen, 1 wesentliche Besserung und nur 1 Misserfolg; letztere beide Fälle sind dabei so frisch operirt, dass durchaus nicht ausgeschlossen ist, dass Abwarten oder eine Wiederholung der Operation, zu der der eine Patient entschlossen ist, noch zu einem günstigen resp. günstigeren Resultate führen wird.

Das sind, wie ich meine, wirklich gute Resultate! Freilich wird man solche Resultate nur dann erzielen, wenn man sich mit Ernst und Eifer dem Studium der Bottini'schen Operation hingiebt, und nicht von vornherein immer etwaige Misserfolge auf das Conto der Operation setzt, statt aus ihnen die Anregung zu einer Revision der eigenen Technik — mitunter auch des eigenen Instrumentariums! — zu entnehmen.

Denn Eins darf man nicht vergessen : So einfach die Bottini'sche Operation scheinbar ist, so muss man doch eine ganze Reihe von Einzelheiten bei ihr genau beachten, um günstige und vor allen Dingen volle Resultate zu erzielen. Dahin gehört eine immer erneuerte sorgfältige Controle des Instrumentariums auf seine Tadellosigkeit; sodann die richtige Lagerung des Schnabels resp. der Schnabelspitze, die genau dort liegen muss, wo die Prostata aufhört und die Blasenwandung beginnt; ferner die Anwendung einer genügenden Glühstärke — ich nehme jetzt immer Weissglut — von der es abhängt, dass die Schnitte auch wirklich in der beabsichtigten Tiefe und Länge ausfallen; endlich die genügende Zahl, die zweckmässigste Richtung, die nothwendige Länge der Schnitte u. A. m. Für Zahl und Richtung der Schnitte betrachte ich die vorausgeschickte kystoskopische Untersuchung als massgebend : ich mache die Schnitte dorthin, wo ich Hervorwölbungen sehe; die Länge der Schnitte messe ich nach dem Befunde der Prostata per rectum bei, mit dem Schnabel nach hinten, liegendem Instrumente ab : von der so mit dem Zeigefinger ermittelten Länge der Prostata, nehme ich für einen Schnitt nach hinten etwa vier Fünftel, für seitliche und den, sehr selten nothwendigen oder zweckmässigen, Schnitt nach vorn 1/2 bis 1 Cm. weniger. Grade die richtige Länge der Schnitte halte ich übrigens für ausserordentlich wichtig. Es ist durchaus irrig, anzunehmen, dass nur in die Blase hineinragende Wulstungen der Prostata ein Hinderniss für die Urinentleerung abgeben; auch Vergrösserungen, die ausschliesslich die Pars posterior Urethræ betreffen, können durch Compression oder Abknickung der Urethra eine mehr oder weniger vollständige Retention zu Stande bringen (Demonstration der Abbildung eines solchen Praeparates). Und in solchen Fällen muss man den Schnitt bis dicht an die Pars membranacea — freilich aber auch nicht weiter — heranführen, um einen Erfolg zu erzielen.

Aus diesem Grunde und aus der Erfahrung heraus, dass bei besonders grosser Prostata die alte Schnittlänge von höchstens 5,6 Cm. nicht ausreicht, habe ich auch seit längerer Zeit[1] ein neues Modell meines Incisors angegeben, das längere Schnitte bis zu 6,6 Cm. ge-

---

1. Die erste Veröffentlichung darüber findet sich in meiner Arbeit in der *Deutschen Medizinalzeitung*, Nr. 1-6, 1900.

stattet. Ich glaube, dass dies selbst für die mächtigsten Prostataver
grösserungen ausreicht; die grösste Schnittlänge, die ich wirklich
angewendet, war bisher 5 Cm. — Dass man auch Schnitte von
solcher Länge nur in sehr seltenen Fällen machen darf und in der
grossen Mehrzahl der Fälle mit wesentlich kleineren von 2 1/2 bis
5 1/2 Cm. Länge auskommt, ist selbstverständlich. Ich brauche ja
wohl kaum hier zu betonen, dass man bei geringern Graden von Pros-
tatavergrösserung durch so lange Schnitte natürlich die schwersten,
in ihren Folgen unberechenbaren Verletzungen der Pars membranacea
oder anterior, ja selbst des Perinaeums hervorrufen würde.

*b*) Ich gestatte mir dann noch, Ihnen ein von mir in Gemeinschaft
mit Herrn Dr Bierhoff construirtes Instrument vorzulegen, einen kys-
toskopischen Prostata-Incisor, bestimmt in geeigneten Fällen die
Bottini'sche Operation unter Controle des Auges zu ermöglichen,

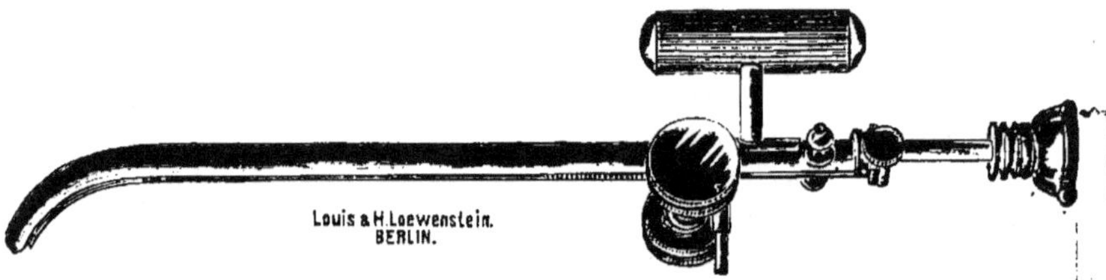


Fig. 1.

entsprechend einem schon von verschiedenen Seiten aufgestellten
Desiderate. Das Instrument ist von der bekannten Firma Louis und
H. Löwenstein in Berlin nach unseren Angaben angefertigt.

Das auf der Grundlage des Nitze'schen Operationskystoskopes auf-
gebaute Instrument (s. Abbildungen) zeigt an der hintern Fläche des
Schaftes eine Röhre, in welcher ein vollkommen gerades Kystoskop
drehbar und verschiebbar liegt, während die Zuleitung zu dem Platini-
ridiummesser in einer Rinne an der vordern Fläche des Schaftes
gleitet. Diese Zuleitung trägt an dem peripheren Ende eine kleine
gezähnte Platte, in welche ein Zahnrad eingreift, welches durch zwei
seitliche grössere Räder gedreht werden kann. Die Drehung dieser
Räder bewegt also das Messer hin und zurück; an der Peripherie
dieser Räder angebrachte Zahlen gestatten, die erreichte Schnittlänge direct abzulesen.

Man führt das Instrument in geschlossenem Zustande ein (s. Fi 1),
wobei das Kystoskop als Obturator dient. Nachdem der Schnabel voll
in die Blase eingetreten, schiebt man das Kystoskop vor, und kann

nun, indem man den Schnabel zur Seite dreht und so aus dem Gesichtsfelde bringt, Blase und Prostata kystoskopisch exploriren. Man stellt sich die Stelle der Prostata, durch welche man schneiden will, genau ein, bringt dann den Schnabel an diese Stelle, wobei man deutlich sehen kann, dass der Schnabel an der betreffenden Stelle auch wirklich liegt und dort die Prostata vorschriftsmässig fest anhakt[1]. Dann stellt man Kystoscop und übrigen Teil des Instruments in dieser Stellung durch eine am peripheren Ende gelegene, eine Muffe dirigirende Schraube fest, und kann nun die Incision in der gewünschten Ausdehnung machen (s. Fig. 2). Die grösste Schnittlänge, welche das Instrument gestattet, ist gut 4 3/4 Cm.

Blutet es bei oder nach einem Schnitte stärker, so dass es wünschenswerth erscheint, vor dem folgenden Schnitt eine neue Ausspülung zu machen, oder ist die Glühlampe während der Operation

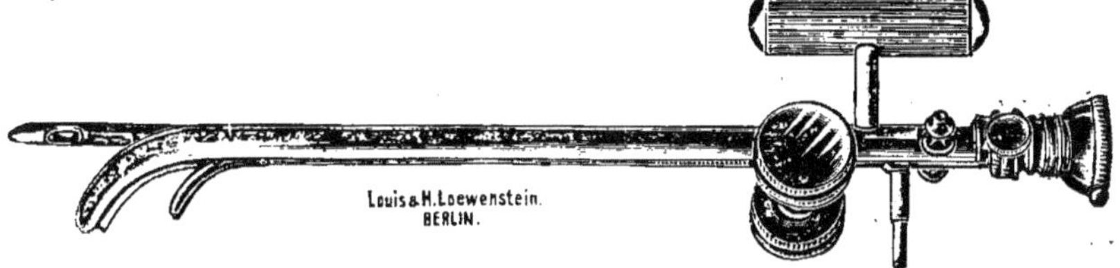


Fig. 2.

durchgebrannt, so entfernt man einfach das Kystoskop durch herausziehen, und kann nun direct durch die sonst das Kystoskop beherbergende Röhre in der einfachsten Weise die Blase entleeren, ausspülen und wieder anfüllen[2], worauf man das Kystoskop wieder einschiebt; — Alles ohne dass man nöthig hätte, das ganze Instrument aus der Blase zu entfernen.

Das Instrument trägt die übliche Wasserheilung. Es ist bis auf das Kystoskop, welches einer Desinfection durch flüssige Desinficienten oder Formaldehyddämpfe keinerlei Schwierigkeiten entgegensetzt — durch einfaches Kosten zu sterilisiren. Zum Festhalten desselben dient ein zum Schafte parallel befestigter geriffter cylindrischer Griff, entsprechend dem Griffe meines alten Incisors.

1. Sicherheitshalber controlire ich aber trotzdem die richtige Lage der Schnabelspitze mit dem Zeigefinger per rectum, was ja auch schon zur Bestimmung der nothwendigen Schnittlänge erforderlich ist.

2. Es ist dabei zweckmässig, dass man auf den Ansatz der zur Ausspülung benutzten Spritze einen der bekannten Gummikeile, wie sie z. B. für die Janet'schen Spülungen benutzt werden, aufsteikt.

Das Instrument hat sich bisher in 2 Fällen vollständig bewährt. Dass es freilich in allen Fällen das alte typische Instrument und das alte typische Verfahren verdrängen wird, glaube ich nicht.

## DEMONSTRATION OF INTRA-VESICAL PHOTOGRAPHS

### by Dr F. BIERHOFF

(New-York)

### Assisted by Dr R. KNORR

(Berlin).

1. Normal Bladder-wall.
2. Air-bubble in bladder.
3. Ureter.
4. Ureter, serted upon a proeminence, at the margin of a " pocket ".
5. " Bladder-Pocket ".
6. Trigone, ureter and " pocket ".
7. Convoluted (inflamed) sphincter-margin, ureter, pocket.
8. Encroachment of gravid uterus cast on bladder.
9. Same as above, with cystoscope nearer.
10. Perivesical strands.
11.      —           —
12.      —           —
13. Vessie à colonnes, with diverticulum.
14.      —           —
15. Polypi at sphincteral margin.
16.      —           —
17.      —           —
18. OEdema bullosum.
19. Blood-clot, in wide ureteral orifice.
20. Papillomatous granulations in a case of cystitis colli gonorrhoica.
21.      —           —           —
22. Carcinoma at the trigone.
23.      —      —      — dans veas wall.
24. Exostosis and symphisis.
25.      —      —      — showing pubic synchondrosis.
26. Ureter catheter being in the ureter.
27. Foreign body.
28.      —
29.      —
30. Calculi.

# SIXIÈME SÉANCE

## MARDI 7 AOUT

*à 2 heures et demie du soir.*

### Présidence de M. le professeur POSNER

(de Berlin).

---

## COMMUNICATIONS DIVERSES

### PROSTATE — GÉNÉRALITÉS

---

### LÉSIONS BLENNORRAGIQUES DE LA PROSTATE

#### von Dr. ERNST R. W. FRANK,

de Berlin.

In einer Arbeit, die vor 5 Jahren erschienen ist, hatte ich auf die ausserordentliche Häufigkeit derjenigen Complicationem der Gonorrhoe hingewiesen, die man als Lésions blennorrhagiques de la Prostate bezeichnet, und seitdem habe ich meine Ansicht durch eine Reihe von Arbeiten bestätigt gesehen, die über diesen Gegenstand veröffentlicht worden sind, besonders auch in der 4. Sitzung des französischen Urologen Congresses. Da besonders die Arbeiten von Desnos, Goldberg, Hogge, Janet, v. Frisch, Jadassohn und zuletzt von Casper sehr ausführliche Angaben über die Symptomatologie der in Rede stehenden Erkrankungen gegeben haben so darf ich mich auf einige Daten beschränken.

Die Häufigkeit der gonorrhoischen Erkrankungen der Vorsteherdrüse erwähnte ich bereits. Ich möchte hinzufügen, dass die Complication häufig sehr früh auftritt, viel früher, als meistens angenommen wird. In vielen Fällen findet man schon innerhalb derersten 8 Tage nach Auftreten der ersten Symptome einer Gonorrhoe trotz fehlender subjectiver Anzeichen und trotz absoluter Klarheit der zweiten Urinportion die Drüse erkrankt. Wenn ich am dritten à bi fünften Tage einer frisch in Behandlung gekommenen und bis dahin uncompliciert gebliebenen Urethritis ant. gon. noch Gonococcen finde, so besteht für mich der Verdacht, wenn paraurethrale Gänge und angeborene Missbildungen der Harnröhrenschleimhaut nicht vorhanden sind, dass es sich um das Weitergreifen des Processes auf die Vorsteherdrüse handelt, ganz gleich ob die zweite Urinportion klar ist oder nicht.

Wenn wir auch das Uebergreifen des gonorrhoischen Processes auf die Prostata durch die Therapie nur in bestimmten Fällen mit Sicherheit verhüten können, worauf ich bei Besprechung der Therapie kurz zurückkommen werde, so können wir sicher durch geeignete therapeutische Massnahmen die Häufigkeit der Urethritis post. gon. überhaupt, wie sie aus den neuesten Statistiken hervorgeht, entschieden erheblich einschränken.

Ich habe aus meinem poliklinischen Material 651 Fälle von gonorrhoischer Urethritis daraufhin zusammen gestellt. Eine Urethritis post. war in 210 Fallen, also in 52 1/4 % der Fälle zu verzeichnen. Dabei muss ich auf die Thatsache hinweisen, dass in einer nicht geringen Zahl dieser Fälle die Patienten mit bereits bestehender Urethritis post. zur Behandlung kamen.

In sämtlichen 210 Fallen war die Prostata erkrankt, also in 100 % der Fälle von Urethritis post.

In 96 Fällen der gonorrhoischen Prostatitis bestand die gon. Erkrankung überhaupt erst seit 8 Tagen oder weniger als 8 Tagen.

Was die Diagnose betrifft, so wurde dieselbe gestellt, einmal auf Grund des mikroskopischen und bacteriologischen Befundes im Prostatasekret, dann auf Grund der digitalen Untersuchung vom Rectum aus. Beide Untersuchungen sind unerlässlich zur Stellung einer klaren Diagnose.

Auf die Palpations-Befunde selbst, auf die Haufigkeit des Befallenseins eines oder beider Lappen, auf die Mitbeteiligung der Samenblasen will ich heute nicht näher eingehen.

Dagegen ist mir vielfach aufgefallen, dass manche Autoren nur in einer sehr geringen Zahl der Fälle Gonococcen im Prostatasekret gefunden haben, dass auch die Ansicht vertreten ist, der Nachweis im Prostatasekret sei schwieriger als im Harnröhrensekret.

Ich habe bei der mikroskopischen Untersuchung des Sekrets bei einfacher Färbung mit Methylenblau überaus häufig das Vorhandensein der Gonococcen nachweisen können. In zweifelhaften Fällen wurde stets das Verfahren nach Gramm und zuweilen das Culturverfahren angewendet.

Es fanden sich bei der Untersuchung des Prostatasekrets der
210 Fälle :

Gonococcen . . . . . . . . . . . . . . . . . . . 179 mal.
Andere Bacterien. . . . . . . . . . . . . . . . 20  —

Aseptisches Sekret mit zahlreichen Leukocythen wurden 11 mal
gefunden. Ich teile durchaus die Ansicht, dass das Vorhandensein
reichlicher Leukocythen im Sekret der Prostataund der Samenblasen
auch bei negativem bacteriologischem Befund als pathologisch und
als bezeichnend für das Bestehen einer Prostatitis oder Vesiculitis
anzusehen ist.

In solchen Fällen, in denen Gonococcen im Harnröhrensekret
dauernd fehlen, wird man vielfach auch im Prostatasekret solche
nicht mehr finden, wie das in 12 von Cohn, — Berlin, zusammenges-
tellten Fällen der Fall ist.

Bei lange bestegenden Prostatitiden kann der Nachweiss der.

Gonococcen sehr schwierig sein, und es bedarf wiederholter Untersuchungen und sehr gründlichen Mikroskopierens, ev. nach provoca-
torischen Massnahmen, um zu der für den Patienten so wichtigen
Diagnose zu kommen.

Auf die sich hieran knüpfende Frage des Eheconsenses und ähn-
liche Dinge kann ich heute nicht weiter eingehen. Kurz erwähnen
will ick eine Beobachtung, welche einen Patienten betrifft, der 5
Jahre nach ärztlich erklärter Heilung einer Gonorrhoe seine Braut
inficierte. Trotz Fehlens von Ausfluss und von Fäden in dem absolut klaren Urin, waren in der Prostata 2 Erweichungsheerde vorhanden und das Expressionssekret enthielt reichliche Leukocythen, und
zwar spärliche, aber deutlich erkennbare Gonococcen.

Sekundäre Infectionender prostatischen Drüsenschläuche können
Jahrzehnte lang bestehen und viele Falle von Nekrospermie und
Sterilität in der Ehe erklären sich auf diese Weise. Um die mikroskopischen Befunde des Prostatasekrets möglichst einwandsfrei zu ge-
stalten, verfuhr ich nach gründlicher Waschung der hinteren und
vorderen Harnröhre mit Protargollösung so, dass ich einen sterilen
Tubus bis zum Ende der Pars membranacea einführte, das Gesi-
chtsfeld mit sterilen Wattetampons bis zur absoluten Trockenheit
säuberte und das durch die Massage erhaltene Sekret aus dem Tubus
zur Untersuchung entnahm.

In den anderen Fällen beschränkte ich mich auf die gründlichte
Waschung beider Harnröhrenabschnitte, und hütete mich, was vielfach geschieht, das durch die Massage gewonnene Sekret durch

Druck auf die Pars pendula nach aussen zu befördern. Durch letztere Manipulation drückt man den Inhalt der Drüsen und Lacunen der Urethra ant. aus und die gewonnenen Resultate sind nicht einwandsfrei. Auch ohne dieses Drücken gelingt es fast stets einige Augenblicke nach Vornahme der Massage das Prostatasecret am Orif. ext. zu sehen.

Der Tubusuntersuchung hat stets eine Waschung der vorderen und hinteren Harnröhre zu folgen. Die Thatsache, dass ich unter 57 so untersuchten Fällen einmalund zwar 14 Tage nach erfolgter Untersuchung eine Epididymitis auftreten sah, beweist, dass eine Gefahr für den Patienten mit diesen Untersuchungen kaum verknüpft ist.

Entsprechend dem anatomischen Bau der Vorsteherdrüse sind die durch den gonorrhoischen Process herbeigeführten pathologischen Zustände complicierter Natur und daraus ergeben sich die Schwierigkeiten der Therapie. Ich schliesse mich vollständig der überaus klaren und sachgemässen Darstellung dieser Verhältnisse an, die Janet in seinem Vortrag « Traitement des Prostatites chroniques » auf dem letzten Urologen Congress gegeben hat.

Je nachdem die Drüsenschläuche durch den bestehenden Katarrh mehr oder weniger kystisch verändert sind, je nachdem die Mündungen derselben durchgängig sind oder nicht, wird der Erfolg der Therapie ein mehr oder weniger schneller sein.

Virulente Gonococcen unterhalten eine starke Sekretion und halten die Mündungen der erweiterten Drüsenschläuche offen, so dass die Evacuation in solchen Fällen auffallend schnell gelingt. In ihrer Virulenz abgeschwächte Gonococcen oder andere Bacterien, z.B. das Bact. coli, können jahrelang in den Drüsenshläuchen vorhanden sein, ohne starke Sekretion hervorzurufen.

Die Drüsenmündungen werden durch den Entzündungsprocess allmählig verengert oder gar verlöthet und setzen der Evacuation erheblichen Widerstand entgegen. Aus diesen anatomisch-pathologischen Verhältnissen ergiebt sich ohne veiteres, dass eine erfolgreiche Therapie der katarrhalischen Erkrankungen der Vorsteherdrüse nur in der mechanischen Entleerung der Drüsenschläuche bestehen kann und diese erreicht man durch die Massage der Drüse vom Rectum aus. Da es sich um ein Organ handelt, dessen Configuration eine sehr vielgestaltige ist, da es ferner von grösster Wichtigkeit ist, die verschiedenen Heerde genau abzutastenund je nach dem Grad der vorhandenen Entzündung sehr verschieden stark zu massieren, so ist das einzig zulässige Instrument der Finger des

Arztes. Alle starren zu diesem Zwecke angegebenen Instrumente, wie die von Feleki und Finger halte ich für unprak tisch und in vielen Fallen für schädlich. Ich bin ferner der Ansicht, dass diese Art der Massage nicht von Masseureh sondern vom Arzt selbst vorgenommen werden soll. Da dem massierenden Finger besonders die ganz peripher gelegenen Drüsenschläuche nicht zugängig sind, so haben Hogge und Janet die Wirkung des faradischen Stromes zu Hülfe genommen, um durch die Elektro-Massage eine energische Contraktion auch dieser Teile zu bewirken. Da diese Instrumente das Tastgefühl des Fingers erheblich einschränken, habe ich ein kleines Instrument anfertigen lassen, das neben der Application des faradischen Stromes ein feines Tastgefühl ermöglicht. Der Massage hat stets eine Spülung der vorderen und hinteren Harnröhre zu folgen, um das exprimierte Sekret, das oft teilweise in die Blase gelangt, gründlich zu entfernen. Die Spürflüssigkeit ist eine verschiedene, je nach dem jeweiligen mikroskopischen Befund. Handelt es sich um das Vorhandensein von Gonococcen im Sekret, so empfehle ich die Lösung der Silber-Eiweiss Präparate, in erster Linie des Protargols. Handelt es sich um andere Bacterien, so spült man mit schwachen Sublimatlösungen, ist das Sekret aseptisch, so bedient man sich adstingirender Lösungen.

Unterstützt wird die Behandlung durch medicamentöse Therapie, wobei es empfehlenswert ist die Medicamente in wässriger Lösung ins Rectum einzuspritzen, Regelung der Diät, heisse Bäder, Application von Hitze direct auf die Vorsteherdrüse. Sehr wichtig ist, besonders bei Vorhandensein von anderen Bacterien als Gonococcen, sein Angenmerkaufeine gründliche Antisepsis des untersten Darmabschnittes zu richten. In erster Linie muss man immer darauf bedacht sein, dass die Therapie, worauf Guyon und seine Schüler, besonders Noguès, hingewiesen haben, eine Decongestionirung des Beckens herbeiführt. Ganz acut entzündliche Processe der Vorsteherdrüse, die die Tendenz zur schnellen Abscedirung haben, bilden eine absolute Contraindication gegenjede active Therapie. Ebensohalte ich es für absolut schädlich bei Temperatursteigerung zu massieren; in solchen Fällen ist absolute Bettruhe notwendig. Sonst aber kann durch eine sachgemässe Massagetherapie dem Patienten nie ein Schaden erwachsen. Man hat vielmehr den Eindruck, dass durch ein rechtzeitiges Beginnen der Massage und Spülung weitere Complicationen vermieden werden. In den 651 Fällen von Gonorrhoe trat 17 mal im Laufe der Behandlung eine Epididymitis auf, also in 2,5 % der Fälle.

Ist die Prostata gonorrhoisch erkrankt gewesen, und meist handelt es sich in solchen Fällen um mannigfaltige anatomische Laesionen der Harnröhrenschleimhaut, so sind nachdem die Harnröhre und ihre Adnexe keimfrei geworden sind, die anatomischen Laesionen mit Hülfe der Endoskopie, der Tastsonde und der Rectalpalpationen genau festzustellen, und immer wieder und wieder muss die so sehr berechtigte Forderung Janet's betont werden, dass durch geeignete mechaniche und chemische Behandlung auch diese aseptischen anatomischen Laesionen ausgeheilt werden müssen; Die bis zu diesem Ziel fortgesetzte chemische und instrumentelle Behandlung hat noch den grossen Vorteil, dass in tieferen Gewebsschichten oder in Drüsenschläuchen der Prostata liegende Bacterien an die Oberfläche befördert werden, dass solche, die in Rundzelleninfiltraten eingeschlossen sind, mobil und der Behandlung zugängig werden, und dass die Recidive auftreten *bevor* man den Patienten geheilt entlassen hat.

## DISCUSSION

M. Georges Berg (de Francfort-sur-le-Mein)). — Dans sa communication, si je l'ai bien comprise, M. Frank affirme avoir remarqué déjà huit jours après l'infection dans beaucoup de cas des lésions prostatiques de nature blennorragique, sans que les malades aient senti aucun symptôme subjectif. Permettez que j'en doute absolument. C'est un symptôme principal de la prostatite aiguë, d'avoir quelques sentiments sinon de douleur, du moins de brûlure ou de piqûre et de l'urgence d'uriner. Quoiqu'il en soit, M. Frank veut avoir constaté la présence des gonocoques dans la prostate par l'examen microscopique. Il lave l'urètre avec du protargol, — et exprime la prostate. Je ne regarde pas que l'opinion de l'effet extraordinairement vite et sûr du protargol est vaincue. Je ne comprends pas, comment il peut différencier exactement les microbes, qui proviennent de la prostate des microbes qui proviennent de l'urètre. Car avant d'arriver à la prostate, il faut que les microbes passent par l'urètre postérieur. Car ce n'est pas bien prouvé, comme je crois, que les microbes entrent dans la prostate par les voies de la lymphe ou du sang. Il est bien possible de constater par la palpation et l'examen microscopique du secret, que la prostate est enflammée ou non. Mais la recherche, si elle contient des gonocoques, sera toujours incertaine, parce que les gonocoques trouvés peuvent provenir aussi bien de l'urètre que de la prostate. Au contraire, il y a des auteurs qui croient que les inflammations de la prostate, même si une blennorragie persiste, est produite par une infection mixte.

Dans les premières phases de la prostatite blennorragique, s'il n'y a pas beaucoup de pus dans la glande, il n'y a pas d'écoulement. Il s'agit dans cette phase d'une congestion. Et à cause de cela tout acte chirurgical aussi petit soit-il, comme le massage par le rectum, loin d'être utile, est nuisible. Je fais une exception si la prostate est atteinte d'un abcès. En ce cas il faut recourir aussi vite que possible à l'incision. A l'exception de ce cas, le traitement de la prostatite aiguë ne doit pas différer du traitement des autres inflammations. L'état aigu ayant fini sous un traitement rationnel, il faut profiter du massage rectal suivi d'un lavage de l'urètre — ou des instillations de Guyon si bien éprouvées. Pour ce qui est du massage, je suis d'avis qu'il n'y a pas un meilleur instrument pour les pratiquer que le doigt. On peut ainsi faire le diagnostic, se rendre compte des progrès du traitement. Enfin il sera nécessaire de faire des dilatations. Le traitement doit être continué assez longtemps, pour faire disparaître les microbes, non seulement les gonocoques, mais encore les autres microbes, et les lésions, conséquences de la maladie. Il faut examiner de temps en temps la sécrétion et provoquer, s'il n'y en a plus, un nouvel écoulement soit par un lavage de sublimé ou de nitrate d'argent, soit par des excès d'alcool. Car je suis persuadé que les foyers restants de la prostate sont la cause principale de l'opiniâtreté d'une urétrite blennorragique, parce que le risque existe pour la muqueuse urétrale d'être infectée de nouveau, quand même elle était reconnue comme guérie par l'examen endoscopique.

En résumé : 1. La prostate est dans beaucoup de cas de blennorragie atteinte par l'infection.

2. Dans les états aigus il y a toujours des symptômes subjectifs.

3. Il est difficile de différencier exactement les microbes de prostate des microbes de l'urètre.

4. Pendant la période aiguë de la prostatite blennorragique il faut s'abstenir absolument d'aucune excitation, excepté l'incision d'un abcès.

5. Le traitement de la prostatite doit être continué aussi longtemps que possible.

M. A. Freudenberg (de Berlin). — Je recommande pour l'électro-massage de la prostate une méthode que j'emploie depuis plus d'un an dans certains cas et qu'on pourrait appeler : « Électro-massage de la prostate avec le doigt électrique ». Comme dans « l'électrisation par la main électrique » on met en communication l'un des pôles du courant électrique avec le médecin par une pelote qui prend l'articulation de la main ; l'autre pôle est représenté par une grande pelote plate à l'hypogastre du malade. En introduisant l'index dans le rectum du malade et en établissant le courant, celui-ci ira par la main et le doigt du médecin à la prostate et transversalement par elle à l'abdomen. Naturellement, il est nécessaire d'isoler le courant pour l'empêcher de passer de la main aux fessiers, sphincter, etc., et produire des sensations très désagréables et non nécessaires. On se sert d'un doigtier en gomme qui se continue avec un capuchon en gomme également. On applique ce doigtier sur l'index avant de l'introduire dans le rectum ; on fait sortir la pointe de l'index par un orifice ménagé dans le doigt de gomme quand on est arrivé à la prostate ; on peut électriser ainsi et masser en même temps sans avoir un corps étranger entre doigt et prostate, qui pourrait être gênant pour la sensation.

Naturellement, on ne peut employer que des courants relativement faibles, parce que le doigt du médecin éprouvera une sensation douloureuse avant le malade. Mais ce n'est pas un inconvénient, parce que chez des malades avec une prostatite chronique on doit éviter tout ce qui pourrait produire de la douleur.

La méthode n'a été employée qu'avec le courant faradique. Pour e courant galvanique, très vraisemblablement elle ne serait pas praticable.

## LA PHAGOCYTOSE AU POINT DE VUE PRATIQUE

### par M. le docteur J. DORST,

d'Amsterdam.

Vous connaissez tous, messieurs, la théorie du célèbre savant russe de l'Institut Pasteur! Je crois presque inutile de vous rappeler qu'il y a divers groupes de phagocytes, des phagocytes fixes et des phagocytes mobiles et que ce sont surtout les leucocytes polynucléaires qui défendent l'organisme contre les microbes pathogènes, ces microbes sécrétant des substances qui développent une chimiotaxie positive vers les leucocytes.

D'après M. Metchnikoff, il y aurait aussi des produits microbiens qui manifestent une chimiotaxie négative.

En faisant des expériences en 1896 sous la direction de M. le professeur Tavel, à Berne, je suis devenu partisan de la théorie cellulaire. J'ai injecté à des lapins des staphylocoques dans des hématomes artificiels, et lorsque l'animal résistait, j'ai vu des leucocytes remplis de staphylocoques se colorant mal. Mais quant à la chimiotaxie négative je ne puis partager l'opinion de M. Metchnikoff. La chimiotaxie positive ou négative ne serait alors qu'une question de virulence. Les microbes de petite virulence donneraient une chimiotaxie positive, les mêmes microbes mais d'une virulence plus forte donneraient une chimiotaxie négative; je dis les mêmes puisque l'on peut diminuer ou augmenter artificiellement la virulence des microbes : le bactériologiste n'est-il pas le jardinier des microbes, comme l'a dit l'immortel Pasteur? Mais je ne crois pas que la question de chimiotaxie positive ou négative puisse être une différence de virulence et cela parce que la formation d'un abcès est non seulement due au degré de virulence, mais aussi bien au *nombre* des microbes pathogènes, à condition que ces microbes aient un certain degré de virulence; telle est mon opinion toujours d'après mes expériences.

Du reste, ce qui se passe quand on injecte des microbes pathogènes

dans l'organisme d'un animal non réfractaire, sous la peau par exemple,
est bien connu : si la virulence est faible, il ne se produit qu'une
hyperémie; si elle est assez forte, l'on verra se développer un abcès;
enfin, si elle est très forte, l'animal meurt presque sans réaction locale.
Dans les deux premiers cas, les leucocytes polynucléaires sont attirés;
dans le dernier cas, suivant l'opinion de M. Metchnikoff, ils seraient
repoussés. Mais si au lieu d'augmenter la virulence des micro-organismes, on augmente leur nombre, qu'arrive-t-il? Le résultat est à peu
près le même. Je crois donc que dans le cas de virulence forte comme
dans celui de virulence faible les leucocytes polynucléaires sont
attirés, mais que dans le premier cas ils sont plus facilement détruits,
de sorte que les microbes plus virulents peuvent se répandre plus
vivement et alors l'abcès ne se formera pas.

Entre ces deux conditions extrêmes se trouve celle dans laquelle
se forme un abcès, c'est-à-dire la *concentration* des leucocytes polynucléaires. C'est cette concentration qu'il faudrait favoriser en traitant
les malades infectés et c'est sur ce point que je reviendrai dans un
instant.

A l'exclusion de la chimiotaxie négative, je suis donc partisan de la
doctrine de M. Metchnikoff et je me suis demandé, il y a déjà longtemps, s'il n'y aurait pas à tirer des conclusions pratiques de cette
théorie et c'est surtout à ce sujet, que je vous demande, messieurs, de
bien vouloir m'accorder quelque attention.

Voyons la chose à trois points de vue : du diagnostic, du pronostic
et du traitement.

Si nous avons affaire à une urétrite naturelle, débutante mais déjà
franchement purulente, est-il en général encore besoin de chercher
le diplocoque de Neisser pour faire le diagnostic bactériologique?
Quand le malade nous rend compte, que son écoulement urétral
purulent s'est tout d'un coup comme arrêté — ce qui peut arriver,
quoique ce soit contesté — est-ce que le diagnostic d'une complication
n'est pas déjà fait? Et pourquoi cet écoulement diminue-t-il brusquement? Assurément parce que les leucocytes polynucléaires sont
concentrés ailleurs. Vous connaissez l'expression dans le monde : la
blennorragie est tombée dans les bourses.

Quant au pronostic d'une infection purulente, la quantité relative
des leucocytes polynucléaires et des microbes pathogènes est très
importante; je ne parle pas ici des inflammations à la surface ou dans
es cavités du corps humain en communication avec l'extérieur, où
l'on peut trouver une quantité énorme de micro-organismes avec peu
ou point du tout de leucocytes, parce que ces microbes ne sont que

des saprophytes; mais en dehors de cela, si l'on voit dans le pus beaucoup de leucocytes polynucléaires et peu de microbes pathogènes, l'on peut *ceteris paribus* faire un pronostic favorable. Les anciens n'ont-ils pas déjà parlé d'un pus louable?

D'un autre côté, quand il y a encore des leucocytes polynucléaires dans l'écoulement urétral, il faut se méfier. M. Finger[1] défend même le mariage tant qu'il rencontre encore des leucocytes, même s'il n'y a plus aucun écoulement.

Abordant maintenant le point de vue du traitement, le plus important de tous, je reviens sur la concentration des leucocytes polynucléaires. C'est elle, qu'il faut favoriser et le remède par **excellence** est la chaleur, chose bien reconnue non seulement par nous médecins, mais aussi par les gens moins compétents. Je me souviens d'une ancienne cliente, qui me disait : « Moi, quand j'ai mal au doigt, je le mets dans l'eau bouillante ». Cela est un peu exagéré, mais elle n'était pas loin de la vérité. Et qu'est-elle la vérité? C'est que la chaleur jusqu'à un certain degré fait mûrir le mal, détermine un abcès si c'est *nécessaire*. Et cet abcès, c'est la concentration des leucocytes polynucléaires, que nous essayons de provoquer en traitant les para-urétrites, les prostatites subaiguës et chroniques, les épididymites, etc. Ce sont surtout les prostatites blennorragiques chroniques, qui se prêtent au traitement par la chaleur locale, appliquée par l'instrument d'Arzberger-Finger. Pour que l'action soit encore plus locale, j'ai modifié le modèle de Winternitz, de sorte que la chaleur n'est appliquée qu'à la paroi antérieure du rectum; je ne dis pas que la chaleur ferait du mal aux parois latérales et postérieure, mais ce n'est pas là que les leucocytes polynucléaires doivent être attirés.

J'ai traité aussi des urétrites subaiguës et chroniques par la chaleur; j'ai fait de grands lavages d'après M. Janet avec des solutions de permanganate de potasse chaudes et j'en ai été satisfait; je crois seulement qu'en général, il ne faut pas dépasser 45 degrés: les températures plus hautes peuvent provoquer des contractions des muscles ischio- et bulbo-caverneux et donner lieu à des urétrorragies. En traitant ainsi le malade, je le fais uriner d'abord, puis je remplis la vessie avec la solution de permanganate de potasse et aussitôt après je le fais pisser dans un verre; je répète ce procédé deux ou trois fois dans la même séance jusqu'à ce que le liquide rendu soit clair, de sorte que deux litres de solution sont à peu près nécessaires. J'ai remarqué

1. **Finger.** Die Blennorrhöe der Sexualorgane. 4. Aufl. S. 180.

que le pronostic est d'autant plus favorable, que la solution est plus tôt
rendue claire, tout cela à condition qu'on ne laisse pas s'écouler plus de
temps que celui juste nécessaire entre les diverses actions de l'opération. A part la durée de chaque séance, je règle le traitement suivant les
circonstances : plus l'inflammation est chronique, plus je prends la
solution forte et surtout plus chaude. Je crois qu'une amélioration
dans le pronostic d'une maladie aussi difficile à traiter que la blennorragie est d'une réelle importance; je suis convaincu que souvent
seul ce pronostic pourra nous encourager à continuer encore le
même traitement; pour moi enfin les grands lavages au permanganate
de potasse chauds sont de beaucoup le meilleur traitement de la
blennorragie subaiguë et chronique, donnant non seulement une
guérison à la surface, une guérison temporaire, mais une guérison
aussi bien à la profondeur des tissus, une guérison définitive, qui met
le malade à l'abri des conséquences mauvaises souvent de l'avenir.
Pour moi, ce procédé est aussi le meilleur moyen pour juger la
question du mariage : il faut ajourner tout projet de mariage jusqu'à
ce que le premier verre de permanganate rendu soit tout à fait clair.

Quant à *la couleur* du liquide rendu je continue le traitement jusqu'à ce qu'elle soit tout à fait violette. Si même le premier verre
rendu n'arrive pas à être plus ou moins violet, il y a une complication
(27 novembre 1900).

M. Finger[1] a bien dit que la blennorragie ne guérit que par l'intermédiaire des leucocytes polynucléaires, quoique je ne sois partisan
de la doctrine cellulaire qu'au sens de M. Metchnikoff et cela par
analogie des autres maladies infectieuses. Cependant les leucocytes
polynucléaires ne pouvant digérer les bacilles de Koch, j'accepte pour
une part la doctrine cellulaire dans le sens de M. Finger pour la
tuberculose.

En dehors de la chaleur nous avons encore d'autres moyens pour
provoquer la leucocytose locale. C'est avant tout la teinture d'iode,
qui peut être de grand service. Les arthropathies blennorragiques
guérissent aussi bien par l'application de la teinture d'iode que par le
cataplasme chaud. Seulement, comme il faut changer souvent un
traitement quelconque à cause de l'accoutumance des leucocytes
polynucléaires, j'ai regretté une fois d'avoir fait suivre l'application
de teinture d'iode sur la peau par un cataplasme dans le sens de
Priessnitz : j'avais provoqué une dermatite aiguë intense.

Je veux encore attirer votre attention sur un fait en faveur de la

---

1. FINGER. Die moderne Therapie der Gonorrhœ, 1900, S. 2.

guérison de la blennorragie par l'intermédiaire des leucocytes polynucléaires, c'est que le traitement de la blennorragie aiguë d'emblée
par les balsamiques échoue pour de beaucoup la plupart des cas; il y
a des exceptions, mais elles sont rares.

Quant au traitement abortif de la blennorragie aiguë chez l'homme,
je suis en général de l'opinion de M. Guiard; les solutions fortes
peuvent devenir dangereuses, nuisant aux phagocytes fixes et mobiles.
La réaction séreuse, à laquelle M. Janet a voulu attribuer une action
microbicide, n'est pour moi que la conséquence de l'amélioration du
canal; elle nous indique que les leucocytes polynucléaires ne sont
plus nécessaires. « Si le permanganate est employé, dit M. Janet, à
doses trop fortes, en lavages trop prolongés ou trop rapprochés, il
détermine une réaction séreuse intense, qui ne tarde pas à devenir
purulente[1]. » Vous voyez, messieurs, que les leucocytes polynucléaires sont redevenus *nécessaires*.

Pour la même raison que je préfère les solutions faibles comme
traitement abortif de la blennorragie, je ne puis approuver de
toucher les plaies en faisant la néphrotomie et la taille hypogastrique à
l'eau phéniquée forte, surtout quand le rein et la vessie sont infectés.
Les antiseptiques faibles peuvent encore donner une leucocytose
locale, les antiseptiques forts nuisent plus qu'ils ne font de bien. Il faut
garder les antiseptiques forts loin des plaies et surtout loin des plaies
infectées. Ce ne sont que les chirurgiens sales, qui ne rasent pas et
qui ne lavent pas, ou ceux qui opèrent dans des circonstances des
plus défavorables, qui ont besoin des antiseptiques pour protéger les
plaies contre une infection *nouvelle*.

Je crois qu'il faut faire plus ou moins exception pour le nitrate
d'argent au-dessous de 5 pour 100; son action alors est plutôt cathé-
térique, elle devient caustique au delà d'après notre maître M. le professeur Guyon[2]. Dernièrement, j'ai enlevé un calcul d'un rein infecté; le
calcul siégeait à la bifurcation d'un des calices supérieurs et avait
donné lieu à une rétention locale incomplète avec infection; quelques
jours après, j'ai voulu laver la plaie au nitrate d'argent au millième;
seulement l'infirmière me donnait une solution à 40 pour 1000, donc
40 fois la dose voulue; j'avais employé un litre entier et le résultat
fut des plus désirables : la fièvre est tombée tout de suite sans
reparaître. La solution forte du nitrate d'argent doit avoir enlevé la
membrane pyogène dans toute son épaisseur; tandis qu'avant l'opéra-

1. JANET. Ann. de derm. et de syph., 1895, p. 1034.
2. GUYON. Leçons cliniques sur les maladies des voies urinaires, 3ᵉ éd., t. III,
p. 406.

tion il y avait une toute petite quantité d'albumine dans l'urine, l'albumine a tout à fait disparu après ce lavage; par le cathétérisme urétéral du rein sain avant l'opération, je m'étais assuré que l'albumine ne venait que du rein affecté. Même si la solution de nitrate d'argent n'avait pu annihiler toute l'infection, elle n'aurait pas fait beaucoup de mal, parce qu'elle était au-dessous de 5 pour 100. Morale : il ne faut pas garder dans son service des solutions de nitrate d'argent au-dessus de 5 pour 100.

Encore une question intéressante quant à la phagocytose : l'infection chez le vieillard. M. Albarran[1] a attiré l'attention dernièrement sur ce point. A mon avis, l'absence des fièvres hautes chez les vieillards et les cachectiques est due au fait que les leucocytes polynucléaires chez eux sont moins forts que chez les gens plus jeunes et plus résistants, de sorte qu'il se formera *plus tôt* un abcès si le malade ne meurt pas avant; la concentration des leucocytes polynucléaires est déjà *nécessaire*, tandis que la même virulence et le même nombre des microbes pathogènes ne seraient pas encore suffisants pour provoquer un abcès chez les jeunes et les plus résistants; quand la virulence ou le nombre des microbes ou tous les deux augmentent, le vieillard meurt avant la formation de l'abcès.

**Infection urinaire et infection générale**, par M. Posner (de Berlin). — Après injection de microbes différents dans l'uretère et le bassinet rénal, les animaux se comportent d'une manière différente au point de vue de l'infection générale. Tandis que le *bacillus anthracis*, les streptocoques, les staphylocoques causent une infection générale peu rapide, les animaux injectés avec le *bacterium coli* ne montrent pas plus de bacilles dans le sang et les organes que les animaux injectés avec le *bacillus prodigiosus*. Il semblerait donc que le danger de l'infection générale est beaucoup plus grand dans les pyélites d'origine streptococcique ou staphylococcique que chez les malades infectés de coli-bacille.

## DES INFECTIONS URINAIRES ANAÉROBIES

### par J. ALBARRAN et J. COTTET.

En 1898, nous avons présenté à l'Association française d'Urologie une *Note sur le rôle des microbes anaérobies*. Nous avons publié alors trois observations détaillées de pyonéphrose et d'infection vésicale et nous faisions allusion aux recherches sur les abcès urineux et l'in-

---

1. Albarran. Maladies chirurgicales du rein et de l'uretère, p. 755, 769.

filtration d'urine[1], à la suite desquelles l'un de nous, Cottet, publiait en 1899 douze observations de suppuration péri-urétrales dans lesquelles on trouvait des micro-organismes anaérobies. En 1900, l'un de nous, Albarran, étudiant les suppurations péri-urétrales, signale neuf nouveaux cas d'infection anaérobie. Nous vous apportons aujourd'hui le détail de ces neuf dernières observations et dix-huit nouveaux cas concernant des abcès urineux et des infiltrations d'urine, des cystites et des pyonéphroses.

L'ensemble de nos recherches comprenant quarante-trois observations démontre aujourd'hui d'une manière indiscutable la fréquence des infections urinaires, anaérobies pures ou à la fois anaérobies et aérobies. L'importance même du rôle des germes anaérobies ressort clairement de la lecture de plusieurs de nos observations, mais des recherches ultérieures seules pourront nous renseigner sur bien des points, que nos travaux n'ont pas réussi à élucider.

Nous étudierons successivement les infections anaérobies dans les abcès urineux et infiltrations d'urine, dans les prostatites, dans les infections vésicales et les infections rénales.

I. *Abcès urineux circonscrits et phlegmons urineux diffus.* — Le tableau suivant résume l'ensemble de nos observations sur les abcès urineux circonscrits et sur les phlegmons urineux comprenant 25 cas. Les 12 observations numérotées de 1 à 7 et de 18 à 22 ont été publiées dans la thèse de Cottet. Les 9 observations comprenant les numéros 8 à 14, les 23 et 24 ont été étudiées par Albarran et mentionnées dans le *Traité de chirurgie* de le Dentu et Delbet. Les quatre autres cas sont complètement inédits.

Avant d'étudier dans leur ensemble ces observations d'abcès circonscrit et d'infiltration d'urine, nous devons écarter deux de nos cas : ce sont les observations 8 et 11.

Dans l'observation 8, nous avons observé à l'examen sur lamelles un grand nombre de microbes de différentes formes, mais nos cultures sont restées stériles aussi bien en milieux aérobies qu'en milieux anaérobies. Ce fait trouve son explication dans l'ensemencement trop tardif du pus et serait plutôt en rapport avec l'existence de micro-organismes anaérobies, dont la culture est plus difficile que celle des aérobies.

Dans l'observation 11, il s'agit d'un malade qui, avec un abcès circonscrit, présenta des phénomènes généraux graves et mourut d'infection sanguine. Le pus de l'abcès périnéal ne fut pas cultivé. Le sang du

---

[1]. J. COTTET. Recherches bactériologiques sur les suppurations péri-urétrales. Thèse Paris, 1899.

Tableau comprenant 23 cas d'abcès urineux circonscrits et diffus.

| | AÉROBIES SEULS | ANAÉROBIES SEULS | AÉROBIES COEXISTANT AVEC ANAÉROBIES | | |
| --- | --- | --- | --- | --- | --- |
| | | | ANAÉROBIES PRÉDOMINANTS | AÉROBIES PRÉDOMINANTS | PROPORTION NON ÉTABLIE |
| Abcès circonscrits. . . . . . . . . . . . . . . . . | 1 | 6 | 7 | 0 | 1 |
| Infiltration . . . . . . . . . . . . . . . . . . . . | 2 | 1 | 4 | 0 | 1 |

Espèces isolées.

| AÉROBIES | DANS LES ABCÈS CIRCONSCRITS | DANS L'INFILTRATION | TOTAUX | ANAÉROBIES | DANS LES ABCÈS CIRCONSCRITS | DANS L'INFILTRATION | TOTAUX |
| --- | --- | --- | --- | --- | --- | --- | --- |
| Le streptocoque commun . . . | 7 | 3 | 10 | Le micrococcus fœtidus . . . . | 7 | 3 | 10 |
| Le colibacille. . . . . . . . | 3 | 4 | 7 | Le bacillus fragilis. . . . . . . | 4 | 2 | 6 |
| Le staphylocoque. . . . . . . | 3 | 0 | 3 | Le bacillus funduliformis . . . | 3 | 1 | 4 |
| Le streptocoque non pathogène | 0 | 1 | 1 | Le diplococcus reniformis . . . | 3 | 2 | 5 |
| Le proteus vulgaris . . . . . . | 0 | 1 | 1 | Le staphylococcus parvulus . . | 4 | 0 | 4 |
| Le bacille pseudo-diphtérique . | 0 | 1 | 1 | Le bacillus nebulosus . . . . . | 2 | 0 | 2 |
| Le coccus indéterminé. . . . . | 1 | 0 | 1 | Le bacillus bifidus. . . . . . . | 1 | 0 | 1 |
| Le bacille indéterminé. . . . . | 0 | 1 | 1 | Le bacillus aerogenes . . . . . | 0 | 1 | 1 |
| | | | | Le bacille indéterminé . , . . . | 4 | 1 | 5 |
| | | | | Le coccus indéterminé. . . . . | 2 | 0 | 2 |

cœur, examiné après la mort, contenait des steptrocoques et des staphylocoques. Nous ne pouvons rien conclure de ce fait incomplètement étudié.

*Espèces microbiennes trouvées dans les suppurations péri-urétrales circonscrites et diffuses.* — Nous avons résumé dans le tableau suivant, qui permettra de mieux se rendre compte de l'ensemble de nos observations, le résultat de nos examens bactériologiques portant sur vingt-trois cas, défalcation faite de nos deux observations incomplètes.

Ces chiffres, considérés dans leur ensemble, nous disent la *très grande fréquence* des microbes anaérobies dans les suppurations péri-urétrales : sur vingt-trois observations, vingt fois il existait des anaérobies et trois fois seulement on trouvait dans le pus exclusivement des microbes aérobies.

Notre tableau démontre encore le rôle pathogène important des microbes anaérobies. Tous les microbes anaérobies, que nous avons rencontrés, sont pathogènes et capables de déterminer expérimentalement des abcès. A côté de cette propriété de virulence se place une considération importante : sur vingt-trois cas, nous en avons sept dans lesquels on ne trouvait que des microbes strictement anaérobies et onze autres cas où ces mêmes microbes prédominaient beaucoup par rapport aux organismes aérobies.

Dans les cas où seuls les anaérobies existaient, nous sommes autorisés à dire que ces microbes sont ceux qui déterminèrent la suppuration. Lorsque chez d'autres malades nous voyons ces mêmes espèces anaérobies être beaucoup plus abondantes que les micro-organismes aérobies, nous pouvons encore dire qu'ils jouèrent, dans la formation du pus, le rôle prépondérant.

Si d'un autre côté nous remarquons que, sur vingt-trois malades, nous n'en trouvons que trois dont le pus ne contenait que des microbes aérobies, que dans aucun autre cas ces organismes n'étaient en prédominance et que seulement deux fois nous les avons vus mélangés aux anaérobies en proportion indéterminée, nous pensons pouvoir conclure : *Dans les abcès urineux circonscrits ou diffus du périnée, le rôle pathogène des microbes anaérobies est plus important que celui des micro-organismes aérobies.*

*Espèces microbiennes isolées.* — Depuis les premières recherches bactériologiques sur les abcès urineux (Albarran et Hallé, 1888) jusqu'à nos premières publications, on n'avait étudié dans les suppurations péri-urétrales que les microbes qui se cultivent à l'air.

**Résumé bactériologique des cas d'abcès urineux circonscrits et diffus.**



| NUMÉROS DES OBSERVATIONS | NOMS | DIAGNOSTIC | DÉBUT DES ACCIDENTS | CARACTÈRE DU PUS | EXAMEN SUR LAMELLES | CULTURES | | PROPORTION DES AÉROBIES ET DES ANAÉROBIES |
|---|---|---|---|---|---|---|---|---|
| | | | | | | MICROBES AÉROBIES | MICROBES ANAÉROBIES | |
| 1 | Paul L. | Abcès urineux. | 2ᵉ poussée, 10 jours. | Pus sanguinolent, bien lié, fétide. | Pas de microbes nets. | 0 | Bacillus fragilis (peu abondant). | Aérobies et anaérobies (anaérobies prédominent. |
| 2 | Henri M. | Abcès urineux fistuleux et réchauffé. | Un mois. | Pus fétide. | Nombreux microbes de formes variées. | 0 | Staphylococcus parvulus; bacillus nebulosus; bacillus funduliformis; micrococcus fœtidus. | Id. |
| 3 | Rou. | Abcès périnéal. | 15 jours. | Pus jaunâtre, assez épais, non fétide. | Nombreux bacilles décolorés par le Gram, quelques cocci colorés par le Gram. | 0 | Micrococcus fœtidus; bacillus fragilis. | Id. |
| 4 | Forw. | Abcès urineux. | 3 semaines. | Pus jaunâtre fétide. | Très nombreux microbes: cocci et bacilles plus ou moins longs. | Coli-bacille, streptocoque. | Staphylococcus parvulus; diplococcus reniformis; bac. funduliformis; bac. nebulosus; bacilles indéterminé. | Id. |
| 5 | Joseph F. | Abcès urineux. | 8 jours. | Sanie purulente, très fétide. | Très nombreux microbes: cocci et bâtonnets. | Coccus indéterminé. | Micrococcus fœtidus; bacillus fragilis. | Id. |
| 6 | Eugène M. | Abcès urineux. | 5 jours. | Pus jaunâtre, épais et très fétide. | Très nombreux microbes: cocci et bâtonnets. | Coli-bacille. | Staphylococcus parvulus; strepto-bacille indéterminé. | Id. |
| 7 | Lon. | Abcès urineux. | 15 jours. | Pus très fétide. | Cocci en chaînettes et fins bacilles. | Streptocoque. | Micrococcus fœtidus; bacille indéterminé. | Id. |
| 8 | Ch., VELPEAU, 27 | Abcès urineux grave. Infection générale. Mort. | 26 jours. | Sang du cœur après la mort. | Diplocoque très abondant, prenant mal le Gram. | Streptocoque (virulent). Staphylocoque bl. Staphylocoque doré. | 0 | Aérobies seuls. |
| 9 | B., VELPEAU, 23 | Abcès urineux à évolution bénigne. | 8 jours. | Pus. | Cocci très abondants, en amas et en chaînettes, colorés par le Gram. | 0 | Micrococcus fœtidus; bacillus bifidus. | Anaérobies seuls. |

Résumé bactériologique des cas d'abcès urineux circonscrits et diffus (*suite*).

| NUMÉROS DES OBSERVATIONS | NOMS | DIAGNOSTIC | DÉBUT DES ACCIDENTS | CARACTÈRE DU PUS | EXAMEN SUR LAMELLES | CULTURES | | PROPORTION DES AÉROBIES ET DES ANAÉROBIES |
|---|---|---|---|---|---|---|---|---|
| | | | | | | MICROBES AÉROBIES | MICROBES ANAÉROBIES | |
| 10 | L., Velpeau, 50 | Abcès urineux, guérison assez lente. | 6 jours. | Pus. | Bacilles prenant le Gram, très abondants. Cocci en amas rares. | Staphylocoque blanc, très rare, streptocoque rose. | Bacille gros, court, trapu, coloré par le Gram, ne donnant pas de gaz, non identifié. | Anaérobies prédominent. |
| 11 | K., Velpeau, 17 | Abcès urineux bénin, guérison rapide. | 3 semaines. | Pus. | Microbes très abondants : cocci et bacilles. | Cultures restées stériles (ensemencement tardif. | 0 | Id. |
| 12 | A., Velpeau, 13 | Abcès urineux multiples, guérison en un mois. | Id. | Pus. | Streptocoque gardant le Gram, rare. Bacille très abondant, crochu, variable, gardant le Gram. | Streptocoque, staphylocoque blanc. | Bacillus funduliformis. | Id. |
| 13 | R., Velpeau, 11 | Abcès urineux bénin. | 8 jours. | Bas fétide. | Cocco-bacille ténu, assez abondant, décoloré par le Gram. | 0 | Cocco-bacille non identifié. | Anaérobies seuls. |
| 14 | B., Velpeau, 18 | Abcès urineux avec fistules. | Ancien. | Pus. | Cocci variés ; souvent en forme de gonocoques. abondants. Bacilles rares. | Staphylocoque blanc, streptocoque, coli-bacille. | Micrococcus fœtidus. Micrococcus petit, en amas, décoloré par le Gram, non identifié. | Aérobies et anaérobies. |
| 15 | V., service du Dr Routier. | Abcès urineux. | 4 jours. | Pus bien lié, non fétide. | Cocci très rares. | 0 | Diplococcus reniformis. Staphylococcus parvulus. | Anaérobies seuls. |
| 16 | V., Velpeau. | Abcès urineux. | 10 jours. | Pus. | Microbes abondants, bacilles fins ; cocci en chaînettes et en diplocoques. | Streptocoque. | Micrococcus fœtidus. Diplococcus reniformis. Bacillus fragilis. | Anaérobies prédominent. |
| 17 | R., Velpeau, 29 | Abcès urineux bénin. | * | Pus. | Streptocoques gardant le Gram. | Streptocoque. | 0 | Aérobies seuls. |
| 18 | Georges J. | Infiltration d'urine. Abcès sous-cutané métastatique. | 6 jours. | Pus séreux très fétide. Pus de l'abcès métastatique bien lié, non fétide. | Très nombreux bacilles décolorés par le Gram. Quelques bacilles décolorés par le Gram. | Coli-bacille (très petite quantité). 0 | Bacillus funduliformis très abondant. Bacillus funduliformis. | Aérobies (très peu), anaérobies abondants. Anaérobies seuls. |

Résumé bactériologique des cas d'abcès urineux circonscrits et diffus (*suite et fin*).

| NUMÉROS DES OBSERVATIONS | NOMS | DIAGNOSTIC | DÉBUT DES ACCIDENTS | CARACTÈRE DU PUS | EXAMEN SUR LAMELLES | CULTURES | | PROPORTION DES AÉROBIES ET DES ANAÉROBIES |
|---|---|---|---|---|---|---|---|---|
| | | | | | | MICROBES AÉROBIES | MICROBES ANAÉROBIES | |
| 19 | Rev…. | Infiltration d'urine. | 3° poussée, 3 jours. | Pus jaunâtre, assez bien lié, très fétide. | Nombreux bacilles décolorés par le Gram. Streptocoques gardant le Gram. | 0 | Micrococcus fœtidus ; bacillus fragilis. | Aérobies (très peu), anaérobies abondants. Anaérobies seuls. |
| 20 | Armand B. | Infiltration d'urine. | 2° poussée, 10 jours. | Pus fétide. | Nombreux microbes : cocci et bâtonnets. | Coli-bacille (très peu abondant). | Micrococcus fœtidus ; bacillus fragilis. | *Id.* |
| 21 | Paul S. | Infiltration d'urine. | 8 jours. | Sérosité purulente, horriblement fétide. | Nombreux microbes de formes variées. | Coli-bacille. | Nombreux anaérobies. | *Id.* |
| 22 | Ernest C. | Infiltration d'urine. | 10 jours. | Sérosité purulente inodore. | Assez nombreux cocci et diplocoques. | Streptocoque. | 0 | Aérobies seuls. |
| 23 | A., VELPEAU, 20 | Rétrécissement infranchissab. Infiltration d'urine très étendue(pubis, périnée,verge), incisions multiples, guéri. | » | Pus. | 0 | Streptocoque, bacille pseudo-diphtérique proteus vulgaris. | 0 | Aérobies seuls, très peu abondants. |
| 24 | B., VELPEAU, 31 | Infiltration d'urine très étendue (verge, flanc droit, fosse iliaque et région lomb.), incisions, mort en 8 jours. | 8 jours. | Pus fétide et gangreneux. | Cocci extrêmement abondants et polymorphes ; bacilles grèles, bacilles trapus, tous gardant le Gram. | Coli-bacille, petit bacille gardant le Gram, streptocoque. | Micrococcus fœtidus. Diplococcus reniformis. | Aérobies et anaérobies extrêmement abondants. |
| 25 | X., VELPEAU. | Infiltration d'urine avec gangrène gazeuse. Mort. | 8 jours. | Sérosité louche, roussâtre, très fétide. | Cocci variés et bacilles décolorés par le Gram. | Streptocoque ne prenant pas le Gram, non pathogène. | Diplococcus reniformis. Bacillus aerogenes anaerobius | Anaérobies prédominent. |

Aujourd'hui, il nous faut étudier, à côté de ceux-là, les variétés de micro-organismes anaérobies.

*Espèces aérobies*. — Réunissant cinquante cas d'abcès urineux et d'infiltration d'urine étudiés au point de vue des microbes aérobies, l'un de nous a trouvé vingt-six fois le coli-bacille seul ou associé à d'autres microbes : venaient ensuite, par ordre de fréquence, le staphylocoque, le streptocoque pyogène et le proteus.

Sur les vingt-trois cas que nous présentons aujourd'hui, nous trouvons le plus souvent le streptocoque (10 fois) et le coli-bacille (7 fois); beaucoup moins fréquemment les staphylocoques (5 fois) et d'autres microbes.

Lorsque les suppurations péri-urétrales n'étaient étudiées qu'au point de vue des aérobies, on pouvait attribuer un grand rôle dans leur production au coli et au streptocoque : aujourd'hui, tout en croyant que ces micro-organismes ont une certaine importance, nous sommes conduits à penser que, dans la plupart des cas, leur rôle est secondaire.

Pour établir que les micro-organismes aérobies sont capables de donner naissance à des abcès urineux circonscrits ou diffus, il est nécessaire de négliger toutes les observations, dans lesquelles on n'a pas fait en même temps les deux espèces de cultures aérobies et anaérobies. En ne tenant compte que de ces faits, au nombre de vingt-trois, nous trouvons trois cas de suppuration exclusivement aérobie, et dans les trois le streptocoque se trouvait deux fois seul et une fois associé à d'autres microbes.

Ces faits sont trop peu nombreux pour permettre de conclure, mais si on les rapproche de la grande fréquence du streptocoque associé aux microbes anaérobies, il semble qu'on puisse dire que, parmi les microbes aérobies, celui qui paraît jouer le rôle le plus important dans les abcès urineux est le streptocoque; après lui vient le coli-bacille.

*Espèces anaérobies*[1]. — Parmi les nombreuses espèces anaérobies que nous avons isolées, les plus fréquentes sont : le micrococcus fœtidus de Veillon (10 fois), le bacillus fragilis de Veillon et Zuber (6 fois) et le diplococcus reniformis de Cottet (5 fois); viennent ensuite le bacillus funduliformis de J. Hallé et le staphylococcus parvulus de Veillon et Zuber.

Si nous ne considérons que les sept cas de suppuration strictement anaérobie, nous voyons encore le micrococcus fœtidus (4 fois) et le

1. Pour la description de ces espèces anaérobies, voir Cottet : Thèse de Doctorat, Paris, 1899, et communication à la Soc. de biologie (5 mai 1900).

bacillus fragilis (4 fois). Il semble bien que, parmi les anaérobies ces deux espèces soient plus fréquentes que les autres dans les suppurations péri-urétrales.

L'importance que prend ainsi le micrococcus fœtidus doit être notée et on doit se rappeler que, au point de vue morphologique, ce microbe est un streptocoque anaérobie. Dans une préparation sur lamelle du pus d'un abcès urineux, le fœtidus et le streptocoque pyogène aérobie sont si ressemblants qu'ils ne peuvent être distingués l'un de l'autre que par la double culture en milieux aérobies et anaérobies.

Nous devons encore remarquer la grande ressemblance que présente, à l'examen sur lamelles, le diplococcus reniformis de Cottet avec le gonocoque. La disposition en diplocoque et le volume des deux microbes est semblable et tous deux se décolorent par la méthode de Gram. La distinction ne peut ici encore être faite que par les cultures en milieu spécial.

*Rapport entre la forme circonscrite ou diffuse de l'abcès et les microbes trouvés dans le pus.* On ne peut, aujourd'hui, établir un rapport constant entre les microbes du pus et la forme circonscrite ou diffuse de la suppuration. Cela ressort de la comparaison établie, d'une part, entre les observations où nous avons trouvé des microbes aérobies et celles qui contenaient des anaérobies, d'autre part, de la comparaison dans chacun de ces deux groupes, des variétés des microbes.

Sur 15 abcès circonscrits nous trouvons : 13 fois des anaérobies seuls ou prédominants, 86 pour 100; 1 fois des aérobies seuls, 6 pour 100.

Sur 8 phlegmons diffus : 6 fois des anaérobies seuls ou prédominants, 75 pour 100; 2 fois des aérobies seuls, 25 pour 100.

A ne considérer que les chiffres on pourrait croire que les anaérobies se trouvent plus fréquemment dans les formes bénignes circonscrites que dans les suppurations diffuses. L'analyse des observations ne permet pas cette conclusion.

Sur nos huit cas considérés comme des infiltrations d'urine, il en est deux dans lesquels nous n'avons trouvé que des microbes aérobies. Or, dans un de ces deux cas, il s'agit d'infiltration limitée et d'allure bénigne, et le second est absolument exceptionnel.

Dans l'observation 22, il s'agissait d'une infiltration d'urine avec collection périnéale, œdème du scrotum et de la verge et tuméfaction des régions inguginales. Le liquide séro-purulent qui s'écoula par l'incision périnéale était inodore, les tissus n'étaient pas sphacelés, et la guérison fut rapidement obtenue.

Dans l'observation 25, le malade fut opéré quelques heures après le début des accidents; la verge seule était infiltrée et le pubis empâté. La sérosité louche qui s'écoula par l'incision n'était pas fétide et au moment de l'intervention il n'existait pas encore de sphacèle. Dans les jours suivants, le malade élimina de larges lambeaux sphacélés. Dans ce cas la rapidité de l'intervention conjura seule des accidents graves. Nous ne trouvâmes dans ce cas que des microbes aérobies, ce qui ne cadre guère avec tout l'ensemble de nos autres observations. Avons-nous fait une erreur de technique? En tous cas, ce fait constitue une véritable exception.

Les huit observations d'infiltration d'urine que nous avons étudiées sont trop peu nombreuses pour nous permettre de conclure, mais elles suffisent à démontrer que si dans la grande majorité des cas la diffusion des lésions est en rapport avec l'existence de microbes anaérobies, d'un autre côté la diffusion des lésions a été observée par nous dans deux cas où les procédés de culture que nous employons d'ordinaire ne nous ont permis d'isoler que des microbes aérobies.

Nos observations démontrent aussi que l'existence exclusive ou prédominante dans le foyer des microbes anaérobies est compatible avec les formes limitées et bénignes des abcès urineux.

Si on considère les *différentes variétés de microbes aérobies ou anaé-robies* on verra les mêmes organismes se retrouver sans préférence marquée dans les cas simples comme dans les cas graves. Parmi les microbes aérobies, nous voyons le streptocoque sept fois dans les abcès circonscrits et trois fois dans les infiltrations; le coli-bacille se trouvant trois fois dans les premiers et quatre fois dans les secondes. Parmi les anaérobies, le micrococcus fœtidus se voyait dans sept abcès circonscrits et dans trois phlegmons diffus et ainsi des autres espèces.

Si nous considérons les associations microbiennes, nous aboutissons encore à des résultats semblables.

Ces faits montrent bien que la variété microbienne n'est pas seule responsable de la plus ou moins grande diffusion des lésions. Il faut encore, en ce qui regarde les microbes eux-mêmes, tenir compte de leur virulence et de leur quantité et considérer par ailleurs le rôle de la lésion urétrale primitive.

*Rapports des variétés microbiennes avec les phénomènes gangreneux.* Nous trouvons signalée dans huit de nos observations l'existence de phénomènes gangreneux plus ou moins intenses dans le foyer périnéal ou dans les parties voisines infiltrées. Dans tous ces cas, les microbes anaérobies existaient seuls ou étaient en prédominance.

Dans cinq autres cas, il n'existait pas de phénomènes gangreneux primitifs et parmi eux nous en trouvons deux qui ne contenaient que des microbes anaérobies et trois ayant, seuls ou en prédominance, des micro-organismes anaérobies. Parmi ces cinq observations figure le cas de ce malade, dont nous avons déjà parlé, chez lequel le foyer purulent ne contenait au moment de l'incision que des aérobies et qui les jours suivants présenta des phénomènes gangreneux de la plaie. S'agit-il dans ce cas d'une infection secondaire ou n'avons-nous pas su voir les anaérobies?

En ce qui regarde la *fétidité* du pus, nous trouvons treize cas à pus fétide et dans les treize, seuls ou en prédominance, des microbes anaérobies.

Chez trois malades le pus n'était pas fétide : une fois il ne contenait que des aérobies et deux fois des anaérobies.

D'après nos observations on peut dire que *la fétidité du pus et les phénomènes gangreneux dans les abcès périnéaux circonscrits ou diffus ont, dans tous les cas, été observés en même temps que l'extrême abondance des microbes anaérobies qui, parfois, existaient seuls dans le foyer infectieux.* Cette constatation importante est bien en rapport avec le rôle que jouent ces organismes anaérobies dans les suppurations fétides et gangreneuses, rôle si bien établi par Veillon et Zuber et par les élèves de Veillon.

Mais si toutes, ou presque toutes les suppurations gangreneuses et fétides paraissent être d'origine microbienne anaérobie, il faut savoir que l'existence des anaérobies dans le foyer n'entraîne nécessairement ni le sphacèle des tissus, ni la fétidité du pus. Ces espèces de micro-organismes peuvent se trouver même à l'exclusion de tout microbe aérobie sans que le pus soit fétide ni le foyer gangreneux.

*Infection sanguine dans les abcès urineux.* — Nous possédons deux observations démontrant que l'infection sanguine peut être due soit aux microbes anaérobies soit aux microbes aérobies.

Dans l'observation 18 (obs. 1, thèse Cottet) on trouvait dans le foyer périnéal du coli-bacille en petite quantité et en grande abondance le bacillus funduliformis. Dans un abcès métastatique ce dernier microbe, strictement anaérobie, existait seul.

Nous n'avons pas examiné le pus de l'abcès périnéal du malade de l'observation 11, mais deux heures après la mort, nous ne trouvons dans le sang du cœur que des streptocoques et des staphylocoques, espèces aérobies.

De l'ensemble de nos observations concernant les abcès urineux circonscrits et les phlegmons diffus péri-urétraux, se dégagent les conclusions suivantes, déjà formulées dans la thèse de l'un de nous :

Les microbes anaérobies seuls ou en grande prédominance par rapport aux aérobies se rencontrent dans la proportion de 86 pour 100 des cas examinés. Ils existent seuls dans un tiers des cas.

Ces microbes sont la cause la plus fréquente des suppurations péri-urétrales : parmi leurs différentes variétés, le *micrococcus fœtidus*, le *bacillus fragilis* et le *diplococcus reniformis* sont ceux qu'on observe le plus fréquemment.

Les formes diffuses des suppurations péri-urétrales (infiltration d'urine) sont le plus souvent en rapport avec l'existence dans le foyer des microbes anaérobies seuls ou associés aux aérobies. Ces formes cliniques peuvent exceptionnellement être déterminées par des microbes aérobies seuls et paraissent alors d'allure plus bénigne.

Les phénomènes gangreneux et la fétidité du pus ont paru, dans tous les cas, être en rapport avec les espèces anaérobies.

Les microbes anaérobies peuvent déterminer l'infection sanguine.

Ces mêmes microbes peuvent se rencontrer, même à l'exclusion des espèces aérobies, dans les formes d'abcès circonscrits bénins, sans phénomènes gangreneux et sans fétidité du pus.

Les suppurations péri-urétrales peuvent être exclusivement dues à des espèces de microbes aérobies (15 pour 100), et ces mêmes microbes sont, dans les deux tiers des cas, associés aux anaérobies.

Parmi les microbes aérobies, les plus importants sont le *streptocoque pyogène*, le *coli-bacille* et les *staphylocoques*.

## II. *Abcès de la prostate.*

Nous n'avons étudié que quatre cas de cette catégorie déjà publiés dans la thèse de Cottet (5 cas) et dans les *Annales génito-urinaires*, 1900 par Cottet et Duval. Trois fois, il n'existait que des microbes aérobies, coli-bacille, streptocoque, staphylocoque et gonocoque.

Dans une quatrième observation de suppuration prostatique et péri-prostatique, avec pus très fétide et sphacèle des tissus, on trouvait associé à un staphylocoque, un bacille anaérobie de grande virulence, le *bacillus perfringens* de Veillon et Zuber. L'existence dans le pus de ce bacille doit être rapprochée d'une ancienne observation de Guyon et Albarran, où l'on trouva, dans un cas de gangrène urinaire avec infection urinaire, aussi bien dans la plaque gangreneuse que dans les viscères, un microbe probablement anaérobie, qui présentait avec le perfringens la plus grande ressemblance morphologique.

De nouvelles observations pourront seules nous apprendre l'importance des microbes anaérobies dans les prostatites : nous ne pouvons pour le moment que faire remarquer que, contrairement à ce qui se voit dans les abcès périnéaux, les prostatites suppurées ne contiennent pas souvent des anaérobies, au moins dans les formes circonscrites. Le seul cas de prostatite diffuse et gangreneuse étudié paraît avoir été déterminé par un bacille strictement anaérobie.

### III. *Infections vésicales.*

Nous n'avons méthodiquement étudié que trois cas d'infection vésicale.

Chez notre premier malade, dont nous avons publié l'observation en 1898 à la Société française d'urologie, il s'agit d'un néoplasme secondaire de la vessie. Les urines de la malade présentaient cette odeur repoussante, véritablement infecte, qu'on observe dans certaines tumeurs vésicales; dans ces cas la tumeur présente souvent un aspect macéré et des portions sphacélées. Dans l'urine de notre malade, il y avait, non seulement des coli-bacilles et des streptocoques, mais on y trouvait aussi un micrococque anaérobie, dont l'inoculation aux animaux détermine la formation d'un abcès; il s'agissait probablement du diplococcus reniformis.

Voici nos trois observations inédites :

Obs. XXX. — Mill..., cocher, âgé de 44 ans, soigné à Necker pour une cystite le 1ᵉʳ mai 1900 (consultation).

Il y a 25 ans, blennorrhagie qui n'a pas été complètement guérie. Depuis 11 ans, le malade a des urines troubles. Il y a 4 ans, quelques hématuries terminales; à cette époque il a été soigné à l'hôpital Ricord.

Il y a 1 mois et demi, nouvelles hématuries; en même temps les troubles de la miction s'accentuent.

Actuellement mictions toutes les cinq minutes, même pendant la nuit, impérieuses, douloureuses. Les urines sont troubles à l'émission et il vient du sang à la fin de la miction.

*Examen.* — Urètre : normal; vessie : très sensible. Épididyme gauche : induration très ancienne. Prostate : induration du lobe gauche. L'examen microscopique de l'urine montre : rares leucocytes, phosphates ammoniaco-magnésiens, nombreux microcoques, pas de bacilles de Koch. Un cobaye inoculé se portait bien trois mois après.

*Examen bactériologique.* — L'examen direct sur lamelles montrait de nombreux microcoques et quelques bacilles fins.

*Cultures : Deux tubes aérobies.* — Il pousse dans le tube 1, trois colonies contenant un microbe ressemblant à une levure (sans doute un saprophyte). Le tube 2 reste stérile.

*Trois tubes anaérobies.* — Ils n'ont poussé presque que dans la zone anaérobie; on y trouve :

Diplococcus reniformis repiqué et obtenu en culture pure.

Un strepto-bacille, à articles fins, se décolorant par le Gram, qui n'a pas été repiqué, mais qui était anaérobie parce que : 1° il n'a pas poussé sur les tubes aérés; 2° il n'a poussé que dans la zone privée d'air des tubes de gélose sucrée en couche profonde.

Obs. XXXI. — M. C..., âgé de 55 ans, arthritique, aucun passé uréthral; pas de blennorrhagie, pas de cathétérisme avant l'apparition de la cystite.

Il y a deux ans phénomènes de cystite qui apparaissent spontanément. Soigné pendant deux ans par divers traitements, lavages de vessie, balsamiques, etc., sans amélioration notable. Les mictions restent fréquentes et douloureuses et les urines sont troubles. Vient consulter M. Guyon en mai 1900. Dans un premier examen microscopique du dépôt purulent, on constate, presque à l'état de pureté, des cocci en amas ou en diplocoques qui se décolorent par le Gram.

*Examen de l'urine.* — L'urine, examinée le 25 mai, est recueillie en recevant dans un ballon stérilisé la dernière portion de la miction spontanée.

Cette urine est trouble avec un dépôt un peu glaireux; son odeur est ammoniacale et sa réaction alcaline.

Examen *direct sur lamelles.* — Cocci en amas et en diplocoques presque tous décolorés par le Gram. Quelques bacilles assez volumineux qui gardent le Gram.

Cultures aérobies sur gélose ordinaire et sur gélose-ascite :

Staphylocoque doré;

Streptocoque décoloré par la méthode de Gram (non pathogène pour le lapin);

Un bacille gardant le Gram qui a donné deux ou trois colonies orangées.

Cultures anaérobies : *diplococcus reniformis.*

Le microbe anaérobie est de beaucoup le plus abondant. On peut même dire que les aérobies sont négligeables tant ils sont en infime minorité : ils ont pu d'ailleurs être introduits par les défauts de la technique employée pour recueillir l'urine.

Ce diplococcus reniformis a été inoculé sous la peau d'un cobaye : il a déterminé la formation d'un abcès dans le pus duquel le diplocoque se trouvait, soit à l'état libre, soit intra-cellulaire. Ce pus expérimental avait une grande ressemblance avec un pus blennorrhagique.

Un *deuxième examen* bactériologique de l'urine de ce malade, pratiqué quelques jours après, a donné les mêmes résultats au point de vue du microbe anaérobie (diplococcus reniformis).

L'inoculation à un cobaye est restée négative au point de vue de la tuberculose.

Deux analyses postérieures de l'urine ont été faites en cours de traitement.

19 *mai* 1900. — Les cocci anaérobies paraissent sur les lamelles plus abondants que les bacilles. En culture, diplococcus reniformis et colibacille.

15 *juin* 1900. — Cette fois les cultures n'ont pas montré de microbes strictement anaérobies; par contre il existe plusieurs espèces aérobies : cocci associés à des bacilles.

Obs. XXXII. — François A..., âgé de 42 ans, entré, le 16 juin 1900, salle Velpeau n° 27, à l'hôpital Necker.

A l'âge de 21 ans, blennorrhagie qui dure 11 jours. Syphilis en 1882; gommes cutanées en 1890. En 1889, orchite du côté gauche, sans cause apparente; elle dura trois jours et céda par les compresses humides. En 1891, sans aucun trouble préalable, crise de rétention aiguë qui dura deux jours; le malade vint alors à Necker et M. Guyon constata un rétrécissement laissant passer le n° 12 : dilatation consécutive.

En 1896, nouvelle crise de rétention, puis phénomènes de cystite avec quelques gouttes de sang à la fin de la miction. Nouvelle dilatation du canal.

Le 13 juin 1900, nouvelle crise de rétention complète; le lendemain et le surlendemain il rendit un peu d'urine très sanglante; il souffrait vivement dans le périnée et du côté du rein droit.

17 juin. Il vient à Necker avec près de 40° de fièvre et souffrant beaucoup. M. Albarran passe facilement une sonde bougie n° 14 qui laisse écouler de l'urine très sanglante et d'odeur repoussante. La sonde est laissée à demeure. On constate à ce moment une légère induration du périnée. Rien dans la prostate ni dans les reins.

18 juin. On place une sonde n° 20; l'hémorragie vésicale continue et le 22 on doit faire une aspiration des caillots.

23 juin. Incision d'un abcès périnéal, l'hématurie a cessé.

Jusqu'au 7 juillet, les urines, d'odeur infecte, charrient des débris pseudo-membraneux; à plusieurs reprises ces débris bouchent la sonde, même la sonde métallique n° 26, et cela malgré des lavages répétés et l'aspiration. Pendant ce temps température oscillante de 37°5 à 39°.

7 *juillet*. Taille hypogastrique par M. Albarran, toute la muqueuse vésicale formant une énorme fausse membrane est enlevée d'un seul bloc. La fausse membrane représente le moule de la vessie entière; on voit deux orifices au niveau des uretères. La face externe de la fausse membrane présente de nombreuses fibres musculaires faisant relief.

Dès le lendemain de l'opération, les urines sont devenues presque claires. Six semaines après, le malade est parti guéri, l'orifice hypogastrique complètement fermé.

*Examen bactériologique*. — Urine recueillie le 7 juillet, immédiatement avant l'opération.

L'*examen sur lamelles* montre une multitude de microbes polymorphes : des cocci en amas et en chaînettes prenant le Gram; des bacilles grêles, moins abondants, ne prenant pas le Gram.

Les cultures n'ont réussi à isoler aucune espèce strictement anaérobie; dans les tubes, malgré les dilutions successives, il poussa toujours en grande abondance des aérobies variés dont nous avons pu isoler :

Des staphylocoques;
Streptocoque;
Coli-bacille;
Un petit cocco bacille prenant le Gram.


Dans l'observation 30 nous ferons remarquer que l'infection vésicale avec cystite ne peut être attribuée qu'au microbe anaérobie, seul organisme pathogène que l'urine contenait.

L'action des anaérobies sur le développement de la cystite se retrouve encore chez le malade de l'observation 31. Nous trouvons dans l'urine trois espèces aérobies très peu abondantes, dont deux non pathogènes, et le diplococcus reniformis, qui lui est pathogène, en grande prépondérance. Il importe en outre de faire remarquer comment dans le cours du traitement s'est modifiée chez ce malade la teneur microbienne de l'urine : un troisième examen pratiqué quinze jours après le premier montre encore le diplococcus reniformis en abondance, mais déjà le coli-bacille pousse abondamment dans les tubes. Lors d'un quatrième examen, pratiqué trois semaines après le second, on ne trouve plus les anaérobies, mais seulement des aérobies : cocci associés à des bacilles.

Cette infection secondaire aérobie prépondérante explique que nous n'ayons pu isoler des anaérobies dans le cas de cystite exfoliante (obs. 32). Il existait chez ce malade une telle quantité de microbes de toutes formes que nous n'avons pu isoler que quatre espèces aérobies ; sur les lamelles il existait d'autres microbes que nous n'avons pu cultiver et qui, très probablement, étaient des anaérobies.

Le nombre restreint des infections vésicales que nous avons étudiées nous permet uniquement de dire : l'infection de la vessie, avec production de cystite, peut être due à des microbes aérobies ou anaérobies ou à ces deux variétés associées.


#### IV. *Suppurations rénales et péri-rénales.*


Nous avons étudié, au point de vue de leur teneur en microbes aérobies et anaérobies, le pus de dix malades atteints de suppuration rénale ou péri-rénale, opérés par Albarran. Dans tous ces cas, le pus a été pris au moment même de l'opération et les ensemencements faits rapidement en milieux ordinaires et suivant le procédé de Veillon pour la recherche des anaérobies.

Les deux observations portant les numéros 1 et 8 ont été publiées par nous, à l'Association française d'urologie. Les huit autres sont inédites : nous les résumons dans le tableau suivant :

Tableau comprenant 10 cas de suppurations rénales et périrénales.

| NUMÉRO | OBSERVATION | DIAGNOSTIC | EXAMEN DU PUS SUR LAMELLES | CULTURES AÉROBIES | CULTURES ANAÉROBIES |
|---|---|---|---|---|---|
| 33 | M., publiée en 1898 (Association d'Urologie). . . . . . . | Pyonéphrose à pus fétide. | Streptocoques; coccobacilles ; bacilles et diplocoques. | Colibacille, streptocoque. | Micrococcus fœtidus. |
| 34 | Giroud . . . . . . . . | Pyonéphrose à pus fétide. | Bacille (probablement le coli). | Colibacille. | o |
| 35 | Galabert . . . . . . | Pyonéphrose calculeuse ouverte. Abcès périnéphrétique. | Staphylocoques. | Staphylocoque doré. | o |
| 36 | Filliaux, publiée in extenso par Albarran (Congrès, 1900). Fistules rénales et sonde à demeure, obs. 5. . . . . . . | Pyonéphrose calculeuse. | Cocci, bacilles. | Staphylocoque blanc, rare. | Diplococcus reniformis et bacillus fusiformis. |
| 37 | Marg... . . . . . . . | Pyonéphrose calculeuse à pus fétide. | Bacilles, streptobacilles, diplocoques. | o | Bacillus fragilis, diplococcus reniformis et bacillus ramosus. |
| 38 | François . . . . . . . | Pyonéphrose calculeuse. | Cocci, bacilles. | Colibacille, streptocoque. | Diplococcus reniformis et fusiformis. |
| 39 | Publiée en 1898 (Associat. d'Urologie). | Abcès rénal tuberculeux. | o | o | Bacille anaérobie, rare. |
| 40 | Guérin, publiée in extenso par Albarran (Société de chirurgie, 1900, p. 844), obs. 12 . . . . . . | Pyonéphrose tuberculeuse. | o | Bacille indéterminé Staphylocoque . . Streptocoque . . . } non pathogène. | o |
| 41 | Vanereau. . . . . . | Pyonéphrose tuberculeuse. | o | o | o |
| 42 | Gibert . . . . . . . . | Abcès périnéphrétique. | Bacille (probablement coli). | Colibacille. | o |

Nos observations ont porté sur des cas de pyonéphrose, de tuberculose rénale et d'abcès périnéphrétique. Nous n'avons pas eu l'occasion d'étudier les pyélo-néphrites banales des urinaires, dont la bactériologie aérobie, commencée par les travaux d'Albarran et Hallé (1888) et la thèse d'Albarran (1889) est assez bien connue, mais qui n'ont jamais été étudiées au point de vue des microbes anaérobies.

## A. *Pyonéphroses*

Sur 6 cas de pyonéphrose simple ou calculeuse (obs. 33 à 38) nous trouverons :

2 cas ne contenant que des microbes aérobies.
1 —        —                — anaérobies.
3 — ayant à la fois des aérobies et des anaérobies.

1° *Pyonéphroses aérobies.* — Nos deux cas de pyonéphrose aérobie pure étaient tous deux monomicrobiens.

Dans l'observation 34 il s'agit d'une malade ayant une très grosse pyonéphrose consécutive à la pression déterminée sur l'uretère par une tumeur pelvienne : cette malade avait des accidents fébriles intenses et graves. Le liquide uro-purulent du rein contenait à l'état de pureté le coli-bacille.

Dans l'observation 35 il s'agit d'une pyonéphrose calculeuse à pus fétide en même temps que d'un abcès périnéphrétique. L'abcès périrénal avait déjà été ouvert, mais le pus n'avait pas été examiné, lorsque nous incisâmes la poche rénale. Dans le pus du rein nous n'avons trouvé que le staphylocoque doré.

Ces deux observations démontrent nettement que des pyonéphroses graves, fébriles, peuvent être uniquement dues aux staphylocoques ou au coli-bacille.

Si à ces deux observations nous ajoutons les trois autres cas où on trouvait à la fois des microbes aérobies et anaérobies nous constatons que, au point de vue de leur fréquence, les aérobies se classent ainsi :

> Coli-bacille. . . . . . . . . . . . . . . . . . . . . . . . 3 fois.
> Staphylocoques . . . . . . . . . . . . . . . . . . . 2 —
> Streptocoques . . . . . . . . . . . . . . . . . . . . 2 —

Nous devons pourtant ajouter que d'autres examens du pus des pyonéphroses, au point de vue exclusif des aérobies, nous ont souvent montré l'existence de staphylocoques, tandis que dans les pyélonéphrites simples sans pyonéphroses le coli est plus fréquent (Albarran).

### B. *Pyonéphroses anaérobies*

Notre observation 37 démontre qu'une pyonéphrose peut être exclusivement anaérobie.

Chez notre malade il s'agissait d'une pyonéphrose calculeuse : nous recueillîmes dans le bassinet, par le cathétérisme urétéral, plus de 200 grammes de pus épais et fétide, qui ne contenait que des espèces microbiennes strictement anaérobies : le diplococcus reniformis, le bacillus fragilis et le bacillus ramosus de Veillon et Zuber.

Dans trois autres cas, nous avons trouvé des anaérobies associés aux aérobies : deux fois ils étaient plus abondants que ces derniers et une fois il y avait très peu de microbes des deux ordres.

Les espèces anaérobies trouvées dans ces pyonéphroses se classent ainsi :

> Diplococcus reniformis. . . . . . . . . . . . . . 2 fois.
> Micrococcus fœtidus. . . . . . . . . . . . . . . . 1 —

Micrococcus fragilis . . . . . . . . . . . . . . . . . . 1 fois.
—      perfringens . . . . . . . . . . . . . . . 1 —
—      ramosus . . . . . . . . . . . . . . . . . 1 —
—      fusiformis . . . . . . . . . . . . . . . 1 —

Nous ne pouvons établir aucune relation entre les variétés microbiennes rencontrées dans les pyonéphroses et la gravité des accidents. Notons toutefois que parmi nos malades opérés, seul celui de l'observation 53 est mort avec des accidents généraux très graves ; localement c'est le seul de nos cas dans lequel nous avons observé des phénomènes gangreneux avec nécrose des pyramides et sphacèle de la plaie. Chez ce malade le pus rénal contenait en abondance le micrococcus fœtidus et le coli-bacille et de rares streptocoques.

### C. *Tuberculose rénale.*

Deux fois nous avons examiné le pus de pyonéphroses tuberculeuses et une fois celui d'un abcès tuberculeux ne communiquant pas avec le bassinet. Dans ces trois observations, on est frappé de voir la rareté des microbes contenus dans le pus : c'est ainsi que dans aucun de nos trois cas nous n'avons pu voir des microorganismes en faisant l'examen direct du pus étalé sur des lamelles.

Dans un de nos cas (obs. 5) les cultures sont restées stériles aussi bien en milieux aérobies que dans les tubes anaérobies ; ce pus était en réalité stérile. Il s'agissait dans ce cas d'une femme ayant une très grosse pyonéphrose tuberculeuse ancienne et opérée par la néphrostomie dans un état très grave.

Chez une autre malade, atteinte elle aussi de pyonéphrose, tuberculeuse le pus du bassinet ne contenait pas des microbes anaérobies. En milieux aérobies nous avons isolé des bacilles, des micrococques et un streptocoque qui ne correspondent pas aux espèces pathogènes connues.

Dans un troisième cas nous avons isolé d'un abcès parenchymateux d'un rein tuberculeux, sans communication avec le bassinet, un bacille anaérobie indéterminé. Ce microorganisme se trouvait en petite quantité. L'existence de ce microbe dans un foyer sans communication avec le bassinet présente de l'intérêt au point de vue du mode d'inoculation du rein par les anaérobies. Il est en effet fort probable que l'infection, chez cette malade, s'est faite par la voie sanguine. Nous avons vu d'ailleurs, à propos des abcès périnéaux, que les microbes anaérobies peuvent pénétrer dans la circulation générale et se fixer dans une autre partie de l'organisme pour constituer un foyer secondaire.

Nous noterons enfin que dans aucun de nos trois cas de tuberculose, nous n'avons trouvé dans le pus le bacille de Koch et que dans tous les trois les inoculations du pus aux cobayes sont restées négatives les animaux n'étant pas devenus tuberculeux.

### D. *Abcès périnéphrétique*

Nous n'avons pu examiner qu'un seul cas d'abcès périnéphrétique. Chez notre malade (obs. 42) l'abcès était consécutif à l'infection du rein. Le pus de cet abcès contenait, à l'état de pureté, le coli-bacille en abondance.

L'ensemble de nos observations sur les suppurations rénales et péri-rénales ne nous permet pas de conclusions définitives. Nous pouvons pourtant dire que ces suppurations peuvent être dues à des microbes aérobies seuls (coli, staphylocoques, streptocoques), à des organismes exclusivement anaérobies, ou aux associations de ces deux ordres de microbes. Le rôle des anaérobies paraît ici moins important que dans les suppurations péri-urétrales, mais il paraît probable que ces microbes ont une action prépondérante, lorsqu'il existe des phénomènes gangreneux. En ce qui regarde la fétidité du pus nous ferons observer que, deux fois, cette fétidité existait sans organismes anaérobies : dans un cas l'agent pathogène était le coli-bacille et dans l'autre le staphylocoque doré.

Nous avons jusqu'à ce jour étudié 42 cas d'infections urinaires à localisations variées et nous sommes arrivés à cette conviction, que de l'urètre au rein l'étude des infections urinaires est à refaire en tenant compte des infections anaérobies à côté de celles déterminées par les microbes aérobies, seules étudiées avant nos travaux.

Dans toutes les parties de l'appareil urinaire, les infections anaéro-bies, seules ou associées aux infections aérobies, peuvent jouer un rôle important, souvent même prépondérant ou exclusif. Des recher-ches ultérieures pourront seules nous apprendre le rôle, dans chaque variété d'infection, des différentes espèces de chaque groupe aérobie et anaérobie et de leurs différentes asociations.

D'une manière très générale on peut dire aujourd'hui :

1° Les microbes anaérobies peuvent déterminer seuls ou associés aux aérobies des infections urinaires bénignes.

2° Ils jouent un rôle prépondérant ou exclusif dans presque toutes, sinon dans toutes les infections graves, surtout dans les infections diffuses, à tendance gangreneuse.

# DES NÉVROPATHIES ET PSYCHOPATHIES URINAIRES

par M. le docteur Barthélemy GUISY,

Professeur agrégé à la Faculté de Médecine d'Athènes.

Comme vous savez, savants confrères, l'état physique et l'anatomie physiologique des organes génitaux et urinaires contribuent beaucoup à maintenir l'équilibre entre les facultés intellectuelles et corporelles ; cet équilibre entre les deux systèmes chez les personnes des deux sexes, héréditairement prédisposées aux névroses ou à l'hystérie, peut, mais pas toujours, se rompre dès qu'une affection quelconque des organes urinaires ou génitaux apparaît. Alors on voit éclater des accès d'hystérie ou des crises nerveuses très caractéristiques tandis qu'elles n'avaient jamais eu de manifestations nerveuses ou hystériques jusqu'au moment même, où la maladie s'est déclarée.

Permettez-moi de vous dire quelques mots seulement sur les névropathies et psychopathies, qui peuvent se développer chez les urinaires prédisposés, dès qu'une affection des organes urinaires, des deux sexes, a lieu. Les urinaires donc peuvent être atteints des diverses névroses et surtout d'hystérie, ou d'hystéro-neurasthénie, des attaques convulsives complètes ou incomplètes, des convulsions générales ou partielles avec ou sans prodromes, des troubles psychiques et d'hallucinations, des troubles de la motilité, c'est-à-dire de tremblements, de secousses, des contractures et des paralysies.

*Chez les urinaires*, les manifestations nerveuses éclatent plutôt brusquement et souvent sans prodromes. Au contraire, chez les individus atteints d'une maladie génitale, les manifestations nerveuses, ou des crises hystériques se développent plutôt progressivement, sauf quelques cas rares, dans lesquels on voit des accès éclater brusquement.

Chez les prédisposés urinaires, les manifestations nerveuses consistent en un changement du caractère, en une mélancolie, mais souvent l'affection urinaire et surtout de la vessie provoque, chez les personnes prédisposées, des accès nerveux, ou hystériques, ou des désordres psychiques, brusques et subits, de sorte que nous voyons des accès ou des crises violentes, ou délirantes pendant lesquelles elles peuvent involontairement commettre des actions méchantes, des crimes même, des accidents funestes, ou enfin le suicide. Au contraire, chez les personnes d'origine névropathe ou hystérique une lésion des organes génitaux peut provoquer des troubles des facultés

intellectuelles ou psychiques produisant ordinairement un changement de caractère variable selon la personne, une répugnance, une
négligence dans la besogne habituelle, ou dans la mise, une mélancolie sans cause apparente, une agitation, une humeur querelleuse et
quelquefois, mais rarement, une vraie folie sympathique.

Chez les urinaires, les troubles nerveux ou psychiques disparaissent
ordinairement avec l'affection urinaire; au contraire, chez les malades
des organes génitaux, les manifestations nerveuses ou hystériques
ordinairement durent un peu plus après la guérison de la maladie
génitale et quelquefois même ne disparaissent pas complètement, ou
pas du tout.

Chez les urinaires, une lésion insignifiante quelquefois, peut commettre des accidents funestes et graves.

Comment peut-on se rendre compte de l'apparition des troubles
nerveux ou des psychopathies chez les urinaires?

On peut accepter que ces manifestations nerveuses ou psychiques
se développent chez les urinaires à cause de leur état mental, à cause
de la crainte que leur inspire leur maladie, ne pouvant uriner qu'à
l'aide d'une sonde, ou à cause de leur dysurie, qui les contraint à
éviter la société et les amusements, etc. On peut accepter que
l'apparition des troubles nerveux et surtout ceux de forme convulsive, s'expliquent mieux par la toxicité des urines (Tison, Barré,
Bouchard, Voisin et Cathelineau). Mais pour expliquer mieux toutes
les manifestations nerveuses, hystériques, les accès psychiques délirants et hallucinatoires je crois qu'il faut faire la conclusion suivante.
Une excitation des filets nerveux sensitifs de la muqueuse des voies
urinaires et surtout de la muqueuse vésicale se transmet de celle-ci
au grand sympathique et par les branches communiquant à la moelle
épinière, d'où l'incitation se transmet à la moelle allongée, où comme
vous savez bien, se trouve le centre des convulsions générales; de là
donc s'explique la production des convulsions générales épilepti-
formes chez les urinaires. Ou il peut arriver que l'incitation de la
moelle allongée se porte aux hémisphères cérébraux, à la zone psychique; de là s'explique la production des troubles psychiques, des
accès délirants, hallucinatoires, etc. Ou il peut arriver aussi que l'incitation se porte jusqu'à la zone motrice ou corticale de l'encéphale,
où comme vous savez bien, se localisent les divers centres corticaux
*psychomoteurs* et *psychosensoriels*. L'excitation donc de cette zone
motrice peut provoquer des convulsions partielles, ou générales, épi-
leptiformes, des contractions, des tremblements, etc. (*Guisy, Rhigas
Nicolaïdès.*)

### Névroses et psychopathies chez les calculeux.

1ᵉʳ Cas. Un calculeux d'origine névropathique, âgé de 45 ans, célibataire; il fut atteint d'une amyosthénie des membres inférieurs et surtout du côté gauche. Après la taille suspubienne fut complètement guéri. Ce malade jusqu'à la déclaration de sa maladie n'avait jamais eu de manifestations nerveuses.

2ᵉ Cas. Une femme mariée, âgée de 52 ans, calculeuse, n'ayant jamais eu des manifestations nerveuses avant sa maladie; elle fut prise d'une mélancolie passagère, qui disparut complètement après l'enlèvement de la pierre.

5ᵉ Cas. Un enfant d'origine névropathe, âgé de 15 ans, calculeux, fut pris des accès du délire maniaque, pendant lesquels il frappait sa mère avec tout ce qui se trouvait devant lui. Un jour pendant l'accès, a pris un couteau de table et a blessé sa mère à la jambe. Après la taille pour enlever la pierre tout est disparu, l'enfant est devenu calme, sombre.

4ᵉ Cas. Un enfant, âgé de 14-15 ans, italien, calculeux aussi et d'origine hystérique, fut atteint d'une pseudo-méningite tuberculeuse hystérique, c'est-à-dire nous avons observé céphalagie intense, vomissements, constipation et surtout convulsions partielles, avec perte de connaissance, des contractions du bras gauche et des convulsions des globes oculaires, la température variait entre 37-37². Après l'enlèvement de la pierre par la taille le petit malade fut complètement débarrassé de l'accès hystérique.

5ᵉ Cas. Un jeune homme, âgé de 22 ans, étudiant, calculeux; il est tombé dans une mélancolie complète et il a laissé ses études scientifiques. Après l'opération pour enlever la pierre le malade fut complètement guéri.

6ᵉ Cas. Un calculeux, âgé de 65 ans, célibataire, fut atteint d'*une paraplégie complète flasque*, de sorte qu'il ne pouvait plus se lever de son lit. Après la cystotomie le malade a repris ses forces progressivement et il a pu après marcher comme s'il n'avait rien eu.

7ᵉ Cas. Un prêtre, calculeux, âgé de 59 ans, fut atteint subitement d'une attaque convulsive épileptiforme. Après l'enlèvement de la pierre le malade fut complètement guéri. Le malade avant l'accès, n'avait jamais rien eu. Sa fille mariée était très hystérique. Le malade lui-même était hystérique l'examen ophtalmoscopique a démontré un rétrécissement bilatéral du champ visuel.

### Manifestations nerveuses et psychopathies chez les malades atteints de la tuberculisation de la vessie.

8ᵉ Cas. Un grand et riche négociant d'éponges, âgé de 37 ans, marié, atteint de tuberculose vésicale, fut plongé dans une mélancolie profonde pendant laquelle il avait des crises maniaques avec des idées de suicide. Le malade après la cystostomie fut guéri de ses accès nerveux.

9ᵉ Cas. Un garçon de brasserie, âgé de 52 ans, atteint de la cystite tuberculeuse, fut pris des accès mélancoliques et délirantes (délire hallucinatoire) et surtout la nuit. Je lui proposai la cystostomie, mais malheureusement depuis ce jour je ne l'ai plus revu. Un cousin du malade était mort fou.

### Névropathies et psychopathies chez les rétrécis urétraux.

10° Cas. Un vieillard, âgé de 65 ans, maçon, rétréci (rétrécissement traumatique) fut pris d'un *tremblement fort et continuel* durant pendant la journée du *bras droit*, ainsi que du membre inférieur du même côté (forme hémiplégique) qui a duré jusqu'au jour même de l'opération (urétrotomie externe). Ce malade était hystérique avéré, il avait une hémianesthésie droite. L'épouse du malade me raconta que dès qu'il a été blessé au périnée (chute à califourchon) son mari fut plongé dans une mélancolie avec accès de délire hallucinatoire qui a disparu après le rétablissement de son urètre.

11° Cas. Un vieillard, âgé de 69-70 ans, vieux marin, rétréci traumatique fut atteint progressivement de la maladie de Parkinson (paralysie agitante). Malheureusement malgré l'urétrotomie externe, ces troubles nerveux n'ont pas été améliorés.

12° Cas. Un vieux rétréci, âgé de 59 ans, fut atteint des évanouissements avec perte de connaissance de courte durée. Par la dilatation de l'urètre tout a disparu. Le même malade trois ans après, le rétrécissement étant revenu, a commencé de nouveau à avoir les mêmes troubles nerveux, la dilatation de l'urètre a fait disparaître ces accès nerveux.

13° Cas. Un italien, âgé de 37 ans, grand buveur, d'origine névropathe, rétréci (rétrécissement blennorrhagique), après un grand abus de bière, fut atteint d'une ischurie complète ; en même temps il fut pris d'un accès de délire maniaque pendant lequel il prit le rasoir pour s'ouvrir le ventre afin de donner issue à l'urine. Mais heureusement un de ses amis lui enleva le rasoir par lequel il avait déjà coupé profondément la peau sur une étendue oblique de 7 centimètres. Je fus invité et immédiatement je lui ponctionnai la vessie, laquelle était assez distendue. Tout de suite après, le malade s'est calmé et il est tombé dans un état léthargique, qui a duré quelques heures. Après l'urétrotomie interne le malade se portait très bien.

14° Cas. Un mécanicien, âgé de 55 ans, hystérique et syphilitique, rétréci aussi, fut pris subitement, au moment même où nous voulions faire passer une bougie fine par le point rétréci, du délire hallucinatoire. Il se leva brusquement debout sur le lit et se mit à parler à haute voix pendant quelques minutes croyant sans doute se trouver devant le public. Après étant descendu du lit il se mit à arpenter le bureau en marchant très vite et parlant toujours. Enfin quelques jours après, l'ayant chloroformé je lui ai fait l'urétrotomie interne qui fit complètement guérir le malade de ses accès psychiques et hallucinatoires.

15° Cas. Un homme, âgé de 52 ans, italien, rétréci aussi, fut atteint des manifestations de pseudo-ataxie, consistant dans une difficulté à marcher et dans une incontinence d'urine, qui coulait par goutte involontairement ; les réflexes rotuliens étaient normaux. L'urétrotomie interne a fait disparaître cet état nerveux.

16° Cas. Un jeune homme, âgé de 37 ans, garçon café, ayant été blessé au-dessus du pubis par une balle de revolver, qui a traversé la paroi abdominale et vésicale, fut plongé dans une profonde mélancolie avec accès hallucinatoires nocturnes. Après l'enlèvement de la balle du fond de la vessie par la taille suspubienne, le cerveau a repris son état normal. Le frère du malade s'est suicidé pendant un accès du délire.

17° Cas. Un célibataire, âgé de 44 ans, atteint d'une chaude-pisse très aiguë, s'est plongé dans une mélancolie avec des idées de suicide et même un jour pendant l'accès du délire il a voulu se jeter dans un puits. Après la guérison de la blennorrhagie le malade fut complètement débarrassé de ses troubles psychiques.

18° Cas. Une femme, mariée, âgée de 31 ans, hystérique avérée, pendant une cystite douloureuse blennorrhagique, fut atteinte d'une monoplégie brachiale droite, l'avant-bras et le poignet se contracturent en flexion, elle avait des points hyperesthésiques sur l'épaule droite et en même temps des points anesthésiques surtout à l'avant-bras du même côté. Cette femme était d'une famille hystérique avec la diathèse de contracture. La sœur aussi de ladite malade, pendant une commotion morale vive, fut prise d'un évanouissement avec perte de connaissance et immédiatement après d'une paralysie contracturée sous forme hémiplégique du membre supérieur ainsi que du membre inférieur droit avec hémianesthésie.

19° Cas. Une femme mariée, âgée de 35 ans, atteinte d'une cystite intense blennorrhagique, contractée de son mari, fut plongée dans une profonde mélancolie avec accès de suicide. Un jour même pendant un accès du délire elle prit du fard, mais heureusement elle fut sauvée par nous. La malade après la guérison de la cystite n'avait plus rien.

20° Cas. Un homme âgé de 56 ans, libraire, atteint d'une cystite du col de la vessie de cause blennorrhagique, fut pris subitement du *blépharospasme tonique non douloureux, monolatéral* droit, après une instillation par une solution de nitrate d'argent 1 : 50 au col vésical, le malade fut atteint du spasme clonique facial, continuel du même côté, de sorte que la commissure droite de la bouche se tirait fortement en arrière, l'aile du nez aussi se relevait fortement du côté droit. Le malade après quelques instillations et un traitement général s'est complètement débarrassé de sa maladie et de ses accès nerveux.

21° Cas. Dernièrement un homme, âgé de 45-48 ans, d'Égypte, marié depuis 18 ans et père des deux enfants, ayant contracté la chaude-pisse fut pris d'une jalousie de sa femme, de sorte qu'il croyait que celle-ci avait des amants, et de plus il s'en doutait de la paternité de son dernier enfant. Et bien le malade d'origine névropathique, jusqu'au moment même de sa blennorrhagie il n'avait jamais eu des manifestations nerveuses.

22° Cas.-Dernièrement aussi nous avons observé trois individus, atteints de la gravelle urique. Chez l'un nous avons observé un seul changement du caractère

23° Cas. Chez l'autre une mélancolie alternée des accès du délire hallucinatoire surtout nocturne.

24° Cas. Chez le troisième cas, qui était un enfant de 15 ans, prêté par le docteur Gianniris, d'Athènes, avéré hystérique, s'étaient remarqué des troubles nerveux, déclarés par des accès rhythmiques choréiformes, alternés des accès d'aphonie, d'astasie (ἀστασίας) et d'abasie (ἀβασίας). Les mêmes accès hystériques avaient trois ans avant sa gravelle, lorsqu'il était enfermé dans une maison de santé.

---

## TOXICITÉ DE L'URINE ET IMMUNISATION. RECHERCHES EXPÉRIMENTALES

### par M. le docteur C. BRUNI,

de Naples.

Depuis quelque temps nous poursuivons dans le laboratoire de M. de Giaxa des recherches pour voir si avec des injections répétées et progressivement croissantes il est possible d'arriver à faire supporter à des animaux des doses d'urine, mortelles pour des animaux neufs de la même espèce.

Comme animaux d'expériences nous nous sommes servis de lapins auxquels nous injections leur propre urine, que nous avons eu soin de recueillir avec des sondes stérilisées. Toutes les fois que nous avions besoin de grandes quantités d'urines nous pratiquions le cathétérisme toutes les deux ou trois heures, et nous avions soin de garder à la glacière les quantités d'urines retirées jusqu'à ce que nous eussions la dose nécessaire. Il est bien entendu qu'avant de faire l'injection, l'urine était filtrée et portée à la température de 57-58°.

Nous avons fait des expériences soit en injectant l'urine dans les veines, soit dans le péritoine. En moyenne la dose mortelle pour l'injection intraveineuse varie entre 16-24 c. c. par kilogr. de lapin : quand on injecte l'urine dans la cavité péritonéale, la dose mortelle varie entre 60 et 90 c. c. par kilogr. Par la voie intra-veineuse il est extrêmement difficile d'arriver à faire supporter aux animaux une dose mortelle d'urine. A la suite des injections de doses progressivement croissantes faites en vue de les accoutumer, les animaux maigrissent considérablement, présentent dans la presque totalité des cas une paralysie du train postérieur et meurent avant d'être arrivés à supporter la dose mortelle.

Sur 50 lapins qui ont reçu des injections intra-veineuses, 7 seulement sont arrivés à supporter des doses variables entre 20 et 25 c. c.

c'est-à-dire des doses de 2 à 7 c. c. supérieures à la dose mortelle moyenne. Aucun de ces lapins n'a survécu définitivement. Tous ceux qui étaient arrivés à supporter des doses mortelles et supérieures ont fini, après un temps plus ou moins long, par mourir cachectiques et en présentant la paralysie caractéristique.

Sur 40 lapins injectés par la voie intra-péritonéale, 9 seulement sont morts avant d'être arrivés à supporter la dose mortelle ; parmi les 31 qui ont résisté, il y en a qui sont arrivés à supporter des doses de 120 à 150 c. c., c'est-à-dire presque deux fois la dose mortelle. Les animaux témoins qui recevaient de pareilles doses de 120 à 150 c. c. mouraient très rapidement après quelques heures.

A la suite des injections intra-péritonéales, quand il s'agit des petites doses jusqu'à 10 ou 20 c. c. les animaux ne présentent aucun trouble apparent ; pour des doses plus élevées ils présentent de la dyspnée, de la somnolence, des secousses, refusent la nourriture, mais un ou deux jours après ils sont complètement rétablis. La diminution de poids n'est pas considérable ; seulement les animaux qui ont succombé en voie d'immunisation ont présenté la cachexie et la paralysie qui est à peu près la règle générale, quand on injecte l'urine dans les veines.

Les animaux habitués aux injections intra-péritonéales supportent facilement les injections intra-veineuses des doses une fois et même une fois et demie mortelles sans présenter que des accidents très légers et très passagers. Le sérum des animaux ainsi traités est capable de préserver des lapins neufs contre une injection intra-veineuse de la dose mortelle d'urine. Trois lapins qui avaient reçu préalablement et respectivement dans le péritoine 12, 15, 18 c. c. de sérum ont parfaitement et définitivement résisté à l'injection intra-veineuse d'une dose d'urine, qui a tué les animaux témoins dans quelques heures.

Les faits que nous venons d'exposer démontrent que des lapins habitués peu à peu, par des injections répétées et progressivement croissantes d'urine, peuvent arriver à supporter des doses une fois et même deux fois mortelles pour des animaux neufs de la même espèce. Cette accoutumance, cette immunité, difficile à obtenir quand on injecte l'urine directement dans les veines, on l'obtient au contraire assez facilement par les injections intra-péritonéales. Le sérum des lapins immunisés contre des doses mortelles d'urine est capable de préserver les lapins neufs contre l'injection des doses mortelles. Nos expériences ne nous permettent pas pour le moment d'aborder la question du mécanisme biologique de l'action antitoxique du sérum anti-urineux. Il est certain que dans l'urine doivent se trouver des produits toxiques variés et la mort des animaux est probablement due à l'action combinée de ces différents produits. On peut donc admettre que certains de ces produits toxiques provoquent chez les animaux immunisés la formation d'antitoxine spécifique et par conséquent le sérum préserve les animaux en neutralisant une partie de ces produits et en diminuant par cela la toxicité générale de l'urine.

Les recherches ultérieures nous permettront, nous voulons l'espérer, de résoudre cette question.

---

## LES PROGRÈS DE LA PETITE CHIRURGIE DES VOIES URINAIRES

### par M. le docteur LAVAUX.

Ancien interne des hopitaux. Professeur libre de pathologie des voies urinaires à l'Université de Paris.

Messieurs,

Permettez-moi tout d'abord d'adresser mes sincères félicitations aux organisateurs du XIIIᵉ Congrès international de médecine et tout particulièrement à l'éminent président de ce Congrès, M. le professeur Lannelongue. C'est une heureuse idée d'avoir créé une section de chirurgie urinaire, ce qui permet aux chirurgiens compétents de mieux montrer l'état actuel de cette chirurgie.

Je regrette seulement que la petite chirurgie des voies urinaires n'ait pas eu l'honneur d'un rapport; car, si le commencement du xixᵉ siècle a vu apparaître la lithotritie, cette merveilleuse opération de Civiale, si la deuxième moitié de ce siècle a vu commencer, avec Gustave Simon (de Heidelberg) et se développer ces audacieuses et heureuses opérations sur le rein et les voies urinaires supérieures, on peut dire que la fin du xixᵉ siècle a vu surtout le triomphe de la petite chirurgie des voies urinaires.

Des progrès considérables ont été, en effet, réalisés en France depuis une quinzaine d'années dans la pratique de cette petite chirurgie, ce qui a permis d'en étendre beaucoup les indications. Aujourd'hui, elle peut revendiquer l'immense majorité des interventions dans le traitement des rétrécissements organiques de l'urèthre et la presque totalité des interventions dans le traitement des diverses variétés de la cystite, même de la cystite tuberculeuse.

La petite chirurgie des voies urinaires, quoi qu'en pensent certains chirurgiens s'occupant principalement de chirurgie générale, reste encore le traitement de choix dans la grande majorité des cas où une intervention est nécessaire chez les prostatiques.

Unie au traitement médical, elle réduit de plus en plus le nombre des cas où une opération sanglante est nécessaire dans les affections rénales, surtout dans la tuberculose des voies urinaires supérieures et dans les diverses variétés de l'urétéro-pyélo-néphrite.

Inutile de dire que les interventions nécessitées par l'inflammation de l'urèthre sont entièrement de son domaine, en dehors de quelques complications, d'ailleurs exceptionnelles, lorsque les malades sont soumis dès le début de l'affection à un traitement rationnel.

Cette question présente donc un grand intérêt au point de vue pratique. Aussi, je vous prie, messieurs, de vouloir bien m'accorder toute votre bienveillante attention.

C'est le lavage méthodique de l'urèthre antérieur, pratiqué avec ma petite sonde à double courant, puis l'anesthésie directe des voies urinaires inférieures et le lavage de la vessie sans sonde, réalisés par les procédés que j'ai décrits, qui ont été le point de départ des progrès obtenus dans la petite chirurgie des voies urinaires. Les beaux travaux de Pasteur trouvaient dès lors une application simple et facile, même chez les rétrécis, dans le traitement des infections des voies urinaires. En même temps, le traitement préventif de la fièvre urineuse, cette redoutable complication des affections des voies urinaires, qui avait causé jusque-là tant de déceptions aux chirurgiens les plus habiles et les plus compétents, était désormais établi sur des bases scientifiques solides et réalisé, même chez les rétrécis, par des moyens d'une extrême simplicité. L'antisepsie directe des voies urinaires inférieures peut, en effet, depuis 1886, grâce aux lavages antiseptiques de la cavité uréthro-vésicale pratiqués sans sonde, être effectuée chez les rétrécis comme chez les urinaires dont le calibre de l'urèthre est normal.

Chez tous ces malades, aucun point de la muqueuse de l'urèthre et de la muqueuse de la vessie ne peut échapper au contact du liquide antiseptique injecté par ce procédé.

C'est également ce procédé des injections uréthro-vésicales pratiquées sans sonde qui m'a permis de réaliser, en 1887, d'une façon simple et absolument inoffensive l'anesthésie directe de la muqueuse des voies urinaires inférieures, considérée jusque-là par les chirurgiens les plus habiles et les plus compétents comme irréalisable. Aussi le traitement local des cystites, même les plus douloureuses, est-il devenu dès lors d'une grande simplicité et d'une merveilleuse efficacité.

La fréquence des mictions dues à une hyperesthésie de la muqueuse des voies urinaires inférieures a pu aussi être diagnostiquée d'une façon précise et traitée d'une manière rationnelle, car il suffisait de rechercher ensuite pour la combattre la cause de cette hyperesthésie.

En supprimant les réflexes ayant pour point de départ la sensibilité superficielle de la muqueuse des voies urinaires inférieures, l'anesthésie de cette muqueuse a permis encore de faire cesser un grand nombre de spasmes de l'urèthre et de la vessie. Ce résultat, si précieux dans le diagnostic et le traitement de diverses affections des voies urinaires inférieures, avait tout particulièrement frappé M. le professeur Alfred Richet, membre de l'Institut, qui ne me ménagea point, à cette époque, ses flatteurs et bien sincères éloges.

C'est une étude plus approfondie de la physiologie du sphincter uréthral qui m'a permis, tout en réalisant le lavage méthodique de l'urèthre antérieur, de diagnostiquer d'une façon précise le siège des lésions dans l'uréthrite aiguë et dans l'uréthrite chronique. J'insiste sur ce point, car le procédé auquel je fais allusion est le seul qui donne une réelle précision au diagnostic et aux indications opératoires. Le traitement de l'uréthrite chronique postérieure nécessite, en effet, un manuel opératoire tout différent de celui auquel on a recours pour guérir l'uréthrite chronique antérieure.

On sait avec quelle rapidité se sont vulgarisés les travaux que j'ai publiés sur cette question, avec quelle facilité on obtient aujourd'hui la guérison de l'uréthrite chronique dans la grande majorité des cas. Mais on oublie encore quelquefois de faire un diagnostic précis, de recourir au manuel opératoire logiquement indiqué, d'où une longueur insolite du traitement et parfois de véritables échecs.

Les progrès de la petite chirurgie des voies urinaires appliquée au traitement des rétrécissements organiques de l'urèthre méritent également une mention toute spéciale.

En effet, le lavage de l'urèthre et le lavage de la vessie sans sonde, en permettant de réaliser chez les rétrécis l'antisepsie directe des voies urinaires inférieures, a considérablement simplifié le traitement des strictures uréthrales.

Dès 1889, au IV^e Congrès français de chirurgie, j'ai prouvé que presque tous les rétrécissements organiques de l'urèthre peuvent être dilatés jusqu'au n° 10 ou 11, d'où la suppression presque totale des indications des interventions sanglantes d'urgence chez les rétrécis. Ainsi s'est trouvé notablement agrandi le champ de la dilatation, en même temps que se perfectionnaient deux procédés puissants, qui se partagent aujourd'hui la presque totalité des indications opératoires dans le traitement des strictures organiques de l'urèthre : la divulsion progressive et l'électrolyse linéaire double.

Mais c'est le traitement de la cystite qui a surtout bénéficié des progrès de la petite chirurgie des voies urinaires. Quelle merveilleuse simplicité il présente aujourd'hui, ce traitement! Quelle efficacité! Quel contraste avec le vieux traitement du catarrhe vésical et même avec le traitement par le procédé des instillations, procédé douloureux et si peu efficace dans les cas graves que l'on était obligé, à l'époque où j'ai soutenu ma thèse, de pratiquer la taille pour apporter un peu de soulagement à ces malheureux malades!

L'anesthésie directe de la muqueuse de l'urèthre postérieur et de la muqueuse de la vessie rend d'autant plus de services dans le traitement de la cystite, surtout de la cystite dite douloureuse, qu'elle ne supprime pas le besoin d'uriner, comme je l'ai montré, en 1889, au Congrès de thérapeutique.

Il en résulte que le lavage de la vessie sans sonde peut être pratiqué après cette anesthésie sans que l'on ait à redouter la distension du réservoir urinaire. Or, on sait combien il est important, chez les malades atteints de cystite, surtout de cystite douloureuse, d'éviter la distension vésicale lorsqu'on a recours, pour obtenir la guérison de cette affection, aux lavages vésicaux, mode de traitement reconnu depuis plus d'un siècle comme le seul logique.

Mais je ne veux pas abuser, messieurs, de votre bienveillante attention.

Je ne rappellerai pas comment les progrès réalisés dans la pratique de la petite chirurgie des voies urinaires ont permis de rendre inoffensif le cathétérisme chez les prostatiques à la troisième période; comment ils ont rendu possible le diagnostic précoce de l'uretéro-pyélo-néphrite; comment ils ont contribué à obtenir la guérison de cette affection dans des cas considérés, il y a quelques années à peine, comme incurables; comment ils ont permis d'améliorer le traitement palliatif des néoplasmes vésicaux; comment ils ont restreint les indications opératoires dans le traitement de la tuberculose urinaire, indications aujourd'hui exceptionnelles lorsque les malades sont soumis de bonne heure à une médication rationnelle.

En terminant, je crois pouvoir, messieurs, sans manquer à la courtoisie, insister sur ce fait que tous les progrès qui viennent d'être rappelés ont été réalisés en France et affirmer catégoriquement sur ce point la supériorité de la science française.

## SUR LES PRINCIPES DU TRAITEMENT DES NEURASTHÉNIQUES GÉNITO-URINAIRES

par M. le docteur BERTHOLD GOLDBERG,

de Wildungen et Cologne.

Quant au traitement, il faut faire une différence entre trois catégories de maladies nerveuses fonctionnelles des organes génito-urinaires.

### I

Dans la première il faut ranger ceux qui ont, outre la neurasthénie, une maladie sérieuse, par exemple une blennorragie encore infectieuse, un rétrécissement très serré, une rétention d'urine. Dans ces cas-là il faut traiter la maladie principale en ne prenant regard de la neurasthénie que pour s'abstenir des méthodes trop énergiques, des méthodes douloureuses, des méthodes épuisantes. La guérison de la maladie, soit causale de la neurasthénie, soit concomitante, soit accidentelle, sera d'une influence heureuse aussi pour la guérison de la neurose.

### II

Dans le deuxième groupe je mets les malades, qui ont seulement un état anormal ou un reste insignifiant d'une maladie antérieure: neurasthénie urinaire, avec prostatite chronique légère, pas plus infectieuse, ou avec une infiltration sous-muqueuse de l'urètre non rétrécissante; ou pollakiurie psychopathique chez un homme ayant une prostate un peu plus enveloppée; ou impuissance relative chez un mari, qui avait à propos de sa chaudepisse ancienne une spermatocystite, etc.

Vu que dans la plupart des cas ces abnormités et ces restes existent sans aucune trace de neurose, vu que souvent guérissent les restes sans que guérisse néanmoins la neurose, vu qu'enfin la maladie nerveuse passe sans aucune amélioration des états abnormes: je ne suis point d'avis 'qu'il faut traiter localement ces petites affections chez les neurasthéniques. C'est la règle que nous ne pouvons pas faire évanouir les flocons urétraux ou les bosselures prostatiques ou les petites irrégularités du jet absolument; l'échec d'un traitement local, surtout longtemps continué, aggravera la neurasthénie d'une manière malheureuse.

Seulement si nous sommes sûrs d'un succès visible pour le malade, nous sommes autorisés de faire un traitement local de ces affections concomitantes de la neurose uro-génitale. Si nous pouvons faire s'éclaircir les urines contenant des microbes subitement par l'urotropine si nous pouvons faire s'évanouir une goutte matinale par une série de grands lavages, eh bien, la fin de la neurose ne sera pas loin.

N'oublions jamais qu'il y a toujours *deux* causes d'une neurose génito-urinaire : l'une, c'est la lésion locale existante, l'autre c'est la faiblesse du système nerveux, soit congénitale, soit acquise ; cette dernière est la cause principale.

Enfin on me dira, ces faux urinaires *veulent* être traités localement.

Eh bien : ou c'est un hystérique ; plus vous lui dilaterez l'urètre, plus vous lui masserez la prostate, plus il aura le désir de la méthode la plus nouvelle pour sa maladie très intéressante ; ou c'est un hypocondriaque : alors il sera mieux de lui prendre les auto-suggestions toujours dirigées vers le point génito-urinaire par une suggestion lente opposée que de lui donner encore plus l'occasion d'observer les accidents et l'échec d'un traitement dirigé vers les organes en question. Encore je rappelle les cas, où ces malades ont fait l'abus des dilatations et d'autres procédés intra-urétraux faits par les médecins comme aphrodisiaques.

## III

Dans la troisième catégorie il faut ranger les neurasthénies génito-urinaires « pures » des hommes ayant des voies urinaires saines.

Vous avez là le jeune homme se croyant impuissant, après s'être masturbé beaucoup et après avoir échoué dans ses tentatives premières du coït ; vous avez le malade qui ne peut jamais pisser en présence de quelqu'un : spasme du muscle sphincter urétro-vésical ; vous avez les individus affectés de la pollakiurie psychopathique ; vous avez là enfin les malades qui ne présentent que des symptômes des nerfs sensitivo-génito-urinaires.

Tous ces faux urinaires et tous ces faux impuissants, vous les pourrez traiter localement, contrairement à la deuxième catégorie. Car par un traitement bien fait, doucement, soigneusement, aseptiquement, vous ne pourrez nuir en rien ; j'ai guéri une partie de ces malades, c'est-à-dire ceux qui n'avaient pas encore des irradiations graves dans la sphère cérébro-spinale, par la suggestion pure en faisant la faradisation recto-abdominale ou lumbo-abdominale.

En somme je ne suis pas partisan pour ces cas-là des méthodes compliquées ou d'une durée longue, c'est-à-dire des distensions de la vessie dans la pollakiurie psychopathique, ou des électrisations intra-urétrales ou intra-vésicales ; enfin j'ai observé des aggravations terribles des neurasthénies urétro-prostatiques — fonctionnelles purement — par des cautérisations endoscopiques de l'urètre prostatique faites par des médecins très habiles dans les artifices endoscopiques ; ce n'était donc point la conséquence d'une faute dans la technique.

---

## DES TROUBLES VÉSICAUX D'ORIGINE NEURASTHÉNIQUE
## ET DE LEUR TRAITEMENT PAR L'ÉLECTRICITÉ

### par M. le docteur DENIS COURTADE,

de Paris.

Le système nerveux peut déterminer dans le fonctionnement des voies urinaires des troubles de plusieurs sortes.

1. Les uns tiennent à une affection organique du système nerveux cérébro-médullaire (ataxie locomotrice, myélite syphilitique.)

2. Les autres sont de nature purement dynamique et se rencontrent dans les différentes névroses (neurasthénie, épilepsie, hystérie.)

Ces maladies occupent une grande place dans les affections des voies génito-urinaires et les sujets qui en sont atteints forment la majeure partie des malades que M. le professeur Guyon a si bien étudiés sous le nom de *faux urinaires*.

Nous aurons à nous occuper dans cette communication des malades du deuxième groupe, surtout de ceux que l'on désigne sous le nom de neurasthéniques.

Il convient d'abord de faire ressortir que, parmi les maladies du système nerveux à siège non encore déterminé et pouvant avoir une localisation génito-urinaire, la neurasthénie occupe de beaucoup le premier rang : l'hystérie ne vient que de très loin à sa suite. Cette différence si grande est facile à expliquer si on considère l'état psychique si différent de ces deux maladies. Le caractère du neurasthénique n'est pas du tout le même que celui de l'hystérique. Ce dernier n'a que peu ou pas de préoccupations mentales : il est anesthésique sans le savoir ; s'il est paralysé ou contracturé cela ne le préoccupe en général que médiocrement et les diverses affections se portant sur les organes génito-urinaires n'agissent pas défavorablement sur son esprit.

Il n'en est pas de même pour le neurasthénique. Le moindre symptôme l'inquiète ; son attention psychique est constamment tournée vers les symptômes physiologiques anormaux, et souvent des phénomènes tout naturels sont pris par lui pour pathologiques. Tout ce qui se passe dans sa sphère génito-urinaire a surtout le don d'attirer vivement son attention et il n'est pas étonnant qu'avec un caractère aussi pessimiste, des symptômes, quelquefois insignifiants, ne prennent tout à coup dans son esprit une importance considérable. Les préoccupations qui en sont la suite entretiennent ou même augmentent l'état neurasthénique déjà existant et, chez certains sujets prédisposés, on peut même voir la névrose jusque-là latente, faire son apparition, comme, par exemple, à la suite d'une blennorragie tardant à guérir complètement.

La neurasthénie peut se localiser sur chacune des parties de l'arbre urinaire. Je ne m'occuperai que de ses déterminations vésicales. J'ai pu, soit dans le service d'électrothérapie de la clinique, soit dans ma clientèle, en étudier un grand nombre et on peut les diviser en deux groupes, suivant que la *sensibilité* ou *la motilité* sont en cause.

Je ne saurais en donner ici une description complète qui ferait double emploi avec les études publiées sur ce sujet par M. le professeur Guyon et ses élèves, en particulier les docteurs Janet et Genouville. J'insisterai seulement sur certaines particularités présentées par les troubles moteurs vésicaux.

Ces derniers consistent le plus souvent dans une parésie vésicale plus ou moins accusée, mais allant rarement jusqu'à la paralysie. Cette parésie se dénote surtout :

*a*. Par la mise en action difficile de la miction ;

*b*. Par le peu de force du jet ;

*c*. Par des phénomènes manométriques particuliers, très bien étudiés par le D$^r$ Genouville et sur lesquels j'insisterai un instant.

Chez l'individu à l'état normal, les envies d'uriner, les douleurs à la distention et la pression manométrique intra-vésicale marchent de pair et sont en raison directe. Dans les cas de neurasthénie vésicale il n'en est plus de même. Le D$^r$ Genouville a trouvé une dissociation presque constante, d'une part entre les envies d'uriner et les douleurs de l'autre contre la pression vésicale examinée au manomètre. Cette dernière peut être presque nulle alors que les premières sont quelquefois exagérées.

Quelle est la cause de cette dissociation ?

La dissociation entre les phénomènes fonctionnels et les phénomènes sensitifs doit être considérée comme un fait général chez les neurasthéniques, et correspond à la distinction que l'on fait en physiologie entre les réflexes de sensibilité spéciale ou fonctionnelle, et les réflexes de sensibilité générale. Chez les neurasthéniques il y a très souvent augmentation de ces derniers et au contraire diminution des réflexes fonctionnels : de là la dénomination de *faiblesse irritable* donnée autrefois comme caractérisant les phénomènes que présentaient les malades que nous appelons maintenant neurasthéniques. Si nous prenons, par exemple, les symptômes se produisant du côté du cerveau, nous voyons une émotivité particulièrement vive jointe à une incapacité quelquefois absolue du travail cérébral. Il en est de même du côté des fonctions digestives. L'estomac et les intestins sont paresseux ; les digestions longues et difficiles ; il y a affaiblissement des réflexes fonctionnels, tandis que l'on observe une exagération des réflexes douloureux caractérisée par de la douleur à la pression au creux épigastrique, des coliques, de la gastralgie, etc. Les mêmes phénomènes s'observent pour la vessie : il y a diminution des réflexes fonctionnels alliée à une exagération des réflexes de sensibilité générale : de là les douleurs quelquefois très vives observées en pratiquant la manométrie vésicale, alors que la pression ne monte pas ou presque pas.

La diminution des réflexes fonctionnels a ceci de spécial : c'est qu'elle n'est pas toujours accompagnée d'atonie vésicale vraie. La vessie ne réagit que peu à la distension, mais ne présente pas de résidu ; l'organe fonctionne d'une manière très paresseuse, mais se vide en général complètement. Lorsqu'il existe un résidu, il faut penser plutôt à une myélite commençante qu'à de la neurasthénie. Mes recherches manométriques sont sur ce point tout à fait d'accord avec celles de M. Genouville.

Ce défaut d'atonie vraie s'observe d'ailleurs aussi pour les maladies de l'estomac symptomatiques de la névrose. La dilatation proprement dite, celle qui persiste après la digestion terminée, ne se rencontre pas dans les formes légères de la neurasthénie stomacale, et dans les formes graves elle ne survient que tardivement (Proust et Ballet, *hygiène du neurasthénique*). Mais si la parésie vésicale neurasthénique n'arrive jamais d'elle-même jusqu'à la paralysie complète, cette dernière peut cependant survenir lorsque certaines causes viennent troubler le fonctionnement d'un organe aussi mal innervé. Ces paralysies, en général facilement curables, s'observent après un traumatisme local (accouchement) ou une distension exagérée des fibres musculaires soit à la suite d'une intervention thérapeutique (lavages) soit après une rétention volontaire trop longtemps prolongée. Elles peuvent aussi survenir à la suite d'une rétention aiguë dans le cours d'une maladie de la prostate ou de l'urètre (prostatite, congestion de la prostate, rétrécissement et spasme de l'urètre). Enfin elles peuvent être d'origine réflexe et succéder à un traumatisme accidentel ou opératoire portant sur un organe plus ou moins éloigné des voies génito-urinaires (neurasthénie traumatique.)

La diminution des réflexes fonctionnels et l'exagération des réflexes psychiques et de sensibilité générale interviennent encore comme facteurs de certaines pollakiuries. Le col de la vessie présente en effet une tonicité normale moindre. Par suite, l'urine entre plus facilement dans la portion prostatique de l'urètre, et, grâce à l'hyperexcitabilité habituelle de cette région chez ces malades, détermine par réflexe sensitif une contraction de la vessie.

Cette forme de pollakiurie peut s'accompagner le jour de fausses incontinences, car souvent le malade n'a pas le temps de contracter en temps voulu son sphincter externe. Cette pollakiurie cesse pendant le sommeil, parce que pendant sa durée, les réflexes psychiques et de sensibilité générale disparaissent.

On a signalé chez les neurasthéniques des incontinences nocturnes coïncidant ou non avec une pollakiurie diurne. Ces incontinences sont rares et il pourrait bien se faire que certaines d'entre elles ne fussent que des cas d'affection médullaire commençante compliquée d'état neurasthénique.

*Quel est le traitement électrique que l'on doit employer?*

1° Il faut agir d'abord d'une manière générale et donner le bain statique avec souffle sur la colonne vertébrale et la tête : on se trouvera bien de faire respirer l'air ozonisé qui se dégage des pointes. Les étincelles ne seront employées qu'avec ménagement, à moins d'avoir affaire à un neurasthénique déprimé. On peut aussi se servir avec·fruit des courants de haute fréquence.

2° On agira ensuite localement. Dans le cas de phénomènes douloureux le courant galvanique sera appliqué avec pôle positif actif sur le périné et une large plaque formant électrode indifférente, appliquée soit sur la région abdominale antérieure, soit au niveau des dernières vertèbres dorsales.

Dans le cas de phénomènes paralytiques, on peut électriser directement la vessie en employant le courant faradique de la bobine à gros fil, avec des intermittences lentes et le pôle négatif placé dans l'intérieur de la vessie remplie médiocrement d'eau salée à 7 pour 1000. Mais il est préférable, surtout en raison de la susceptibilité de ces malades à l'infection, d'agir d'une manière réflexe, en employant le courant faradique à fil fin et intermittences rapides, avec un pôle indifférent placé sur le ventre ou les dernières vertèbres dorsales et un pôle actif porté successivement sur le périnée et la paroi abdominale antérieure, au niveau des fosses iliaques droite et gauche. La même technique s'applique aux malades pollakiuriques.

Il est bien entendu que le traitement électrique doit être associé au traitement neurasthénique général (hydrothérapie, fer et arsenic).

*Quel est le résultat du traitement?* Les phénomènes soit moteurs, soit douloureux guérissent en général rapidement dans la neurasthénie simple. Les troubles moteurs sont ceux qui cèdent le plus rapidement et le plus sûrement, en particulier les pollakiuries et les rétentions dont nous avons expliqué plus haut la pathogénie. Les difficultés pour entamer la miction sont aussi vite améliorées. Les phénomènes douloureux résistent plus longtemps, mais finissent cependant par guérir.

Si les résultats sont, comme nous venons de le voir, excellents dans la neurasthénie simple, il est loin d'en être de même dans la forme constitutionnelle ou héréditaire de la névrose. On voit dans ce cas les stigmates ordinaires de la neurasthénie s'accompagner des stigmates dits de dégénérescence. Des préoccupations hypocondriaques, de véritables obsessions viennent alors compliquer le complexus symptomatique et prennent le pas soit sur les phénomènes moteurs, soit sur les phénomènes douloureux. Ces cas relèvent en grande partie du domaine de la pathologie mentale et l'électricité ne donne que de médiocres résultats, surtout dans les cas invétérés.

## COMMUNICATIONS RÉSUMÉES

### Un cas de bactériurie,

#### par M. NANU (de Bucarest).

Il s'agit d'une femme de 40 ans qui se plaignait uniquement de l'odeur pénétrante et repoussante de ses urines, sans autres troubles fonctionnels du côté des voies urinaires. La fétidité des urines datait depuis trois mois. Dans les antécédents, on trouve une constipation opiniâtre datant depuis l'enfance et des ménorragies. Enfin, il y a quatre ans la malade a eu une pyélo-néphrite calculeuse pour laquelle j'ai dû faire la néphrectomie. Détail important, elle n'a jamais été sondée depuis cette opération.

Un examen minutieux de cette femme m'assura que tous les organes étaient sains. Du côté des organes génitaux, il y avait seulement une métrite fongueuse. La vessie avait une capacité de 300 grammes, et, examinée au cystoscope, elle ne présentait pas le moindre indice d'inflammation.

L'urine récemment émise était nauséabonde. Au premier abord elle paraissait claire et ne présentait aucun trouble ; mais en l'examinant plus attentivement et en pleine lumière, on s'apercevait facilement qu'elle était légèrement troublée par d'innombrables corpuscules, comparables à des particules d'une poussière fine qui nageaient dans le liquide.

Les recherches microscopiques et bactériologiques ont démontré que les corpuscules scintillants n'étaient que des agglomérations de colibacilles. Il n'y avait pas d'autres microbes.

Comme traitement, je me suis adressé d'abord à la métrite et j'ai fait un curettage de la matrice. Ensuite, contre la fétidité des urines, j'ai administré du salol à l'intérieur et des lavages vésicaux avec le nitrate d'argent.

Après un mois de traitement, cette malade est sortie de l'hôpital manifestement améliorée, presque guérie.

Relativement à la cause de cette bactériurie, je pense que c'est la métrite qu'on doit incriminer.

Les microbes ont pris probablement la voie des vaisseaux lymphatiques pour arriver à la vessie. Ce serait le premier cas de bactériurie d'origine métritique.


## Traitement de la bactériurie par l'urotropine,

### par M. JULES JANET (de Paris).


La bactériurie est constituée par une fuite microbienne à travers le rein sa source est le plus souvent dans l'intestin ; elle est plus fréquente qu'on ne le croit généralement, on ne peut la reconnaître que par l'analyse immédiate de l'urine par centrifugation en ajoutant quelques gouttes d'ammoniaque à l'urine à centrifuger.

Elle est rebelle à tous les traitements chirurgicaux, lavages vésicaux et instillations, puisque sa source est en dehors de la vessie ; seuls les médicaments pris par la bouche peuvent la modifier, le salol à haute dose semble avoir une heureuse influence, mais on ne peut continuer longtemps son usage car il est trop irritant pour l'estomac et les reins.

L'urotropine, même à faible dose, 0$^{gr}$,25 à 0$^{gr}$,75 par cachets de 0$^{gr}$,25 pris aux repas, éclaircit immédiatement les urines bactériuriques et cela pendant aussi longtemps que dure la médication, le trouble reparaît du reste aussitôt qu'on en cesse l'usage. Mais ce médicament présente sur le salol l'avantage d'être parfaitement toléré par l'estomac et les reins.

Pour arriver à la guérison complète de la bactériurie il ne faut pas négliger le traitement de l'intestin, car ces malades sont en général des constipés ou sont atteints d'entérocolite muco-membraneuse. Le massage de l'intestin rend de bons services en pareil cas.

Grâce à la réunion de ces deux moyens : urotropine à l'intérieur d'une part et soins de l'intestin d'autre part, il nous est permis d'espérer que nous arriverons à combattre efficacement cette affection si rebelle, mais mon expérience est encore trop courte pour pouvoir l'affirmer. Je pourrais citer des améliorations persistantes pendant des mois, mais je n'oserais encore affirmer que j'ai obtenu des guérisons définitives.

M. A. HOGGE (Liége). — La bactériurie proprement dite (c'est-à-dire à coli-bacilles, par opposition à la microburie) est une affection très banale chez nos malades, si on se donne la peine de la rechercher et si on en connaît les symptômes. Plus j'observe ce trouble si particulier et si intéressant des urines, plus je trouve qu'une distinction fondamentale s'impose : il y a des cas très vite et facilement curables (tant par les remèdes internes que par les lavages antiseptiques) et des cas à peu près incurables, tant ils sont rebelles. Dans ces derniers la source infectieuse est manifestement en dehors des voies urinaires.

J'ai employé l'urotropine dans de très nombreux cas de bactériurie depuis plus d'un an C'est un remède qui agit bien, à peu près comme le salol et que l'on peut administrer (jusqu'à 3 et 4 grammes par jour) quand le salol est mal supporté, ce qui est très rare.

Que la bactériurie résulte de sondages (prostatiques, etc.), ou qu'elle ait sa cause en dehors des voies urinaires, cette affection doit conserver son nom aussi longtemps qu'il n'y a pas de pus dans l'urine : il n'y a pas de cystite sans pus.


## Des névralgies urétrales,

### par M. PASTEAU (de Paris).


Il persiste souvent après les uréthrites chroniques douloureuses, surtout chez la femme, des douleurs uréthrales à forme névralgique. Comme la cause première est l'infection, il faut employer un agent antiseptique; comme la douleur est le symptôme principal, il faut chercher à anesthésier l'urèthre; enfin, comme il existe ordinairement de la contracture du sphincter, il faut dilater, et je conseille de dilater progressivement.

J'ai employé dans 12 cas un béniqué cannelé pourvu d'un canal central disposé de façon à ce que la substance médicamenteuse utilisée puisse venir déboucher au fond des cannelures de l'instrument. J'ai fait construire ainsi des béniqués de grosseur différente qui permettent de faire l'instillation sur dilatation. J'ai utilisé l'huile gaïacolée à 1/20 ou l'huile goménolée à 1/10 ou à 1/5. Il ne faut d'ailleurs pas négliger de traiter l'état général et, en particulier, il est nécessaire d'insister sur l'hydrothérapie.

SEPTIÈME SÉANCE

---

## MERCREDI 8 AOUT

· *à 9 heures.*

Présidence de **M. le professeur SAXTORPH,**
de Copenhague.

*Quatrième question à l'ordre du jour :*

# RÉSULTATS ÉLOIGNÉS DES INTERVENTIONS SANGLANTES
# DANS LES RÉTRÉCISSEMENTS DE L'URÈTHRE

---

## REPORT ON THE REMOTE RESULTS OF SANGUINARY INTERVENTION
## (INTERVENTIONS SANGLANTES) IN URETHROSTENOSIS

### By REGINALD HARRISON,

Fellow and Hunterian Professor of Surgery (1894), Royal College of Surgeons of England.

I have been asked to report on the remote effects of structura
lesions (interventions sanglantes) employed in the treatment of stricture of the urethra.

I think it will be generally admitted that these results are mainly
determined by the nature of the wound and the circumstances under
which it healed. For instance, incised and contused wounds, and
wounds that heal without any or with much inflammation, or with
little or no provision for drainage, may be expected to yield different
results. For this happens in all parts of the body.

But in estimating the results of structural lesions of the urethra we
must never lose sight of the fact that this canal conveys for several
inches, at varying intervals, a compound and complex fluid which
under certain conditions, not very clearly defined, is capable of exercising a highly poisonous effect on the tissues and fluids of the body
with which it may accidentally come in contact. This is evidenced
by the frequency of rigors and fever not unlike a malaria after slight
lesions, such as passing a catheter or dividing a stricture, by the

sudden suppression of urine which is sometimes similarly occasioned, by the happening of serious if not fatal septicæmia later on, and more remotely by the formation of a contractile scar at and about the seat of the wound.  Surely we may say that the pathology of the urethra is an unique one.

To compare their results it will be necessary to define with some accuracy the kinds of wound that preceded and their probable process of healing.  For the purposes of this report the following varieties have been examined and carefully studied both during life and, as opportunity offered, after death :

1.   Lacerated or contused wounds as follow such methods of divulsion as were practised by Perrève[1] in Paris, and Holt[2] in London.

2.   Incised wounds from within the urethra as illustrated by Maissonneuve's[3] and other kinds of internal urethrotomy.

3.   Incised wounds from without inwards as described by Syme[4] of Edinburgh under the name of external urethrotomy or perineal section.

1.   Wounds inflicted by instruments for rapidly causing divulsion or rupture of a stricture are usually of a contused or lacerated character.  When thus employed, unless the stricture is an annular or a ring-like one, a condition which is rare, the canal usually gives way at a point in its circumference where the resistance is least, and this is naturally not the densest portion of the contraction.  Hence these operation-wounds heal not unlike accidental lacerations of the urethra from injury, and in both instances the liability to stricture and to its recurrence is considerable.  This was found to be so in cases examined both during life and after death; and repeated operations by divulsion appear to have been followed by additions to the amount of contractile scar-tissue at or about the seat of stricture.

There is, however, a form of stricture where divulsion is not open to these objections as judged by its more remote effects.  Reference is here made to what are known as peri-urethral or sub-mucous strictures. My attention was first called to them some years ago by examining a patient who died from some other cause shortly after (within a week) a tight stricture in the deep urethra had been divulsed by Holt's method.  The stricture was found to be peri-urethral, and thus com-

<hr>

1. *Traité des rétrécissements organiques de l'urètre*. Emploi méthodique des dilateurs mécaniques dans le traitement de ces maladies. Paris, 1847.

2. On the Immediate Treatment of Stricture. London, 1861.

3. *L'urethrotomie interne*. Paris, 1879.

4. On the Treatment of Strictures by External Incision, 1851.

pressed the mucous coat as a ligature round it would do. The effects of the divulsion had been to rupture the fibres of the stricture whilst it left the mucous lining almost intact. Mr. Christopher Heath[1] has also noted and recorded a similar observation.

I am inclined to think that the consequence of its casual application to this class of cases and the excellence of the results was that Holt's operation attained a position regarding the treatment of strictures generally which it hardly appears to have merited.

No better result relative to the permanency of the cure can be desired than this, and if it were possible to limit divulsion to peri-urethral strictures I believe this operation would still be frequently employed. I have examined several urethras many years after Holt's operation had been performed where the canal had maintained its full measurements, and no trace of a lesion of the mucous membrane could be found. We may claim these as instances of the successful treatment of stricture by subcutaneous, or rather, submucous, methods.

2. The remote effects following internal urethrotomy are of a variable character, arising mainly from the nature of the cicatrix or scar-tissue that follows the operation. In some instances I found from examination after death several years afterwards that no signs of the original stricture were discoverable either in the mucous membrane itself or the submucosa. As far as I could ascertain the incision made by the urethrotome had soundly healed without leaving any mark or contraction.

As illustrating this class of cases I will select one that has recently come under my observation where the previous history was well authenticated throughout. It was that of a man aged 55 whom I saw in February 1900. He was operated upon in 1885 by the late Mr. Berkeley Hill for a stricture in the deep urethra which would only then admit a filiform bougie. Internal urethrotomy was performed. I saw and examined this patient with Mr. Lockwood, who had been personally acquainted with him throughout. I could find no evidence of stricture. The patient had ceased to use a bougie for some years. There could be no question that this man had been permanently cured by the operation.

On the other hand, the majority of instances examined showed in varying degrees that a tendency to relapse occurred within a few weeks or months after the operation, even where patients had endea-

1. *Brit. Méd. Journal*, July 17, 1869.

voured to prevent this by the use of a bougie. In these, for the most part, there were signs that the wound inflicted had probably been an irregular or jagged one, more resembling a lacerated wound than an incised one, and not what would be expected from a well-constructed urethrotome. Further, the resulting cicatrix often presented an appearance not unlike what happens after a burn of the second or third degree, or as I have seen following electrolysis for stricture.

In some instances of recurrence after internal urethrotomy it was apparent that this operation had only partly divided the stricture. From the evidence that was afforded by this class of cases it was concluded that the combination of partial incision of a stricture by internal urethrotomy, followed immediately by stretching of the wound thus made by divulsion or bougies, did not yield good permanent results. It was in some of these cases that recurrence took place most speedily and in an aggravated form.

5. The third group of cases examined were those where the stricture was divided from without inwards on a grooved staff in accordance with Syme's description of external urethrotomy or perineal section. In several instances where this operation had been practised some years previously I found no recurrence had occurred, though the use of a bougie had practically been discontinued.

I have recorded[1] a case where a patient aged 46 had been operated upon by external urethrotomy for stricture and urinary fistulæ by a former colleague of mine in 1867. He died 18 years afterwards, and on examining his urethra I could find no sign of stricture. The dimensions of the canal along the line where the section had been made were larger than the rest. The patient had not been in the habit of using a bougie since the operation.

It will not be necessary to further illustrate the permanent advantages that have followed perineal section in some cases of urethral stricture. In restoring and preserving the normal dimensions of the canal, and in rendering catheterism easy where previously it was difficult, its advantages must be apparent in cases to which it is applicable, and these include some of the worst varieties of stricture. If performed without a guide the prospect of a good result is very small.

Where practised successfully it was not easy to determine how much of the permanent good that resulted was due to the complete

1. Surgical Disorders of the Urinary Organs, 4th Ed. p. 100.

division of the stricture and how much to the drainage which the external wound provided; but it seemed probable that both contributed to this end.

Taken as a whole, these investigations support a conclusion that most strictures treated in the three ways referred to showed a tendency to re-contraction in varying degrees. In some this liability was easily counteracted by the use of bougies after the operation, though practically it could not be said there was any time limit to this expedient. In others the tendency to relapse was so rapid and strong as to require repeated operations to maintain the dimensions of the canal, or even to necessitate the formation of a urinary fistula in place of the urethra.

In a few instances after rapid divulsion, internal urethrotomy, and perineal section, or external urethrotomy, the evidence was conclusive that a permanent cure had resulted, and where the subsequent use of a bougie appeared precautionary rather than necessary.

It must, however, be stated that, compared with the large number of stricture cases which were investigated for this purpose, and where the observations extended over a considerable number of years under favourable circumstances for conducting such an enquiry, the instances last mentioned were extremely rare. These conclusions will, I think, correspond with the experience of most surgeons.

I take it that the object of this report is not merely to reiterate a foregone conclusion, but to explain, if possible, how these variations may have happened, and how both good and indifferent results may alike contribute to advance knowledge in connection with this subject.

In examining the lesions thus made for the treatment of certain forms of stricture by urethrotomy, and I include both varieties under this term, it was evident that some of them had been faulty in their, application and in their construction relative to the process of healing which would follow.

In a few instances appearances indicated that the incision or incisions had not been accurately applied to the constriction, that the urethrotome had lacerated rather than cut, that several wounds had been made in various directions, and thus the obstruction was rather added to than lessened by what had been done. This was probably directly due to faulty instruments in the case of internal urethrotomy, and to want of precision and completeness in carrying out the details of perineal section.

Though some failures may be accounted for in these ways, more were evidently due to the conditions under which healing proceeded after the operation. Many of the incisions that were made for the purposes of internal urethrotomy were inadequately provided with means for proper drainage, having regard to their extent, whilst some cases of perineal section or external urethrotomy were hardly any better off in this respect.

About the time I commenced to make these observations on a somewhat extended scale internal urethrotomy was being practised with a very free hand

Professor Otis of New-York had recently formulated his views relative to the male urethra, which to some extent were responsible for this. Though fully recognising the value of his work in demonstrating the greater capacity of the male urethra and the important influence this had on the new lithotrity or litholapaxy which Bigelow was developing in the wake of Otis's investigations, I could not follow him in the practical application of it, in its entirety, to the treatment of stricture. However, it tended in the direction of increasing the range of internal urethrotomy as well as the size of the wounds thus made, but I cannot say that it proportionately added to the number of cures in chronic stricture of the deep urethra.

It struck me in examining cases which had been thus operated on some years previously by various surgeons where the stricture had recurred, that the size or depth of the wound so made was out of proportion to the facilities for drainage, whilst healing was going on, which the urethra alone afforded. In the absence of the latter condition I recognised one reason for the contractile condition of the scar that resulted. In arriving at this conclusion I was much influenced by what I had observed in connection with the treatment of accidental lacerations of the deep urethra by perineal incision and drainage.

It may be generally stated that the worst forms of strictures are those following laceration of the urethra, and considering the circumstances under which such lesions usually heal this is not to be wondered at. Repair goes on slowly under the irritating influence of constant contact with urine, and excessive exudation about the seat of the wound takes place. This eventually, in conjunction with the irregularity caused by the wound, forms a stricture of the closest and most contractile character.

On the other hand, in cases where perineal section and drainage were applied, this either did not happen at all, or to a much more limited extent. In some instances where this principle was adopted in the case of ruptures of the deep urethra, healing took place just as kindly as it usually does after a median cystotomy, and no stricture followed. This I proved in many instances. It seemed reasonable to conclude that the treatment of stricture by section, or division of the stricture, might be improved by providing better drainage for urine and the discharges from a wound which can only be imperfectly treated antiseptically.

I am not aware that the influence of urine-drainage in relation to the healing of wounds of the urethra and the kind of scar-tissue that results has ever been adequately discussed in connection with the operative treatment of urethral stricture.

With the view of meeting what I consider to be causes of failure and recurrence following some operations, I published[1] a series of cases and observations where I had combined the principles of internal and external urethrotomy in the treatment of certain forms of urethral stricture which on the whole have afforded good results. I shall best illustrate this practice by a typical case I have recorded and watched for a considerable number of years.

A man, aged fifty-one years, whom I saw and operated upon in 1890, had been the subject of a stricture with a strong tendency to contract for some years, and had undergone no less than six operations for it, including a divulsion by Holt's method, and five internal urethrotomies at various intervals and places. For some months before I saw him the stricture had been contracting and closing in spite of the patient's well-directed efforts with suitable bougies to keep it open. Straining to urinate was constant and prevented continuous sleep, and there was some cystitis with probably pyelitis. I performed an internal urethrotomy with Teevan's modification of Maisonneuve's instrument, as I thought that the latter might not stand the strain put upon it by the cartilaginous character of the tissues which had to be divided. This being done, I passed a full-sized grooved staff (No. 12 English) into the bladder. As the staff was evidently gripped in the deep urethra the patient was placed in the lithotomy position, and I divided in the median line from without inwards such contracted tissues as remained. I thus opened the urethra and found by passing my finger first into the bladder and then hooking it forwards along the urethra in the direction of the penile orifice, that the walls of the canal had now been rendered free and unresisting. A full-sized gum-elastic drainage-tube, such as I have

<hr>

1. *Brit. Med. Journal*, July 18th, 1885.

elsewhere described and figured[1] (Fig. 1), in connection with the larger subject of bladder drainage, was passed into the bladder through the wound and retained. The parts were well washed out with a solution of perchloride of mercury (1 in 6000). The stiff drain-

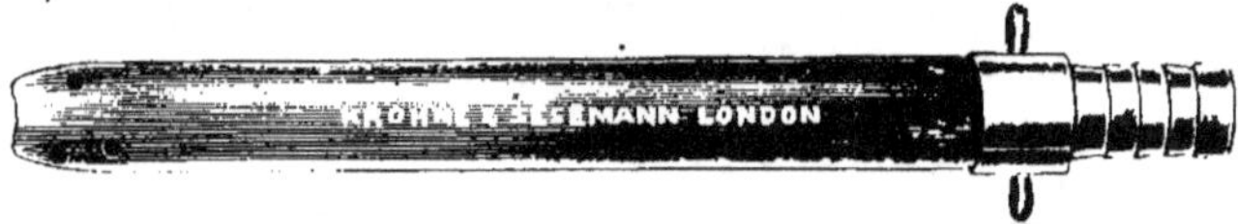

Fig. 1.

age-tube was withdrawn on the sixth day and a soft rubber one (Fig. 2) substituted, which was worn for a fortnight longer and then finally removed, when the wound soon healed. Ten years have now elapsed since this operation was practised. The patient is in fair general health and has suffered no further inconvenience from his urinary organs than having occasionally to pass a full-sized bougie for himself.

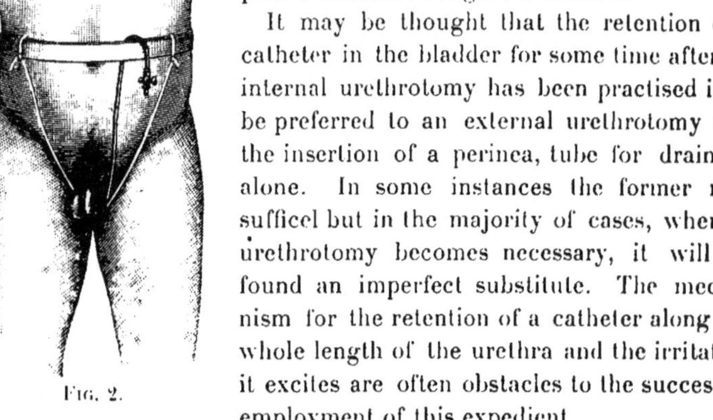

Fig. 2.

It may be thought that the retention of a catheter in the bladder for some time after an internal urethrotomy has been practised is to be preferred to an external urethrotomy and the insertion of a perinea, tube for drainage alone. In some instances the former may suffice: but in the majority of cases, where a urethrotomy becomes necessary, it will be found an imperfect substitute. The mechanism for the retention of a catheter along the whole length of the urethra and the irritation it excites are often obstacles to the successful employment of this expedient.

The conclusions arrived at from the examination of structural lesions used in the treatment of urethral strictures as I have detailed in the foregoing remarks may be summed up as follows :

*First.* That there is evidence to show that in peri-urethral strictures of the deep urethra the effects of divulsion as practised in Perrève's and Holt's operations may be limited to rupturing the dense stricture bands in the submucosa of the urethra, whilst the mucous membrane itself may escape any serious injury or laceration and is merely restored by stretching to its original dimensions. Here a permanent cure may result.

1. Surgical Disorders of the Urinary organs, fourth édition.

On the other hand, where the mucous membrane is in itself the seat of stricture and forms part of the latter structurally, it is necessarily much torn or lacerated by the process of a sudden divulsion, and the pathological condition consequently becomes assimilated with that of traumatisms of the urethra from external violence accidentally applied, which are followed by strictures of the most contractile and recurrent form.

*Second.* That there is evidence to indicate that where the entire thickness of a stricture can be included within an incision of moderaet dimensions made by an internal urethrotome the,normal calibre of the urethra may be completely and permanently restored. Where this happens, it may be concluded that all the fibres of contraction constituting the stricture were divided at the time of operation. And further that the converse is equally true. There is also evidence to show that the absence of recurrence, under such circumstances, is not necessarily dependent on the use of a bougie, though the latter is a precautionary measure which should invariably be advised.

*Third.* That in the case of multiple strictures, or strictures of the deep urethra of considerable dimensions either in their length or thickness treated by an internal incision of corresponding proportions, apart from other considerations, the tendency to recontraction and recurrence, with an additional amount of cicatricial material, is frequent : the latter being probably due to the circumstances under which healing takes place in wounds of these dimensions so situated.

*Fourth.* That lesions of the urethra demonstrate in various ways the poisonous effects that unprotected and confined urine is capable of exercising both on the body generally and on the tissues in constant contact with it, and that the liability to such effects is greatly diminished where drainage renders these conditions of the urine impossible.

*Fifth.* That in the case of recurring strictures previously treated by incision, and in primary strictures of such length or extent as to require an internal section of a correspondieg size, or as to which there might be doubt as to whether it would be safely possible so to include them, that for the purposes of the operation and its results such wounds should be made with due regard to other surgical principles in addition to the one pertaining to the division of the contraction.

*Sixth.* That there is direct evidence to show that the tendency to recontraction and recurrence of stricture after internal urethrotomy is largely diminished by the concurrent employment of systematic and efficient urine-drainage, such as the combination of external urethrotomy, or perineal puncture, affords.

## RÉSULTATS ÉLOIGNÉS DES INTERVENTIONS SANGLANTES
## DANS LES RÉTRÉCISSEMENTS DE L'URÈTRE

### par M. le docteur HÉRESCO,

de Bucarest.

Chargé, un peu tard, de faire un rapport sur la question, j'ai accepté cet honneur non sans une certaine hésitation : car, s'il est difficile en général, de connaître les résultats éloignés de nos opérés, la difficulté devient particulièrement grande, quand il s'agit des rétrécis. Ils forment une classe à part remarquables par leur insouciance.

Malgré toutes les recommandations que nous ne cessons de leur donner, pour venir se faire dilater ; malgré toutes les conséquences nuisibles, qui résultent de leur inconduite et que nous leur signalons à chaque instant, ils ne reviennent plus. Si bien que très souvent lorsqu'ils sont pris d'accidents nouveaux, ils considèrent que c'est le chirurgien qui les a mal opérés et ils s'en vont chez un autre. C'est une entrave au traitement des strictures et en même temps une difficulté pour nous de juger des résultats éloignés de nos interventions sanglantes et je vous avoue être un peu embarrassé de prouver par des statistiques très fournies, les conclusions que je vais formuler.

Mais il faut bien le dire, ce ne sont pas seulement les malades, qui sont cause de cet état de choses, nous autres chirurgiens nous avons aussi notre part de responsabilité. On part, en effet, bien souvent des idées préconçues, on met trop d'amour-propre à soutenir certaines méthodes, de sorte que l'on soumet les faits aux idées et il arrive ainsi de voir des travaux dont les faits sont contraires aux conclusions.

Nous ne chercherons pas à faire un historique des opérations sanglantes pratiquées contre les rétrécissements de l'urètre. Cela nous ferait sortir des limites imposées à ce rapport et vraiment ce serait par trop fastidieux ; mais nous ne pouvons nous empêcher de constater qu'il y a peu d'opérations, qui aient soulevé plus de passions et qui aient suscité plus de querelles que les urétrotomies. Nous ne citerons pour preuve que le fameux prix d'Argenteuil de 1836 ; de combien de discussions et polémiques acerbes n'a-t-il pas été cause à la fin de la première moitié de ce siècle !

Et il est curieux de constater que, pour des opérations comme l'urétrotomie interne et externe, qui datent de près de trois siècles, nous ne soyons pas plus fixés, en ce qui concerne leurs indications et leurs résultats éloignés, alors que des opérations relativement récentes ont pu être jugées d'une manière plus définitive.

Il y a peu de temps encore, que l'on traitait tous les rétrécissements de l'urètre par une et seule méthode et nous nous contentons simplement de rappeler que Reybard faisait et conseillait de faire des incisions internes profondes là où Sayme préconisait l'urétrotomie externe.

Leur exclusivisme a été vivement critiqué et sans parler de Reybard, pour l'opération de Sayme n'a-t-on pas écrit en Angleterre même, que c'est le plus grand opprobre de la chirurgie? N'empêche qu'aujourd'hui, il est généralement admis que l'opération de Sayme est un procédé excellent pour certains rétrécissements.

C'est qu'aujourd'hui nous connaissons mieux l'histologie et l'anatomie pathologique des rétrécissements et à la lumière de ces connaissances on a pu poser des indications plus rationnelles et partant les interventions ont été plus sûres et plus durables.

L'urétrotomie interne et externe, l'urétrectomie partielle et totale, telles sont les interventions sanglantes, dont nous allons étudier les résultats éloignés.

*L'urétrotomie interne* convient, comme on le sait, à la grande classe des rétrécissements blennorragiques.

Avant d'envisager les résultats éloignés de cette opération, avant de faire appel à la clinique, voyons ce que l'anatomie et l'histologie pathologique nous disent sur la nature des rétrécissements blennorragiques et comment se fait la cicatrisation des plaies urétrales par les sections internes. Cette dernière question délaissée un peu de nos jours a beaucoup préoccupé les chirurgiens d'antan.

De l'intéressant travail de Wassermann et N. Hallé sur l'anatomie pathologique des rétrécissements de l'urètre, il ressort que « dans la plus grande partie de sa longueur, l'urètre rétréci est le siège des lésions importantes. L'urétrite chronique, dans les points où elle n'a pas diminué le calibre de l'urètre jusqu'à produire un rétrécissement cliniquement appréciable, a pourtant laissé dans la paroi des traces profondes. Parmi ces lésions diffuses d'urétrite chronique, les modifications épithéliales paraissent être les plus constantes. Avec elle il y a toujours un degré plus ou moins avancé de lésions scléreuses sous-muqueuses ».

Mais il n'y a pas seulement que l'étendue, la profondeur des lésions est aussi remarquable et les auteurs cités continuent : « Aux points rétrécis, en dehors même de ces points, partout où l'urètre a été chroniquement enflammé, on constate la présence de lésions pénétrant profondément le corps spongieux, modifiant sa structure dans toute son épaisseur. Ce sont des lésions profondes, totales atteignant le canal dans toutes les couches de sa paroi. L'urètre atteint de cette *urétrite scléreuse totale*, même en dehors des points rétrécis n'a plus son fonctionnement physiologique. »

Ceci posé, il est bien entendu que l'urétrotomie interne ne peut avoir la prétention de guérir toutes ces lésions. Elle ne fait que sectionner et il ne faut pas lui demander plus qu'elle ne peut donner. C'est la dilatation qui se charge ensuite, sinon de guérir toutes ces lésions, tout au moins de les rendre compatibles avec un bon fonctionnement de l'urètre.

Mais il est d'un intérêt majeur de savoir ce que devient la section faite par l'urétrotomie. Des expériences que Reybard, Voillemier, Mercier et d'autres ont faites, il résulte que, après la section d'un urètre rétréci, il reste une plaie. Cette plaie se cicatriserait, si on n'avait soin de maintenir les deux lèvres de la section écartées l'une de l'autre. Alors seulement ces lèvres se cicatriseront séparément, et elles se trouveront ainsi reliées par un tissu de nouvelle formation, tissu embryonnaire qui constituera la pièce à l'appui, comme l'appelait Reybard, et sur laquelle s'exercera la dilatation.

D'où il résulte qu'il faut toujours : 1° inciser les rétrécissements suffisamment, pour que les deux lèvres restent écartées à l'aide d'une sonde à demeure, et 2° faire des incisions multiples pour avoir plusieurs foyers de tissu embryonnaire, sur lesquels la dilatation sera plus facilement pratiquée.

L'urétrotomie interne n'est pas une opération radicale, elle ne fait que faciliter la dilatation. Ces deux méthodes se complètent, car là où la dilatation qui, soit dit en passant, constitue la vraie base du traitement des rétrécissements blennorragiques, n'est pas possible, l'urétrotomie interne doit être pratiquée, et pour que ses résultats soient durables, ils doivent être soutenus par une dilatation consécutive persévérante. De plus, la dilatation doit être faite d'après certaines règles. J'ai donné mes soins à un malade atteint de rétrécissements blennorragiques multiples, dont le dernier dans la portion périnéo-bulbaire n'admettait que le n° 10. Pendant un mois je n'ai pu gagner que trois numéros, et cela avec grande peine et après lui avoir laissé par deux fois une bougie filiforme à demeure. Je lui ai pratiqué l'urétrotomie interne en juin 1899, puis l'ai dilaté, le malade continuant, sur mes indications, à se passer lui-même, tous les deux jours, les n°ˢ 19 et 20.

Deux mois après il présentait une tendance très marquée au resserrement des rétrécissements et plusieurs rétentions complètes, qui se sont terminées soit spontanément, soit par le cathétérisme.

Je lui ai conseillé les hautes dilatations, je suis arrivé bientôt au n° 50, et depuis que je lui ai fait des hautes dilatations il n'a plus eu de rétention d'urine et la miction est devenue depuis très facile.

Ce cas, pareil à ceux publiés par Guiard dans les *Annales génito-urinaires* de 1899, montre bien l'action bienfaisante des hautes dilatations comme complément de l'urétrotomie interne.

Donc, toute urétrotomie interne doit être suivie de dilatation, car, ainsi qu'on l'a dit depuis bien longtemps, la récidive est la règle et l'urétrotomie interne réduite à ses propres moyens ne constitue qu'une opération palliative.

Il est très intéressant de savoir le temps qu'il faut pour que la récidive se produise. Ceci est très variable et dépend des rétrécissements et de la manière dont on a pratiqué les incisions. Avec des incisions plus profondes, la récidive sera plus tardive, tandis qu'à la uite des incisions superficielles, elle se produira plus rapidement.

La récidive après l'urétrotomie interne sans dilatation est la règle; mais même ceux qui se font dilater ne sont pas toujours exempts de la récidive.

Ces derniers doivent être divisés en deux groupes : ceux qui se sont fait dilater régulièrement et ceux qui ont eu une dilatation irrégulière. Il est bien certain que ce sont les premiers qui fournissent un critérium certain pour juger des bons résultats de l'urétrotomie interne. Mais combien rares sont les malades qui ont suivi une dilatation régulière !

J'ai trouvé que la récidive était survenue chez un malade 5 semaines, chez un autre 4 mois, chez un troisième 6 mois, chez d'autres enfin 1 an 1/2, 2, 3 ans malgré la dilatation.

Je me demande si, dans ces cas, la dilatation n'a pas présenté quelque défaut ou si, chez le premier en particulier, l'urétrotomie interne a été assez méthodiquement pratiquée.

Dans le travail d'Azéma, je trouve que la récidive est survenue, malgré la dilatation, au bout d'un an, 2, 3, 4, 5 jusqu'à 50 ans, et je me demande encore si la dilatation a été assez soignée chez des malades qui ont vu la récidive survenir au bout d'un si long temps.

Pour que la dilatation donne des résultats durables, il faut qu'elle soit poussée jusqu'à des gros numéros.

A Bucarest, sur 21 résultats éloignés que les docteurs Drugesco, Frumusianu et Costin ont obligeamment mis à ma disposition de la pratique du professeur Jonnesco, des docteurs Léonté et Duma, la récidive a été observée dans 15 cas, au bout de 6 mois à 2 ans ; les autres cas ne présentaient pas de récidive 1 an, 2 ans et 2 ans 1/2 après ; et il faut faire remarquer que parmi ces derniers, tous s'étaient fait dilater plus ou moins régulièrement.

L'*urétrotomie externe* a surtout été employée contre les rétrécissements traumatiques ou contre les rétrécissements infranchissables, ou bien alors quand la stricture était compliquée de fistules avec indurations, callosités périnéales.

Sayme, renversant la formule acceptée jusqu'à son époque, avait préconisé l'urétrotomie externe dans les cas où on pouvait introduire un conducteur. Il prétendait que l'urétrotomie externe guérissait mieux les rétrécissements. D'autres chirurgiens après lui ont insisté sur cet avantage. Mais on sait que dans les sténoses blenorragiques les lésions ne sont pas limitées seulement au niveau des rétrécissements.

La chose ne paraît pas possible et c'est en vain que nous avons cherché de meilleurs résultats, en consultant les auteurs qui ont considéré cette opération préférable à l'urétrotomie interne.

Il est incontestable que l'urétrotomie externe présente une grande supériorité sur l'interne, lorsque le périnée est pourvu d'une ou de plusieurs fistules entourées de tissu scléreux, induré. Alors, en effet, ainsi que le professeur Guyon l'a montré, en incisant toutes ces fistules en même temps que le rétrécissement, la guérison est meilleure et plus durable, mais ce bon résultat est obtenu, non pas parce que la section du rétrécissement a été pratiquée de dehors en dedans au lieu du contraire, mais parce qu'en incisant les fistules on dégage mieux l'urètre en faisant ce que l'éminent chef de l'école de Necker appelle la *libération externe du canal.*

A la suite de l'urétrotomie externe, il y a une pièce au canal et si la dilatation n'est pas pratiquée, il en résultera une cicatrice plus serrée qu'antérieurement. Les faits de tous les jours montrent l'exactitude de cette donnée.

Grégory sur 12 opérés de Bordeaux a pu revoir 5 malades 1 an, 2 et 5 ans et chez aucun la récidive n'avait encore eu lieu, mais sur les trois, 2 se sondaient plus ou moins régulièrement.

Eugène Bœckel, de Strasbourg, a observé une récidive 8 ans après l'urétrotomie externe.

Félix Bron de Lyon, sur 24 opérés a constaté le maintien de la cure au bout d'un temps fort long, entre 1 an et 11 ans chez 16 de ses opérés.

Dudon de Bordeaux retrouve 6 de ses malades sur 15 opérés plus de 1 an après et chez tous le canal était parfaitement libre.

Enfin Post, van Buren, Sayre ont observé de leurs opérés 20, 21 et 25 ans après l'urétrotomie externe sans récidive.

De son côté Phélip, dans une série très intéressante d'articles de la *Revue de chirurgie* de 1890 et 1891 donne l'observation de 18 opérés.

Sur ces 18 opérés, 7 ne se sont jamais sondés et 5 n'ont pas vu récidiver leur rétrécissement 14, 15 et 16 ans, après l'opération. Mais, ajoute l'auteur, « leur canal, à cette date, n'avait pas conservé la largeur qu'il possédait, lorsqu'ils prirent congé du chirurgien : à ce moment, en effet, on passait facilement jusqu'aux numéros 25 à 27 suivant le sujet ; à l'époque de notre examen le canal n'admettait que jusqu'aux numéros 15 à 18 et sur un des opérés le cathétérisme ne put être fait que très difficilement et sur un autre, le cathétérisme fut impossible. »

Il nous semble qu'alors cela s'appelle de la récidive et qu'on ne peut les considérer comme exemples de guérison définitive.

Sur 10 urétrotomies externes que j'ai pratiquées, je n'ai pu en revoir qu'une seule : la récidive s'était produite 15 mois après.

Le temps qu'il faut à la récidive pour se produire est tout aussi variable pour l'urétrotomie externe que pour l'interne. Et dans le cas de Bœckel, elle n'a pas mis moins de 8 ans, pour se faire constater.

Pas plus pour l'urétrotomie externe que pour l'urétrotomie interne on n'a pu arriver à faire un pourcentage à cause de l'impossibilité où on se trouve de revoir les malades.

D'ailleurs nous savons combien défectueuse serait une pareille statistique, en rapprochant des cas très dissemblables par la nature des strictures, par les diversités d'opérations et par les conditions diverses dans lesquelles se trouvaient les praticiens au moment de l'opération.

En somme, l'urétrotomie externe ne donne pas une guérison définitive ; elle a besoin d'être secondée par la dilatation, tout comme dans l'urétrotomie interne et puisque celle-ci est d'une exécution plus facile et plus indiquée contre les rétrécissements blennorragiques, c'est à elle qu'on doit donner la préférence, excepté bien entendu lorsque le ou les rétrécissements sont accompagnés de fistules et lorsque le périnée est induré, sclérosé, car alors les résultats de l'urétrotomie externe sont d'une supériorité évidente.

*La résection de l'urètre* est l'opération idéale. Enlever le rétrécissement complètement et suturer les deux bouts c'est de la chirurgie radicale et les résultats ne peuvent en être que très durables.

Malheureusement l'urétrectomie n'est applicable qu'à un nombre restreint de cas. Lorsque le rétrécissement est traumatique, par conséquent unique, lorsqu'il est situé assez bas, dans le périnée, lorsqu'il ne dépasse pas 5 centimètres, c'est à la résection de l'urètre qu'on aura recours.

Elle peut être totale ou partielle, mais qu'elle soit totale ou partielle, la condition essentielle d'une bonne résection suivie de suture c'est que la plaie ne suppure pas, car si la suppuration s'établit, on n'aura plus une réunion primitive, en d'autres termes une cicatrice souple, mais une cicatrice qui diminuera à nouveau le calibre de l'urètre.

Les faits nombreux consignés dans la remarquable thèse de mon ami Noguès et ceux recueillis par Vignard montrent que cette opération est excellente et que ses résultats peuvent être considérés comme permanents. Sur 15 malades la guérison a été observée au bout de 6 mois à 8 ans. Parmi les plus remarquables il y a lieu de citer ceux de Horteloup, de Heussner. Un des réséqués de Heussner mourut 2 ans et demi plus tard d'une affection des reins et à l'autopsie on ne trouva qu'une simple cicatrice linéaire.

Un malade de Horteloup mourut 5 ans et demi après l'opération et l'on trouva que la cicatrice du périnée était très souple et il n'y avait aucune différence entre les muqueuses des portions spongieuses et prostatiques et la muqueuse au niveau du point réséqué.

Nous espérons que notre ami Noguès viendra apporter aux débats les résultats éloignés de ses malades trop récemment opérés au moment de l'apparition de son travail.

Enfin deux opérés d'urétrectomie partielle de Jonnesco n'avaient pas de récidive 1 an et demi et 2 ans après l'opération.

La résection de l'urètre ne peut donner de bons résultats qu'alors que le périnée est souple, car lorsqu'il y a des indurations, des callosités, alors le résultat tant immédiat qu'éloigné ne peut être très brillant.

J'ai opéré, au mois de mai 1899, le frère d'un médecin, homme âgé de 56 ans, dont le périnée était le siège d'une tumeur fibreuse, dure comme le bois, suite de fistules et abcès périnéaux multiples. Le malade souffrait depuis 10 ans de rétrécissements blennorragiques de l'urètre.

Plusieurs essais de cathétérisme avec des bougies fines étant restés infructueux, j'ai fait la résection de toute la partie indurée; malgré une recherche attentive, il ne m'a pas été possible de découvrir l'urètre, que j'ai enlevé sur une longueur de 10 à 12 centimètres. J'ai laissé longtemps une sonde à demeure après avoir suturé les parties molles autour.

J'ai revu ce malade 10 mois après, le périnée était souple à sa partie antérieure, mais vers la partie postérieure il y avait une induration, grosse comme une noix, adhérente à l'urètre. Le malade se dilate lui même tous les 10 ou 15 jours en se passant des sondes des numéros 20 et 21.

Dans ces cas-là, on ne peut demander d'une urétrectomie autre chose qu'une amélioration relative, et par une dilatation persévérante consécutive, le chirurgien doit s'efforcer de maintenir le calibre de l'urètre.

Chez la femme, les rétrécissements de l'urètre sont bien plus rares que chez l'homme. Sur 112 observations que Pasteau a réunies en 1896, la dilatation a été la méthode de choix et elle a suffi dans la plupart des cas.

Dans 15 cas seulement l'urétrotomie interne a été pratiquée et dans ces 15 cas, on ne connaît les résultats éloignés que dans 5 cas : dans un cas d'Otis, la guérison se maintenait 1 an après; dans un autre cas, également d'Otis, la guérison persistait 2 ans après; enfin dans le cas personnel de Pasteau, la malade n'avait pas de récidive 1 an et demi après.

Arrivé aux limites de ce rapport, nous croyons pouvoir formuler les conclusions suivantes :

1° Aucune des méthodes sanglantes, actuellement connues contre les rétrécissements de l'urètre, ne peut donner une guérison définitive, hormis la résection de l'urètre dans certains cas déterminés;

2° L'urétrotomie interne, employée contre les rétrécissements blennorragiques, où il y a une sclérose plus ou moins totale du canal, n'est pas une opération définitive; elle ne fait que faciliter la dilatation.

Toute urétrotomie interne sans dilatation consécutive est vouée à une récidive certaine;

3° Le temps qu'il faut à la récidive pour se produire est variable depuis des semaines jusqu'à des dizaines d'années et dépend de la nature du rétrécissement et de la manière plus ou moins complète dont la dilatation consécutive a été effectuée;

4° L'urétrotomie externe n'obtient pas plus la guérison que l'interne et la récidive se produit comme après l'urétrotomie interne.

Lorsque le périnée se présente avec des fistules, indurations, callosités, l'urétrotomie externe offre un grand avantage sur l'interne par la libération externe du périnée;

5° La résection de l'urètre dans certaines conditions déterminées peut donner la guérison définitive. Ces conditions sont rares;

6° Toutes les interventions sanglantes doivent être secondées par une dilatation consécutive persévérante.

---

## RÉSUMÉ DU RAPPORT SUR LES RÉSULTATS ÉLOIGNÉS DES INTERVENTIONS SANGLANTES DANS LES RÉTRÉCISSEMENTS DE L'URETRE

### par M. J. ALBARRAN.

L'étude comparée des résultats éloignés, obtenus par les différentes méthodes de traitement dans les rétrécissements de l'urètre, conduit à séparer nettement, d'un côté, les rétrécissements dits inflammatoires et, d'un autre côté, les rétrécissements traumatiques. Dans chacune de ces deux catégories, il faudrait encore établir de nombreuses divisions suivant le siège, le nombre, l'étendue et le degré du rétrécissement lui-même. Le même traitement pourra donner des résultats éloignés absolument dissemblables, suivant les cas où il s'applique. Nous ne pouvons que dire d'une manière très générale ce qu'on est en droit d'attendre des différentes méthodes de traitement.

I. *Rétrécissement inflammatoire non compliqué.* — Au point de vue de la fréquence des récidives, on peut classer ainsi les principaux modes de traitement des rétrécissements de l'urètre : électrolyse, dilatation progressive, urétrotomie interne, urétrotomie externe, résection et opérations autoplastiques.

L'*électrolyse* pratiquée par le procédé rapide, en une séance, donne lieu à des récidives d'autant plus rapides que la dilatation consécutive est moins prolongée. Les résultats éloignés de l'électrolyse, par le procédé lent, paraissent un peu meilleurs, mais les documents publiés ne permettent pas de juger le procédé à ce point de vue.

La *dilatation progressive* doit être méthodiquement conduite jusqu'au numéro 60 Béniqué : il faut s'efforcer en outre de rendre au canal sa souplesse, de supprimer les brides que le passage de l'instrument efface, de guérir l'urétrite qui accompagne le rétrécissement et de tarir toutes les sources d'infection urétrale et péri-urétrale. A ces conditions, on peut obtenir de bons résultats éloignés par la dilatation progressive, mais, sauf dans les cas légers, les résultats obtenus ne seront conservés que par l'entretien du calibre du canal au moyen de périodes successives de cathétérisme dilatateur.

L'*urétrotomie interne* ne peut guère être considérée que comme le premier temps de la dilatation progressive. Elle paraît donner de meilleurs résultats lorsqu'on pratique des sections multiples que lorsqu'on ne fait que la section unique; mais, quel que soit le procédé employé, les résultats ne seront durables que si on arrive, après une ou plusieurs opérations et par la dilatation consécutive, à placer l'urètre dans les conditions mentionnées à propos de la dilatation progressive. La récidive est aussi bien à craindre après la dilatation progressive qu'après l'urétrotomie interne.

L'*urétrotomie externe* donne des résultats éloignés supérieurs à ceux des méthodes précédentes, mais cette opération n'est applicable qu'aux rétrécissements limités. Certains malades sont guéris après l'urétrotomie externe sans avoir pris de soins consécutifs : ces exemples sont rares et la récidive n'est guère évitée que par la dilatation régulièrement entretenue après l'opération.

La *résection de l'urètre* dans les rétrécissements inflammatoires limités de la région périnéo-scrotale donne des résultats éloignés comparables ou supérieurs à ceux de l'urétrotomie externe : lorsque le rétrécissement est susceptible d'être extirpé complètement, on peut espérer que la guérison se maintienne sans traitement consécutif. Dans la région pénienne, les résections étendues exposent à l'incurvation de la verge.

II. *Rétrécissements inflammatoires compliqués de tumeurs et fistules urineuses.* — Dans ces cas, la dilatation progressive et l'urétrotomie interne deviennent insuffisantes. L'urétrotomie externe, et mieux encore la résection partielle ou totale de l'urètre donnent les meilleurs résultats éloignés.

Les opérations autoplastiques n'ont guère été pratiquées que dans des cas particuliers peu comparables à ceux dans lesquels ont été faites les autres opérations.

III. *Rétrécissements traumatiques.* — La dilatation progressive est ici insuffisante à assurer une guérison de quelque durée ; il en est de même de l'urétrotomie interne, quel que soit le nombre des sections. Avec ces modes de traitement la récidive est rapide.

L'urétrotomie externe donne de meilleurs résultats, mais expose aussi aux récidives malgré des soins consécutifs réguliers.

La résection de l'urètre est l'opération de choix : elle réussit mieux dans les rétrécissements traumatiques que dans les inflammatoires et peut conduire d'emblée à la guérison définitive.

# RÉSULTATS ÉLOIGNÉS DE L'URÉTROTOMIE INTERNE ET EXTERNE DANS MA PRATIQUE

### par M. le docteur P. HAMONIC,
#### de Paris.

J'ai l'occasion de pratiquer tous les ans un nombre relativement considérable d'*urétrotomies internes*. J'emploie surtout le procédé de Maisonneuve, mais depuis quelque temps je fais usage d'un nouvel instrument que je communiquerai ces jours-ci à la Société et qui me paraît être appelé à rendre des services en perfectionnant la section du canal.

Je ne fais l'*urétrotomie externe* que dans les rétrécissements traumatiques ou dans les rétrécissements inflammatoires inodulaires particulièrement serrés. Dans ces cas-là, je pratique d'habitude la résection de l'urètre avec sutures réunissant les deux segments du canal.

Quel que soit le procédé d'*urétrotomie*, quelque étendue qu'on donne à l'incision du canal, quelque soin qu'on mette à restituer le calibre intégral du conduit, il faut bien se convaincre que la guérison définitive du malade est loin d'être obtenue par l'intervention sanglante.

Ainsi que je l'ai écrit, il y a huit ans, dans mon traité des *rétrécissements de l'urètre*, l'urétrotomie interne ne doit être considérée que comme la *première phase de la dilatation*. L'incision du canal ne fait que préparer la voie au passage de l'instrument dilatateur, qui seul est capable d'amener la guérison durable.

L'*urétrotomie externe* agit de même façon. Même lorsqu'on résèque un segment inodulaire du canal de l'urètre, et qu'on suture entre eux les deux bouts, il n'est pas possible de s'opposer à la formation secondaire d'un rétrécissement cicatriciel qu'on n'évitera que par l'emploi méthodique des instruments de dilatation.

Pour que la dilatation donne son plein effet, il faut la pousser très loin, et sauf les cas où j'ai affaire à des malades pourvus d'une verge très grêle, j'atteins systématiquement le 55 et le plus souvent j'arrive au 60, c'est-à-dire au numéro maximum de la filière.

A ce sujet, je dois dire qu'après une nouvelle année d'expériences, les cathéters que j'ai présentés l'année dernière à la Société me donnent la plus grande satisfaction, en facilitant beaucoup la dilatation et en permettant de l'exagérer sans danger ni inconvénient pour le malade

Mes cathéters, beaucoup plus ouverts que les anciens, et présentant une double courbure latérale calquée sur l'état de nature, ainsi qu'il résulte de mes recherches, glissent aisément sur un conducteur fixe qu'on introduit une fois pour toutes dans la vessie et qui n'en bouge plus jusqu'à la fin de la séance.

Mon conducteur trace sa voie à l'instrument de dilatation, et voudrait-on intentionnellement faire une fausse route que cela ne serait pas possible. Cette assurance donne plus de hardiesse à la main de l'opérateur, en même temps que la régularité de l'introduction du cathéter évite de la douleur au malade, de telle sorte qu'on peut avec mes instruments pousser la dilatation bien plus loin qu'on ne le faisait autrefois.

Plus je vais et plus je suis convaincu de l'importance de la dilatation dans n'importe quel rétrécissement de l'urètre et principalement dans ceux qu'on est obligé d'urétrotomiser.

De telle sorte que pour moi les résultats éloignés de l'urétrotomie interne et externe résident exclusivement dans la façon dont on a dirigé la dilatation secondaire. Un procédé d'incision urétrale peut l'emporter sur tel autre au point de vue de la direction, de l'étendue de la section, du danger qu'il fait ou non courir. Mais le mode d'urétrotomie importe peu pour le résultat ultérieur, si la dilatation n'intervient pas.

Dans mes statistiques, tous mes cas sont très favorables, et tous mes malades guérissent définitivement, parce que je les avertis, dès le début, du rôle de l'urétrotomie et de celui de la dilatation et de la nécessité absolue qu'il y a à recourir à la seconde dès que la première est effectuée.

J'insiste de plus pour que le malade revienne à certaines époques déterminées pour entretenir sa dilatation, c'est à ce prix seulement qu'on obtient une guérison définitive.

En terminant ces quelques observations, je répéterai encore une fois que l'urétrotomie est une opération préparatoire pour la dilatation.

## RÉSULTATS ÉLOIGNÉS DE CENT TRENTE-DEUX URÉTROTOMIES INTERNES

### par M. le docteur PAUL NOGUÈS,

assistant de la Clinique des voies urinaires de l'hôpital Necker.

La discussion ouverte au Congrès a déjà permis de fixer un point important dans l'histoire de l'urétrotomie interne. Tout le monde est d'accord pour admettre qu'elle n'est pas une opération définitive, qu'il ne saurait être question après elle de guérison radicale et que la récidive survient fatalement, si le malade n'entretient pas son calibre par une dilatation régulière. Les rapporteurs sont unanimes, à l'exception de M. Harrison, qui néanmoins recommande l'usage méthodique des bougies.

Ces suites éloignées de l'urétrotomie interne sont encore bien mises en lumière par les chiffres que je vais fournir. J'ai eu, en effet, l'idée de rechercher tous les malades ayant subi l'urétrotomie interne depuis le 1er juillet 1867, dans le service de mon maître, le professeur Guyon ; je n'ai pu en retrouver que 152 ; et si ce chiffre est minime par rapport à celui des malades convoqués, il a cependant une certaine importance. Or, sur ces 152 malades, 64 ayant négligé la dilatation sont revenus en récidive, et parmi les 68 qui se sont présentés avec un calibre suffisant, tous s'étaient astreints à des séances plus ou moins régulières de dilatation faite soit par eux-mêmes, soit à l'hôpital. Il n'y a pas une seule exception à cette règle et nous sommes autorisés à conclure que les résultats éloignés de l'urétrotomie interne, quand ils sont bons, sont bien moins le fait de l'opération que de la dilatation consécutive.

Cette conclusion se dégage manifestement de mes tableaux et s'applique à toutes les variétés d'urétrotomies internes, que la section ait porté uniquement sur la paroi supérieure ou sur les autres parois. J'ai, en effet, divisé mes malades en trois catégories : malades n'ayant subi qu'une urétrotomie à lame courante ; malades ayant, après une urétrotomie à lame courante, subi au bout d'un temps plus ou moins long une urétrotomie complémentaire ; enfin, malades ayant subi d'emblée une urétrotomie à sections multiples. Dans chacune de ces catégories les résultats ont été appréciés de la manière suivante : malades s'étant dilatés et étant restés guéris ; malades ayant récidivé, mais ayant pu être dilatés sans opération nouvelle ; malades ayant récidivé et ayant eu besoin d'une nouvelle uré-

trotomie. Ces diverses catégories sont groupées dans le tableau
suivant :

| | MALADES régulièrement dilatés et restés guéris. | MALADES ayant récidivé et ayant pu être dilatés. | MALADES ayant récidivé et n'ayant pu être dilatés. |
|---|---|---|---|
| Malades n'ayant subi qu'une urétrotomie à lame courante. . . . . . . . . . | 39 | 28 | 6 |
| Malades ayant d'abord subi une urétrotomie à lame courante et plus tard une urétrotomie à sections multiples . . . . . . . | 10 | 17 | 3 |
| Malades ayant subi d'emblée une urétrotomie à sections multiples. . . . | 15 | 10 | 4 |

La conclusion à tirer de ces statistiques est que la proportion des
récidives est à peu près la même pour tous les procédés opératoires ;
ce n'est donc pas sur ces chiffres que l'on peut se baser pour établir
la supériorité de l'une ou de l'autre méthode.

Une seconde question, celle-ci peut être plus discutée, se pose
maintenant : les résultats fournis par l'urétrotomie interne sont-ils
plus durables que ceux que donne la dilatation simple? En d'autres
termes, si nous prenons deux malades théoriquement porteurs de la
même lésion anatomique et si nous soumettons l'un à la dilatation,
l'autre à l'urétrotomie, le premier gardera-t-il moins longtemps le
bénéfice de son traitement? A mon avis, il faut délibérément répondre
par la négative, mais ce point demande quelques explications. Il ne
faut pas oublier, en effet, que, dans quelques cas, l'urétrotomie
interne permet de pousser plus loin la dilatation, et dans ces conditions, il est naturel que le bénéfice acquis soit plus durable et la récidive plus longue à se produire. Mais alors les termes de la comparaison ne sont plus les mêmes et l'on met en parallèle deux malades
dont l'un a sur l'autre une supériorité incontestable.

Ces deux faits bien positifs, d'une part absence de résultat définitif
et d'autre part récidive aussi rapide, me paraissent considérablement
réduire les indications de l'urétrotomie interne. Je n'en vois pour ma
part que deux, l'une tirée des complications, l'autre du rétrécissement
lui-même. La première a depuis longtemps rallié tous les suffrages et

ses mérites ne sont plus à célébrer dans les cas d'infection avec rétention septique; nous comptons tous des malades qui doivent leur vie à notre intervention hâtive.

Quant à l'indication tirée du rétrécissement lui-même, elle existe, mais à mon avis elle se pose très rarement; on peut parfois rencontrer quelques rétrécissements difficilement dilatables et chez lesquels l'urétrotomie interne facilite les premières séances, mais je répète que je considère le fait comme exceptionnel, surtout si je m'en rapporte aux résultats de ma pratique. En effet, depuis sept ans que j'exerce, j'ai déjà soigné un certain nombre de rétrécis et je n'ai eu à intervenir que dans trois cas où la dilatation était difficile. Je reste donc convaincu que la dilatation, quand elle est bien conduite, suffit dans presque tous les canaux, et que le maintien de la bougie à demeure et l'emploi des petits béniqués conduits qu'a fait construire mon ami Janet peuvent avoir raison des cas les plus rebelles.

Je désire, en terminant, dire quelques mots d'une catégorie de malades à canaux tellement durs, tellement scléreux que la dilatation aussi bien que l'urétrotomie ne donnent chez eux aucun résultat. La récidive se produit avec une rapidité désespérante et, après un mois d'absence de soins, ils se retrouvent au même point qu'avant la dilatation ou l'urétrotomie. Chez ces malades, je me suis fort bien trouvé d'une pratique que je tiens de M. Guyon et qui consiste à mettre tous les jours ou tous les deux jours, suivant les cas, une sonde à demeure pendant quelques heures. Grâce à cette précaution facile à prendre, non seulement le résultat immédiat est excellent et la dilatation peut être poussée très haut, mais encore l'amélioration persiste pendant un temps assez long.

---

## RÉSULTATS ÉLOIGNÉS DE L'URÉTROTOMIE INTERNE ET DE LA DILATATION PROGRESSIVE DANS MA PRATIQUE

### par M. le docteur JULES JANET,

de Paris.

J'ai toujours eu une tendance à préférer la simple dilatation à l'urétrotomie interne; peut-être que la grande extension que j'ai donnée dans ma pratique aux traitements ambulatoires, au préjudice des procédés chirurgicaux, m'a conduit à tirer de la dilatation tout ce qu'elle pouvait donner, plutôt que de m'adresser aux méthodes sanglantes.

Mais je dois dire que j'ai été encouragé dans cette manière de faire par les résultats mêmes que j'obtenais et par certaines considérations théoriques que je tiens à développer.

La dilatation pure et simple est, je crois, pour nous tous, le moyen de choix de traitement des rétrécissements : si nous faisons des urétrotomies, c'est parce que la dilatation nous semble impossible, exception faite pour ces cas d'urgence où l'urétrotomie s'impose pour mettre rapidement fin à de graves accidents infectieux. Mais laissons de côté ces derniers cas qui sont, du reste, très peu fréquents, pour n'envisager que les rétrécis qui nous laissent le temps de choisir notre procédé d'intervention. Je dis que ces cas d'urgence sont rares; en effet, j'ai vu bien souvent ces rétrécis infectés, fébriles et rétentionnistes s'améliorer très rapidement sous l'influence de la bougie fine à demeure, des lavages sans sonde à l'eau boriquée et de la dilatation si minime qu'elle pût être. Je ne connais dans ma clientèle qu'un seul cas qui ait nécessité une urétrotomie d'urgence.

Pour en revenir aux rétrécis qui nous laissent le temps de la réflexion, nous préférons tous, je le répète, la dilatation aux urétrotomies. Si nous faisons une urétrotomie, c'est parce que la dilatation nous semble impossible, et, ce faisant, nous savons que cette urétrotomie, pour être efficace, ne nous dispensera pas de séances indéfinies de dilatations consécutives.

L'urétrotomie interne, quelle que soit sa nature, sanglante ou électrolytique, n'est donc pas, même pour ceux qui la pratiquent le plus volontiers, un procédé curatif des rétrécissements, mais simplement un moyen de rendre possible la dilatation. Ceci étant établi, je me suis demandé s'il n'était pas plus simple, en se donnant un peu de mal, de pratiquer tout de suite la dilatation, puisqu'on devait toujours y revenir plus tard. C'est ce que j'ai fait dans ma clientèle et je puis dire que j'y suis presque constamment arrivé, puisque je ne puis noter parmi mes malades que 4 urétrotomies internes depuis 10 ans.

Le point intéressant de la question des urétrotomies est de savoir quel est l'avenir de la section que l'on a pratiquée et si le rétrécissement en bénéficie. Ce point est difficile à élucider, puisqu'on combine la dilatation à l'urétrotomie et que par cela même il n'est pas aisé de savoir ce qui revient à l'un ou à l'autre de ces deux procédés. Je crois pouvoir apporter un élément sérieux à ce problème par la méthode que j'ai suivie jusqu'à ce jour.

Les urétrotomies pratiquées sur mes malades ayant été réservées aux cas réellement indilatables, les résultats qu'elles ont donnés sont absolument purs et toute influence possible de la dilatation en est supprimée.

Quand on urétrotomise un rétrécissement en réalité dilatable, voici ce qui se passe : l'anneau rétréci sectionné est refoulé en un point de la périphérie du nouveau canal dont le reste est constitué par le tissu cellulaire lâche péri-urétral. La dilatation que l'on pratique peu de jours après l'urétrotomie porte uniquement sur ce dernier tissu qui se prête facilement et permettrait d'atteindre sans difficulté les plus énormes numéros, mais l'anneau cicatriciel lui-même n'est nullement influencé par cette dilatation.

On laisse ensuite le malade sans dilatation pendant quelques semaines. Pendant ce temps, la surface sectionnée se réduit peu à peu, ses bords se rapprochent, elle devient moins extensible. La séance suivante de dilatation la trouvera moins docile et la partie cicatricielle ancienne sera forcée de subir un commencement de dilatation. Nouveau repos pendant lequel la plaie de l'urétrotomie se referme complètement et perd toute élasticité. Les dilatations suivantes trouveront l'anneau cicatriciel déjà en partie dilaté par les séances précédentes et porteront désormais sur cet anneau lui-même. A partir de ce moment, tout le bénéfice revient à la dilatation.

L'urétrotomie, dans un cas semblable, n'aura donc eu pour avantage que de faciliter la dilatation en évitant le passage des petits numéros.

Si, au contraire, l'urétrotomie porte sur un rétrécissement absolument indilatable, les premières séances de dilatation sont aussi aisées que précédemment, il n'y a aucune raison, dans ce cas comme dans les précédents, pour ne pas arriver au béniqué 60. Mais il n'en est pas de même plus tard et l'on est bien étonné de constater quinze jours après ce beau résultat que l'on passe péniblement un 15 Charrière. On redilate et l'on a de la peine à gagner quelques numéros, le moindre arrêt dans la dilatation vous fait perdre plus que vous n'avez gagné et, au bout d'un mois à six semaines, le rétrécissement est revenu malgré tous vos efforts au chiffre primitif, 8 ou 9, ou même moins, qu'il avait avant l'urétrotomie.

C'est exactement ce qui s'est passé chez les 4 malades qui ont été urétrotomisés dans ma clientèle ; ils sont revenus chacun à leur ancien numéro de rétrécissement entre un mois et six semaines après leur opération. Et cela malgré les plus vigoureux efforts de dilatation consécutive.

Ceci ne prouve-t-il pas surabondamment que le bénéfice de l'urétrotomie est nul dans l'avenir du rétréci, que s'il gagne quelque chose à son opération, ce n'est pas à l'urétrotomie mais à la dilatation qu'il le doit et que s'il n'a rien à attendre de la dilatation, il ne doit en aucune façon compter sur l'urétrotomie pour élargir son canal?

La dilatation progressive des rétrécissements très durs n'est pas facile; elle est forcément très lente et bien souvent elle s'arrête à un numéro peu élevé, mais il est remarquable de voir combien ces résultats péniblement acquis persistent longtemps. J'ai vu de ces malades ne rien perdre de leur dilatation après avoir passé trois mois sans sondages.

Voici comment je la pratique : j'introduis comme d'habitude une bougie filiforme que je laisse à demeure si je le juge nécessaire, mais cela est rare. Le plus souvent je commence immédiatement la dilatation.

Si l'on voulait pratiquer cette dilatation, comme on le fait d'habitude, avec des bougies de gomme, on ne pourrait y arriver, car ces bougies sont trop flexibles pour vaincre la résistance du rétrécissement; si elles étaient plus rigides, elles seraient dangereuses, n'étant pas conduites.

C'est ce qui détermine d'ordinaire les chirurgiens à pratiquer l'urétrotomie, ne pouvant introduire les bougies coniques au delà du numéro 8 ou 9, ils considèrent la dilatation comme impossible et ils y renoncent. Mais il n'en est pas de même si, au lieu de se servir de bougies de gomme, on se sert de béniqués métalliques très fins. J'ai fait faire une série de ces béniqués à extrémité franchement conique, se continuant directement avec l'armature de la bougie conductrice sans aucun ressaut. Ces béniqués commencent au numéro 16, c'est-à-dire au numéro 8 de la filière Charrière. Il est important de s'assurer que la monture des bougies conductrices n'excède pas ce numéro. J'ai fait, du reste, construire par M. Rondeau des bougies conductrices dont je suis très satisfait. Elles sont plus courtes que les bougies habituelles (28 cm.), elles sont presque rigides et aussi grosses que leur armature dans leur tiers supérieur et leurs deux tiers inférieurs sont, au contraire, extrêmement déliés pour faciliter l'accès du rétrécissement et leur enroulement dans la vessie.

Étant ainsi armé, la dilatation des rétrécissements les plus durs n'est plus illusoire.

J'ai soin de toujours opérer à vessie pleine. La plupart des cas de ruptures de bougies conductrices sont dus à ce que l'on a omis cette précaution.

Si le remplissage de la vessie au siphon est difficile, je recommande au malade de venir avec sa vessie pleine ; si, au contraire, ce remplissage est facile, je préfère le faire uriner d'abord et remplir sa vessie d'eau boriquée qu'il expulse spontanément après la dilatation.

Assez souvent, je fais une petite injection d'huile dans le canal et je graisse soigneusement la bougie conductrice et le béniqué avec la vaseline ; les pommades solubles si avantageuses à d'autres égards ne glissent pas aussi bien que la vaseline et la sonde s'en dégarnit trop vite pendant la traversée urétrale.

Ces précautions prises, j'introduis le béniqué le plus fin et les deux suivants, si c'est possible, et je recommence de même à chaque séance, tous les deux jours.

Il faut souvent déployer une certaine force pour introduire ces béniqués, le tout est de savoir les bien diriger.

Je n'agis jamais autrement en pareil cas que par la pression du pouce de la main droite sur la coudure du béniqué, à travers les parois du périnée, jamais je n'exerce aucune pression sur le manche de l'instrument. On est averti qu'on doit s'arrêter quand le béniqué ne gagne plus de terrain et rebondit en arrière à chaque pression du pouce.

Il est souvent plus difficile de retirer le béniqué que de l'entrer. Je l'extrais en agissant sur la partie concave de la coudure avec l'index de la main droite qui va le chercher au-dessus de la racine de la verge.

En règle générale, le dernier béniqué, si pénible à introduire à une séance, pénètre très facilement à la séance suivante et les mêmes difficultés se représentent pour le suivant ; néanmoins, j'ai eu des cas où il me fallait deux et trois séances pour assurer l'introduction libre d'un numéro. Je ne passe au suivant que quand cette introduction facile est obtenue.

Quand je suis arrivé au numéro 54, par exemple, j'interromps les séances pendant un, deux ou trois mois, suivant la peine que j'ai eue à faire la dilatation. Au bout de ce temps, je recommence la dilatation qui, le plus souvent, n'a rien ou presque rien perdu et je tâche de la pousser plus haut.

Chez quelques malades très récalcitrants et qui reculent devant ces séances trop prolongées, je me contente d'entretenir ce numéro qui leur suffit parfaitement.

Dans quelques cas, je prie le malade de s'introduire lui-même chez lui une petite bougie inférieure au numéro de dilatation, pendant deux ou trois heures, avant la séance.

En tout cas, j'apprends toujours aux malades à se faire eux-mêmes des lavages au siphon à l'eau boriquée, et j'ai toujours remarqué que ceux qui les font régulièrement entre les séances et même pendant la période d'interruption de traitement s'en trouvent fort bien.

De cette description il résulte que ce genre de dilatation un peu forcée des rétrécissements n'est guère applicable que dans la clientèle privée, elle demande beaucoup trop de temps et des soins trop délicats pour être acceptable dans les cliniques. L'urétrotomie interne, qui est une excellente opération, trouve là sa place tout indiquée ; elle facilite les premiers temps de la dilatation et rend facilement dilatables des rétrécissements qui l'étaient fort peu. Elle n'échoue, comme je l'ai dit plus haut, que dans les cas de rétrécissements rigoureusement indilatables qui sont très rares. Et encore, dans ces cas, elle assure à ces malades plusieurs mois de tranquillité, à la suite desquels ils se font pratiquer une nouvelle urétrotomie. Je connais des malades qui se sont fait ainsi opérer tous les ans et qui continueront probablement de même indéfiniment.

L'urétrotomie interne reste donc une opération très précieuse, mais il est bon de savoir que l'on peut, si on le désire, la remplacer par la dilatation progressive avec les béniqués fins.

M. F. LEGUEU (de Paris). — Dans les rétrécissements traumatiques, l'urétrotomie interne n'a que rarement à intervenir, et dans tous ceux qui sont accompagnés d'une virole, d'un calus appréciable extérieurement, la *résection* est l'opération de choix. L'urétrotomie externe n'est que le premier temps de la résection. A la suite de la résection, les meilleurs résultats appartiennent aux cas dans lesquels la réunion a été obtenue par la première intention.

Dans les rétrécissements inflammatoires, la dilatation est le traitement de choix, je dirais volontiers le seul traitement. En effet, l'urétrotomie externe n'est qu'une méthode accessoire, qui permet de pousser la dilatation jusqu'à des limites impossibles sans elle : mais elle ne peut rien sans la dilatation ultérieure. Plus la dilatation sera souvent répétée après l'urétrotomie, et plus le rétrécissement deviendra souple, large et élastique. Dans les urètres durs, pour les rétrécissements très serrés. je fais faire la dilatation tous les jours, et j'ai vu, grâce à cette précaution, des malades recouvrer un canal tel qu'ils ne l'avaient pas eu depuis longtemps.

L'urétrotomie externe n'intervient que dans les rétrécissements compliqués de péri-urétrites; en dehors de cela, elle n'est qu'une méthode de nécessité et dont les indications sont exceptionnelles.

La résection dans ces rétrécissements compliqués est une excellente opération. Je la fais partielle le plus souvent; mais alors même qu'elle est totale, on peut avoir un très bon résultat. Sur un de mes malades, j'ai réséqué au mois de décembre dernier 4 centimètres au moins de l'urètre périnéal; ce malade s'est refait un urètre aux dépens des parties molles; il urine largement, et se sonde de temps en temps et par précaution avec une sonde à béquille n° 21.

M. LAVAUX (de Paris). — Chez l'opéré d'Horteloup dont a parlé M. Heresco, il s'agissait d'une véritable résection de l'urètre. Je rappelle aussi que Horteloup ne plaçait pas de sonde à demeure après cette opération et qu'il ne faisait aucune suture. Ceci tout en reconnaissant qu'il faut aujourd'hui s'efforcer d'obtenir la réunion par première intention.

Je tiens également à protester contre la conclusion du rapport de M. Albarran relative aux résultats éloignés de l'électrolyse linéaire. Je regrette que le rapporteur n'ait pas précisé. Chez les malades dont il a parlé avait-on pratiqué l'électrolyse linéaire simple ou l'électrolyse linéaire *double*, telle que je l'ai décrite? Ce détail a une importance capitale. Les faits que j'ai publiés et qui sont relatifs à des malades que je suis depuis plusieurs années, quelques-uns depuis 1892 ou 1893, prouvent au contraire que les résultats éloignés sont excellents, à condition, bien entendu, de pratiquer le cathétérisme à intervalles réguliers, tous les mois ou toutes les six semaines chez la plupart de ces opérés. Aussi je considère qu'au point de vue des résultats immédiats comme au point de vue des résultats éloignés, l'électrolyse linéaire est bien supérieure à l'urétrotomie interne, à condition de pratiquer l'électrolyse linéaire double.

---

## URÉTROTOMIE EXTERNE

### par M. GOLDBERG,

de Wildungen et Cologne.

M. Albarran et M. Legueu ont dit que la résection totale est le traitement idéal des rétrécissements traumatiques. Mais j'ai pratiqué, en avril dernier, l'urétrotomie externe à un malade qui avait fait, il y avait une année, une chute sur le périnée, après laquelle il avait porté un mois une sonde à demeure. Or, chez ce malade, le tissu scléreux était si étendu en longueur et en largeur, qu'il était tout à fait, à mon avis, impossible de réséquer toute l'étendue de ce tissu, s'étendant du bulbe jusqu'au hile même de la prostate comme une vraie tumeur. Comme je ne pouvais trouver dans ce tissu l'orifice vésical du rétrécissement, M. Cahn, qui opérait avec moi, a fait séance tenante la taille suspubienne; j'ai fait le cathétérisme rétrograde; la vessie fut suturée immédiatement; sonde à demeure périnéale. Après une semaine, sonde à demeure urétrale; après un mois, guérison. Aujourd'hui, le malade se sonde avec un numéro 20 Charrière. S'il se sonde toujours, il restera en bon état.

D'autre part, nous ne pouvons pas, dans certains cas de rétrécissements traumatiques de l'urètre membraneux et prostatique, atteindre l'idéal de la résection, comme l'a déjà dit M. Carlier.

M. William Hingston (de Montréal). — Il me semble que j'avais des idées précises sur cette question, mais les différentes appréciations que je viens d'entendre ont apporté à mes idées beaucoup de confusion. Le temps effacera sans doute cette confusion, comme il a déjà changé mes idées sur le traitement des strictures.

En 1851, le traitement de Stanley (dilatation graduelle et douce) continué pendant des semaines et des années était celui auquel j'avais recours. Plus tard, j'en suis venu à l'opération de Maisonneuve. Plus tard encore, j'ai pratiqué l'opération de Syme. Ensuite, je suis revenu à la dilatation et à la divulsion. Je puis dire que maintenant j'ai abandonné toutes ces méthodes, excepté la division externe de Syme dans des cas tout à fait exceptionnels. Habituellement, je pratique l'extension du rétrécissement, et de suite l'urétrotomie interne. Mais c'est ici où ma pratique se distingue surtout de celle de mes confrères. La division n'est qu'une petite partie du traitement. J'introduis, de suite après la division, la plus grande bougie en acier et si le méat n'a pas un calibre suffisant, je le divise. Je ne la laisse pas à demeure, je la réintroduis le lendemain et les jours suivants pendant trois ou quatre semaines. Au bout de trois ou quatre jours, on est souvent obligé de diminuer un peu d'un numéro. Mais on revient vite au point de départ. Il me semble que c'est l'introduction répétée d'un grand instrument après l'opération qui fait toute la différence dans les résultats. Quelquefois, lorsque les malades ne veulent pas rester à l'hôpital, je vois la récidive. Mais chez les autres, la récidive ne se voit pas habituellement.

# HUITIÈME SÉANCE

## MERCREDI 8 AOUT

*à 2 heures et demie*

---

COMMUNICATIONS DIVERSES

## URÈTRE — ORGANES GÉNITAUX

---

Présidence de M. le Professeur **DE FARKAS**

(de Budapest)

## DU CATHÉTÉRISME RÉTROGRADE DANS LES RUPTURES DE L'URÈTRE

### par F. LEGUEU.

En 1895, dans un mémoire publié dans les Annales des maladies des organes génito-urinaires, j'ai étudié la technique et les indications du cathétérisme rétrograde dans les rétrécissements infranchissables de l'urètre. J'avais à cette époque laissé de côté le cathétérisme rétrograde appliqué aux ruptures de l'urètre. Depuis lors, j'ai eu l'occasion de pratiquer deux fois cette opération pour des ruptures complexes ou compliquées, et je voudrais montrer par ces deux observations nouvelles combien cette ressource peut être précieuse dans des circonstances difficiles.

Dans les ruptures de l'urètre postérieur, surtout dans celles qui sont la conséquence d'une fracture du bassin, l'urétrotomie externe est particulièrement difficile. Les points de repère font défaut; au fond de la plaie périnéale, les recherches manquent de la précision nécessaire et il me paraît difficile de mener à bien par cette voie une restauration utile de l'urètre postérieur. Au contraire, avec le cathétérisme rétrograde, du premier coup on retrouve l'urètre et il est facile de terminer rapidement l'opération dont le but principal est la mise à demeure d'une sonde dans l'urètre.

Je me suis trouvé une fois en présence de ces difficultés chez un enfant de dix ans, et j'ai eu recours d'emblée au cathétérisme rétrograde.

Voici d'ailleurs l'observation de ce malade :

Obs. 1. — *Fracture du bassin. Rupture de l'urètre postérieur. Cathétérisme rétrograde d'emblée. Mort.*

Le 10 octobre 1898, un enfant de 10 ans était écrasé dans la rue par un camion qui lui passait sur le corps. On le relève avec des contusions multiples, et on l'amène à l'hôpital des Enfants-Malades. L'interne de garde constate des lésions multiples : une fracture des deux cuisses, une fracture du bras gauche. En même temps on voit du sang s'écouler par le rectum et non par l'urètre.

On m'envoie chercher.

Je trouve un enfant dans un état de choc assez prononcé : l'accident a eu lieu trois heures avant, le poids est petit à 100, la température à 36°,5, le facies est pâle, les traits tirés, et l'œil fixe. Je constate les contusions multiples signalées, et je porte de suite mon attention sur l'urètre et sur la vessie.

Il n'y a pas eu de miction depuis l'accident, il n'y a pas eu non plus d'urétrorragie. J'introduis cependant une boule dans l'urètre, et je m'aperçois que la sonde s'enfonce à une grande profondeur. Elle ne présente pas cependant la liberté complète qu'elle devrait avoir dans une vessie modérément distendue. Je pratique alors le toucher rectal, et je constate que la bougie a pénétré de l'urètre dans la vessie. Sur la paroi antérieure du rectum, il y a une déchirure étendue, et c'est à travers cette déchirure que la bougie s'est échappée. La vessie semble au palper bimanuel contenir une petite quantité d'urine; sur les branches ischio-pubiennes, je ne trouve pas de fragments mobiles, bien que cependant il doive y avoir une fracture à ce niveau.

Le diagnostic est donc le suivant : rupture de l'urètre postérieur avec déchirure du rectum, par fracture probable du bassin.

Dans ces conditions, je me décide à pratiquer de suite le cathétérisme rétrograde.

Dans ce but, je pratique à la main au-dessus du pubis une incision de 5 centimètres : la vessie est distendue, elle se laisse facilement découvrir et inciser. Par cet orifice, j'introduis ma sonde que je glisse sur le doigt jusqu'au col dans lequel elle s'engage. Elle arrive ainsi jusqu'au niveau du rectum. Alors je reviens au périnée, et je fais à ce niveau une incision verticale et j'ouvre l'urètre : par cet orifice je vais avec une pince chercher la sonde que j'ai introduite par la vessie, et je parviens après quelques tâtonnements à la ramener dans la plaie urétrale.

Alors j'introduis par l'urètre d'avant en arrière une autre sonde-bougie n° 16, qui ressort au périnée, est articulée à ce niveau avec la sonde vésicale et est ramenée par celle-ci jusque dans la vessie.

La vessie est fermée : la plaie périnéale est également fermée. Dans le rectum, je place un tampon de gaze iodoformée.

L'enfant à ce moment est dans un état général assez défectueux, on le remonte avec du sérum. Il mourut quelques heures après.

Dans ce cas, la mort n'est pas due à l'opération, les lésions étaient multiples et complexes, elles étaient irrémédiables.

Quoi qu'il en soit, grâce au cathétérisme rétrograde, j'ai pu dans ce cas terminer l'opération, atteindre le but qu'elle se propose, c'est-à-dire celui de mettre une sonde à demeure dans l'urètre.

Et le cathétérisme rétrograde d'emblée me paraît l'opération de choix dans les ruptures de l'urètre postérieur.

Au contraire, dans les ruptures de l'urètre antérieur, le cathétérisme rétrograde est loin d'être nécessaire. Grâce à l'incision périnéale, on peut faire avec méthode une urétrotomie externe et la suture de l'urètre.

Mais dans quelques cas, alors que la recherche du bout postérieur apparaît très difficile, alors le cathétérisme rétrograde devient une ressource très précieuse pour terminer rapidement l'opération.

C'est dans ces conditions que j'ai procédé au cathétérisme rétrograde sur le malade qui fait le sujet de ma seconde observation.

Obs. II. — *Rupture complète de l'urètre périnéal. Fausse route, cathétérisme rétrograde avec suture totale. Guérison.*

Le 8 mai 1899, un enfant de 8 ans jouait à sauter sur un banc; dans un de ses mouvements, il manque son coup et tombe à califourchon sur le dossier. Il éprouve de suite une vive douleur, et sa chemise est tachée de sang : il y a urétrorragie immédiate.

Il rentre cependant à pied chez ses parents : mais ses douleurs sont plus vives, l'écoulement sanguin continue, on le transporte à l'hôpital Boucicaut.

Là on le sonde : on le dira à la mère plus tard; on parvient à passer la sonde jusqu'à la vessie, ce qui, comme nous le verrons, est inexact.

Mais l'enfant n'a que 8 ans, on ne peut le garder à demeure, et on conseille à la mère de le conduire à l'hôpital des Enfants-Malades.

Il est reçu dans cet hôpital et l'interne de garde, M. Rosenthal, m'envoie chercher.

J'arrivai à cinq heures du soir, l'accident avait eu lieu à midi.

Je constate au niveau du périnée une tuméfaction très légère, et une ecchymose étendue; le gonflement est limité au périnée, le scrotum n'est pas œdématié. L'écoulement de sang par l'urètre s'est arrêté, il y a sur la chemise quelques taches rouges. L'enfant n'a pas uriné depuis l'accident. J'appris alors qu'il avait été sondé, et on m'affirme même que la sonde aurait pénétré jusqu'à la vessie. Pour m'en assurer, je prends moi-même une sonde molle de Nélaton n° 13 : cette sonde traverse sans obstacle l'urètre jusqu'au périnée, et là j'ai l'impression qu'elle s'enfonce dans l'urètre postérieur. Cependant je n'ai pas la sensation de liberté qui indique qu'une sonde est dans la vessie, je ne vois d'ailleurs venir aucune goutte d'urine. Je pratique alors le toucher rectal; et je m'aperçois que la sonde est en avant du rectum, tout au contact de la paroi rectale décollée : il y a donc fausse route, et dans cette fausse route la sonde s'est engagée. Je puis rétablir alors la filiation des accidents : rupture de l'urètre, tentative infructueuse de cathétérisme et création d'une fausse route.

Ces manœuvres avaient été faites sous chloroforme, et tout avait été préparé pour l'opération que j'avais de suite jugée nécessaire. L'enfant étant mis dans la situation de la taille, je pratique sur la ligne médiane une incision de 5 centimètres, je traverse des tissus infiltrés, et j'arrive à l'hématome relativement peu volumineux que j'évacue. Une sonde introduite par ce méat ressort par le périnée et me montre le bout antérieur d'un urètre complètement rompu au niveau du bulbe : la section est nette, non mâchonnée.

Je me mets en devoir de chercher le bout postérieur : j'explore d'abord la région sans rien voir, puis je tâte avec le stylet, avec une sonde et je ne parviens qu'à retomber dans cette fausse route, qui me conduit à droite de l'urètre postérieur, au devant du rectum. Il est incontestable que cette fausse route enlève à mes recherches la précision qu'elles auraient sans elle : aussi bien je me décide très vite pour la taille hypogastrique et le cathétérisme rétrograde.

Au-dessus du pubis, sur la ligne médiane, je pratique une incision de 5 centimètres, et j'arrive vite à la vessie qui est distendue et ouverte. L'urine est évacuée : une sonde bougie est guidée sur mon doigt jusqu'au col au travers d'une boutonnière vésicale, que j'ai faite avec intention assez minime, d'un diamètre un peu supérieur à celui de l'index. Cette bougie ressort par le périnée, et me sert de point de repère.

Je reconnais alors que le bout postérieur de l'urètre était séparé du bout antérieur par une étendue de 2 centimètres au moins; la rupture était totale, et le bout antérieur s'était rétracté en avant, comme il arrive presque toujours, quand il n'y a pas au fond une paroi supérieure pour le retenir en arrière. La rupture avait eu lieu à la partie la plus reculée du bulbe, à l'union du bulbe et de la portion membraneuse ou un peu en avant.

En me servant de la bougie introduite dans la vessie, j'attirai vers celle-ci une sonde introduite dans le bout antérieur de l'urètre en arrière, au niveau du périnée, avec la sonde vésicale : et lorsque la sonde fut placée, je fermai complètement la plaie vésicale par un double étage de sutures : suture de la paroi abdominale, je laissai un petit drain dans l'angle inférieur de la plaie.

Je procédai alors à la suture de l'urètre : celle-ci fut plus délicate. L'écartement des deux bouts tendait les catguts, et plusieurs fils cassèrent. J'eus beaucoup de peine à assurer la suture au niveau de la paroi supérieure, que la sonde rendait moins accessible.

Je parvins cependant à placer circulairement six points de catgut qui adossaient les deux bouts de l'urètre très exactement; je parvins ensuite à ramener autour de l'urètre tout ce que je pus des tissus voisins de façon à fermer le périnée et à faire une suture à étages. Suture complète de la peau.

La sonde à demeure fut laissée huit jours en place; le drain prévésical fut retiré au bout de quatre jours. La vessie s'était réunie.

Au bout de huit jours, la sonde et les fils furent enlevés : il y avait réunion par première intention. L'enfant se levait au quatorzième jour et quittait l'hôpital au bout de vingt jours.

Dans cette seconde observation, le succès de l'opération a été comet ; le cathétérisme rétrograde m'a permis de terminer vite une opération d'urétrotomie externe qu'une fausse route menaçait de prolonger inutilement. Et j'ai fermé complètement la plaie vésicale et la plaie périnéale : j'ai obtenu la réunion par première intention. De sorte que cette observation est bien faite pour plaider la cause du cathétérisme rétrograde dans les ruptures de l'urètre antérieur alors que la découverte du bout postérieur ne se réalise pas facilement.

Il est un autre point que je veux soulever : c'est celui qui a trait aux résultats éloignés de la suture de l'urètre avec réunion première.

J'ai revu cet enfant le 6 février 1900, soit neuf mois après l'accident. Il urine bien, ses urines sont très claires, le jet d'urine est très fort. Une boule n° 14 passe facilement, elle rencontre au fond du périnée un obstacle qu'elle franchit et qui est constitué par une bride mince unique. Une sonde bougie n° 16 est introduite sans difficulté, ce qui représente un fort numéro pour un enfant de dix ans.

En somme, le résultat éloigné est aussi parfait que l'on pouvait le désirer, et la suture, la restauration de l'urètre, a donné dans ce cas, grâce à la réunion primitive, tout ce qu'elle pouvait donner.

Je me demande en terminant ce qui serait advenu si, chez ces malades, j'avais renoncé à terminer l'opération par le cathétérisme rétrograde, et si, renonçant à trouver le bout postérieur j'avais, comme le recommandent encore quelques chirurgiens, tamponné la plaie périnéale.

Il suffit de mettre en présence les deux solutions pour résoudre la question au bénéfice du cathétérisme rétrograde

---

## CORPS ÉTRANGERS DE L'URÉTRE

### par M. CASAMAYOR DE PLANTA

(de Mauléon)

J'ai signalé deux cas de corps étrangers, curieux par leur nature et le but perverti dans lequel ils furent introduits. Dans l'un, il s'agit d'un homme de 64 ans qui, ne pouvant accomplir l'acte sexuel, imagine de creuser un morceau de bois qu'il introduit dans le canal en guise de « tuteur », d'après son expression; il le retirait avec une ficelle fixée à l'un des bouts.

Un jour il ne peut le retirer et le voit descendre jusqu'au niveau du périnée; après huit jours d'essais infructueux, il veut se faire ouvrir l'urètre par une boutonnière périnéale; mais j'essaye d'un autre moyen en attachant le peu de ficelle qui passait à un fil de soie que je passe dans une canule vaginale en verre; j'introduis la canule dans le canal jusqu'au contact du corps étranger, alors je tire avec précaution et le tout suit.

Le tuyau avait 9 centimètres de long, 1 centimètre de diamètre, la ficelle avait 10 centimètres et paraissait à peine au méat après tractions très douloureuses.

Dans le second cas, un jeune homme s'introduisait, d'une manière fréquente, un crayon dans le canal, par perversion morale; il ne peut un jour l'enlever, d'où turgescence, œdème, douleurs et rétention d'urine mécanique; il était au niveau du périnée et sans prise pour les pinces; je pique une longue aiguille entourée d'un tube de caoutchouc sur le crayon, puis j'introduis également une canule en verre dans le canal, en plaçant l'aiguille dans sa lumière, et quand les deux objets se touchent, je tire lentement le tout. Le crayon avait 11 centimètres de long, 8 millimètres de large.

Paralysie consécutive de la vessie durant trois jours.

### De la glace dans les prostatites.

J'ai cité quelques cas de prostatite aiguë consécutive à des excès chez des vieillards et chez un jeune homme tombé accidentellement sur le périnée, améliorés très rapidement par de la glace introduite dans le rectum en guise de suppositoire, par petits morceaux fréquemment renouvelés.

### Accidents urinaires dans la fièvre typhoïde.

J'ai tenu à signaler les accidents urinaires survenus dans les 519 cas de fièvre typhoïde que j'ai soignés en 1898-1899, avec 12 décès seulement, grâce au traitement que j'ai combiné et qui fera l'objet d'une communication spéciale.

Dans bien des cas, j'ai constaté de l'albumine et des phosphates en petite quantité. Dans 6 cas, albuminurie très considérable ayant amené des manifestations urémiques dans deux cas, dont un mortel.

Dans 11 cas j'ai eu de la paralysie vésicale avec rétention complète d'urine ayant une durée de cinq à neuf jours au maximum.

Dans trois cas, de la cystite purulente très intense ayant cédé aux lavages boriqués et aux instillations.

Dans un cas mal déterminé, car le malade était très éloigné, j'ai assisté à une débâcle purulente par les urines. Le malade a des urines claires le matin ; à dix heures, les violentes douleurs lancinantes, qu'il ressent dans les reins du côté gauche, cessent subitement, et, à la première miction, les urines sortent purulentes et avec des traces de sang ; les mictions suivantes sortent troubles, à la fin seulement, pendant quatre jours et la fièvre tombe du coup de 39°,8 à 37°,4. Je l'ai attribué à une rupture d'un abcès infectieux rénal. Le malade guérit.

---

## DU TRAITEMENT DES RÉTRÉCISSEMENTS URÉTRAUX
## PAR L'ÉLECTROLYSE LINÉAIRE

### par M. le docteur J.-A. FORT

(de Paris)

Il y a dix-sept ans que je fis construire par M. Dubois un instrument au moyen duquel je traite les divers rétrécissements, les urétraux et les œsophagiens principalement, par l'*électrolyse linéaire*.

Dans cette communication je ne réfuterai pas les critiques dont mes opérations d'électrolyse linéaire ont été l'objet et je laisserai de côté la question théorique, me cantonnant uniquement sur le terrain chirurgical, sur le terrain pratique.

A mon retour d'Amérique, le baron H. Larrey et le Pr Richet eurent la bienveillance de présenter à l'Académie de médecine, en mon nom, deux mémoires sur un *nouveau procédé pour guérir les rétrécissements de l'urètre, rapidement et sans danger*. Ces deux mémoires furent présentés à quelques mois de distance.

Le Pr Richet ne voulut pas faire la présentation sans s'être rendu compte de l'exactitude des faits annoncés, et, après plusieurs entrevues et plusieurs expériences, il me chargea d'opérer deux hommes de son service chirurgical de l'Hôtel-Dieu, gravement malades de rétrécissement urétral. Le résultat atteint fut tel, que le professeur s'empressa de présenter mon mémoire avec des paroles élogieuses.

Ces mémoires, dont les conclusions étaient basées sur un grand nombre d'observations, se terminaient par ces conclusions :

1° *L'électrolyse linéaire n'est pas douloureuse ;*

2° *Elle est rapide;*

3° *Elle ne s'accompagne pas d'écoulement sanguin;*

4° *Elle ne nécessite pas de séjour au lit;*

5° *Elle ne réclame pas de sonde à demeure;*

6° *Il n'y a jamais d'accidents consécutifs;*

7° *La récidive est rare.*

Douze années se sont écoulées depuis la présentation de ces deux mémoires. Les observations sur lesquelles étaient basées ces conclusions n'avaient pas été prises avec toute la rigueur désirable, mais, depuis douze ans, je les recueille toutes avec le plus grand soin. J'apporte ici, à l'appui de ma communication, un faisceau respectable de 140 observations les plus récentes. J'aurais pu en fournir un plus grand nombre, mais j'ai pensé qu'il était inutile de grossir ce faisceau outre mesure, le nombre de 140 étant bien suffisant pour corroborer les premières conclusions.

Elles n'ont pas varié ; je suis à même de le prouver.

J'en ajouterai cependant une nouvelle :

8° *Pour électrolyser un rétrécissement urétral un faible courant de dix milliampères est suffisant.*

Il résulte de mon expérience de l'électrolyse linéaire qu'il y a moins de rétrécissements durs qu'on ne le croit généralement, et il m'est arrivé fréquemment d'avoir une série de vingt rétrécissements tendres, sans en rencontrer un seul dur.

Sur les 140 observations dont je fournis ici le résumé, y a 66 opérations d'électrolyse linéaire ayant duré 30 secondes ou moins de 30 secondes, 69 ayant duré de 30 à 60 secondes. Donc 135 fois sur 140, l'opération n'a pas duré plus d'une minute.

*a)* L'opération par l'*électrolyse linéaire* ne produit pas une cicatrice dure; celle-ci est parfaitement dilatable, comme on peut s'en assurer en parcourant les 140 observations que je cite.

*b)* Au moment de l'opération, on voit une gouttte de sang perler au méat. Quand on prie le malade de rendre l'injection antiseptique, généralement employée après l'opération, il s'écoule une ou deux gouttes de sang au commencement et à la fin de la miction.

Puis, pendant 24 heures, après chaque miction, il s'écoule deux ou trois gouttes de sang.

Quelques malades ont des rétrécissements qui saignent facilement. Il arrive rarement qu'ils aient une petite hémorragie de quelques grammes de sang. J'ai vu deux cas où l'hémorragie a été assez considérable et pourrait être attribuée à la bougie introduite après l'opération.

Mais, en général, je le répète, il n'y a pas d'écoulement sanguin.

Je n'ai jamais imposé à un malade le séjour au lit, à moins de cas exceptionnel. Il m'est arrivé de maintenir au lit le jour de l'opération quelques sujets pusillanimes qui ont exigé d'être chloroformés. En général, je prie le malade de rester chez lui le jour de l'opération. Mais le lendemain je lui permets de sortir.

c) Jamais je n'ai employé la sonde à demeure, je n'insisterai donc pas sur ce point.

d) Ainsi qu'on peut s'en rendre compte, 7 malades sur mes 140 opérés ont eu un accès de fièvre urineuse. Elle se manifeste, dans les cas où elle survient, le soir même du jour de l'opération, après la miction. Mais dans quelques cas je l'ai observé le lendemain et parfois le surlendemain.

Mais cet accès est généralement unique et je n'en ai jamais vu qui pût inspirer de l'inquiétude.

Je n'ai jamais observé de ces accidents locaux graves dont parlent les auteurs, je n'ai jamais vu un cas d'infiltration d'urine, de phlegmon du pénis, etc. Ces accidents ne peuvent se produire que dans les cas d'opérations mal conduites, où l'on a employé un courant très intense pendant une très longue durée.

e) Dans les observations que je présente et qui sont prises à la suite les unes des autres comme elles se sont présentées, nous trouvons 7 récidives, c'est-à-dire 5 1/2 pour 100. Comme on a l'habitude de comparer l'électrolyse linéaire à l'urétrotomie interne, je fais remarquer que les récidives me paraissent plus fréquentes après l'urétrotomie, ce qui s'explique, d'ailleurs, par la nature de la plaie produite par un instrument tranchant, ensuite par le peu de hauteur des lames généralement employées. Après l'urétrotomie on passe une sonde n° 16 ou 18 tout au plus. Après l'électrolyse on passe le n° 22, le n° 23 ou le 24, et même plus.

Du reste, il faut bien reconnaître que les bases manquent pour établir une statistique comparative.

Je pourrais citer l'observation d'un grand nombre de malades guéris depuis une dizaine d'années, je me contenterai d'en fournir un petit nombre.

f) Il est naturel de penser que la destruction du tissu du rétrécissement est en raison directe de la densité du courant employé et du temps pendant lequel l'instrument électrolyseur reste en contact avec le rétrécissement. Sous ce rapport, mes observations sont très nettes. Je n'emploie que 10 milliampères constatés au galvanomètre apériodique, et l'opération ne dure en moyenne que de 20 à 30 secondes, ce qui me permet d'introduire une bougie n° 22 séance tenante.

Que faut-il donc dire de ces expériences et opérations citées maintes fois, dans lesquelles on a employé jusqu'à 50 milliampères pendant quinze minutes? Avec un tel courant et ce laps de temps, il n'est pas étonnant qu'on observe des accidents graves, comme la perforation de l'urètre, etc.

*g*) Il résulte de la lecture des observations que je présente, que certains rétrécissements opérés par l'électrolyse linéaire restent guéris, pour ainsi dire, indéfiniment. Je ne voudrais pas dire qu'il en est de même dans tous les cas. Au contraire, certains rétrécissements récidivent assez promptement. On peut admettre, selon moi, que les rétrécissements, opérés par l'électrolyse linéaire, lorsque le malade n'a pas recours à un cathétérisme régulier, récidivent après quatre ou cinq ans.

Quant à ces rétrécissements qu'on a dit récidiver à bref délai, ce sont des cas d'opérations mal dirigées dans lesquels la lame de l'électrolyseur a franchi le rétrécissement, sous l'influence d'une trop forte pression, sans qu'il y ait eu opération véritable.

### Conclusions.

Depuis que mon mémoire a été écrit, j'ai été surpris, en même temps qu'attristé, de lire dans une *notice* sur la clinique des voies urinaires de la Faculté de médecine de Paris, publiée par le D<sup>r</sup> Paul Noguès, assistant de la clinique, les lignes suivantes :

« MM. Albarran et Noguès, désireux de se rendre un compte exact de la valeur de l'électrolyse, ont soumis à cette thérapeutique 10 malades atteints de rétrécissements. Grâce aux précautions qu'ils ont prises, ils n'ont pas eu de décès à déplorer, mais quelques accidents locaux immédiats, tels que urétrorragie, péri-urétrites, abcès urineux même, et surtout l'insuffisance chez tous de résultat définitif, ont fait complètement abandonner cette opération. A cette expérience personnelle s'ajoute l'observation d'une série de malades, qui, ayant subi une électrolyse en ville, sont venus à l'hôpital pour se faire soigner soit de complications consécutives, soit d'une récidive rapide. »

Il est étrange que le professeur Guyon, et MM. Albarran et Noguès soient absents de la Section à la séance même où devait avoir lieu ma communication. Il faut, et je demande, que le public médical soit éclairé. Les assertions de MM. Albarran et Noguès sont une véritable charge à fond de train contre l'électrolyse linéaire. Comment concilier ces assertions avec les résultats constants que j'ai obtenus dans les 140 cas que je présente à la Section.

Ou mes observations ne sont pas authentiques, ou mes contradicteurs n'ont pas opéré selon les règles. Or j'affirme que mes observations sont l'expression de la vérité et qu'elles ont été recueillies avec soin. Je demande donc à l'honorable président de la Section, au professeur Guyon, au nom du droit et de la justice, d'avoir l'obligeance de nommer une Commission qui assistera à mes opérations et qui en fera l'objet d'un compte rendu.

## QUELQUES MOTS AU SUJET DE L'ÉLECTROLYSE LINÉAIRE DANS LE TRAITEMENT DES RÉTRÉCISSEMENTS DE L'URÈTRE

### par M. DE GARAY

(de Mexico)

D'après ce que l'on déduit des conclusions des rapporteurs distingués qui ont traité la question du résultat éloigné des traitements sanglants des rétrécissements de l'urètre, ce résultat ne signifie rien pour le choix du procédé à suivre pour traiter un rétrécissement de cette espèce. Par aucun de ces procédés, sauf peut-être quelques cas de résection de l'urètre, on n'obtient une guérison certaine et définitive par la seule opération. Dans tous les cas le cathétérisme dilatateur périodique et perpétuel s'impose, même si le rétrécissement se reproduisait au bout de six mois en suivant un traitement, au bout d'un an, de deux ou plus, en en suivant d'autres. Ceci n'est sujet à aucune formule mathématique ; ce qu'il arrive à un malade n'arrive pas à un autre, et le clinicien ne peut conseiller rien de mieux à un individu opéré d'un rétrécissement, que de continuer toujours à dilater son canal urinaire. Le choix du procédé dépend sans doute de sa bénignité, de sa facilité d'exécution et en général des avantages que le malade peut en retirer. Selon la nature, la place et l'étendue du rétrécissement, la situation et la condition du malade, il faudra varier le procédé choisi. Dans les rétrécissements traumatiques, les rétrécissements très durs et véritablement scléreux, qui sont la plupart du temps la conséquence d'urétrotomies internes antérieures, dans les rétrécissements très étendus ou en chapelet, conviendront en général l'urétrotomie externe ou la résection urétrale partielle ou complète, le méat abdominal ou périnéal, comme le conseille le D^r Poncet, de Lyon. Dans les rétrécissements proprement inflammatoires ou gonococciques, on peut employer l'urétrotomie interne, externe ou mixte, ou l'électrolyse linéaire.

Je ne suis pas partisan de la divulsion urétrale. L'urétrotomie interne peut être simple ou accompagnée au moment opératoire de la dilatation du canal, c'est-à-dire qu'il faut sectionner en dilatant. L'urétrotomie interne n'est pas exempte de dangers, et malgré l'antisepsie qui ne peut pas toujours s'effectuer dans un canal presque fermé, et avec l'urine infectée, on observe parfois des infections diverses dont quelques-unes sont graves, et des hémorragies quelquefois importantes. L'antisepsie du canal urinaire par la voie interne est loin de mériter une confiance absolue. Cette opération occasionne encore des ennuis et des souffrances, et fait perdre au malade plusieurs jours ou semaines.

Pour obtenir le meilleur résultat possible avec l'urétrotomie interne, il faut que le rétrécissement soit sectionné en un point et d'une manière complète. Le tissu sclérosé, toujours plus ou moins élastique, se contracte quand il est sectionné totalement et le calibre de l'urètre s'élargit. C'est sur ceci qu'est basé le procédé américain d'Otis, de New-York. Si le couteau coupait sans dilater, il y aurait besoin de faire une grande incision pour couper toute l'épaisseur du rétrécissement, et si l'incision était petite, le rétrécissement ne serait pas complètement sectionné et le calibre de l'urètre n'aurait pas beaucoup augmenté. Les incisions petites et multiples ont le même inconvénient, et doivent faciliter la reproduction du rétrécissement, à cause du tissu cicatriciel qu'elles occasionnent. Toute blessure faite par un instrument coupant produit une cicatrice dont le tissu est plus ou moins scléreux suivant que la cicatrisation a été primitive ou secondaire. Si cette cicatrice se trouve dans un canal, ce canal perd son calibre normal, et cela d'autant plus que les incisions qu'on y a pratiquées sont plus nombreuses. Dans le cas où il faudrait faire une urétrotomie interne, je préfère le procédé d'Otis, sans donner une exactitude mathématique au rapport entre la circonférence du pénis et le diamètre de l'urètre, comme le fait cet auteur. Je n'aime pas non plus le métrotome de ce chirurgien, parce qu'il produit la dilatation de tout l'urètre. A Mexico, le métrotome d'Otis est modifié dans ce sens qu'il ne dilate l'urètre qu'au point rétréci. Mais chaque fois que je puis substituer à l'urétrotomie interne, l'électrolyse, je le fais sans hésiter. J'ai à ma charge deux services de chirurgie, et aussi bien là que dans ma maison de santé et dans ma clientèle privée, j'ai eu l'occasion de pratiquer tous les principaux procédés pour la guérison des rétrécissements de l'urètre. J'ai pratiqué environ 300 électrolyses, dans des cas divers, et grâce à cette pratique, je crois pouvoir donner ici mon opinion sur ce sujet. Il y a plus de trois ans que j'ai étudié à Mexico, à côté du D<sup>r</sup> Fort, l'électrolyse linéaire.

La manière dont je pratique cette opération est la suivante. J'emploie un électrolyseur dont la largeur de lame est en rapport avec le degré du rétrécissement. J'emploie le nombre de milliampères nécessaire, 5 à 10, et dans quelques cas j'en ai employé jusqu'à 40 sans inconvénient, en les faisant durer jusqu'à 5 minutes, temps maximum que j'aie employé. En général j'opère en moins d'une minute. Je fais immédiatement la dilatation avec les bougies lourdes de Vergne, généralement jusqu'au numéro 21, ou l'un des numéros correspondants des bougies Béniqué ou des dilatateurs du savant professeur Guyon. Les jours suivants, je continue la dilatation, et en 8 ou 10 jours j'arrive jusqu'au numéro 25 ou 58 des bougies de Vergne. Si je ne parviens pas à continuer facilement la dilatation, je fais une ou deux électrolyses secondaires avec des électriseurs à double lame, l'une antérieure et l'autre postérieure et plus larges, et je continue la dilatation jusqu'à atteindre le numéro convenable. Les électrolyses peuvent être répétées sans aucun inconvénient et à des intervalles plus ou moins éloignés. Très souvent je ne puis vaincre un rétrécissement en une séance et je le traite en plusieurs séances. Chez des malades qui, après avoir été opérés, n'ont pas continué la dilatation, j'ai observé que le rétrécissement commence à se reproduire au bout de six mois ou d'un an. Quelques opérés sont restés deux ans sans se sonder et ont conservé toujours leur calibre urétral. Je ne donne pas grande importance à ceci, car je conseille à tous mes opérés la dilatation périodique et continuelle, et qu'en la pratiquant le rétrécissement reste guéri pour toujours et sans qu'il se présente d'accident. Je n'emploie jamais de sonde en permanence; l'opération se fait sans douleur en employant au préalable quelques grammes de solution de cocaïne à 1 pour 100. Je n'ai jamais observé d'accidents graves qui puissent réellement être imputés à l'électrolyse : hémorragies, perforations urétrales, infections sérieuses, etc. Parfois quelques accidents : néphrite, urémie par anurie, etc., sont dus à l'état d'imminence morbeuse de ces organes ou à leur état de septicité préalable. Les malades ne gardent pas le lit et poursuivent leurs occupations habituelles.

Dans les rétrécissements œsophagiens, à la suite de grandes brûlures, par exemple, l'œsophagotomie interne est une opération très grave, presque abandonnée et qui ne guérit pas le rétrécissement.

L électrolyse linéaire, répétée plusieurs fois, guérit complètement ces rétrécissements, en la combinant avec la dilatation; mais une fois que celle-ci est obtenue, les malades peuvent rester plusieurs années sans se sonder et sans que le rétrécissement se reproduise. J'ai vu plusieurs opérés du D<sup>r</sup> Fort dans ces conditions : l'un d'eux avait souffert plusieurs opérations par instrument coupant, et la trachéotomie, car le rétrécissement arrivait jusqu'à l'extrémité inférieure du pharynx. Il fut complètement guéri. J'ai moi-même deux cas dans lesquels jai obtenu aussi des guérisons définitives.

Pourquoi l'électrolyse guérirait-elle ces terribles rétrécissements de l'œsophage et non ceux de l'urètre? Puisque avec l'électrolyse nous détruisons, nous désagrégeons les polypes de l'urètre, pourquoi n'en serait-il pas de même des tissus qui forment le rétrécissement? Dans l'électrolyse l'instrument est froid, il ne cautérise pas, son action est électrochimique et il produit des modifications, qui sont encore peu connues dans les tissus. Un exemple de ceci c'est la guérison de l'ozène par l'électrolyse cuprique.

Je crois juste que l'on fasse occuper à l'électrolyse linéaire la place à laquelle elle a droit. Je prétends non pas qu'elle guérisse tous les cas de rétrécissements de l'urètre, mais qu'elle remplace avantageusement l'urétrotomie interne dans la plupart des cas où cette opération est indiquée.

Le meilleur procédé pour opérer les rétrécissements de l'urètre serait celui qui guérirait ces affections d'une manière radicale, sans grand danger pour les malades et sans nécessiter de dilatations ultérieures de l'urètre, mais ce procédé n'est malheureusement pas encore connu.

M. de KEATING-HATT (de Montréal). — Ayant écouté attentivement la communication que vient de nous faire M. le docteur Fort, je tiens à vous soumettre sur le même sujet quelques observations, à titre de médecin électricien, puisqu'il s'agit en somme d'une des applications de l'électricité à la thérapeutique des voies urinaires.

Tout d'abord, je ne saurais que répéter, après M. Fort, que l'électrolyse donne, dans le traitement de la plupart des rétrécissements urétraux, des résultats parfaits et *définitifs*. Je n'insisterai du reste pas, la statistique de M. Fort ayant une valeur probante plus grande que mes simples affirmations.

Mais où je me sépare complétement de lui, c'est dans le choix de la méthode à suivre et de l'instrument à utiliser.

Je ne crois rien exagérer en affirmant que la presque unanimité des spécialistes électriciens se sert surtout de l'instrument de Newman, n'employant le couteau de Fort qu'à titre d'*urétrotome* électrolytique, dans les cas rares où la méthode de douceur préconisée par Newman n'a pas été suffisante pour guérir leurs patients. Le spécialiste américain se sert, vous le savez, d'une olive et non d'une anse, ce qui permet à l'électrisation d'être moins dense, et par conséquent d'agir comme antispasmodique beaucoup plus que comme agent destructeur.

Les reproches que je ferai à l'instrument de Fort sont de sens inverse, car 1° il augmente la densité du courant, en limitant son contact à une zone restreinte du tissu malade, et 2°, il risque de manquer complètement son but, quand il a affaire par exemple à un rétrécissement en nid de pigeon, parce qu'alors, il peut laisser de côté la lésion, et creuser un sillon en tissu sain.

Dans l'électrolyseur modifié que M. Fort vient de nous présenter, il a diminué les défauts sus-indiqués, en ajoutant un nouvel arc de cercle à l'ancien. En les multipliant à l'infini, il rendrait son instrument parfait, mais alors celui-ci serait à peu près identique à l'olive de Newmann, qui, à mon avis, demeure jusqu'à nouvel ordre l'électrolyseur urétral par excellence.

M. Comanos (du Caire). — Quelques mots seulement pour confirmer les résultats d'électrolyse du docteur J. Fort dans les rétrécissements urétraux. J'ai pratiqué au Caire, dans l'espace de cinq ans, l'électrolyse linéaire sur 52 malades avec des résultats vraiment merveilleux. Je n'ai jamais eu à déplorer d'accidents ou de suites fâcheuses. J'ai eu l'occasion d'examiner 2 et 5 ans après l'électrolyse des malades qui ne s'étaient pas du tout sondés et de constater à ma grande satisfaction que le résultat de l'électrolyse continuait à persister.

---

## TRAITEMENT DE LA BLENNHORRAGIE RÉCENTE CHEZ LA FEMME

### par M. le docteur JULES JANET.

J'ai eu souvent l'occasion de soigner des femmes pour des blennorragies récemment contractées. Il arrive, en effet, assez fréquemment que les blennorragiques, qui se présentent à ma consultation, ont eu peu de temps avant le début de leur écoulement des rapports avec une femme saine et se sont ainsi exposés à la contaminer. Je demande toujours, en pareil cas, à examiner cette femme et le plus souvent je constate chez elle un début de blennorragie.

J'ai acquis, par ces examens, la conviction de l'extrême facilité de l'infection gonococcique chez la femme. Alors qu'un homme peut coïter pendant des mois avec une femme blennorragique sans être infecté, alors qu'il peut avoir des rapports avec un grand nombre de prostituées qui sont, pour la plupart sinon toutes, gonococciques, sans être atteint; une femme, au contraire, est pour ainsi dire forcément contaminée, quand elle a un rapport avec un homme blennorragique, même dans la période d'incubation où les gonocoques sont encore très peu nombreux.

Le traitement de ces blennorragies récentes chez la femme est simple quoiqu'un peu minutieux. Il doit avoir surtout pour but d'empêcher l'infection de s'étendre au delà du col utérin.

On peut, en effet, comparer la blennorragie urétrale, vulvaire et cervicale de la femme à la blennorragie de l'urètre antérieur de l'homme et la blennorragie du corps de l'utérus à celle de l'urètre postérieur. Les grosses complications chez l'homme comme chez la femme ne sont guère à redouter que quand le gonocoque s'étend aux parties profondes : corps de l'utérus chez la femme, urètre postérieur chez l'homme.

Un traitement bien conduit doit donc chercher, avant tout, à empêcher cette extension en profondeur de l'infection. Et cela est encore plus vrai pour la femme que pour l'homme, car les complications de l'infection gonococcique profonde sont infiniment plus graves chez elle que chez lui et peuvent conduire à la persistance presque indéfinie de gonocoques, malgré tous les traitements que l'on peut diriger contre eux, ce qui n'arrive jamais chez l'homme.

Les différents foyers de l'infection gonococcique récente chez la femme sont l'urètre et les glandes para-urétrales, les glandes de Bartholin et le col utérin. Ils peuvent être tous infectés simultanément, mais cela est rare, le plus souvent quelques-uns de ces foyers restent indemnes.

Quelquefois un foyer primitivement indemne s'infecte au cours du traitement. Ils doivent donc être tous surveillés de près à chaque séance.

Pour la facilité de la description, je suppose un cas dans lequel tous ces foyers sont pris simultanément.

Je commence par faire uriner la malade, je lave la vulve avec un tampon imbibé de permanganate de potasse au 1/1000°.

Je lave l'urèthre avec une canule métallique à jet récurrent semblable à celle que M. le D<sup>r</sup> Burkhardt (de Bâle) a proposée pour le même but, mais garnie d'une olive beaucoup plus petite.

J'ai fait construire cet instrument et les suivants par M. Gentile. Cette canule adaptée à une seringue ou au tube d'un siphon est introduite progressivement d'avant en arrière jusqu'au col vésical et retirée de même. 150 à 200 cc. de la solution de permanganate de 0 gr. 50 à 1 gramme pour 1000 suffisent pour ce lavage. Si l'urine est trouble, je remplace la canule par une sonde Nélaton courte n° 16 ; je l'introduis progressivement en lavant l'urètre et je la conduis jusque dans la vessie, je lave la vessie à plusieurs reprises, puis je la remplis : je retire alors la sonde en lavant encore l'urètre et à la fin de l'opération je prie la malade d'uriner la solution de permanganate que j'ai laissée dans sa vessie. En pareil cas, je termine la séance par ce lavage, pour ne pas laisser trop longtemps la solution dans la vessie.

Les glandes para-urétrales ou de Skene sont tantôt placées sur les lèvres du méat, tantôt à l'intérieur de l'urètre, à quelques millimètres de l'orifice.

Dans le premier cas, elles sont très faciles à laver avec une fine canule en platine mousse montée sur une seringue de 10 à 20 grammes. J'emploie pour cet usage une solution de permanganate de potasse au 1/500e.

Dans le second cas, il faut les rechercher avec un petit spéculum bivalve en s'éclairant avec un photophore frontal.

J'ai fait construire par M. Gentile deux de ces spéculums ; le premier a des valves verticales et permet d'explorer les parois supérieure et inférieure de l'urètre, le second a ses valves horizontales et permet d'explorer les parois latérales de l'urètre.

Si les orifices des glandes restent invisibles, je presse légèrement la paroi du vestibule au-dessus du spéculum avec un tampon de coton roulé sur une petite tige de bois, je fais sourdre ainsi une petite goutte de pus qui marque l'orifice cherché.

Autrement, je fais à distance une petite injection de permanganate entre les valves du spéculum quand il est en place. La solution colore souvent en rouge l'orifice de la glande et permet de le découvrir aisément.

Une fois les glandes découvertes je les injecte avec la canule fine dont j'ai parlé plus haut, mais il est préférable de se servir dans ce cas d'une canule plus longue et coudée au niveau de son tiers inférieur. Il faut avoir soin, après ce lavage, d'éponger l'excès de solution qui reste dans l'urètre.

Ces lavages des glandes n'arrivent pas aisément à les débarrasser du pus qu'elles contiennent. Il est bon dans le cours du lavage d'exprimer à plusieurs reprises le vestibule urétral pour expulser ce pus et permettre à la solution de pénétrer jusqu'au fond des culs-de-sac glandulaires.

Si l'on veut s'éviter ces lavages assez pénibles, on peut sectionner la paroi qui sépare les glandes de l'urètre de manière à les faire communiquer aisément avec lui, mais ce procédé ne dispense pas de laver à part le sillon profond qui résulte de cette opération, car le lavage urétral aurait beaucoup de chance de ne pas y pénétrer suffisamment.

Le traitement des glandes de Bartholin se fait de même : on découvre l'orifice très facilement soit à la vue, soit en exprimant le contenu de la glande, soit en déposant un peu de permanganate sur la région occupée par l'orifice, celui-ci se colore aussitôt en rouge.

Je me sers pour laver ces glandes d'une canule fine courbée dans son milieu à angle droit, je l'introduis, après expression du contenu glandulaire, dans le canal excréteur et j'injecte à petits coups, et retirant légèrement la canule après chaque poussée pour laisser le liquide ressortir plus facilement.

J'emploie comme pour les glandes para-urétrales la solution à 1/500e.

Si l'orifice glandulaire est trop étroit pour laisser passer la canule, je le dilate avec des bougies coniques fines.

Grâce à ce traitement, j'ai toujours évité l'abcédation de la glande et obtenu des guérisons très rapides.

Après ce traitement de l'urètre et de la vulve, je lave à l'aide du bock et d'une canule de verre le vagin avec la solution de permanganate à 0,50/1000e. Le doigt que l'on introduit dans le vagin parallèlement à la canule permet de le déplisser et d'extraire les mucosités du col.

Cela fait, j'introduis le spéculum, je lave la surface extérieure du col avec un tampon de coton monté sur une pince et imbibé de la solution à 0,50/1000e.

Le lavage de la cavité cervicale se fait très commodément avec les porte-tampons dont on se sert pour l'endoscopie urétrale, c'est-à-dire des tiges fines de bois d'allumettes ou de stores autour des extrémités desquelles on enroule un peu de coton hydrophile. Ces tiges sont assez souples pour s'accommoder à l'incurvation du col si elle existe.

Je les imbibe de la solution de permanganate à 1/100e, et je réitère l'écouvillonnage jusqu'à ce que toutes les mucosités du col aient été extraites. Je me sers aussi quelquefois pour le même usage d'une sonde métallique à jet récurrent semblable à celle dont je me sers pour l'urètre, mais beaucoup plus longue. Cette sonde est adaptée à une seringue. Je ne laisse aucun tampon vaginal.

La malade doit compléter le traitement chez elle en se lavant la vulve matin et soir avec le permanganate à 0,50/1000e immédiatement après avoir uriné et en prenant ensuite une injection vaginale avec la même solution. Je répète les séances tous les jours au début du traitement, puis tous les deux jours.

Le moment le plus délicat de ce traitement de la blennorragie chez la femme c'est le moment des règles.

D'après tous les faits que j'ai observés, je reste convaincu que le seul moyen de mener à bien un pareil traitement et d'éviter les très graves complications de la blennorragie profonde, c'est de continuer les lavages tels que je viens de les indiquer pendant toute la durée des règles.

Jusqu'à présent j'ai hésité à faire le lavage du col utérin pendant cette période et j'ai vu deux fois le gonocoque pénétrer dans le corps de l'utérus, je crois que j'aurais pu éviter ces deux mauvais cas en continuant régulièrement le traitement du col. Je n'hésiterai pas à le faire dorénavant.

Il n'est pas rare, après la disparition des gonocoques, de voir s'installer à leur suite des microbes secondaires dans les régions qu'ils ont occupées. Je les combats comme chez l'homme par des lavages de sublimé : 1/10000e à 1/20000e pour l'urètre, 1/4000e pour le vagin, 1/2000e pour l'utérus. Ces infections secondaires peuvent, comme le gonocoque, remonter dans le corps de l'utérus, on les y poursuit à l'aide de la sonde de Bozeman. Ces infections secondaires ne présentent, du reste, en général que peu de gravité.

Je n'ai pas voulu dans ce travail qui n'a trait qu'à la blennorragie récente parler du traitement de la blennorragie profonde, utérine et annexielle, qui rentre plutôt dans le chapitre des complications blennorragiques. On doit, du reste, les éviter par un traitement bien conduit.

---

## TRAITEMENT DE LA BLENNORRAGIE DE L'URÉTRE ANTÉRIEUR

par M. le docteur A. SUAREZ DE MENDOZA,

de Madrid.

Le traitement de la blennorragie par la méthode de Janet est aujourd'hui classique. Dès son apparition, je l'adoptai et l'appliquai, me conformant à la technique conseillée par l'auteur, avec laquelle je m'étais familiarisé dans cet hôpital même.

Les inconvénients signalés un peu partout, principalement lorsqu'il s'agit d'infections limitées à l'urètre antérieur, me frappèrent bientôt et j'essayai de modifier le procédé, tout en conservant les principes de la méthode.

Un des plus sérieux inconvénients, le plus sérieux à mon point de vue, du procédé de lavage de M. Janet, c'est que le malade ne peut laver lui-même son urètre d'une façon convenable; l'obligation d'avoir recours au médecin chaque fois que le besoin du lavage se fait sentir, impose à tous deux une servitude dont la moindre conséquence fâcheuse est l'irrégularité du traitement. De plus, il est difficile de faire proprement un lavage de l'urètre avec le procédé de Janet, on se salit les mains, on tache et on mouille le malade, le lit et parfois les objets environnants.

Pour parer à tous ces inconvénients, il fallait modifier l'instrument et disposer d'une canule qui permît au malade de faire lui-même, mécaniquement pour ainsi dire, un bon et complet lavage de l'urètre antérieur; en outre, il était indispensable de limiter le lavage à cette partie de l'urètre, autrement, il eût été dangereux de confier cette petite opération à des mains inhabiles.

Je fis donc construire par la maison Collin la canule que voici; elle se compose de deux tubes concentriques dont l'intérieur est destiné à l'irrigation, pendant que l'évacuation du liquide s'effectue par le tube externe. Le cylindre d'irrigation doit être d'un millimètre et demi plus long que l'externe; autrement, la muqueuse urétrale obstruant celui-ci, le double courant peut s'établir à l'intérieur de l'instrument, donnant l'illusion du lavage de l'urètre, lorsque pas une goutte de liquide n'y aurait pénétré. Cette canule remplit les conditions voulues d'une façon parfaite :

1° Le malade peut faire lui-même les lavages avec toute la perfection désirable;

2° Avec cette canule on lave parfaitement l'urètre antérieur;

3° On ne lave que l'urètre antérieur.

De plus, lorsque le médecin le désire, il peut, sans changer d'instrument, faire pénétrer le liquide dans la vessie, en bouchant simplement, avec le doigt, l'orifice de sortie de la canule.

Pour prouver qu'avec cette canule fonctionnant normalement, c'est-à-dire sans boucher l'orifice de sortie du liquide, on lave très bien l'urètre antérieur, il suffit d'injecter dans celui-ci une solution de ferrocyanure de potassium, le laver à fond avec la canule et chercher dans les dernières parties de l'eau du lavage la présence du ferrocyanure au moyen du perchlorure de fer; la réaction fera défaut.

Pour se convaincre que le liquide employé ne dépasse pas le sphincter externe, on fera un lavage de l'urètre avec une solution de ferrocyanure, après quoi on le lavera à fond, de façon à le débarrasser complètement du sel ferrocyanique et l'on fera uriner le malade dans un verre dans lequel on versera ensuite quelques gouttes de perchlorure de fer ; si l'on constate que la réaction caractéristique (bleu de Prusse) fait défaut, c'est une preuve évidente que la solution de ferrocyanure n'a pas pénétré dans la vessie.

Voici ma technique pour les lavages de l'urètre, qu'ils soient pratiqués dans un but curatif comme dans les urétrites, ou bien qu'ils soient simplement prophylactiques, précédant une intervention instrumentale quelconque dans la vessie.

Le récipient placé à 1 m. 20 de hauteur et le sujet couché, je le couvre d'une alèze imperméable de 60 centimètres carrés environ. Dans les commencements, je me servais d'une alèze en feuille anglaise ; j'y ai renoncé bientôt, cette feuille produisant une très désagréable sensation de froid, j'emploie maintenant une fine toile imperméable, dont une seule face, celle qui ne touche pas le malade, est caoutchoutée. Sur la ligne médiane de cette alèze, et à 15 centimètres du bord supérieur existe un orifice de 5 centimètres et demi de diamètre pour laisser passer le pénis. L'alèze en place, garantissant le malade de toute souillure, on met entre ses cuisses un récipient long et étroit de contenance suffisante et on procède au lavage, qui s'effectue avec une propreté absolue, sans que malade ni médecin soient jamais souillés.

On lave d'abord le gland, puis, séparant les bords du méat, on les lave très soigneusement ainsi que la partie du canal y aboutissant, après quoi on procède au lavage de l'urètre proprement dit.

Il est indispensable de surveiller attentivement la forme du jet de sortie qui doit être plein et former une courbe régulière ; lorsqu'il n'en est pas ainsi, le double courant intra-urétral n'est pas régulièrement établi et le lavage de l'urètre n'est certainement pas bien fait.

C'est pourquoi ceux qui ont imité ou modifié cette canule, ont eu tort d'ajouter un embout à l'orifice de sortie pour y fixer un tuyau de caoutchouc ; tout contrôle est ainsi supprimé et l'on risque de faire souvent de la mauvaise besogne. J'avais fait cela dans les commencements, mais je dus bientôt y renoncer.

Il est mauvais aussi de donner une forme effilée au bout urétral de la canule ; ce bout pénètre trop profondément dans la fosse naviculaire et comme le double courant s'établit à l'extrémité de la canule, la partie terminale de l'urètre auprès du méat se trouve ainsi en dehors de ce courant, elle n'est pas lavée et demeure foyer d'infection.

Quant au liquide employé, ce sont les solutions de permanganate de potasse, le nitrate d'argent et le protargol qui m'ont donné les résultats les plus satisfaisants.

Cette canule et ce *modus faciendi* se sont rapidement généralisés en Espagne. A l'hôpital San Juan de Dios de Madrid, on n'en emploie plus d'autre depuis plus de deux ans. M. le professeur Bombin, médecin en chef de cet hôpital, me disait naguère que les résultats obtenus étaient parfaits et que les accidents observés de temps à autre avec la technique de M. Janet avaient totalement disparu.

Dans ma clinique des voies urinaires, nous nous en servons constamment pour laver l'urètre, soit dans un but curatif, soit pour faire l'asepsie relative, mais cliniquement suffisante du canal, lorsqu'il faut faire pénétrer des instruments dans la vessie; or, nous n'avons jamais eu à déplorer la plus petite infection du réservoir urinaire.

Messieurs, la blennorragie est une véritable calamité sociale; là où on le pense le moins, on trouve le gonoccoque; dans des milieux où l'on ne songerait pas à soupçonner sa présence, on peut trop souvent constater ses ravages: aussi, je crois que son traitement prophylactique est bien plus intéressant que son traitement curatif, et c'est dans ce sens que j'ai voulu diriger mes recherches.

Nous savons aujourd'hui que les gonocoques, avant de pénétrer dans les parties profondes de l'urètre, restent fixés sur l'épithélium pendant un laps de temps, que les expériences Finger ont évalué à trois jours. Or, il me paraît probable qu'en les attaquant vigoureusement pendant les premières vingt-quatre heures, on pourrait avoir des chances d'empêcher l'éclosion de la blennorragie.

Les expériences que j'ai commencées dans ce sens paraissent devoir confirmer mes présomptions; si elles se confirmaient en se multipliant, on aurait en mains un traitement prophylactique facile et inoffensif de la blennorragie; il suffirait de faire, le plus tôt possible après tout coït suspect, un ou plusieurs lavages de l'urètre avec une solution faible de permanganate ou de toute autre substance appropriée, pour détruire les gonocoques qui auraient pu pénétrer dans ce conduit. Le temps utile pour cette intervention, sa modalité et sa limite extrême sont à déterminer; dans tous les cas, comme quelques lavages de l'urètre, dans les conditions que je viens de dire, sont sans aucun danger et qu'en les faisant, le sujet contaminé est certain de n'aggraver en rien sa situation si toutefois il n'échappe pas à l'infection, je n'hésite pas à les conseiller systématiquement, malgré l'insuffisance de mes expériences.

Ces expériences, qui consistent en somme à déposer dans l'urètre de l'homme, en évitant tout traumatisme, une culture pure de gonocoques et à empêcher l'infection du canal au moyen de lavages dont elles auront à préciser le nombre, la durée et le temps utile pour leur administration, sont très délicates et entourées de difficultés de tout ordre, dont la moindre n'est pas de trouver des sujets qui veuillent se prêter aux expériences sachant très bien qu'ils s'exposent à contracter une blennorragie ; aussi, elles ne sont encore ni assez nombreuses, ni assez détaillées, ni assez concluantes pour être communiquées au Congrès.

Mon principal but en vous lisant ces lignes, c'est pour ainsi dire de prendre date, de vous faire connaître la voie où je me suis engagé, espérant que d'autres, mieux armés que moi, voudront m'y suivre, ce qui aplanirait considérablement les obstacles de la route et permettrait d'atteindre bien plus rapidement le but désiré.

---

## TRAITEMENT DES INFLAMMATIONS DE LA PARTIE ANTÉRIEURE DU CANAL DE L'URETRE A L'AIDE DE LAVAGES

par M. le docteur N. A. MIKHAILOFF,

de Saint-Pétersbourg

L'inflammation du canal urinaire chez les hommes appartient au nombre des maladies fréquentes et rebelles des voies génito-urinaires. Parmi les différents moyens intérieurs et extérieurs, proposés pour combattre l'inflammation, le traitement par les injections dans le canal à l'aide d'une seringue en verre est le plus répandu, mais en même temps le moins raisonnable et le plus dangereux par ses suites. Les expériences des docteurs Panin, Guiard et Courtade nous ont démontré depuis longtemps que le liquide injecté même à l'aide d'une grande seringue ne pénètre pas jusqu'au bulbe. Et nous savons très bien que les urétrites aigües siègent seulement pendant le premier temps dans les parties antérieures du canal urinaire, tandis que plus tard on les trouve plus souvent et même presque uniquement dans la partie bulbeuse. Grâce aux injections, l'inflammation se transporte des parties antérieures de l'urètre sur la partie postérieure souvent mécaniquement. Le pus avec les micro-organismes qu'il contient, les gonocoques, est entraîné par le liquide injecté hors du méat extérieur jusqu'aux parties plus profondes et même jusqu'à la partie spongieuse et prostatique. Même la miction avant l'injection n'éloigne pas ce danger. Les injections peuvent même transporter le liquide par le méat jusqu'à la vessie, ce qui a été prouvé par des autorités comme Reliquet, Guyon et beaucoup d'autres.

On recourt aux injections pendant les inflammations en général dans l'intention de détruire l'élément spécifique contagieux, mais cela ne réussit jamais pour la simple raison qu'à mesure que la partie antérieure du canal se remplit du liquide injecté, le pus se détache des parois et pénètre plus profondément jusqu'à la partie bulbeuse où il peut former des colonnes plus ou moins grandes qui obstruent tout à fait l'ouverture du canal. Le remède injecté ne touche et n'influence que la partie antérieure du cône de cette colonne de liquide, tandis que la partie postérieure n'est nullement influencée par le remède. Outre cela une partie de l'écoulement (le pus et le mucus) reste sur les parois de l'urètre, surtout entre ses plis et empêche l'effet du remède sur les muqueuses.

Ainsi nous voyons qu'à l'aide des injections nous ne pouvons ni désinfecter, ni provoquer l'effet du remède sur la grande paroi du canal. Il est clair que dans les cas d'inflammation de la partie antérieure, la maladie siège avant la pars membranatia de l'urètre où le liquide injecté ne pénètre pas : recourir aux injections avec la seringue en verre serait non seulement imprudent mais même nuisible.

En 1892, le docteur Janet a pour la première fois fait part de son nouveau traitement de la blennorragie à l'aide de lavages abondants du canal urinaire avec une dissolution de kali hypermanganicum. Ce traitement original a vite conquis une place de premier ordre au milieu des autres traitements de la blennorragie. De mon côté je puis remarquer que depuis deux ans que j'applique ce traitement à mes malades, sur 52 cas de différentes inflammations blennorragiques du canal urinaire, 20 ont été accompagnés de complications (soit inflammation, soit blennorragie postérieure).

Voici trois ans que je n'ai plus recours à la méthode de Janet parce qu'elle n'empêche pas la maladie de s'étendre sur la partie postérieure du col de la vessie. Ainsi ne trouvant efficaces ni les injections avec une seringue en verre, ni les lavages de kali hypermanganicum sous différentes pressions proposées par le docteur Janet, depuis deux ans j'ai recours à d'autres lavages dans les cas aigus ainsi que dans les formes chroniques d'inflammation de la partie antérieure du canal urinaire. Ce traitement ne présente rien de nouveau, mais il semble être oublié ou tout au moins il ne s'applique plus. Déjà en 1871 Mercière a proposé de faire des lavages de l'urètre, pendant les inflammations chroniques, à l'aide d'un cathéter élastique ayant un orifice de côté et un au bout.

En 1886 le professeur Soubbotin a proposé de pratiquer des lavages avec un cathéter dans les cas d'inflammation de l'urètre. Sur 51 malades qui ont été soumis à ce traitement, 29 se sont entièrement rétablis; chez 2 seulement on a constaté des complications.

N'oubliant pas que généralement et même presque exclusivement les inflammations soit aiguës. soit chroniques siègent dans la partie bulbeuse la plus large, j'emploie un cathéter élastique français ayant 16 centimètres de longueur pour pouvoir l'introduire dans le canal de l'urètre à une distance de 12-14 centimètres du méat extérieur. L'orifice de ce cathéter se trouve au bout, n° 14-16 d'après Charière. L'appareil dont se servent mes malades pour les lavages de toute la pars pendula est très simple. Il se compose d'un cathéter et d'un entonnoir muni d'un petit tube en caoutchouc. L'entonnoir est en verre et a un volume de 200 grammes. Le tuyau en caoutchouc a 1 m. 50 de long et on met à son extrémité un embout de verre auquel on adapte le cathéter élastique. Pour faciliter le fonctionnement de l'appareil, on place avant l'embout en verre un robinet ou une pince. L'emploi de cet appareil n'est pas compliqué. On suspend l'entonnoir à une hauteur d'à peu près 1 m. 50 au-dessus des organes génitaux et on l'emplit de la solution destinée pour le lavage, ensuite on approche des reins un vase pour recevoir le liquide à son retour. Puis on introduit dans le canal de l'urètre un cathéter lavé dans une solution de sublimé et enduit de glycérine. Le cathétérisme a pour effet de faire couler le liquide, puis on pousse le cathéter plus au fond, absolument jusqu'à la partie bulbeuse. Le liquide injecté dans le canal urinaire ressort immédiatement et passe entre le cathéter et les parois du canal en lavant ce dernier. Quand il s'agit d'une blennorragie à gonocoques de la partie antérieure du canal, on emploie avec succès des solutions chaudes de kali hypermanganicum 1 : 4000 jusqu'à 1 : 2000, ou une solution de sublimé de 40 (1 : 10000-1 : 5000) et 1 : 6000 d'argentum nitricum tiède jusqu'à 1 : 2000, en lavant le canal une fois par jour.

Quand j'avais à faire à de simples catarrhes de la partie antérieure du canal urinaire, j'ai employé de la même manière et avec succès des lavages avec une solution physiologique de natrum bicarbonicum et de sel de cuisine (6-1000). En pratiquant les lavages il faut de temps à autre interrompre le traitement pour quelques jours pendant la période de l'irritation mécanique.

Les deux dernières années j'ai recouru à cette méthode de lavages à l'aide d'un cathéter élastique, non seulement dans les cas aigus, mais aussi quand il s'agissait des inflammations chroniques, et je suis très satisfait de mes résultats. Sur 69 malades d'inflammation de la partie antérieure du canal de l'urètre que j'ai observés, il y en a eu 18 chez lesquels l'inflammation était subaiguë, chez les autres il s'agissait de cas chroniques. Sur 18 malades 14 ont été complètement guéris, quant aux 4 autres le résultat du traitement ne m'est pas connu car ils ne sont plus revenus dès qu'une amélioration s'est opérée dans leur état. Sur 51 malades chroniques 39 se sont complètement rétablis, les 9 autres ont aussi interrompu le traitement quand ils étaient en voie de guérison. Dans deux cas seulement le traitement a été suivi de complications (épididymitis et orchitis). Par complète guérison j'entends :

1) absence absolue de tout écoulement du méat ;
2) une urine tout à fait claire ;
3) absence de fils blennorragiques ;
4) résultat négatif de l'analyse microscopique sur les gonocoques après une injection (1 : 4000) de solution d'argentum nitricum.

M'appuyant sur le succès relativement heureux qu'ont obtenu mes lavages à l'aide d'un cathéter élastique dans les cas d'inflammations de la partie antérieure du canal urinaire, je recommande ce procédé à mes collègues et leur conseille d'être prudents, avec les injections à l'aide d'une seringue en verre, dans les cas aigus, subaigus et chroniques. Instruit par une amère expérience je n'en ,veux pas aux injections parce qu'elles sont vieillies, mais parce qu'elles ne sont pas naturelles et que même elles présentent des dangers.

En prescrivant les injections nous violons la muqueuse et permettons au procès blennorragique de s'étendre librement sur les parties plus profondes du canal urinaire et même sur la vessie.

---

## TRAITEMENT ABORTIF DE LA GONORRHÉE

von Dr Ernst R. Z. FRANK

(Berlin)

Angesichts der grossen Häufigkeit der Prostatitis gon., angesichts der grossen Gefahr der von ihr weiter ausgehenden Complikationen und den Consequenzen, angesichts endlich der grossen Schwierigkeiten, die sich so oft der Therapie entgegenstellen, muss das therapeutische Handeln vor allen Dingen darauf ausgehen, zu vermeiden, dass der gonorrhoische Process auf die Drüsenschluche der Prostata übergreift; das wird in allen Fällen möglich sein, die unserer Behandlung zugängig werden, wenn die Infection noch frisch und auf den vorderen Harnröhrenabschnitt beschränkt ist.

Abgesehen von einer erfolgreichen Prophylaxe der Gonorrhoe überhaupt, deren Möglichkeit ich in einer vor 2 Jahren veröffentlichen Arbeit nachgewiesen habe, empfehle ich Ihnen eine Art abortiver Behandlung für die bald nach erfolgter Infection in Ihre Hände gelangenden Gonorrhoeen, die mein College Lewin und ich seit einigen Monaten angewendet haben. Nach gestellter mikroskopischer Diagnose uriniert der Patient. Ist die zweite Portion klar, so wird mittelst einer 1/4 % Protargollösung unter geringem Druck zunächst die vordere Harnröhre gespült, bis die Spüleflussigkeit klar abläuft. Bei grosser Empfindlichkeit des Patienten cocainisiert man sodann die Harnröhre mit einer schwachen Lösung 1 : 200, der man vorsichtshalber etwas Protargol zufügt. Sodann wird genau entsprechend der Janet'schen Vorschriftseine grosse Spülung beider Harnröhrenabschnitte mit der gleichen Protargollösung vorgenommen. Man lässt die Spülflüssigkeit so lange einlaufen, bis der Patient Urindrang verspürt, also etwa 1/4 bis $\frac{1}{2}$ ltr. Sodann enleert der Patient seine Blase. Die gleiche Prozedur wird an den beiden folgenden Tagen wiederholt. Schon nach 24 Stunden ist der vorher abundante, eitrige Ausfluss minimal und serös, und meist sind Gonococcen nicht mehr nachzuweisen. Im gleichen Masse schwinden die Leucocythen, während das Präparat reichlich Epithel und Fibrin enthält. Sind am dritten Tage noch Gonococcen vorhanden, so ist das ein Zeichen dafür, dass die Abortivkur nicht gelungen ist. Der Grund liegt entweder darin, dass bereits die Vorsteherdrüse inficiert war, dass paraurethrale Gänge vorhanden sind, in welchen die Gonococcen der Therapie nicht zugängig sind, oder dass Missbildungen der Harnröhrenschleimhaut, Falten oder Klappen vorhanden sind. In den letzteren Fällen führt ein entsprechender chirurgischer Eingriff sofortige Heilung herbei.

Ich habe in dieser Weise 60 Fälle behandelt. In 27 Fällen, also in 45 %, war der Erfolg ein positiver, d.h. nach 3 Spülungen, und in 3 dieser Fälle nach einer einzigen Spülung, blieben die Gonococcen definitiv verschwunden., trotz vielfacher provocatorischer Reizungen. Ich habe die Patienten fast sämtlich noch Wochen und Monate nachher beobachtet. In 26 Fällen waren nach 3 Tagen noch Gonococcen vorhanden. In drei von diesen Fällen waren gonorrho

isch inficierte paraurethrale Gange vorhanden. Nach Inciscion derselben mitte Ist des Janet'schen Trajectotoms genügten weitere 2-3
Spülungen um die Gonococcen zum definitiven Verschwinden zu
bringen.

In 2 Fällen handelte es sich um angeborene Klappen und Fälten-
bildung bei sehr engem Meatus. Nach Entfernung des Hindernisses
verliefen die Fälle wie die oben beschriebenen.

In 21 Fällen war trotz zweiten klaren Urins bereits eine gonorrhoische Infection der Prostata nachzuweisen, und ich habe Gründe,
anzunehmen, dass diese Infection bereits vor Einleitung der Abor-
tivbehandlung vorhanden war.

In 7 Fällen, welche poliklinische Patienten betrafen, blieben die
Patienten aus der Beobachtung fort, einige stellten sich gelegentlich
später vor, um zu berichten, sie sien gesund. Da aber diese Fälle
nicht genau beobachtet sind, habe ich sie nich als positiv betrachtet.

Jedenfalls beweisen diese Thatsachen, dass in einer grossen Anzahl
von Fällen, nämlich wenn der Patient früh genug die ärztliche
Behandlung aufsucht die geschilderte Abortivmethode, die in keinem
Falle sich als schädlich erwiesen hat, zu schnellem Verschwinden der
Gonococcen führt, wodurch das Uebergreifen des Processes auf die
Vorsteherdrüse und auch tiefergehende Laesionen der Harnröhren-
schleimhaut vermieden werden können.


## COMMUNICATIONS RÉSUMÉES

### Blennorragie chronique d'un urètre surnuméraire,
#### par M. PERKOWSKI (de Varsovie).

Le nommé Jacob G..., âgé de 25 ans, remarqua dès son enfance que son
gland avait un autre orifice en outre du méat normal. Il ne commença
à s'en inquiéter, que depuis un an, quand il contracta la blennorragie
de ce canal anormal surnuméraire; à la suite d'injections, l'écoulement disparaissait par instant, pour revenir à chaque nouveau rapport
sexuel. *La chose digne à remarquer est que l'urètre normal dont le méat se
trouvait au sommet du gland ne s'en infecta jamais.*

Le gland présentait deux ouvertures : l'une était celle du méat au sommet du gland, l'autre supérieure anormale était située à la surface supérieure du gland, à 13 millimètres en arrière.

On pouvait introduire facilement le n° 18 Béniqué dans l'urètre normal,
tandisque le n° 16 entrait avec peine dans le canal anormal, dont la longueur totale était de 12 centimètres.

Après l'introduction d'une sonde cannelée, je fis l'incision de l'urètre
surnuméraire; c'est un canal sous-cutané, placé à la superficie des deux

corps caverneux non séparés qui, après un parcours de 9 centimètres, s'enfonçait à la base du pénis entre les couches des muscles de la paroi abdominale, pour finir en trou borgne à la symphyse du pubis. Cette partie profonde de ce canal anormal avait la longueur de 3 centimètres. *Si on compare cet urètre surnuméraire avec l'urètre normal on trouve qu'il ne lui manquait que la partie membraneuse et prostatique.*

Son incision montra que la muqueuse avait une teinte rouge foncé, sa surface était striée par place, il restait des plis longitudinaux sur toute sa longueur ; ces plis disparaissaient par l'extension. Le diamètre de cette surface incisée était analogue aux dimensions des différentes régions de l'urètre normal ; car après un rétrécissement normal du méat succédait l'élargissement comparable à la fosse naviculaire, ensuite ce canal se rétrécissait pour s'en élargir à son extrémité du côté du pubis.

Comme il y avait des fortes adhérences de cette muqueuse malade avec les corps caverneux, sa dissection était presque impossible et demandait des larges incisions des muscles abdominaux, je me bornai à l'application de simples sutures entre les bords de la peau et de la muqueuse incisées ; sachant qu'après un court espace de temps, la muqueuse devait acquérir les caractères de la surface cutanée.

Grâce aux cautérisations employées sur la surface de la muqueuse incisée et aux injections d'iode dans la partie profonde du canal, la cicatrisation et l'oblitération de l'urètre anormal se firent en peu de temps.

---

## PATHOGÉNIE ET PROPHYLAXIE DES GÉNITALITES FÉMININES POST-MATRIMONIALES

par M. GUIARD,

de Paris

On peut les diviser en deux catégories absolument distinctes :

Les unes sont *virulentes* et résultent d'une transmission conjugale qui a son point de départ dans la persistance, chez l'homme, d'une urétrite, le plus souvent subaiguë ou chronique. Celle-ci peut encore être gonococcique ; elle est alors éminemment contagieuse. D'autres fois, elle ne contient plus que des microbes variés sans gonocoques ; parfois même, elle est aseptique ; dans ces conditions, il n'est pas absolument démontré qu'elle soit transmissible. En aucun cas cependant, il n'est prudent d'autoriser le mariage sans s'être assuré par des examens bactériologiques réitérés, notamment après les réactions hygiéniques et thérapeutiques en usage, qu'il n'y a plus à compter avec le gonococcisme latent, et sans avoir consciencieusement employé tous les moyens rationnels qui peuvent procurer la guérison radicale.

Mais on observe, chez les jeunes mariées, d'autres génitalites *non virulentes*. Ce qui fournit la preuve péremptoire qu'elles ne relèvent pas de la contagion, c'est : 1° que la recherche du gonocoque soit dans la sécrétion urétrale, soit dans celle du col utérin, soit dans celle du cul-de-sac vaginal postérieur, est constamment négative ; 2° que l'examen direct du mari par les moyens d'investigation les plus méticuleux, alors même qu'il est pratiqué le plus près possible du début, ne permet aucune constatation suspecte ; 5° enfin, que les injections vaginales antiseptiques à base de sublimé sont incomparablement plus efficaces que dans les formes virulentes, à condition pourtant qu'elles soient utilisées sans retard.

Ces génitalites non virulentes ont pour facteur essentiel les microbes saprophytes qui pullulent normalement dans tous les vagins. Longtemps et parfois indéfiniment inoffensifs, ces agents sont néanmoins la grande cause et des pertes blanches dont tant de jeunes filles sont affectées et de la métrite des vierges qui n'est pas absolument rare. Mais, aussitôt après le mariage, la congestion dont s'accompagnent inévitablement les premiers rapports, plus ou moins immodérés, favorise puissamment leur action pathogène. C'est ainsi qu'apparaissent les inflammations génitales que l'on appelait autrefois « balistiques », et que l'on attribuait exclusivement à l'action mécanique réitérée de l'acte vénérien.

Dans leur pathogénie, on le comprend sans peine, aucune part de responsabilité ne saurait incomber au mari, contre lequel il serait souverainement injuste de laisser planer des soupçons ou des accusations qui peuvent compromettre gravement et pour toujours le bonheur du jeune ménage, quand ils ne servent pas de préface à un prochain divorce. Il importe donc au plus haut point que le médecin sache reconnaître, dès le début et avec la précision absolue qui résulte des recherches bactériologiques, la véritable nature du processus morbide.

Pour l'enrayer et aussi pour le prévenir, il suffit de détruire les microbes autochtones du vagin. On y arrive aisément par l'emploi régulier d'injections vaginales antiseptiques à base de sublimé. Quoi qu'on en ait dit, les solutions variant de 1 pour 10 000 à 1 pour 5000, sont absolument inoffensives, en dehors de l'état puerpéral, et possèdent une indiscutable efficacité, à condition que l'on ait recours à une technique spéciale. Il faut, en effet, que le liquide antiseptique imprègne toute l'étendue des parois vaginales et, pour cela, qu'il en produise le déplissement. C'est ce qu'il est impossible d'obtenir à moins de le soumettre à une retenue intermittente, grâce à la constriction de la vulve autour de la canule avec la main, constriction qui l'empêche de sortir. La tension vaginale ainsi déterminée doit nécessairement être modérée, c'est-à-dire ne mettre en jeu qu'une différence de niveau de 1 mètre à 1 m. 25 entre le réservoir et le vagin; alors elle ne comporte jamais le moindre inconvénient.

Il serait à désirer, suivant moi, que ces soins d'hygiène antiseptique fussent systématiquement adoptés non seulement par toutes les femmes, mais même par les jeunes filles : ils seraient une précieuse garantie de santé pour leur appareil génital. Ainsi seraient prévenues nombre de leucorrhées interminables et de métrites, chez les femmes comme chez les vierges, de génitalites chez les jeunes mariées. J'ajoute que ces injections devraient aussi être régulièrement conseillées au cours de la grossesse; elles sont inoffensives et constituent le meilleur moyen de préparer un milieu génital stérile pour l'époque de l'accouchement et d'empêcher ainsi les accidents puerpéraux.

Elles ont malheureusement contre elles des préjugés populaires invétérés et puissants, surtout en ce qui concerne les jeunes filles. On craint vaguement que leur innocence immaculée et peut-être même les signes physiques de leur virginité subissent une atteinte quelconque de pratiques de ce genre. Cependant, convenablement effectuées, avec une canule assez petite, elles sont incapables d'agrandir l'orifice de l'hymen; quant au point de vue moral, je ne vois vraiment pas pourquoi les injections vaginales seraient plus contraires à la pudeur que l'administration des lavements. Il n'en est pas moins probable qu'il faudra encore beaucoup de temps et de luttes pour en obtenir la vulgarisation; car elles sont énergiquement combattues par quelques-uns de nos maîtres les plus éminents, professeurs à la Faculté ou membres de l'Académie de médecine. Ils attribuent aux injections vaginales de sublimé des dangers formidables. Je crois qu'ils prennent l'exception pour la règle et qu'en dehors de l'état puerpéral ces dangers sont purement imaginaires. Sans doute, après l'accouchement, des injections mercurielles intra-utérines abondantes, même d'un faible titre, peuvent à la rigueur provoquer les phénomènes toxiques les plus sérieux. Néanmoins, dans les cas d'accidents infectieux graves des suites de couches, un certain nombre d'accoucheurs des hôpitaux fort distingués continuent encore d'y recourir, en employant, il est vrai, des procédés chirurgicaux particuliers, qui rendent impossible la retenue indéfinie du liquide injecté et ils obtiennent ainsi les cures les plus merveilleuses. En tout cas, on ne saurait oublier qu'il existe alors une vaste plaie utérine largement ouverte à toutes les résorptions. S'il est sage, en pareil cas, de s'abstenir des injections de sublimé sous pression telles que je les préconise, j'estime qu'il est absolument irrationnel de les condamner indistinctement d'une façon générale; j'estime surtout que c'est rétrograder que de méconnaître les propriétés pathogènes des microbes autochtones du vagin, aussi bien chez les jeunes filles et les femmes exemptes de grossesse que pendant le cours de la gestation.

Quoi qu'il en soit, au point de vue des génitalites non virulentes post-matrimoniales dont il est ici question, une expérience assez étendue m'autorise à soutenir que ces injections constituent un moyen préventif et curatif à la fois très simple et très efficace.

# NEUVIÈME SÉANCE

## JEUDI 9 AOUT

*à 9 heures du matin.*

### Présidence de M. le professeur GUYON.

---

#### PRÉSENTATION DES INSTRUMENTS

---

#### UN NOUVEL URÉTROTOME
par M. le docteur P. HAMONIC,
de Paris.

L'instrument que j'ai l'honneur de présenter poursuit le but de sectionner le tissu pathologique formant le rétrécissement en même temps qu'il incise la paroi supérieure de l'urètre à la façon de l'urétrotome de Maisonneuve.

Je ne m'attarderai pas à montrer l'avantage de la section supérieure dans l'urétrotomie interne.

On sait que le plafond de l'urètre est la région qui est la moins susceptible de donner lieu à des hémorragies en même temps qu'elle est la plus propre à fournir au canal rétréci une rallonge lorsqu'on l'incise.

Mais l'urétrotomie de Maisonneuve a toujours été passible du reproche de laisser intact ou à peu près le tissu du rétrécissement. En effet ce dernier occupe le plus souvent d'une façon exclusive le plancher du canal. Quand il l'entoure circulairement, c'est en bas qu'il présente son maximum de développement.

La section médiane supérieure atteint donc des parties saines ou présentant des lésions minima. Elle a l'inconvénient de donner lieu à une cicatrice nouvelle d'autant plus large que le canal est plus serré et aux dépens de laquelle va se faire la dilatation ultérieure.

J'ai pensé qu'il y aurait intérêt à sectionner le tissu du rétrécissement dans la partie où il est le plus développé en même temps qu'on incise le plafond de l'urètre.

Mon procédé d'urétrotomie conserve tous les avantages de la méthode de Maisonneuve en même temps qu'il échappe au reproche de respecter le tissu strictural. Ce dernier se trouve sectionné complètement dans sa partie la plus développée.

Cette section n'encourt pas le reproche de créer une cicatrice nouvelle puisqu'elle s'exerce sur un tissu déjà sclérosé.

Par contre, elle offre l'avantage de donner une place relativement considérable en coupant directement l'obstacle urétral et d'empêcher ainsi l'incision du plafond du canal, de mordre aussi profondément qu'elle le fait, lorsqu'elle est seule et isolée.

En résumé, mon procédé d'urétrotomie interne dérive de celui de Maisonneuve, mais, au lieu de créer la rallonge circulaire aux dépens seulement de la paroi supérieure, il le fait aux dépens du plafond et du plancher du canal. En coupant l'obstacle lui-même, il évite de mordre profondément sur la paroi supérieure qui, le plus souvent, est saine, et de déterminer ainsi une cicatrice opératoire large et épaisse.

Mon instrument se compose d'un *conducteur* et d'un *couteau*.

Le *conducteur* est formé de deux longues *valves* juxtaposées présentant chacune une rainure. Les deux valves sont retenues au contact l'une de l'autre à l'aide d'un *bouton terminal* qui se visse sur leur extrémité.

Ce *bouton* est parcouru par un petit *canal* allant obliquement de son extrémité vers sa base et dans lequel on insinue un de mes *conducteurs*.

L'année dernière, j'ai communiqué au Congrès d'urologie mon nouveau mode de conducteur sur lequel je crois inutile de revenir aujourd'hui.

Les deux valves étant rapprochées, leurs rainures se juxtaposent, formant une coupe perpendiculaire à l'axe, une fente transversale s'élargissant à chacune de ses deux extrémités.

A leur terminaison externe, les deux valves sont reliées entre elles par une *petite pièce mobile* qui les empêche de s'écarter.

Le *couteau* est formé de deux *lames tranchantes* ayant, la supérieure 6, 7 ou 8 millimètres d'élévation, tandis que l'inférieure n'en a constamment que deux.

Chacune des *lames* présente à son point culminant une partie mousse, *un dos d'âne* à la façon de l'instrument de Maisonneuve. Elle est tranchante en avant et en arrière de ce point à partir duquel elle s'abaisse progressivement dans un sens et dans l'autre.

Ces *lames* sont soudées, la plus large en haut, la plus mince en bas sur un *mandrin* aplati qui s'insinue dans la rainure formée par les deux valves du cathéter conducteur.

Pour retenir ces valves au contact intime l'une de l'autre, le mandrin présente de distance en distance, sur ses parties latérales, de petites saillies qui pénètrent dans les parties latérales renflées de la rainure formée par les valves du conducteur. Ces dernières s'accolent de la sorte d'autant mieux entre elles que le couteau progresse davantage.

Ce simple exposé suffit pour faire comprendre ce qui se passe dans mon nouveau procédé d'*urétrotomie interne*.

Une fois ma longue bougie conductrice introduite dans l'urètre, je fais glisser sur elle mes deux valves, réunies ainsi qu'il a été indiqué, et elles viennent prendre naturellement la position qu'elles doivent occuper.

Cela fait, j'insinue le mandrin qui porte les lames et, avant de l'engager à fond, je fixe l'une à l'autre les extrémités extérieures des valves conductrices à l'aide de la *pièce mobile*.

Je pousse alors le couteau et le retire aussitôt.

La partie mousse de chaque lame écarte l'une de l'autre la paroi supérieure et la paroi inférieure de l'urètre, de telle sorte que dans les régions saines toute section est impossible.

Mais, dès que le rétrécissement se présente, le tissu strictural résiste, et la partie antérieure des lames tranchantes entre en action, celle d'en bas pour inciser le tissu pathologique, et celle d'en haut pour mordre sur la paroi supérieure et rétablir le calibre normal de l'urètre.

Grâce à sa faible saillie, la *lame inférieure* ne doit et ne peut que sectionner le tissu fibreux pathologique. Il ne lui est pas possible de pénétrer très avant dans le corps spongieux et d'amener les hémorragies qu'on serait en droit de redouter si on incisait largement de ce côté.

Le débridement du tissu strictural dans son point le plus accusé donne beaucoup de place et s'oppose à ce que la section supérieure soit aussi profonde qu'elle l'est dans les autres procédés d'urétrotomie.

Il résulte de cela que mon instrument expose moins à l'hémorragie que n'importe quel autre.

Je n'ai pas encore pratiqué un nombre suffisant d'opérations pour pouvoir faire ressortir la supériorité de mon urétrotome sur les autres. J'espère pouvoir revenir sur ce sujet à la prochaine session, mais, dès maintenant, je puis certifier que l'urétrotomie est plus facile et moins dangereuse avec mon instrument qu'avec celui de

Maisonneuve ; que la voie créée est beaucoup plus large ; que la cicatrice de la paroi supérieure est sensiblement plus restreinte, et qu'enfin la dilatation consécutive est plus aisée et plus rapide.

La logique fait supposer que les résultats lointains seront meilleurs puisqu'on coupe le tissu strictural lui-même et que la dilatation subséquente s'opère aussi bien aux dépens de la paroi supérieure que de la paroi inférieure.

J'espère avoir l'honneur, l'année prochaine, de donner à la Société une statistique opératoire qui permettra de mieux apprécier la valeur de l'instrument que je présente aujourd'hui.

---

## UN NOUVEAU MÉATOTOME-MÉATOMÈTRE

### par M. le docteur P. HAMONIC,

de Paris.

Malgré sa bénignité, la *méatotomie* est une opération qui doit solliciter l'attention du chirurgien en raison de sa fréquence et parfois des accidents hémorragiques auxquels elle peut donner lieu. Nombreux sont les spécialistes qui ont eu des ennuis de ce genre.

L'hémorragie m'a paru provenir de ce que les instruments à bascule qu'on emploie mordent trop profondément au niveau de la base du gland. C'est surtout à quelques centimètres du méat que l'incision *profonde* est dangereuse à ce point de vue, et cependant, dans l'opération qui nous occupe, il importe de sectionner sur une étendue de plusieurs centimètres si l'on veut avoir un résultat suffisant et durable.

Le *méatotome* de Civiale et autres instruments à bascule qui sont d'un usage courant me paraissent avoir d'autres inconvénients. Quand on presse sur la pédale pour faire saillir la lame tranchante, celle-ci donne tout d'un coup son maximum de profondeur d'incision, de telle sorte qu'entre l'urètre proprement dit et sa région antérieure incisée, il existe une sorte d'angle saillant, d'éperon en avant duquel le conduit est largement béant, tandis qu'en arrière il devient tout à coup beaucoup plus restreint.

Dans ces circonstances, quand on introduit un cathéter après la méatotomie, l'instrument accroche cet éperon saillant qui parfois gêne beaucoup sa progression et est susceptible de saigner et d'amener divers accidents dont le moindre est la douleur.

Un autre point à faire ressortir, c'est que, dans certains cas, il importe, en même temps qu'on incise la face supérieure de la fosse naviculaire et du méat, de débrider la partie inférieure de cet orifice pouvant former une véritable valvule.

Le *méatotome* que j'ai l'honneur de présenter a pour but de réaliser ces divers desiderata. Il peut devenir de plus un *méatomètre* permettant de mesurer le calibre de l'orifice du canal comme les bijoutiers mesurent leurs bagues. Pour cela, il n'y a qu'à enlever les lames tranchantes fixées sur l'axe de l'instrument. Ce dernier est conique et présente une graduation qui lui permet cet usage.

En haut et en bas, il présente sur chacun de ses diamètres opposés une rainure dans laquelle on introduit les lames. Ces dernières sont

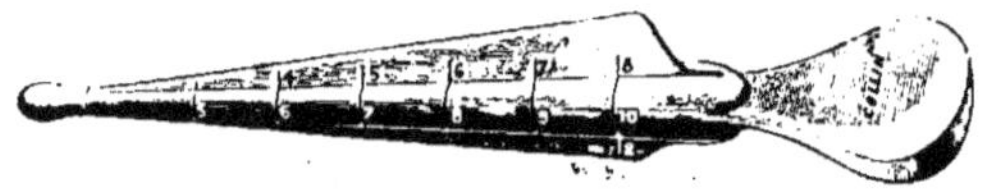

Nouveau méatotome-méatomètre.

retenues en place à l'aide d'un bouton olivaire terminal qu'on visse à l'extrémité de l'instrument.

La lame inférieure fait une saillie régulière de 2 millimètres. Elle n'est en effet destinée à couper que le bord inférieur du méat lorsqu'il présente la disposition valvulaire signalée ci-dessus. On peut, du reste, la supprimer à volonté.

La lame supérieure fait une saillie de plus en plus considérable. Elle présente 8 millimètres dans sa partie la plus large. Cette dernière répond au point de l'axe de l'instrument pourvu d'un centimètre de diamètre, de telle sorte qu'à ce niveau, en comprenant la saillie de la lame inférieure qui est de 2 millimètres, l'instrument présente un diamètre total de 20 millimètres de haut en bas. Cette dimension est la plus grande qu'il soit nécessaire de donner à la région du méat.

Il suffit de jeter les yeux sur mon instrument, pour se rendre compte qu'il ouvre le méat en *entonnoir régulier* et qu'avec lui il est impossible de déterminer l'éperon brusque dont j'ai parlé et qui résulte d'une section immédiate trop profonde des tissus.

Pour opérer la *méatotomie*, je soutiens l'extrémité de la verge avec la main gauche, tandis que de la droite je fais pénétrer mon instrument à telle distance que je veux, m'arrêtant dès que j'ai atteint le degré convenable que je lis sur la graduation.

A l'inverse du méatotome à bascule, je sectionne *d'avant en arrière en poussant*. J'obtiens de la sorte un conduit en entonnoir, régulier, qui se fusionne peu à peu, en pente douce avec l'urètre proprement dit.

Ma section est d'autant plus profonde qu'elle est plus voisine de l'orifice du méat. J'évite de la sorte de mordre trop avant au niveau de la base du gland, c'est-à-dire dans la région la plus vasculaire et de former ainsi un éperon préjudiciable à tous les points de vue.

Je puis enfin avec mon méatotome débrider la partie inférieure du méat en même temps que je sectionne sa région supérieure.

## CYSTOSCOPE

### par M. CASPER.

Le grand intérêt que le cathétérisme urétéral a provoqué était très vraisemblablement la cause que plusieurs de nos confrères, qui n'avaient pas vu mon instrument à ma première communication, m'ont prié d'en faire une démonstration.

Mon instrument permet : 1° de pouvoir changer et diriger à volonté la courbure et la direction du cathéter urétéral, ce qui est indispensable pour pouvoir l'introduire dans l'embouchure de l'uretère, et pour pouvoir après son introduction dans l'uretère lui faire suivre facilement son parcours;

2° Après avoir fait le cathétérisme d'un côté, l'instrument permet de laisser la sonde en place, tourner facilement l'instrument et faire le cathétérisme du côté opposé sans retirer le cystoscope de la vessie.

J'obtiens les divers mouvements de la sonde urétérale par un mécanisme très simple : le glissement de la paroi supérieure de la gouttière par laquelle passent les sondes.

Si l'on veut introduire dans l'uretère une sonde, on emploie le couvercle avec des tubes qui permettent de faire passer une grosse ou une fine sonde suivant le cas.

Si l'on veut introduire deux sondes *en même temps* dans les deux uretères, on prend un couvercle qui a deux tubes. La partie métallique de l'instrument, on la peut ou non laisser dans l'urètre.

## DEUX OBSERVATIONS SUR MON STÉRILISATEUR PAR LE FORMOL

### par le docteur P. HAMONIC

(de Paris)

L'appareil formolateur que j'ai eu l'honneur de présenter l'année dernière au Congrès d'urologie continue à me donner les plus grandes satisfactions, et j'ai eu ces jours-ci, à maintes reprises, le plaisir de constater que nombre de confrères en sont très satisfaits.

J'ai annoncé l'année dernière qu'on peut obtenir en 10 minutes environ une stérilisation complète.

Quelques confrères, qui ont expérimenté mon appareil, m'ont fait remarquer qu'il leur avait fallu un temps un peu plus long, les uns une demi-heure, d'autres même une heure.

C'est à propos de ce fait que je tiens à faire deux petites observations. Si vous voulez obtenir une stérilisation très rapide, il importe :

1º De ne pas trop chauffer le réservoir contenant l'aldéhyde formique. En donnant trop de lumière, on transforme le formol en carbure, et on affaiblit son pouvoir antiseptique ;

2º D'employer un aldéhyde formique aussi chargé que possible en formol. Le commerce fournit des aldéhydes formiques extrêmement variables au point de vue de leur teneur en gaz formolé. Le triformométhylène me paraît supérieur à l'aldéhyde formique ordinaire.

Il faut tenir compte de ces deux remarques si l'on veut exiger de mon appareil son maximum de rapidité.

---

## MICRO-ENDOSCOPE

### par le professeur LÉONE LÉVY

(de Gênes)

L'instrument que j'ai l'honneur de présenter a été par moi-même nommé *micro-endoscope*, parce qu'il présente sur les autres l'avantage de faire voir les lésions organiques les plus détaillées d'une manière très précise avec un agrandissement. Il consiste en une chambre qui

porte deux petites lampes qui projettent la lumière dans le tube endoscope et en un système de lentilles qui sert à donner l'agrandissement
des images. Du reste, si M. le professeur Guyon le permet, je vais
vous montrer le fonctionnement de l'appareil. Je ne parle pas des
avantages que me semble présenter cet appareil sur les autres. Voir
avec une grande précision tous les détails des altérations, c'est déjà
un grand pas vers une thérapie prompte et efficace. Comme l'instrument n'a besoin d'aucun courant d'eau réfrigérant et permet une
vision très exacte, il me semble unir le côté pratique à la simplicité.


## SONDE DIVARICATRICE

par le docteur ADOLPHE LISCIA

(de Livourne)


Je crois devoir donner quelques brèves indications pour mieux faire
comprendre le fonctionnement de ma sonde divaricatrice.

D'abord je dirai que j'ai été amené à introduire cette modification
aux sondes communes métalliques par les fréquents incidents désagréables où chacun peut se trouver dans les cas de rétention par rétrécissement de l'urètre, particulièrement dans les cas de rétention
aiguë. Qui ne sait que, dans ces cas-là, le praticien se trouve bien
souvent dans un fort embarras? et, pour arriver promptement à aider
le malade, il est plus que nécessaire de pratiquer la ponction hypogastrique.

Comme on le voit, ma sonde de petit calibre a une courbe à peu
près semblable à celle du conducteur cannelé de l'urétrotome de
Maisonneuve, son extrémité est légèrement arrondie en olive et percée,
afin de donner le passage à la bougie filiforme de baleine (mandrin
du Corradi modifié par Montenovesi pour son divulseur) préalablement introduite dans la vessie. Cette bougie, qui a l'avantage d'être
mince et résistante, peut aisément se redresser à l'aide de l'eau très
chaude, chaque fois qu'elle vient à fléchir dans les diverses tentatives
d'introduction. Aussitôt que l'on aura fait glisser la sonde sur la
bougie en vertu de la faible divulsion que l'on vient à effectuer grâce
à l'extrémité en forme d'olive, il n'est pas difficile de surmonter un ou
plusieurs rétrécissements, de manière qu'à peine a-t-on pénétré dans

la vessie il ne reste qu'à retirer la bougie et donner libre passage à l'urine, à la plus grande satisfaction du malade.

Je ne dois pas manquer d'ajouter que, avec ma sonde, le chirurgien n'a pas besoin d'être aidé, et qu'il réussit non seulement à apporter soudain au malade le soulagement presque sans le moindre versement de sang, mais qu'il obtiendra dans un bref espace de temps la guérison radicale de la maladie, complétant la cure avec la dilation graduelle.

Un autre avantage de ma sonde divaricatrice serait le suivant : il arrive quelquefois dans les formes de graves rétrécissements que, après avoir introduit la bougie et vissé le conducteur cannelé de l'urétrotome, celle-ci ne réussit pas à surmonter le rétrécissement, et pour peu que l'on insiste l'on peut risquer de fléchir à angle la vis de manière à blesser l'urètre et à produire des fausses routes. En présence de pareils accidents, avant d'opérer l'urétrotomie, l'on peut pratiquer une légère divulsion avec ma sonde.

Tout le monde se rappelle les paroles que l'illustre professeur Guyon prononça dans une de ses magistrales leçons :

« Vous ne pouvez, sans grande gêne pour votre patient, laisser la sonde métallique à demeure. »

J'ai fait des expériences de ma sonde sur un grand nombre de malades, soit dans mon service à l'hôpital, soit sur mes clients particuliers, et je suis vraiment satisfait de pouvoir affirmer qu'elle m'a toujours servi le plus avantageusement, même quand je l'ai laissée à demeure, y ajoutant le tube-siphon pour vingt-quatre heures, bien rarement pour quarante-huit, et jamais je n'ai eu à constater qu'on ne pouvait pas la tolérer.

---

## NOUVELLE BOUGIE BÉNIQUÉ

### par le docteur G. NANU.

#### (de Bucarest)

Résumé de la communication faite au XIIIe Congrès international de médecine (Paris 2-9 août).

On sait que la bougie Béniqué avec conducteur présente quelques inconvénients.

On éprouve assez souvent des difficultés pour visser la bougie et il est malaisé de nettoyer la cavité de l'écrou. Enfin, ce qui est plus grave, la bougie conductrice peut se détacher de l'embout métallique qui la fixe au Béniqué. Cela nous expose à blesser le canal, à faire fausse route et à perdre la bougie dans l'urèthre ou la vessie.

Pour remédier à ces inconvénients, on a cherché à perfectionner l'instrument. En effet, les fabricants, mettant à profit les conseils de M. Guyon, ont modifié le pas de vis et se sont ingéniés d'une part à fixer solidement le raccord à la bougie conductrice, d'autre part à renforcer le talon de celle-ci sur une étendue de plusieurs centimètres, de manière à le rendre inflexible.

Néanmoins j'ai pensé qu'il serait préférable, pour rendre cet instrument réellement commode et surtout non dangereux, de supprimer le raccord du conducteur.

Un de mes internes, M. Busila, a cherché à répondre à ce desideratum, et fit construire par la maison Broëhm, de Bucharest, la bougie que j'ai l'honneur de vous présenter.

Le conducteur est une simple bougie molle, de longueur double de celles dont on se sert habituellement, et est effilée à ses deux extrémités. La bougie métallique est parcourue, d'un bout à l'autre, par un canal dont le calibre est tel qu'il permet d'enfiler aisément le conducteur. Au niveau du manche elle est pourvue d'une petite plaque creusée d'une gouttière qui continue le canal à l'extérieur. L'autre extrémité est arrondie et mousse au niveau de l'orifice.

Pour cathétériser, on introduit dans l'urèthre le conducteur par l'une des extrémités et on fait passer l'autre par le canal de la bougie. Il ne reste qu'à présenter au méat la bougie et à parcourir le canal, en ayant soin de fixer le conducteur dans la rainure du manche, ce qui se fait aisément en pressant avec le pouce sur la plaque du manche.

Le Béniqué ainsi construit me semble être commode, facile à stériliser et surtout non dangereux.

## URÉTROSCOPE

### par le docteur VALENTINE.

(de New-York)

M. Noguès, remplaçant M. Janet, présente l'urétroscope du docteur Valentine, de New-York. Cet instrument comporte une boîte faci-

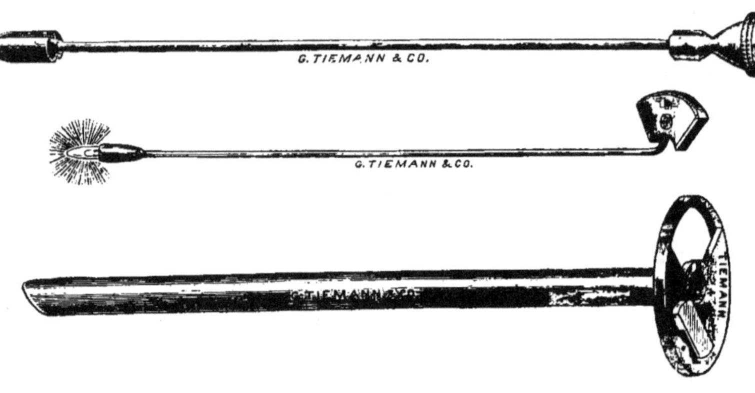


lement portative qui renferme la source lumineuse et les tubes et mandrins de calibre et de longueur différents.

Le tube est introduit dans l'urètre à l'aide d'un mandrin : après retrait du mandrin on glisse dans l'intérieur du tube une tige métallique qui porte à son extrémité une petite lampe qui projette une vive lueur sur le champ d'observation. L'appareil ne porte pas de système de réfrigération.

---

## NOUVEAUX INSTRUMENTS POUR LE TRAITEMENT DES RÉTRÉCISSEMENTS DE L'URÈTRE ET LE CATHÉTÉRISME

### par le docteur PAOLETTI

(de Florence)

Ayant fait une large pratique, comme assistant dans la clinique de chirurgie de Florence, dirigée par le professeur Corradi, j'ai pu m'appliquer sérieusement à l'étude des maladies des voies urinaires.

M'occupant d'une manière spéciale du traitement des rétrécissements de l'urètre, j'ai observé que quelques-uns des instruments que l'on emploie le plus généralement, présentent certains inconvénients que j'ai pu facilement éviter dans les instruments que j'ai l'honneur de présenter à ce Congrès de Chirurgie des voies urinaires.

Les inconvénients que j'ai observés se rapportent spécialement à l'instrument de Maisonneuve (Fig. 1) et aux autres qui ont en commun avec lui la petite bougie en gomme avec armature à vis.

Dans la plupart des cas, l'instrument de Maisonneuve peut s'introduire facilement dans l'urètre, mais quelquefois le passage dans l'urètre profond en est assez difficile, et, en quelques cas, impossible. Je crois que la cause principale de cette difficulté, consiste dans la façon avec laquelle la bougie est unie à la sonde.

L'armature à vis qui unit la bougie à la sonde, est nécessairement rectiligne (Fig. 1, $a$... $a'$) ce qui enlève à la courbure de la sonde la régularité nécessaire afin que l'instrument, selon les règles du cathétérisme, puisse glisser au contact de la paroi supérieure de l'urètre.

Une autre cause de cette difficulté se trouve aussi dans la différence de grosseur, parfois notable, qui se trouve entre la bougie, l'armature à vis, et la sonde. En outre, l'armature fixée sur l'extrémité extérieure de la bougie, rend l'instrument peu solide, en ce que la bougie peut s'user dans le point où elle se greffe à l'armature, ou l'armature même peut se rompre dans le pas de vis qui la tient fixée à l'extrémité de la sonde. Pareil accident peut survenir spécialement quand on introduit dans l'urètre, sur la sonde conductrice de Maisonneuve, une sonde élastique, comme on le fait ordinairement après l'uréthrotomie ou dans le cathétérisme à la suite. La sonde élastique à uréthrotomie est rectiligne et en glissant sur la sonde conductrice, elle en suit la courbe, jusqu'au point de l'armature, mais à ce point, à cause de la flexibilité de la bougie, la sonde élastique tend à reprendre la position rectiligne, et ainsi, en forçant dans l'armature, elle peut la rompre et la pousser avec la bougie dans la vessie.

Pour obvier à cet inconvénient, j'ai tâché d'éviter l'attache à vis de la bougie avec la sonde, en employant de minces bougies de tissu élastique ou en baleine (construites à Paris en 1896) d'une longueur double de celle de Maisonneuve, et qui peuvent glisser dans une fine sonde d'acier dont l'extrémité vésicale est conique ou légèrement olivaire (Fig. 2, Fig. 3).

Après avoir d'abord introduit la moitié de la longue bougie dans l'urètre, je fais glisser sur la partie de bougie qui reste dehors, la mince sonde d'acier, puis je pousse dans l'urètre sonde et bougie à la fois. Par cette disposition on n'altère aucunement la direction de la courbure de la sonde, et la différence de grosseur entre sonde et bougie est insignifiante, spécialement quand on emploie la sonde à extrémité conique : on comprend facilement que l'instrument ainsi construit est beaucoup plus solide que la bougie armée de Maisonneuve.

J'ai pu, dans tous les cas, introduire facilement dans l'urètre la mince sonde métallique, principalement celle à extrémité conique : je me suis servi de préférence des sondes à extrémité olivaire, quand j'ai voulu exécuter une légère dilatation dans l'urètre, pour rendre plus facile l'introduction d'autres instruments, comme l'uréthrotome, ou les sondes communes de gomme pour la dilatation forcée ou pour le cathétérisme.

Sur le même système de la petite sonde, j'ai construit d'autres cathéters de différents diamètres, avec extrémité conique ou olivaire, quelques-uns ressemblant aux sondes communes métalliques à cathétérisme (Fig. 4). Ils peuvent aussi, guidés sur les longues bougies, servir à pratiquer la dilatation urétrale, ou le cathétérisme dans le cas où il devient difficile avec les sondes ordinaires; ils peuvent aussi remplacer les sondes de Béniqué et même les sondes plus ingénieuses du professeur Guyon, avec l'avantage de la plus grande solidité dans le point d'attache de la bougie avec la sonde.

J'ai imaginé et construit moi-même un uréthrotome qui pénètre dans l'urètre, guidé sur la sonde métallique; à la différence de l'uréthrotome de Maisonneuve et de bien d'autres uréthrotomes, la lame tranchante, au lieu de glisser dans la sonde cannelée, glisse sur la surface extérieure de la sonde. Il se compose principalement de trois parties : d'une lame tranchante, qui ressemble à celle de l'uréthrotome Maisonneuve : d'une gaine qui protège la lame jusqu'au moment d'exécuter l'incision, et d'une tige qui sert de manche à l'instrument et sur laquelle se meuvent ensemble et lame et gaine, guidées dans l'urètre sur la petite sonde métallique.

La lame est soudée à l'extrémité d'une canule d'acier (Fig. 5 *a*) dans laquelle peut glisser la petite sonde métallique : une fente longitudinale, sur presque toute la longueur de la canule, en rend facile le nettoyage.

La gaine. dans laquelle est cachée la lame, est aussi une canule ouverte aux deux extrémités (Fig. 5 *c*), et son calibre intérieur est tel, que la canule de la lame peut facilement y glisser : elle est aussi fendue longitudinalement sur toute sa longueur.

A l'extrémité opposée de la lame, la fente longitudinale de la gaine

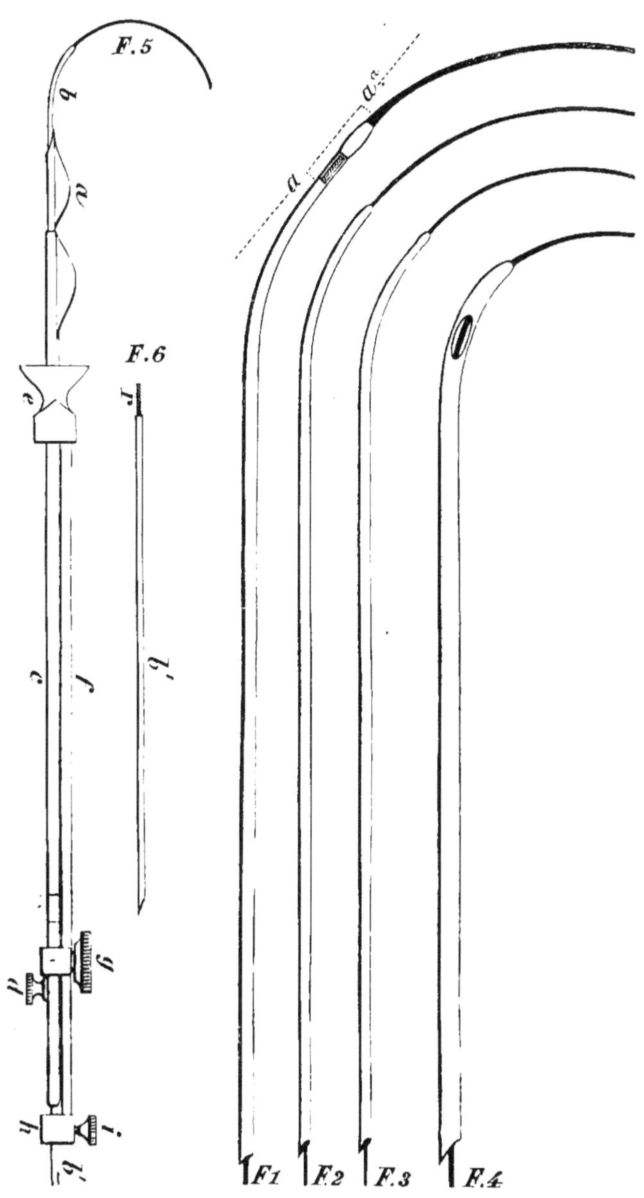
F.5
F.6
F.1
F.2
F.3
F.4

sert à guider la vis *d* au moyen de laquelle la lame est tenue ferme dans la gaine, ou peut en être retirée au moment d'exécuter l'incision urétrale.

La gaine et la lame glissent ensemble dans le pavillon *e* guidées sur la tige *f* au moyen de la vis *g* qui sert aussi à l'y fixer en un point quelconque. La tige, à l'extrémité opposée au pavillon, porte un petit étau à vis *h* qui sert à la fixer solidement au prolongement *b′* de la petite sonde.

Pour exécuter l'uréthrotomie, après avoir introduit la sonde dans l'urètre, on ajoute à celle-ci le prolongement *b′* (Fig. 6) moyennant le pas de vis *r* qui se greffe au pas de vis que se trouve à l'extrémité extérieure de la sonde. Le prolongement et la sonde unis ensemble, forment la tige *b*, *b′* sur laquelle glisse l'uréthrotome. On pousse l'uréthrotome sur la tige jusqu'à ce que le pavillon *e* soit en contact avec la glande. La tige est alors sortie du petit étau *h* qui, serré au moyen de la vis *i*, fixera solidement l'instrument à la tige.

L'uréthrotome ainsi disposé sur la tige. on soutient avec la main gauche la verge et l'uréthrotome ensemble, tenant la verge avec les derniers doigts et fixant avec les deux premiers le pavillon *e*. Alors avec la main droite, on ouvre d'un demi-tour la vis *g* et sans la laisser, on pousse au moyen de celle-ci la gaine dans l'urètre : gaine et lame glissent alors ensemble sur la tige. Quand la gaine a rencontré la résistance d'un rétrécissement, on serre la vis *g* qu'on laisse ensuite pour ouvrir la vis *d* qu'on pousse en avant; ainsi la lame sort de la gaine, pénètre dans le point rétréci et l'incise. L'incision exécutée, on porte en arrière la lame au moyen de la même vis *d* que l'on serre après, pour maintenir de nouveau la lame ferme dans l'urètre.

L'opération accomplie, ayant répété la manœuvre décrite dans le cas de rétrécissements multiples, on lève l'instrument de la tige en ouvrant la vis *i* du petit étau *h*, tandis que les premiers doigts de la main gauche ont cessé de soutenir le pavillon, pour tenir ferme la tige, afin qu'elle ne sorte point de l'urètre en retirant l'instrument. Sur la tige, qui reste alors disposée comme au premier moment de l'opération, on fait glisser jusque dans la vessie une sonde élastique à uréthrotomie, de laquelle enfin on retire la tige, pour laisser dans l'urètre la sonde en permanence.

# INSTRUMENTS POUR L'URÉTROSCOPIE

## par M. DESNOS.

(de Paris)

L'appareil présenté conserve la disposition générale de l'urétroscope d'Otis ; les tubes endoscopiques à lumière externe sont mats ou
brillants à l'intérieur. Dans le premier cas, la muqueuse urétrale est
mal éclairée ; dans le second, des reflets gênent la vue. Aussi ai-je fait
construire ce tube qui peut être de verre ou de métal, brillant dans la

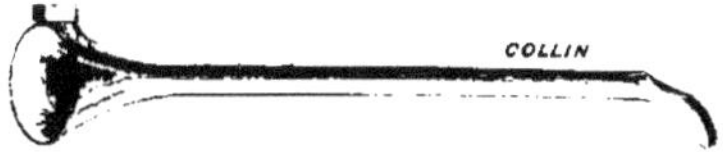


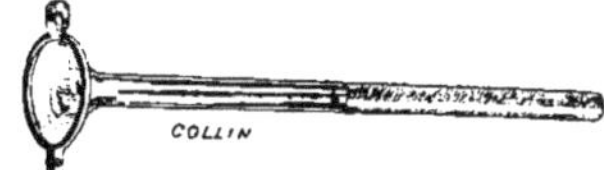


moitié attenante à l'entonnoir, mat dans sa moitié postérieure ; on
réunit ainsi les avantages des deux procédés.

Pour l'urètre postérieur, l'introduction d'un tube droit est difficile
et toujours un peu offensive ; un instrument de ce genre est cependant nécessaire pour voir toute la périphérie de l'urètre, mais dans
l'immense majorité des cas, c'est la paroi inférieure et surtout la région du verumontanum qui est atteinte. On peut donc, quand on a
fait le diagnostic, se servir d'un instrument courbe ou coudé dont la
partie courbe se loge presque d'elle-même dans la région prostatique

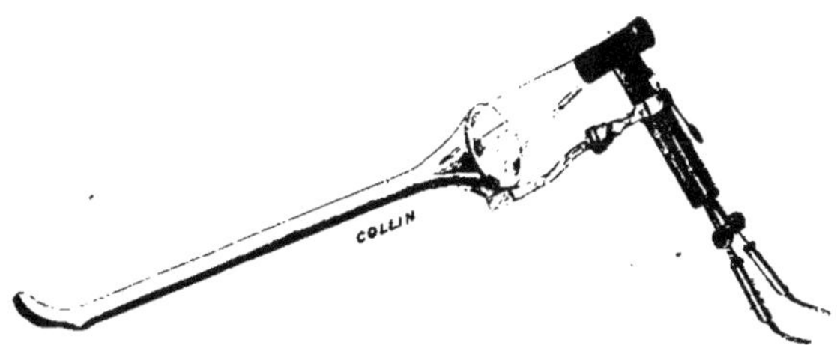


et qui présente au niveau du coude une large fenêtre : celle-ci est
oblitérée au moment de l'introduction par un mandrin qu'on retire
dès que l'instrument est en place. La région du verumontanum est
alors largement découverte dans l'axe de la partie rectiligne de l'instrument, et accessible à la vue et aux porte-topiques.

A ces endoscopes, je joindrai dans mes présentations divers instruments qui m'ont rendu des services.

Un porte-topiques, porte-ouate, bien en main, dont le manche est

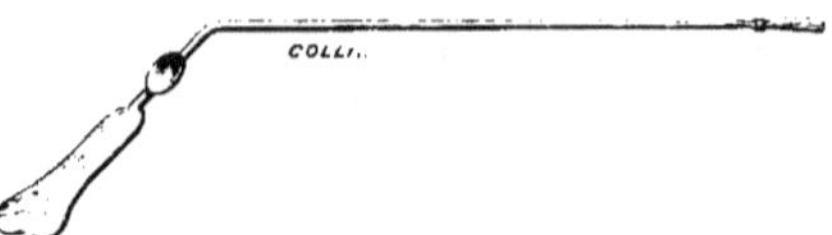

coudé et qui permet de surveiller la position et de suivre l'action du topique au fond de l'urétroscope.

Une pince à mors articulés, très petite, se mouvant facilement à l'intérieur du tube endoscopique, disposés comme ceux de la pince à

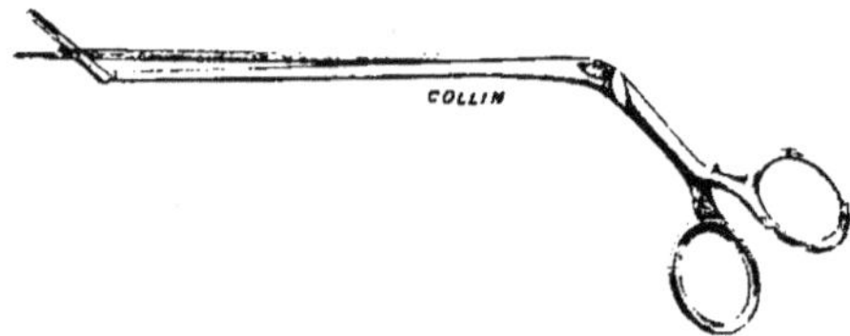

corps étrangers de Collin. Elle est très utile pour retirer un fragment d'ouate échappé, un corps étranger, un petit calcul ou fragment calculeux, etc.

Un sécateur à lame arrondie, mobile dans une glissière, se logeant dans une branche femelle à extrémité courbe, concave, inférieure-

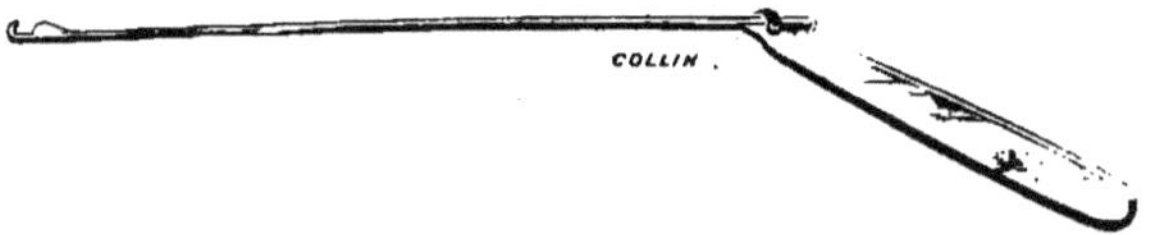

ment; cette dernière est munie de deux petits crochets qui permettent, l'instrument étant ouvert, de saisir et de fixer un polype ou une tumeur de l'urètre; en poussant la lame dans la concavité, la saillie se trouve sectionnée. M. Collin en a construit deux modèles sur nos indications, l'un à manche long pour l'homme, l'autre plus court, d'un usage plus fréquent, pour la femme.

# TABLE DES MATIÈRES

## TROISIÈME SÉANCE



## QUATRIÈME SÉANCE

# TABLE DES AUTEURS

# TABLE ANALYTIQUE DES MATIÈRES

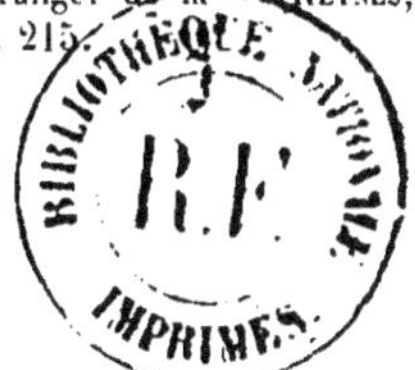

44150. — PARIS, IMPRIMERIE LAHURE
9, rue de Fleurus.

# Masson et C^{ie}, Éditeurs

*Libraires de l'Académie de Médecine*

120, Boulevard Saint-Germain, Paris (VI^e)

---

EXTRAIT

DU

# CATALOGUE MÉDICAL

Décembre 1900

La librairie Masson et C^{ie} envoie gratuitement et franco de port les catalogues suivants à toutes les personnes qui lui en font la demande.

— **Catalogue général** contenant, classés par subdivisions, tous les ouvrages publiés à la librairie ainsi que la liste de ses différents journaux et revues.

— **Catalogues de l'Encyclopédie scientifique des Aide-Mémoire**
I. *Section de l'ingénieur.*
II. *Section du biologiste.*

— **Catalogue des ouvrages d'enseignement.**

Des prospectus spéciaux des différents grands Traités publiés par la librairie sont également adressés sur demande.

# Traité
## de
# Pathologie générale

PUBLIÉ PAR

## CH. BOUCHARD

MEMBRE DE L'INSTITUT
PROFESSEUR DE PATHOLOGIE GÉNÉRALE A LA FACULTÉ DE MÉDECINE DE PARIS

SECRÉTAIRE DE LA RÉDACTION
### G.-H. ROGER
Professeur agrégé à la Faculté de médecine de Paris, Médecin des hôpitaux.

*COLLABORATEURS* :

MM. ARNOZAN — D'ARSONVAL — BENNI — R. BLANCHARD — BOULAY — BOURCY — BRUN — CADIOT — CHABRIÉ — CHANTEMESSE — CHARRIN — CHAUFFARD — COURMONT — DEJERINE — PIERRE DELBET — DEVIC — DUCAMP — MATHIAS DUVAL — FÉRÉ — FRÉMY — GAUCHER — GILBERT — GLEY — GUIGNARD — LOUIS GUINON — J.-F. GUYON — HALLÉ — HÉNOCQUE — HUGOUNENQ — LAMBLING — LANDOUZY — LAVERAN — LEBRETON — LE GENDRE — LEJARS — LE NOIR — LERMOYEZ — LETULLE — LUBET-BARBON — MARFAN — MAYOR — MENETRIER — NETTER — PIERRET — G.-H. ROGER — GABRIEL ROUX — RUFFER — RAYMOND TRIPIER — VUILLEMIN — FERNAND WIDAL.

*6 vol. grand in-8°, avec figures dans le texte.*

Sous la puissante impulsion du professeur Bouchard, la pathologie générale a pris une place prépondérante dans les études du monde médical. C'est qu'elle fournit des enseignements indispensables à toutes les branches de la médecine : elle fixe les idées sur les grands problèmes que soulève l'étude de l'homme ; elle éloigne le médecin des changeantes données de l'empirisme et lui apprend à réfléchir sur les phénomènes qu'il observe, à discuter et à comprendre les interventions qu'il doit faire.

Pour être véritablement utile, la pathologie expérimentale doit constamment s'efforcer de réunir et de synthétiser les données de la clinique et de l'expérimentation. C'est dans cet esprit qu'est conçu l'enseignement du professeur Bouchard; c'est dans cet esprit qu'a été écrit le livre dont il dirige la publication. Si tous les collaborateurs ont conservé leur indépendance, tous cependant ont suivi la même idée directrice qui assure à l'œuvre son unité.

Le plan adopté est d'ailleurs fort simple. Il consiste à rechercher par quel mécanisme agissent les causes pathogènes, par quels procédés l'organisme répond à l'attaque, par quels moyens le médecin peut apprécier à leur juste valeur les troubles morbides, les rattacher à leur cause et modifier leur évolution.

C'est la première fois, croyons-nous, qu'une pléiade de savants s'est groupée autour d'un maître illustre, pour élever un pareil monument à l'étude de la pathologie générale. L'intérêt qu'a soulevé cet ouvrage dans le monde scientifique étranger montre que nulle part n'existait l'équivalent d'une telle œuvre, et dès à présent, deux traductions, l'une en italien, l'autre en espagnol, ont été publiées.

Tome V. Fig. 65. Facies myopathique.

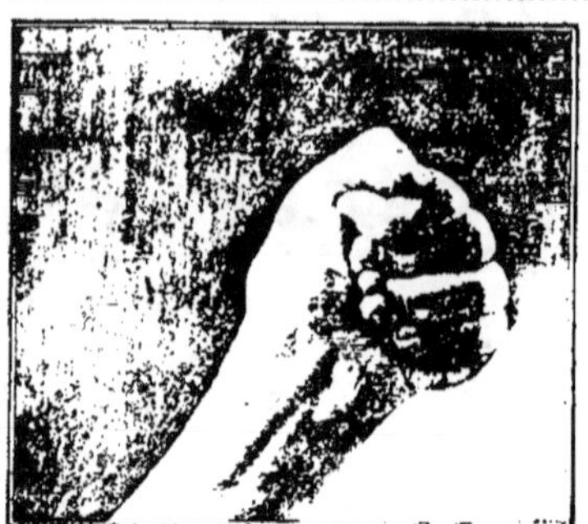

Tome V. Fig. 179. — Déformation de la main par contraction excessive dans un cas de maladie de Parkinson.

## DIVISION DE L'OUVRAGE

**TOME Iᵉʳ.** — *1 vol. grand in-8° de 1018 pages avec figures dans le texte :* **18 fr.**

Introduction à l'étude de la pathologie générale, par G.-H. Roger, professeur agrégé à la Faculté de médecine, médecin de l'Hôpital de la porte d'Aubervilliers. — Pathologie comparée de l'homme et des animaux, par G.-H. Roger et P.-J. Cadiot. — Considérations générales sur les maladies des végétaux, par P. Vuillemin, chargé de cours à la Faculté de médecine de Nancy. — Pathogénie générale de l'embryon. Tératogénie, par Mathias Duval, professeur à la Faculté de médecine de Paris. — L'hérédité et la pathologie générale, par Le Gendre, médecin des hôpitaux. — Prédisposition et immunité, par Bourcy, médecin des hôpitaux. — La fatigue et le surmenage, par Marfan, professeur agrégé à la Faculté de médecine de Paris, médecin des hôpitaux. — Les Agents mécaniques, par Lejars, professeur agrégé à la Faculté de médecine de Paris, chirurgien des hôpitaux. — Les Agents physiques. Chaleur. Froid. Lumière. Pression atmosphérique. Son, par Le Noir. — Les Agents physiques. L'énergie électrique et la matière vivante, par d'Arsonval, membre de l'Institut, professeur au Collège de France. — Les Agents chimiques. Les caustiques, par Le Noir. — Les intoxications, par G.-H. Roger.

**TOME II.** — *1 vol. grand in-8° de 940 pages avec figures dans le texte :* **18 fr.**

L'Infection, par Charrin, professeur agrégé à la Faculté de médecine de Paris, médecin des hôpitaux. — Notions générales de morphologie bactériologique, par Guignard, membre de l'Institut, professeur à l'École de pharmacie. — Notions de chimie bactériologique, par Hugounenq, professeur à la Faculté de médecine de Lyon. — Les microbes pathogènes, par Roux, professeur agrégé à la Faculté de médecine de Lyon. — Le sol, l'eau et l'air agents des maladies infectieuses, par Chantemesse, professeur à la Faculté de médecine de Paris, médecin des hôpitaux. — Des maladies épidémiques, par Laveran, membre de l'Académie de médecine. — Sur les parasites des tumeurs épithéliales malignes, par Ruffer. — Les parasites, par L. Blanchard, professeur à la Faculté de médecine de Paris, membre de l'Académie de médecine.

**TOME III.** — *1 vol. in-8° de plus de 1400 pages avec fig. dans le texte, publié en deux fascicules :* **28 fr.**

Fasc. I. — Notions générales sur la nutrition à l'état normal, par E. Lambling, professeur à l'Université de Lille. — Les troubles préalables de la nutrition, par Ch. Bouchard, professeur à la Faculté de médecine, membre de l'Institut. — Les réactions nerveuses, par Ch. Bouchard et G.-H. Roger, professeur agrégé à la Faculté de médecine de Paris, médecin de l'Hôpital de la porte d'Aubervilliers. — Les processus pathogéniques de deuxième ordre, par G.-H. Roger.

Fasc. II. — Considérations préliminaires sur la physiologie et l'anatomie pathologiques, par G.-H. Roger. — De la fièvre, par Louis Guinon, médecin des hôpitaux de Paris. — L'hypothermie, par J.-F. Guyon. — Mécanisme physiologique des troubles vasculaires, par E. Gley, professeur agrégé à la Faculté de médecine de Paris. — Les désordres de la circulation dans les maladies, par A. Charrin, professeur agrégé à la Faculté de médecine de Paris, professeur remplaçant au Collège de France, médecin des hôpitaux. — Thrombose et embolie, par A. Mayor, professeur à la Faculté de médecine de Genève. — De l'inflammation, par J. Courmont, professeur agrégé à la Faculté de médecine de Lyon, médecin des hôpitaux.

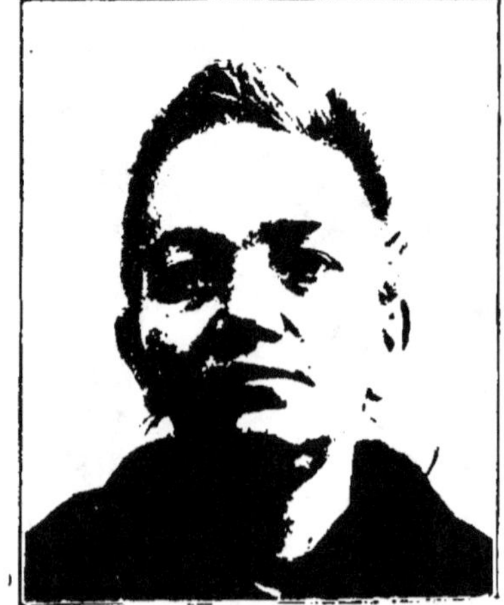

Tome V. Fig. 17. Paralysie bulbaire par névrite périphérique, avec participation du facial supérieur.

— Anatomie pathologique générale des lésions inflammatoires, par M. Letulle, pro-

fesseur agrégé à la Faculté de médecine de Paris, médecin de l'hôpital Boucicaut. —
Les altérations anatomiques non inflammatoires, par P. LE NOIR, médecin des hôpitaux.
— Les tumeurs, par P. MENETRIER, professeur agrégé, médecin de l'hôpital Tenon.

TOME IV. — 1 vol. in-8° de 719 pages avec figures dans le texte : 16 fr.

Évolution des maladies, par DUCAMP, professeur à la Faculté de médecine de Montpellier. — Semiologie du sang, par A. GILBERT, professeur agrégé, médecin de l'hôpital
Broussais. — Spectroscopie du sang. Sémiologie, par A. HÉNOCQUE, directeur-adjoint
du Laboratoire de physique biologique du Collège de France. — Semiologie du cœur
et des vaisseaux, par R. TRIPIER, professeur à la Faculté de médecine de Lyon et
DEVIC, agrégé à la Faculté de Lyon, médecin des hôpitaux. — Sémiologie du nez et
du pharynx nasal, par M. LERMOYEZ, médecin de l'hôpital Saint-Antoine, et M. BOULAY,
ancien interne des hôpitaux. — Sémiologie du larynx, par M. LERMOYEZ et M. BOULAY.
— Sémiologie des voies respiratoires, par M. LEBRETON, médecin des hôpitaux. —
Sémiologie générale du tube digestif, par P. LE GENDRE, médecin de l'hôpital Tenon.

TOME V. — 1 vol. in-8° de 1180 pages avec nombreuses figures dans le texte : 28 fr.

A. CHAUFFARD, professeur agrégé à la Faculté de médecine de Paris, médecin des hôpitaux : Pathologie générale et Sémiologie du foie. — X. ARNOZAN, professeur à la
Faculté de médecine de Bordeaux : Pancréas. — C. CHABRIÉ, sous-directeur du

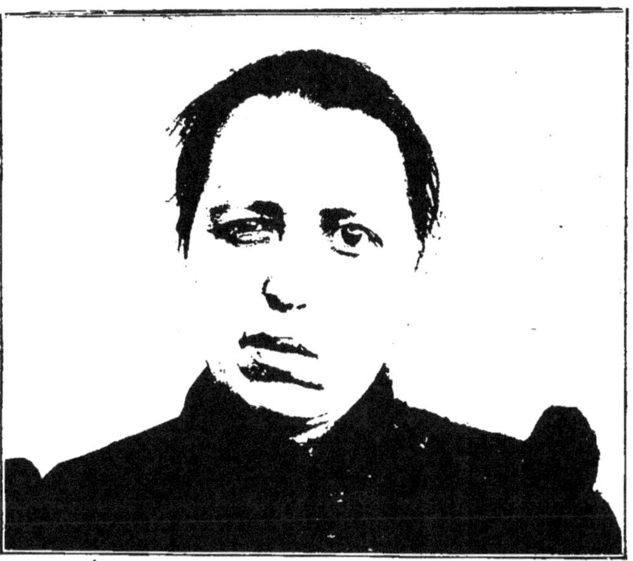

Tome V. Fig. 148. — Paralysie faciale gauche par lésion du rocher.

Laboratoire de Chimie appliquée à la Faculté des Sciences de Paris : Analyse chimique
des urines. — NOEL HALLÉ : Analyse microscopique des urines (histo-bactériologique). —
A. CHARRIN, professeur remplaçant au Collège de France : Le rein, l'urine et l'organisme.
— PIERRE DELBET, professeur agrégé à la Faculté de médecine de Paris, chirurgien des
hôpitaux : Sémiologie des organes génitaux. — J. DEJERINE, professeur agrégé à la
Faculté de médecine de Paris, médecin des hôpitaux : Sémiologie du système nerveux.
Cet article comprend plus de 800 pages et est illustré de très nombreuses photogra-
phies, schémas et dessins.)

## *CONDITIONS DE LA PUBLICATION* (Décembre 1900)

Le Traité de Pathologie générale est publié en six volumes. Chaque volume est
vendu séparément, et le prix en est fixé suivant l'étendue des matières.
Les tomes I et II sont vendus chacun. 18 fr. | Le tome IV est vendu. . . . . . . 16 fr.
Le tome III forme 2 part. et est vendu. 28 fr. | Le tome V est vendu . . . . . . . 28 fr

Il est accepté des *souscriptions* au Traité de Pathologie générale à un *prix à forfait*, quels que soient l'étendue et le prix de l'ouvrage complet.
*Ce prix à partir de ce jour a été élevé de 112 francs à 120 francs, et restera tel,
dans tous les cas, jusqu'à la publication du tome VI.*

## CHARCOT — BOUCHARD — BRISSAUD

BABINSKI — BALLET — P. BLOCQ — BOIX — BRAULT — CHANTEMESSE — CHARRIN
CHAUFFARD — COURTOIS-SUFFIT — DUTIL — GILBERT — GUIGNARD — L. GUINON
GEORGES GUINON — HALLION — LAMY — LE GENDRE — MARFAN
MARIE — MATHIEU — NETTER — ŒTTINGER — ANDRÉ PETIT
RICHARDIÈRE — ROGER — RUAULT — SOUQUES — THOINOT
THIBIERGE — FERNAND WIDAL

# TRAITÉ DE MÉDECINE

## DEUXIÈME ÉDITION

(Entièrement refondue.)

PUBLIÉE SOUS LA DIRECTION DE MM.

| **BOUCHARD** | **BRISSAUD** |
|---|---|
| Professeur à la Faculté de médecine de Paris, Membre de l'Institut. | Professeur à la Faculté de médecine de Paris, Médecin de l'hôpital St-Antoine. |

**10 volumes grand in-8°, avec figures dans le texte**

En Souscription.. . . . . . . . . . . . . . . . . . . . . . 150   francs

*La deuxième édition du TRAITÉ DE MÉDECINE a été entièrement revisée et augmentée dans de notables proportions. En outre, et pour la commodité des lecteurs, les matières sont réparties en dix volumes qui paraissent successivement.*

*Chaque volume est vendu séparément.*

*Jusqu'à ce jour le prix de l'ouvrage reste fixé pour les souscripteurs à 150 francs.*

DÉCEMBRE 1900.

Le succès de la première édition du **Traité de Médecine** de MM. Charcot, Bouchard et Brissaud, a rendu nécessaire une seconde édition, et loin de se borner à une réimpression les auteurs ont voulu présenter au public un ouvrage nouveau, gardant le plan et les idées qui avaient assuré le succès sans précédent du traité, lors de son apparition, mais complétant et remaniant la plupart de ses parties et corrigeant les quelques imperfections qui s'étaient glissées dans la première édition. Comprenant désormais 10 volumes, dont 6 déjà ont été publiés, le **Traité de Médecine** reste le plus complet, le plus documenté des livres de ce genre et l'autorité croissante qui s'attache aux noms de ceux qui y collaborent en confirme et en assure le succès persistant.

### TOME I<sup>er</sup>

1 vol. grand in-8° de 845 pages, avec figures dans le texte : **16 fr.**

*Les bactéries*, par L. GUIGNARD, membre de l'Institut et de l'Académie de médecine, professeur à l'Ecole de Pharmacie de Paris. — *Pathologie générale infectieuse*, par A. CHARRIN, professeur remplaçant au Collège de France, directeur du Laboratoire de médecine expérimentale (Hautes-Études), médecin des hôpitaux. — *Troubles et maladies de la nutrition*, par PAUL LEGENDRE, médecin de l'hôpital Tenon. — *Maladies infectieuses communes à l'homme et aux animaux*, par G.-H. ROGER, professeur agrégé, médecin de l'hôpital de la Porte d'Aubervilliers.

## TOME II

1 vol. grand in-8° de 896 pages, avec figures dans le texte : 16 fr.

*Fièvre typhoïde*, par A. CHANTEMESSE, professeur à la Faculté de médecine, médecin des hôpitaux de Paris. — *Maladies infectieuses*, par
F. WIDAL, professeur agrégé, médecin des hôpitaux de Paris. — *Ty-
phus exanthématique*, par L.-H. THOINOT, professeur agrégé, médecin
des hôpitaux de Paris. — *Fièvres éruptives*, par. L. GUINON, médecin
des hôpitaux de Paris. — *Erysipèle*, par E. BOIX, chef de laboratoire
à la Faculté. — *Diphtérie*, par A. RUAULT. — *Rhumatisme articulaire
aigu*, par ŒTTINGER, médecin des hôpitaux de Paris. — *Scorbut*, par
TOLLEMER, chef de laboratoire à la Faculté.

## TOME III

1 vol. grand in-8° de 702 pages, avec figures dans le texte : 16 fr.

*Maladies cutanées*, par G. THIBIERGE, médecin de l'hôpital de la Pitié. —
*Maladies vénériennes*, par G. THIBIERGE, médecin de l'hôpital de la
Pitié. — *Maladies du sang*, par A. GILBERT, professeur agrégé, médecin des hôpitaux de Paris. — *Intoxications*, par H. RICHARDIÈRE,
. médecin des hôpitaux de Paris.

## TOME IV

1 vol. grand in-8° de 680 pages, avec figures dans le texte : 16 fr.

*Maladies de l'estomac*, par A. MATHIEU, médecin de l'hôpital Andral. —
*Maladies du pancréas*, par A. MATHIEU, médecin de l'hôpital Andral.
— *Maladies de l'intestin*, par COURTOIS-SUFFIT, médecin des hôpitaux
de Paris. — *Maladies du péritoine*, par COURTOIS-SUFFIT, médecin des
hôpitaux de Paris. — *Maladies de la bouche et du pharynx*, par
A. RUAULT, médecin honoraire de la Clinique laryngologique de l'institution nationale des Sourds-Muets.

## TOME VI

1 vol. grand in-8° de 612 pages, avec figures dans le texte : 14 fr.

*Maladies du nez et du larynx*, par A. RUAULT, médecin honoraire de la
Clinique laryngologique de l'Institution nationale des Sourds-Muets. —
*Asthme*, par E. BRISSAUD, professeur à la Faculté de médecine de Paris,
médecin de l'hôpital Saint-Antoine. — *Coqueluche*, par P. LE GENDRE,
médecin des hôpitaux. — *Maladies des bronches*, par A.-B. MARFAN,
professeur agrégé à la Faculté de médecine de Paris, médecin des
hôpitaux. — *Troubles de la circulation pulmonaire*, par A.-B. MARFAN,
professeur agrégé à la Faculté de médecine de Paris, médecin des
hôpitaux. — *Maladies aiguës du poumon*, par NETTER, professeur
agrégé à la Faculté de médecine de Paris, médecin des hôpitaux.

## TOME VII

1 vol. grand in-8° de 550 pages, avec figures dans le texte : 14 fr.

*Maladies chroniques du poumon* par A.-B. MARFAN, professeur agrégé à
la Faculté de médecine de Paris, médecin des hôpitaux. — *Phtisie
pulmonaire*, par A.-B. MARFAN, professeur agrégé à la Faculté de médecine de Paris, médecin des hôpitaux. — *Maladies de la plèvre*, par
NETTER, professeur agrégé à la Faculté de médecine de Paris, médecin
des hôpitaux. — *Maladies du médiastin*, par A.-B. MARFAN, professeur
agrégé à la Faculté de médecine de Paris, médecin des hôpitaux.

### Le TOME V sera publié ultérieurement

# Traité
# de Chirurgie

Publié sous la direction

DE MM.

**Simon DUPLAY**

Professeur de clinique chirurgicale à la Faculté
de médecine de Paris
Chirurgien de l'Hôtel-Dieu
Membre de l'Académie de médecine

**Paul RECLUS**

Professeur agrégé à la Faculté de médecine de Paris
Secrétaire général de la Société de chirurgie
Chirurgien des hôpitaux
Membre de l'Académie de médecine

PAR MM.

BERGER. — BROCA. — Pierre DELBET. — DELENS. — DEMOULIN
J.-L. FAURE. — FORGUE. — GÉRARD-MARCHANT
HARTMANN. — HEYDENREICH. — JALAGUIER. — KIRMISSON. — LAGRANGE
LEJARS. — MICHAUX. — NÉLATON
PEYROT. — PONCET. — QUÉNU. — RICARD. — RIEFFEL. — SEGOND
TUFFIER. — WALTHER

**DEUXIÈME ÉDITION, ENTIÈREMENT REFONDUE**

8 forts volumes grand in-8° avec nombreuses figures dans le texte. . .   **150** fr.

Plus de neuf ans se sont écoulés depuis le jour où fut arrêté le programme du *Traité de Chirurgie*, et, des vingt-quatre collaborateurs du début, aucun, par un rare bonheur, ne manque encore à l'entreprise. Les portes de l'Hôpital et de l'Agrégation se sont ouvertes devant les plus jeunes, le Professorat et l'Académie de médecine en ont élu de plus âgés; tous ont vu s'étendre leur sphère d'activité professionnelle. Aussi pouvons-nous affirmer que ce nouvel ouvrage porte la marque d'une expérience plus mûre et d'une plus grande autorité.

**TOME PREMIER.** 1 fort vol. de 912 pages avec 218 figures. . .   **18** fr.

Reclus. Inflammations. — Traumatismes. —
Maladies virulentes.
Quénu. Des Tumeurs.

Broca. Peau et tissu cellulaire sous-cutané.
Lejars. Lymphatiques, muscles, synoviales
tendineuses et bourses séreuses.

**TOME II.** 1 fort vol. de 996 pages avec 361 figures. . . . . . .   **18** fr.

Lejars. Nerfs.
Michaux. Artères.
Quénu. Maladies des veines.

Ricard et Demoulin. Lésions traumatiques
des os.
Poncet. Affections non traumatiques des os.

**TOME III.** 1 fort vol. de 940 pages avec 285 figures . . . . . .   **18** fr.

Nélaton. Traumatismes, entorses, luxations,
plaies articulaires.
Lagrange. Arthrites infectieuses et inflammatoires.

Quénu. Arthropathies. Arthrites sèches. Corps
étrangers articulaires.
Gérard Marchant. Maladies du crâne.
Kirmisson. Maladies du rachis.
Simon Duplay. Oreilles et Annexes.

**TOME IV.** 1 fort vol. de 896 pages avec 354 figures. . . . . . .   **18** fr.

Delens. Œil et annexes.
Gérard-Marchant. Nez, fosses nasales, pharynx nasal et sinus.

Heydenreich. Mâchoires.

TOME V. 1 fort vol. de 948 pages avec 187 figures. . . . . . .  **20** fr.

**Broca**. Vices de développement de la face et du cou. Face, lèvres, cavité buccale, gencives, langue, palais et pharynx.
**Hartmann**. Plancher buccal, glandes salivaires, œsophage et larynx.

**Broca**. Corps thyroïde.
**Walther**. Maladies du cou.
**Peyrot**. Poitrine.
**Delbet**. Mamelle.

TOME VI. 1 fort vol. de 1127 pages avec 218 figures. . . . . .  **20** fr.

**Michaux**. Parois de l'abdomen.
**Berger**. Hernies.
**Jalaguier**. Contusions et plaies de l'abdomen. Lésions traumatiques et corps étrangers de l'estomac et de l'intestin.
**Hartmann**. Estomac.

**Jalaguier**. Occlusion intestinale. Péritonites. Appendicite.
**Faure et Rieffel**. Rectum et Anus.
**Quénu**. Mésentère. Rate. Pancréas.
**Segond**. Foie.

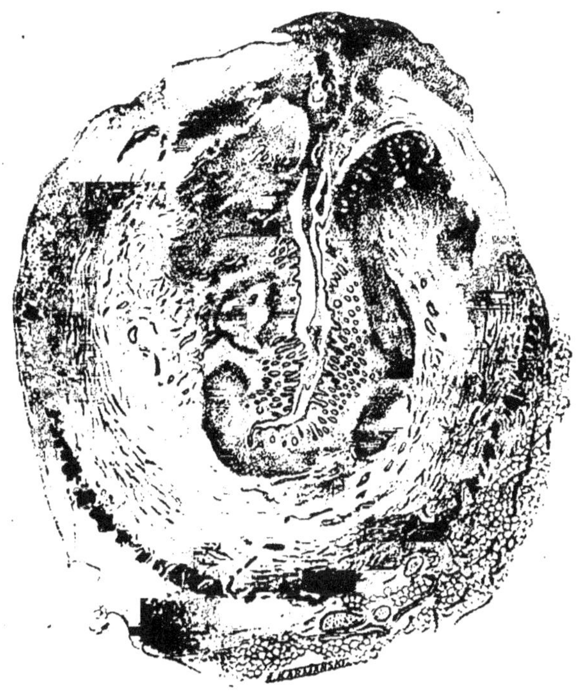

Tome VI. Fig. 116. — Appendicite folliculaire perforante.

TOME VII. 1 fort vol. de 1272 pages avec 297 figures dans le texte.  **25** fr.

**Walther**. Bassin.
**Rieffel**. Affections congénitales de la région sacro-coccygienne.

**Tuffier**. Rein. Vessie. Uretères. Capsules surrénales.
**Forgue**. L'urèthre et prostate.
**Reclus**. Organes génitaux de l'homme.

TOME VIII. 1 fort vol. de 971 pages avec 163 figures dans le texte.  **20** fr.

**Michaux**. Vulve et Vagin.
**Pierre Delbet**. Maladies de l'utérus.

**Segond**. Annexes de l'utérus, ovaires, trompes, ligaments larges, péritoine pelvien.
**Kirmisson**. Maladies des membres.

TABLE ALPHABÉTIQUE des 8 volumes du *Traité de Chirurgie*.

# La Pratique Dermatologique

## Traité de Dermatologie appliquée

PUBLIÉ SOUS LA DIRECTION DE MM.

### ERNEST BESNIER, L. BROCQ, L. JACQUET

PAR MM.

AUDRY, BALZER, BARBE, BAROZZI, BARTHÉLEMY, BÉNARD, ERNEST BES-
NIER, BODIN, BROCQ, DE BRUN, DU CASTEL, J. DARIER, DEHU, DOMINICI,
W. DUBREUILH, HUDELO, L. JACQUET, J.-B. LAFFITTE, LENGLET, LE-
REDDE, MERKLEN, PERRIN, RAYNAUD, RIST, SABOURAUD, MARCEL SÉE,
GEORGES THIBIERGE, VEYRIÈRES.

*4 volumes richement cartonnés toile formant ensemble environ 3600 pages, très
largement illustrés de figures en noir et de planches en couleurs. En souscription
jusqu'à la publication du Tome II. . . . . . . . . . . . . . . . . . . . . .* **140 fr.**
*Chaque volume sera vendu séparément.*

---

## EXTRAIT DE LA PRÉFACE

..... A tous les titres, il y a intérêt majeur à résumer l'état présent de
la dermatologie à la fin de ce siècle scientifique si fécond et si brillant, et
à l'aube de celui qui le suit, quelque grand qu'il doive être !

Notre but le plus essentiel est, avant tout, de faire œuvre de clinique et de thérapeutique.

Nous voulons fixer les types morbides par des descriptions sobres et précises, appuyées sur des représentations graphiques aussi nombreuses et aussi parfaites que possible, et réaliser ainsi une œuvre de toute utilité, destinée à la grande masse des praticiens.

La thérapeutique des maladies de la peau sera exposée avec une ampleur au moins égale : nous nous sommes attachés à donner place, dans la *Pratique dermatologique*, à tout ce qui peut être utile au médecin praticien pour le traitement de chaque maladie en particulier.

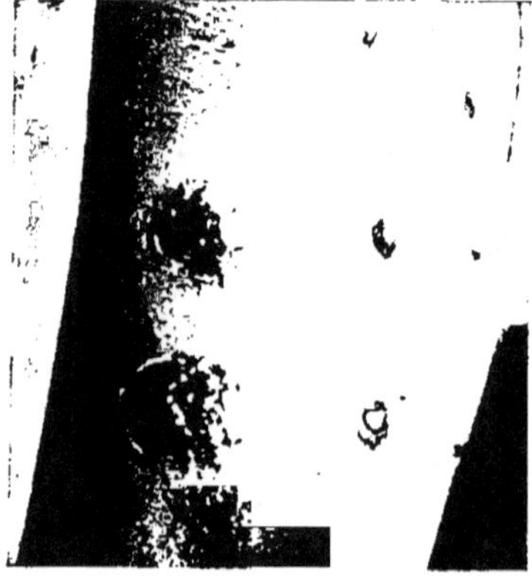

Fig. 225. — Ecthyma.

Que l'on ne se méprenne pas cependant. La *Pratique dermatologique*
ne sera pas un simple manuel illustré renfermant seulement, à propos de
chaque dermatose, un abrégé symptomatologique suivi de formules banales et non contrôlées ; notre but est beaucoup plus élevé. A l'exposé de
chaque question, le médecin dermatologiste trouvera toujours les indications scientifiques principales sur la matière. L'histologie, la bactério-

logie, l'histochimie et l'hématologie seront traitées dans la mesure indiquée par l'état actuel de ces connaissances et par leur importance relative aux dermatoses en particulier. Les plus grands développements seront réservés à la description clinique basée sur l'observation précise et minutieuse des faits, assurés que nous serons, en cela, de faire œuvre durable.

Afin de mieux fixer les types dermatologiques, et pour permettre aux

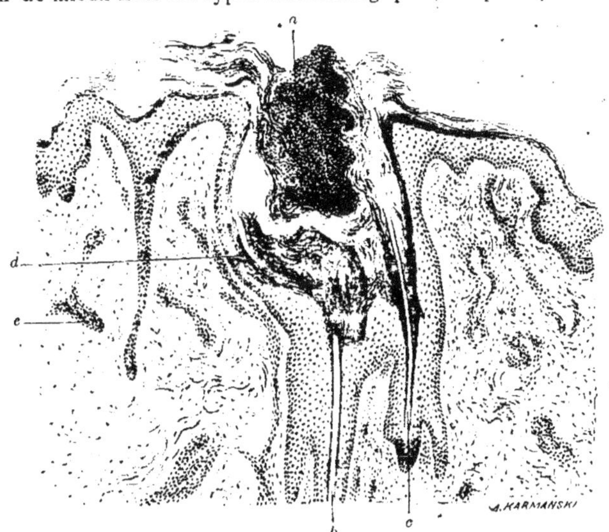

Fig. 23. — Coupe d'acné pustuleuse passant par le comédon.

praticiens de médecine générale de les connaître à coup sûr, nous annexerons au texte, en grand nombre, des planches coloriées et des dessins en noir, aussi exacts que l'on peut actuellement les réaliser.

Et, à titre complémentaire, nous indiquerons, toutes les fois où cela pourra être utile, les numéros correspondants des magnifiques reproductions *ad naturam* accumulées dans le merveilleux musée de l'hôpital Saint-Louis, et dues au talent de Baretta.

## TOME PREMIER

1 fort vol. in-8º avec 230 figures en noir et 24 planches en couleurs.
Richement cartonné toile.   **36 fr.**

**Anatomie et Physiologie de la Peau. — Pathologie générale de la Peau. — Symptomatologie générale des Dermatoses. — Acanthosis nigricans. — Acnés. — Actinomycose. — Adénomes. — Alopécies. — Anesthésie locale. — Balanites. — Bouton d'Orient. — Brûlures. — Charbon. — Classifications dermatologiques. — Dermatites polymorphes douloureuses. — Dermatophytes. — Dermatozoaires. — Dermites infantiles simples. — Ecthyma.**

SOUS PRESSE : Tome II contenant les articles : *Eczéma*, par ERNEST BESNIER.— *Électricité*, par BROCQ. — *Electrolyse*, par BROCQ. — *Éléphantiasis*, par DOMINICI. *Eosinophilie*, par LEREDDE. — *Épithélioma*, par DARIER. — *Eruptions artificielles*, par THIBIERGE. — *Erythème*, par BODIN. — *Erythrodermie*, par BROCQ. — *Favus*, par BODIN. — *Folliculites*, par HUDELO. — *Furonculose*, par BAROZZI. — *Gale*, par DUBREUILH. — *Greffe*, par BAROZZI. — *Herpès*, par DU CASTEL. — *Icthyose*, par THIBIERGE. — *Impétigo*, par SABOURAUD. — *Kératodermie*, par DUBREUILH. — *Kératose pilaire*, par VEYRIÈRES. — *Langue*, par BÉNARD. — *Lèpre*, par MARCEL SÉE. — *Leucokératose*, par BÉNARD. — *Lichens*, par BROCQ.

# Traité d'Anatomie Humaine

PUBLIÉ SOUS LA DIRECTION DE

### P. POIRIER                    et                    A. CHARPY

Professeur agrégé à la Faculté
de médecine de Paris
Chirurgien des hôpitaux

Professeur d'anatomie
à la Faculté de médecine
de Toulouse

AVEC LA COLLABORATION DE

O. AMOEDO — A. BRANCA — B. CUNÉO — P. FREDET
P. JACQUES — TH. JONNESCO — E. LAGUESSE — L. MANOUVRIER
A. NICOLAS — M. PICOU
A. PRENANT — H. RIEFFEL — CH. SIMON — A. SOULIÉ

### 5 vol. grand in-8° avec figures noires et en couleurs

---

### ÉTAT DE LA PUBLICATION (Décembre 1900)

Tome I. — *(Deuxième édition, revue et augmentée.)* — **Embryologie**. Notions d'embryologie. **Ostéologie**. Considérations générales. Des membres. Squelette du tronc. Squelette de la tête. **Arthrologie**. Développement des articulations. Structure. Articulations des membres. Articulations du tronc. Articulations de la tête. *Un volume grand in-8°, avec 807 figures* . . . . . **20 fr.**

Tome II. — 1<sup>er</sup> Fascicule : **Myologie**. Embryologie. Histologie. Peauciers et aponévroses. *Deuxième édition revue et augmentée. Un volume grand in-8°, avec 331 figures* . . . . . . . . . . . . . . . . . . . . . . . . . . **12 fr.**

2<sup>e</sup> Fascicule : **Angéiologie** (Cœur et Artères). Histologie. *Un volume grand in-8°, avec 145 figures.* . . . . . . . . . . . . . . **8 fr.**

3<sup>e</sup> Fascicule : **Angéiologie** (Capillaires. Veines). *Un volume grand in-8°, avec 75 figures* . . . . . . . . . . . . . **6 fr.**

Tome III. — 1<sup>er</sup> Fascicule : **Système nerveux**. Méninges. Moelle. Encéphale. Embryologie. Histologie. *Un volume grand in-8°, avec 201 figures*. . **10 fr.**

2<sup>e</sup> Fascicule : **Système nerveux**. Encéphale. *Un volume grand in-8°, avec 206 figures.* . . . . . . . . . . . . . . . . . . **12 fr.**

3<sup>e</sup> Fascicule : **Système nerveux**. Les Nerfs. Nerfs crâniens. Nerfs rachidiens. *Un volume grand in-8°, avec 205 figures* . . . . . . . . . . . . . . **12 fr.**

Tome IV. — 1<sup>er</sup> Fascicule : **Tube digestif**. Développement. Bouche. Pharynx. Œsophage. Estomac. Intestins. *Deuxième édition, revue et augmentée. Un volume grand in-8°, avec 201 figures.* . . . . . . . . . . . . . . . **12 fr.**

2<sup>e</sup> Fascicule : **Appareil respiratoire**. Larynx. Trachée. Poumons. Plèvre. Thyroïde. Thymus. *Un volume grand in-8°, avec 121 figures*. . . . . **6 fr.**

3<sup>e</sup> Fascicule : **Annexes du tube digestif**. Dents. Glandes salivaires. Foie. Voies biliaires. Pancréas. Rate. **Péritoine**. *Un volume grand in-8°, avec 361 figures.* . . . . . . . . . . . . . . . . . . . **16 fr.**

---

### IL RESTE A PUBLIER

**Les Lymphatiques** qui termineront le tome II.

**Les organes génitaux-urinaires** et les **organes des sens** qui formeront le tome V.

Le prolongement caudé du lobule de Spigel dans le lobe droit du foie adulte (colliculus . caudatus de Haller) obture en partie la fente de Winslow.

Récemment Klaatsch a donné une interprétation tout à fait spéciale de l'hiatus de Winslow. (Voy. *Bibliographie*, p. 1005; ou le premier travail de Brachet (cf. p. 945) et le *Traité d'em-*

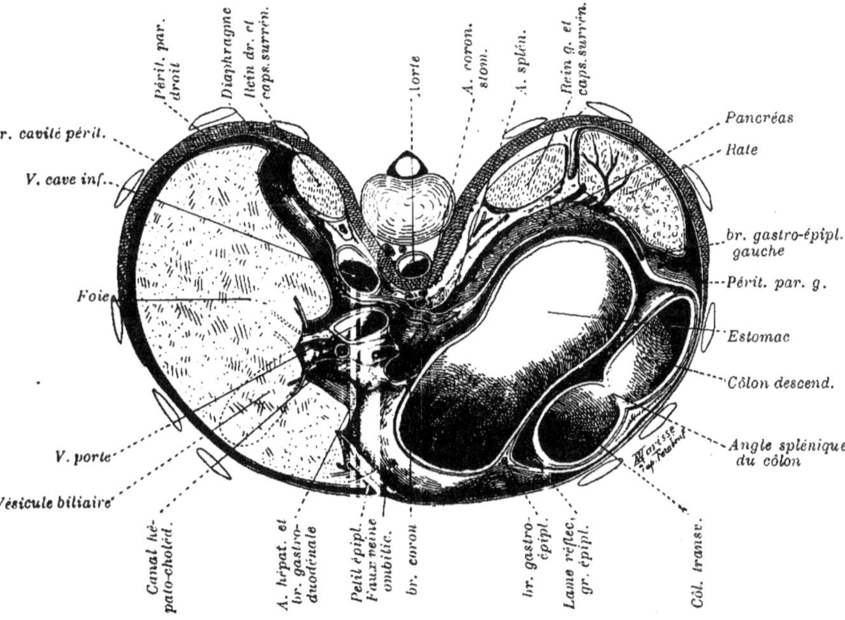


Fig. 577. — Coupe transversale de l'abdomen, au-dessus du seuil de l'hiatus de Winslow, et vue perspective des organes sous-jacents. Reproduction d'un dessin inédit, d'après nature, du Prof. L.-H. Farabeuf. La disposition de l'estomac relativement au côlon est expliquée par le schéma 577 *bis*.

La flèche qui traverse l'hiatus de Winslow, entre la veine cave et la veine porte, franchit l'arc de l'hépatique. Elle peut pénétrer, en arrière de l'estomac, à gauche de la faux de la coronaire (poche rétro-stomacale) ou descendre dans le sac épiploïque.

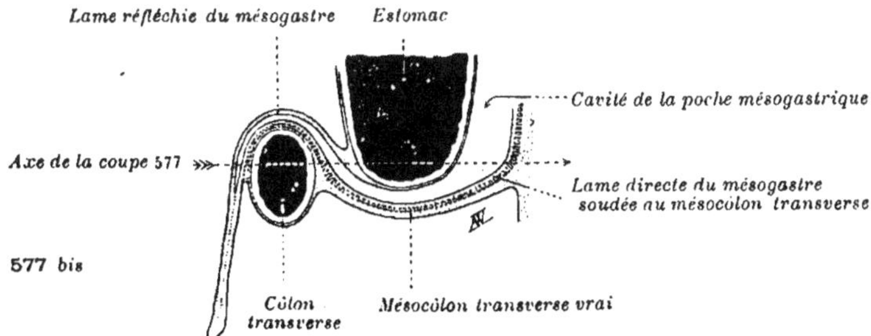


*bryologie* de Prenant (liv. II. p. 780-781 et 784-785). — Ses théories ont été réfutées par Toldt (*l. c.*, 1893, p. 63), et par Brachet et Swaen.

Pour pénétrer dans l'hiatus de Winslow, il suffit de reconnaître la vésicule biliaire et de suivre son bord droit. On est conduit au niveau du plafond de l'hiatus et on y pénètre aisément, en arrière du ligament hépato-duodénal. On

[*FREDET.*]

# *Traité*

## DES

# *Maladies de l'Enfance*

### PUBLIÉ SOUS LA DIRECTION DE MM.

## J. GRANCHER

PROFESSEUR A LA FACULTÉ DE MÉDECINE DE PARIS
MEMBRE DE L'ACADÉMIE DE MÉDECINE, MÉDECIN DE L'HOPITAL DES ENFANTS-MALADES

## J. COMBY

MÉDECIN DE L'HOPITAL DES ENFANTS-MALADES

## A.-B. MARFAN

AGRÉGÉ, MÉDECIN DES HOPITAUX

5 forts volumes grand in-8°, avec figures dans le texte . . . . . . . **90 francs**

Ce *Traité des Maladies de l'Enfance* comble une lacune, et les médecins attendaient avec impatience l'apparition de cet ouvrage. Il existait déjà en effet, traitant des maladies de l'Enfance, plusieurs manuels dont quelques-uns sont fort appréciés, mais nous n'avions pas de traité complet dans lequel les questions de pédiatrie fussent étudiées d'une façon complète. Cet ouvrage paraît en cinq beaux volumes, et la notoriété qui s'attache aux noms des directeurs de cette publication et à ceux des collaborateurs suffit pour lui assurer un plein succès. Les maladies qui y sont traitées ont été confiées, en effet, aux pédiatres qui les ont étudiées d'une façon spéciale. Cette œuvre est pour ainsi dire une œuvre internationale, et parmi les noms des collaborateurs nous trouvons ceux des pédiatres les plus renommés de tous les pays, qui nous font ainsi profiter de l'expérience qu'ils peuvent avoir d'affections qu'ils rencontrent plus que d'autres dans leur champ d'observation. Bien plus, la Médecine et la Chirurgie, ces deux sœurs jumelles qu'on tend bien à tort à séparer sans cesse, ont trouvé le moyen de se retrouver côte à côte au grand profit des lecteurs.

Les 5 volumes se vendent séparément :
Tome I, **18** fr.   Tome II, **18** fr.   Tome III, **20** fr.   Tome IV, **18** fr.   Tome V, **18** fr.

# Traité élémentaire

## DE

# Clinique Thérapeutique

## Par le Dʳ Gaston LYON

Ancien chef de clinique médicale à la Faculté de médecine de Paris.

### TROISIÈME ÉDITION REVUE ET AUGMENTÉE

1 *volume grand in-8 de* VIII-1332 *pages. Relié peau*.. . . . . . **20** *fr.*

La seconde édition de ce livre a reçu du public médical le même accueil favorable que la première. Nous trouvant par suite dans l'obligation agréable de préparer une troisième édition, nous avons considéré comme un devoir strict d'y apporter tous nos soins et de justifier ainsi la faveur soutenue dont notre ouvrage a été l'objet.

Un certain nombre de chapitres nouveaux ont été ajoutés avec tous les développements que comporte leur importance ; citons notamment ceux consacrés aux cardiopathies infantiles, aux sténoses du pylore, aux angiocholites infectieuses, aux péritonites aiguës, aux méningo-myélites aiguës, aux polio-myélites, à la peste, etc.

Le chapitre consacré anx dyspepsies a été récrit en entier. Tous les autres chapitres de notre ouvrage ont été l'objet de modifications de détails, quelques-uns même ont été presque entièrement refondus (blennorragie, syphilis, neurasthénie, infections gastro-intestinales infantiles, etc.)

Sur la demande d'un grand nombre de nos lecteurs, une table alphabétique a été ajoutée, qui facilitera les recherches.

Le rôle du médecin change en même temps que se modifient les médications. La mise en œuvre des soins antiseptiques, l'emploi des injections de sérum, tout cela fait que le rôle actif du médecin grandit, sans cesse. Nous avons tenu, dans cette édition, à insister sur les détails de direction des traitements, en un mot à justifier, mieux encore que par le passé, notre titre de *Traité de clinique thérapeutique.*

# Traité
## de Physiologie

PAR

**J.-P. MORAT**

PROFESSEUR A L'UNIVERSITÉ DE LYON

ET

**Maurice DOYON**

PROFESSEUR AGRÉGÉ A LA FACULTÉ DE MÉDECINE DE LYON

*Ce Traité de Physiologie formera 5 volumes dont voici le détail :*

I. — **Fonctions élémentaires.** — Prolégomènes. — Nutrition en général. — Physiologie des tissus en particulier (moins le système nerveux).

II. — **Fonctions d'innervation et du milieu intérieur.** — Système nerveux. — Sang; lymphe; liquides interstitiels.

III. — **Fonctions de nutrition.** — Circulation; calorification.

IV. — **Fonctions de nutrition** (suite). — Digestion; respiration; excrétion.

V. — **Fonctions de relation.** — Sens. — Langage; expression; locomotion.
**Fonctions de reproduction**, à l'exception du développement embryologique.

Ces volumes ne seront pas publiés dans l'ordre ci-dessus, mais le seront dans celui de leur achèvement.

Chaque volume sera, pendant tout le cours de la publication, vendu séparément à des prix qui varieront selon l'étendue de chacun.

Toutefois, les éditeurs acceptent, dès à présent, au prix à forfait de **50 francs**, des souscriptions à l'ouvrage complet.

Les souscripteurs payeront en retirant chaque volume le prix marqué; mais le tome V et dernier leur sera fourni gratuitement ou à un prix tel qu'ils n'aient, en aucun cas, payé plus de 50 francs pour le total de l'ouvrage.

## *Volumes publiés :*

III. — **Fonctions de nutrition.** — Circulation, par M. DOYON; calorification par J.-P. MORAT. 1 volume grand in-8 avec 173 figures noires et en couleurs **12 fr.**

IV. — **Fonctions de nutrition** (suite et fin). — Respiration; excrétion, par J.-P. MORAT; Digestion; absorption, par M. DOYON. 1 volume grand in-8 avec 167 figures en noir et en couleurs.. . . . . . . . . . . . . . . . . . . . **12 fr.**

C'est un grand traité de physiologie, tel qu'il n'en était pas paru depuis la troisième édition (1888) de l'ouvrage classique de Beaunis, que les auteurs ont eu le courage d'entreprendre et qu'ils mèneront certainement à bien, si l'on en juge par le remarquable spécimen qui forme le premier volume.

E. GLEY (*Archives de physiologie*).

... En résumé, à en juger par le spécimen que nous avons sous les yeux, MM. MORAT et DOYON sont en train de doter nos bibliothèques d'un ouvrage précieux et très bien fait en ce sens qu'ils savent le rendre complet sans le grossir démesurément. Leur *Traité de physiologie* conviendra au débutant, à l'étudiant avancé et à toutes les personnes qui ont besoin de prendre une idée générale ou de remonter à l'origine des faits qui ont permis de la dogmatiser.

D' ARLOING (*Lyon médical*).

# TRAITÉ
### DE
# Physique Biologique

PUBLIÉ SOUS LA DIRECTION DE MM.

**D'ARSONVAL**
Professeur au Collège de France
Membre de l'Institut et de l'Académie des sciences

**CHAUVEAU**
Professeur au Muséum d'histoire naturelle
Membre de l'Institut et de l'Académie de médecine

**GARIEL**
Professeur à la Faculté de médecine de Paris
Membre de l'Académie de médecine

**MAREY**
Professeur au Collège de France
Membre de l'Institut et de l'Académie des sciences

SECRÉTAIRE DE LA RÉDACTION

**M. WEISS**
Professeur agrégé à la Faculté de médecine de Paris

Le **Traité de Physique Biologique** sera publié en trois volumes :
Tome   I. *Mécanique. Actions moléculaires. Chaleur.*
Tome  II. *Radiations. Optique.*
Tome III. *Électricité. Acoustique.*
Chaque volume sera vendu séparément.
Le tome I est vendu **25** fr. On souscrit dès maintenant à l'ouvrage complet au prix de **60** fr. — Ce prix restera tel jusqu'à la publication du tome II.

## EXTRAIT DE LA PRÉFACE

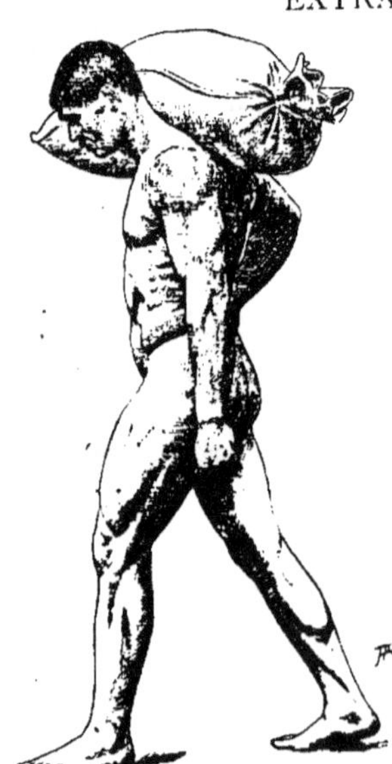

Tome 1. Fig. 180. — Marche avec un fardeau sur l'épaule. Moment du double appui.

Au moment où dans les facultés de médecine il s'est produit un changement considérable dans l'enseignement de la physique. il a semblé utile de réunir en un ouvrage tous les matériaux qui pouvaient faire le fond de cet enseignement.

Déjà les maîtres qui ont pour ainsi dire fondé la Physique biologique, les Weber, Helmholtz, du Bois-Reymond, Chauveau, Marey, Paul Bert, d'autres encore, ont écrit sur certains points spéciaux des traités importants. — Mais si l'on en excepte les manuels et les traités élémentaires à l'usage des étudiants, il n'a encore paru aucun ouvrage d'ensemble sur la physique biologique. — Il y avait là, semble-t-il, une lacune à combler . . . . . . . . . . . . . . . . . . . .

La Physique pure ne tient dans cet ouvrage qu'une place excessivement réduite. — Sa lecture exige la connaissance des notions générales, toutefois il a paru nécessaire de faire précéder chaque partie d'une sorte d'aide-mémoire rappelant brièvement les principaux faits sur lesquels il pouvait être nécessaire de s'appuyer dans la suite. . .

L'ouvrage complet comprendra trois volumes.

Nous avons cru devoir placer en tête du premier un court article sur les diverses espèces d'erreur que l'on est exposé à commettre dans les sciences expérimentales, car nous avons remarqué trop souvent que beaucoup de physiologistes ne faisaient pas la distinction convenable entre elles.

Contrairement à notre principe de passer rapidement sur les questions de physique pure, nous avons aussi donné quelque développement à la mécanique et aux actions moléculaires. Il est, en effet, souvent difficile pour le physiologiste de lire des traités de mécanique générale, et nous avons cherché à en exposer les notions les plus indispensables.

Dans ce même volume, se trouve tout ce qui a rapport à la mécanique animale, à la chaleur et aux actions moléculaires, cependant une grande partie des phénomènes de la contraction musculaire a été renvoyée au troisième volume qui contient l'électrophysiologie.

Ce premier volume sera suivi prochainement, nous l'espérons, par un deuxième volume contenant toutes les applications de l'optique géométrique et des radiations.

Enfin le troisième volume est réservé à l'Electricité et à l'Acoustique.

Nous avons fait tous nos efforts pour mener cet ouvrage à bonne fin ; il nous semble avoir réuni pour cela les meilleures conditions, il suffit pour s'en convaincre de lire la table de noms de nos collaborateurs et de se rappeler celui de notre éditeur dont l'éloge n'est plus à faire ; puissions-nous avoir fait œuvre utile.

## TOME PREMIER

1 fort volume in-8° avec 591 figures dans le texte : **25 fr.**

**Ce volume contient** : Des erreurs dans les mesures. Principes généraux de mécanique, par M. G. WEISS. — Propriétés des solides. Résistance des matériaux. Architecture des os, par M. GARIEL. — Architecture des muscles. Principes généraux de méthode graphique. La contraction musculaire, par M. G. WEISS. — Locomotion humaine, par M. PAUL RICHER. — La locomotion animale, par M. MAREY.
— Principes généraux d'hydrostatique et d'hydrodynamique, par M. WEISS. — Cœur. Cardiographie, par M. WERTHEIMER. — Circulation du sang dans les vaisseaux. Pression et vitesse, pouls et sphygmographie, par M. E. MEYER. — Pléthysmographie, par M. HALLION. — Capillarité et tension superficielle. Solubilité des solides. Imbibition, par M. A. IMBERT. — Filtration, par M. GARIEL. — Osmose, par M. A. DASTRE. — Propriétés des gaz. Analyse des gaz. Gaz du sang. Phénomènes physiques de la respiration, par M. J. TISSOT. — Principes généraux de la chaleur, par M. WEISS. — Thermométrie, par M. GARIEL. — Température, par M. J.-P. LANGLOIS. — Calorimétrie. Etuves et régulateurs de température, par M. C. SIGALAS. — Chaleur animale, par M. LAULANIÉ. — Travail fourni par les animaux. Rendement des moteurs animés. Propagation de la chaleur. Protection des animaux, par M. GARIEL.
— Influence de la pression sur la vie, par MM. P. REGNARD et P. PORTIER. — Influence des

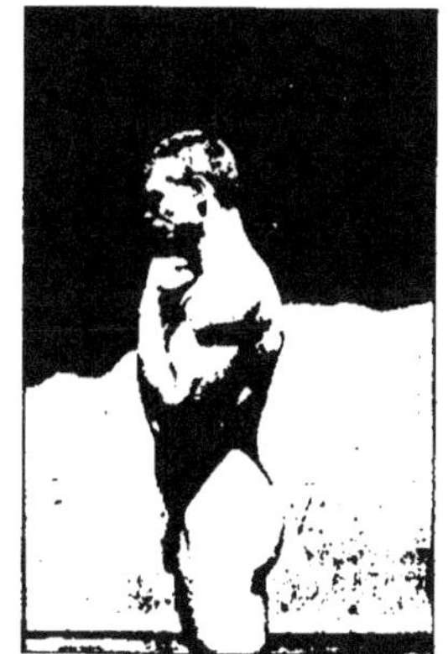

Tome I. Fig. 143. III. — Mouvement rapide. Flexion.

agents atmosphériques sur les éléments cellulaires, par M. A. CHARRIN. — Actions hygrométriques sur les végétaux. Influence de la chaleur sur les végétaux. Actions mécaniques sur les végétaux, par M. MANGIN.

# Précis d'Obstétrique

PAR MM.

**A. RIBEMONT-DESSAIGNES**
Agrégé de la Faculté de médecine,
Accoucheur de l'hôpital Beaujon,
Membre de l'Académie de médecine

**G. LEPAGE**
Professeur agrégé à la Faculté de médecine
de Paris,
Accoucheur de l'hôpital de la Pitié

CINQUIÈME ÉDITION

AVEC 590 FIGURES DANS LE TEXTE DONT 437 DESSINÉES PAR M. RIBEMONT-DESSAIGNES

1 vol. grand in-8° de XXIV-1405 pages, relié toile. . . .   30 fr.

Le Précis d'Obstétrique est un bel et bon ouvrage, appelé à rendre de grands services aux praticiens par son plan et son exécution qui sont parfaits. Tenant le milieu entre les Manuels qui tentent les étudiants, mais ne leur apprennent pas grand' chose, et les traités magistraux qu'ils n'ont guère le temps ni les moyens d'aborder, cet ouvrage nous paraît réaliser parfaitement le but des auteurs d'être un livre d'enseignement proprement dit. Et cet enseignement, c'est, dans ses grandes lignes, celui de M. Tarnier et de M. Pinard.

*(Revue scientifique.)*

Cet ouvrage est appelé à rendre de grands services, non seulement à l'étudiant qui prépare ses examens, mais aussi au praticien, abandonné qu'il est, la plupart du temps, au milieu des multiples difficultés de la clinique et avec une instruction pratique souvent insuffisante....

.... Nous devons aussi parler de la partie Iconographique de l'ouvrage; tous les dessins qui sont l'œuvre personnelle de M. Ribemont - Dessaignes joignent à une exactitude photographique un

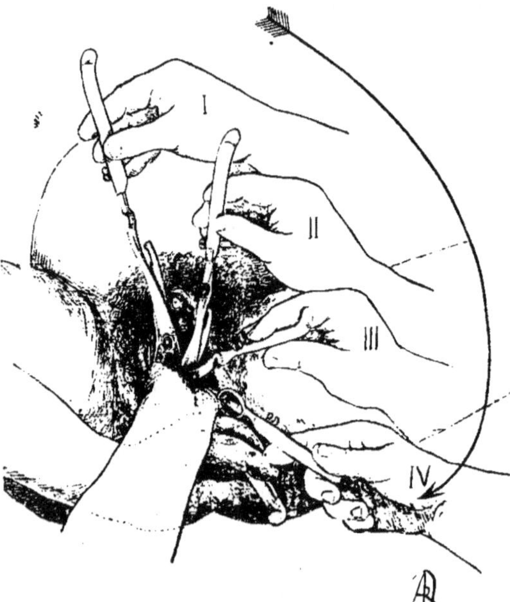

Fig. 489. — Introduction et placement de la cuiller droite sur le sommet en position gauche (variété antérieure).

caractère artistique qui donne au livre un aspect particulier.— Ce précis est donc le résumé très complet et très clair de l'art des accouchements; il est pratique pour le clinicien et l'étudiant, en même temps qu'intéressant pour le savant, et les auteurs seront récompensés de leur travail considérable par le succès qu les attend.

*(Revue de chirurgie.)*

# Traité
## de Gynécologie

### CLINIQUE ET OPÉRATOIRE

### Par le Dᵣ Samuel POZZI

Professeur agrégé à la Faculté de médecine, Chirurgien de l'hôpital Broca.
Membre de l'Académie de médecine

TROISIÈME ÉDITION, REVUE ET AUGMENTÉE

1 vol. in-8° de xxii-1270 pages, avec 628 fig. dans le texte. Relié toile. 30 fr.

...... L'ordonnance générale du traité n'est pas changée, mais de nombreuses additions et des figures multiples sont venues l'enrichir. La thérapeutique chirurgicale des opérations pelviennes, en particulier, a été complètement revisée, et M. Pozzi, tout en restant laparotomiste convaincu, reconnaît à l'hystérectomie vaginale la large place qui lui est due.... Au point de vue thérapeutique, je mentionnerai, comme nouvelles, les pages relatives aux différents procédés d'hystéropexie vaginale recommandés ces derniers temps, celles qu sont consacrées au traitement chirurgical du prolapsus, enfin, et surtout, un petit chapitre relatif à la chirurgie conservatrice des ovaires. — L'anatomie pathologique et la bactériologie tiennent une grande place ; de nombreuses figures originales inédites viennent très heureusement compléter des descriptions qui seraient un peu ardues à la simple lecture.

Partout l'auteur a cherché à être aussi complet que possible, de là une abondance d'indications bibliographiques et de courtes analyses bien fondues ensemble, dont le chercheur tirera grand profit. Mais M. Pozzi a eu soin également de donner toujours son opinion personnelle, permettant ainsi aux jeunes de bénéficier de sa longue expérience. Nous retrouvons ainsi dans cette troisième édition toutes les qualités des deux premières ; il est facile d'en prédire le grand succès.

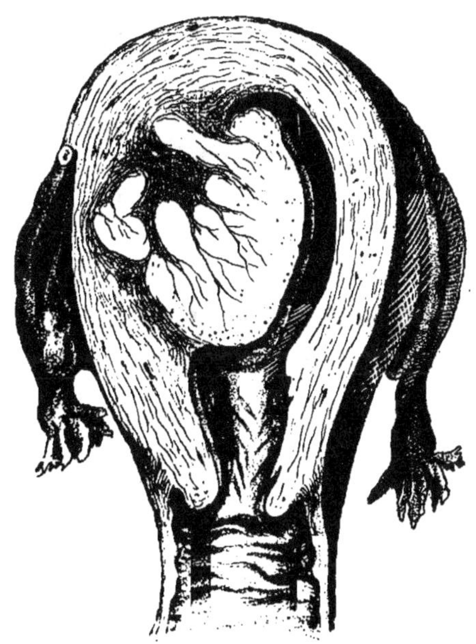

Fig. 251. — Sarcome de la muqueuse utérine.

E. BONNAIRE (*Presse médicale*).

# Traité de Chirurgie d'urgence

## PAR

### FÉLIX LEJARS

Professeur agrégé à la Faculté de médecine de Paris,
Chirurgien de l'hôpital Tenon
Membre de la Société de chirurgie

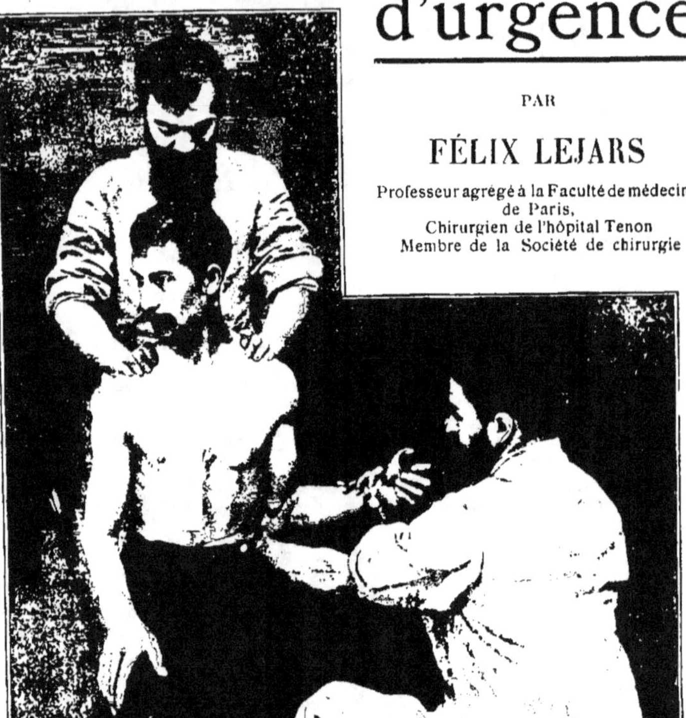

Fig. 431. — Luxation intra-coracoïdienne — Essai de réduction par le procédé de Kocher.
*1ʳᵉ manœuvre complémentaire: Le coude est reporté le plus loin possible en arrière.*

**TROISIÈME ÉDITION, REVUE ET AUGMENTÉE**

Plus de 670 figures dont la plupart dessinées d'après nature par le Dʳ E. DALEINE
et environ 170 photographies originales.

*1 volume grand in-8⁰, d'environ 950 pages. Relié toile.* **25 francs**

Le succès de deux éditions enlevées en quelques mois prouve mieux que tout éloge la valeur et l'utilité du *Traité de Chirurgie d'urgence* du Dʳ F. Lejars.

Fidèle à la méthode qui lui a assuré le succès, le Dʳ Lejars s'est contenté de rendre cette nouvelle édition à la fois plus complète et plus pratique.

Des additions considérables, des remaniements importants ont été faits au texte et des dessins inédits et des photographies originales ont enrichi encore l'illustration déjà hors de pair et universellement appréciée qui fait de cet ouvrage un véritable album.

Ainsi amélioré, le *Traité de Chirurgie d'urgence* se présente pour la troisième fois au public. Il trouvera auprès de lui l'accueil élogieux et empressé qu'il a déjà rencontré et dont les extraits suivants de la presse scientifique ne donnent qu'une incomplète expression.

... Par cette courte analyse, j'aurai voulu engager praticiens et étudiants à lire cet excellent traité. Tous y puiseront avec avantage des notions d'une utilité éminemment pratique et la multiplicité des figures leur facilitera merveilleusement à chaque pas la compréhension du texte.. .

*(Presse médicale.)*

... L'auteur a voulu offrir au public un traité essentiellement simple et pratique, permettant à tout médecin, en présence d'un cas de chirurgie d'urgence, de poser une médication thérapeutique et d'être à même de la remplir; c'est dire l'immense service que cet ouvrage est appelé à rendre partout où le chirurgien de profession fait défaut....

*(Revue de Chirurgie.)*

... Non e inopportuno aggiungere che alla bonta del libro corrisponde la bellezza dell' edizione, nella quale disegni originali e fotografie sono ritratti con esattezza e finezza non comuni.

*(La Clinica Chirurgica.)*

Ohne theoretische Auseinandersetzung und ohne viel Gelehrsamkeit führt uns Lejars unmittelbar aus Krankenbett und schildert uns den — vielfach selbsterlebten — Krankheitsfall mitt einer Anschaulichkeit und Klarheit, dass wir glauben, die Gefahr vor unseren Augen zu sehen....

*(Klinisch-therapeutische Wochenschrift.)*

Der Werth des Buches ruht nicht allein in dem reichem Inhalt, sondern ganz besonders in den vortrefflichen Darstellung, welche vollendet klar, obendrein durch ein Fülle instructivster neuer Zeichnungen ergäntz wird, dann durch den modernen, fortgeschrittenen Standpunkt, welche der Verfasser in allen klinischen und technischen Fragen einnimmt. Die neuesten Erfahrungen und Vorschläge sind berücksichtigt : die Serumtherapie wie die Gelatineinjection, die moderne Hirnchirurgie wie die Fortschritte der Bauchchirurgie und die Naht der Herzwunden; die deutsche Litteratur ist fleissig mit verwerthet.

HELFERICH.

*(Zeitschrift für Chirurgie.)*

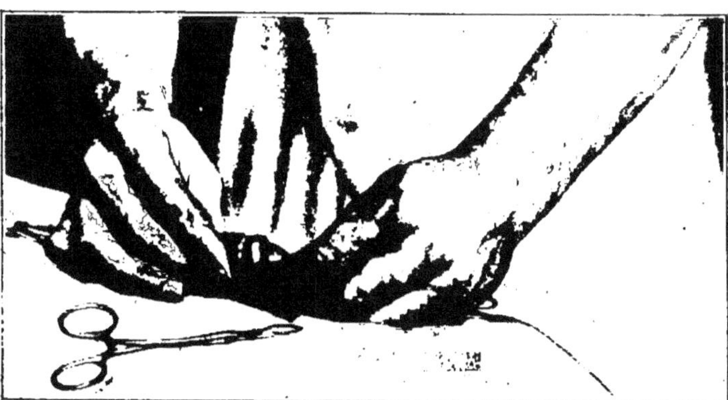

Fig. 259. — Réunion intestinale par le bouton de Murphy (4ᵉ *temps*). *Emboîtement à fond des 2 moitiés.*

**ARTHUS**. — *Éléments de Chimie physiologique*, par MAURICE ARTHUS, professeur de physiologie et de chimie physiologique, à l'Université de Fribourg (Suisse). *Troisième édition*, revue et corrigée. 1 vol. in-16 diamant, avec figures dans le texte, cartonné toile. . . . . . . . . . . . . . . . . . . **4 fr.**

**BARD**. — *Précis d'anatomie pathologique*, par M. L. BARD, professeur à la Faculté de Médecine de Lyon, médecin de l'Hôtel-Dieu. *Deuxième édition, revue et augmentée*. 1 volume in-16 diamant, avec 125 figures, cart. à l'anglaise, tranches rouges. . . . . . . . . . . . . . . . . . . **7 fr. 50**

**BAZY**. — *Maladies des Voies urinaires, Urètre, Vessie*, par le Dʳ BAZY, chirurgien des hôpitaux, membre de la Société de chirurgie. 2 vol. petit in-8° de l'*Encyclopédie des Aide-Mémoire*.
    I. *Moyens d'exploration et traitement.* 2ᵉ édition.
    II. *Séméiologie*
    III. *Thérapeutique générale. Médecine opératoire.*
    IV. *Thérapeutique spéciale.*
Chaque volume séparément. . . . . . . . . . . . . . . . . . . **2 fr. 50**

**BERLIOZ**. — *Manuel de Thérapeutique*, par le Dʳ BERLIOZ, professeur à la Faculté de médecine de Grenoble, avec une préface par M. BOUCHARD, professeur à la Faculté de médecine de Paris. 4ᵉ édition revue et augmentée. 1 vol, in-18 diamant, cartonné toile anglaise, tranches rouges. . . . . . . . . . . . . **6 fr.**

**BLOCQ ET LONDE**. — *Anatomie pathologique de la moelle épinière.* 45 *planches en héliogravure*, avec texte explicatif, par PAUL BLOCQ, ancien interne des hôpitaux, chef des travaux anatomo-pathologiques à la Salpêtrière et ALBERT LONDE, directeur du service photographique à la Salpêtrière. Ouvrage précédé d'une préface de M. le professeur CHARCOT. 1 vol. in-4° relié toile. . . . **48 fr.**

**BONNIER**. — *L'Oreille*, par PIERRE BONNIER, 5 vol. petit in-8° de l'*Encyclopédie des Aide-Mémoire*.
    I. *Anatomie de l'oreille.*
    II. *Pathogénie et mécanisme.*
    III. *Physiologie : Les Fonctions.*
    IV. *Symptomatologie de l'oreille.*
    V. *Pathologie de l'oreille.*
Chaque volume séparément. . . . . . . . . . . . . . . . . . . **2 fr. 50**

**BOTTEY**. — *Traité théorique et pratique d'hydrothérapie médicale*, par le Dʳ F. BOTTEY, médecin de l'Établissement hydrothérapique de Divonne. 1 volume grand in-8° . . . . . . . . . . . . . . . . . . . . . . . . **10 fr.**

**BOUCHARD (CH.)** — *Leçons sur la thérapeutique des maladies infectieuses.* — (*Antisepsie*), professées à la Faculté de médecine de Paris, par M. CH. BOUCHARD. membre de l'Institut. 1 vol. grand in-8°. . . . . . . . . . . . . . . **9 fr.**

**BRAULT**. — *Les Artérites*, par A. BRAULT, médecin de l'hôpital Tenon, chef des travaux pratiques d'anatomie pathologique à la Faculté de médecine. 2 vol. petit in-8° de l'*Encyclopédie des Aide-Mémoire*.
    I. *Les Artérites, leur rôle en pathologie.* 1 vol.
    II. *Les Artérites et les Scléroses.* 1 vol.
Chaque volume séparément. . . . . . . . . . . . . . . . . . . **2 fr. 50**

**BRISSAUD**. — *Anatomie du cerveau de l'homme.* — *Morphologie des hémisphères cérébraux ou cerveau proprement dit.* Texte et figures par le Dʳ E. BRISSAUD, professeur agrégé à la Faculté de médecine. 1 atlas grand in-4°, de 43 planches gravées sur cuivre, représentant 270 préparations, grandeur naturelle, avec explication en regard de chacune ; et 1 volume in-8° de 580 pages, avec plus de 200 figures schématiques dans le texte. 2 vol. reliés toile anglaise. . . **80 fr.**

— *Leçons sur les maladies nerveuses* (Salpêtrière, 1893-1894), recueillies et publiées par HENRY MEIGE. 1 vol. gr. in-8° avec 240 fig. (schémas et photographies). . . . . . . . . . . . . . . . . . . . . . . . . **18 fr.**

— *Leçons sur les maladies nerveuses* (*Deuxième série* ; hôpital Saint-Antoine), recueillies et publiées par Henry Meige. 1 vol. grand in-8° avec 165 figures dans le texte . . . . . . . . . . . . . . . . . . . . . . . . . . **15** fr.

BROCA (A.). — *Traitement des tumeurs blanches.* Ostéo-arthrites tuberculeuses des membres chez l'enfant, par A. Broca, chirurgien de l'hôpital Trousseau, professeur agrégé à la Faculté de médecine. 1 vol. in-8° de l'*Encyclopédie des Aide-Mémoire.* . . . . . . . . . . . . . . . . . . . . . **2** fr. **50**

BROUSSES. — *Manuel technique de massage*, par le D<sup>r</sup> J. Brousses, médecin-major de 2<sup>e</sup> classe. 2<sup>e</sup> édition. 1 vol. in-16, avec nombreuses figures, cartonné toile, tranches rouges. . . . . . . . . . . . . . . . . . . . . . **4** fr.

*Centenaire de la Faculté de médecine de Paris* (1794-1894), par le D<sup>r</sup> A. Corlieu. 1 vol. in-4°, imprimé par l'Imprimerie Nationale et accompagné d'un album in-4° de 130 portraits des professeurs de la Faculté reproduits d'après des documents authentiques. Les 2 volumes. . . . . . . . . . . . . . . . . . **100** fr.

CHARRIN. — *Leçons de pathogénie appliquée. Clinique médicale, Hôtel-Dieu* (1895-1896), par A. Charrin, professeur agrégé, médecin des hôpitaux, directeur adjoint au laboratoire de Pathologie générale, assistant au Collège de France, Vice-président de la Société de Biologie. 1 vol. in-8° . . . . . . . . . **6** fr.

— *Poisons de l'organisme*, par le D<sup>r</sup> A. Charrin. 3 vol. petit in-8° de l'*Encyclopédie des Aide-Mémoire.*

 I. *Poisons de l'urine*, Paris, 1893.
 II. *Poisons du tube digestif*, Paris, 1895.
 III. *Poisons des tissus*, Paris, 1897.
Chaque volume séparément. . . . . . . . . . . . . . . . . . **2** fr. **50**

— *Les Défenses naturelles de l'organisme : Leçons professées au Collège de France*, par A. Charrin. 1 vol. in-8°. . . . . . . . . . . . . . . . **6** fr.

CHAUVEL ET NIMIER. — *Traité pratique de Chirurgie d'armée*, par J. Chauvel, médecin-principal de 1<sup>re</sup> classe, professeur à l'École du Val-de-Grâce, et H. Nimier, médecin-major de 2<sup>e</sup> classe, professeur agrégé à l'École du Val-de-Grâce. 1 vol. in-8° avec 126 figures dessinées par le D<sup>r</sup> J.-E. Pesmes, médecin aide-major de 1<sup>re</sup> classe. . . . . . . . . . . . . . . . . . . . . . . . . . **12** fr.

DASTRE. — *Les Anesthésiques. Physiologie et applications chirurgicales*, par M. Dastre, professeur de physiologie à la Sorbonne. 1 vol. in-8°. . . . . . **5** fr.

DIEULAFOY. — *Manuel de Pathologie interne*, par G. Dieulafoy, professeur de clinique médicale de la Faculté de médecine de Paris, médecin de l'Hôtel-Dieu, membre de l'Académie de médecine. *Treizième édition entièrement refondue et considérablement augmentée.* 4 vol. in-16 diamant avec figures en noir et en coul., cart. à l'anglaise, tranches rouges **28** fr.

— *Clinique médicale de l'Hôtel-Dieu de Paris*, par le professeur G. Dieulafoy. 3 vol. gr. in-8°, avec figures dans le texte.
 I. 1896-1897, 1 vol. in-8°. . . . **10** fr.
 II. 1897-1898, 1 vol. in-8°. . . . **10** fr.
 III. 1898-1899, 1 vol. in 8°. . . . **10** fr.

Figure extraite du *Manuel de Pathologie interne*, de M. G. Dieulafoy.

DUCLAUX. — *Pasteur. Histoire d'un esprit*, par E. Duclaux, membre de l'Institut, directeur de l'Institut Pasteur, professeur à la Sorbonne et à l'Institut Agronomique. 1 vol. gr. in-8° avec 22 figures dans le texte. . . . . . . . . . . **5** fr.

— *Traité de microbiologie*, par E. Duclaux.
 Tome I *Microbiologie générale.* 1 vol. gr. in-8° avec figures . . . . . **15** fr.
 Tome II. *Diastases, toxines et venins.* 1 vol. gr. in-8° avec figures . . **15** fr.
 Tome III. *Fermentation alcoolique.* 1 vol. gr. in-8° avec figures . . . **15** fr.
L'ouvrage formera 7 volumes qui paraîtront successivement.

**DUFLOCQ.** — *Leçons sur les bactéries pathogènes, faites à l'Hôtel-Dieu annexe*, par P. DUFLOCQ. 1 vol. in-8°. . . . . . . . . . . . . . . **10 fr.**

**DUPLAY.** — *Cliniques chirurgicales de l'Hôtel-Dieu*, par SIMON DUPLAY, professeur de clinique chirurgicale à la Faculté de médecine de Paris, membre de l'Académie de médecine, chirurgien de l'Hôtel-Dieu. Recueillies et publiées par les Dʳˢ M. CAZIN, chef de clinique chirurgicale à l'Hôtel-Dieu, et L. CLADO, chef des travaux gynécologiques à l'Hôtel-Dieu.

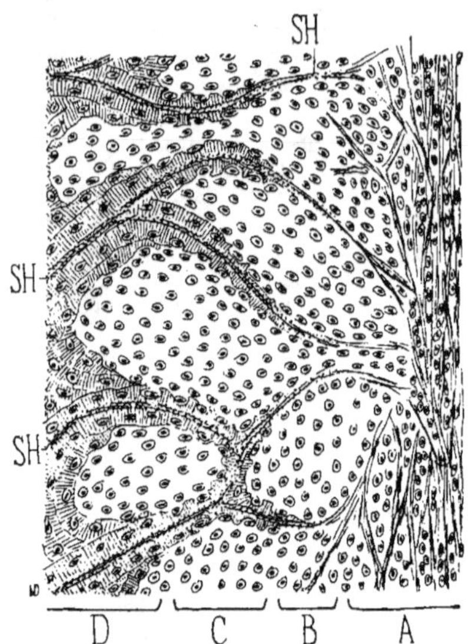



Figure extraite du *Précis d'Histologie*, de M. MATHIAS DUVAL. — Schéma de l'ossification périostique.

1ʳᵉ SÉRIE. 1 vol. in-8° avec figures dans le texte. **7 fr.**
2ᵉ SÉRIE. 1 vol. in-8° avec figures dans le texte. **8 fr.**
3ᵉ SÉRIE. 1 vol. in-8° avec figures dans le texte. **8 fr.**

**DUVAL.** — *Atlas d'embryologie*, par M. MATHIAS DUVAL, professeur d'histologie à la Faculté de médecine de Paris, membre de l'Académie de médecine. 1 vol. in-4°, avec 40 planches en noir et en couleurs, comprenant ensemble 652 figures. Cartonné toile . . . . . . . . **48 fr.**

— *Précis d'histologie*, par M. MATHIAS DUVAL, professeur à la Faculté de médecine de Paris, membre de l'Académie de médecine. *Deuxième édition, revue et augmentée.* 1 vol. gr. in-8° avec 427 figures dans le texte. **18 fr.**

**FAISANS.** — *Maladies des organes respiratoires. Méthodes d'exploration, signes physiques*, par LÉON FAISANS, médecin de la Pitié. *Deuxième édition.* 1 vol. petit in-8°, de l'*Encyclopédie des Aide-Mémoire*. . . . . . . . **2 fr. 50**

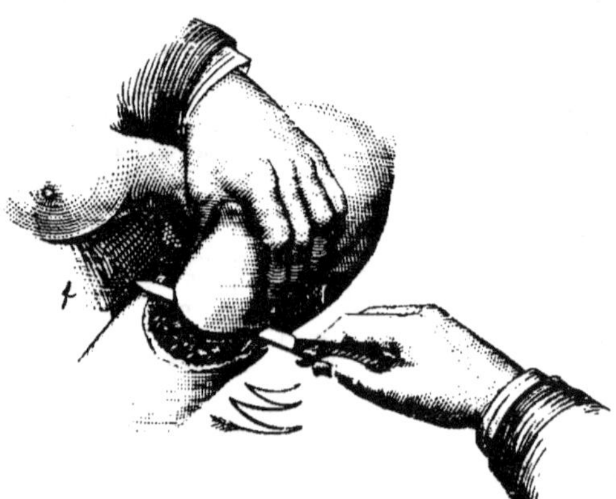

Figure extraite du *Précis de Manuel opératoire*, de M. L.-H. FARABEUF.

**FARABEUF.** — *Précis de manuel opératoire. Ligatures, Amputations, Résections, Appendice*, par M. L.-H. FARABEUF, professeur à la Faculté de médecine de Paris, membre de l'Académie de médecine. *Quatrième édition entièrement revue.* 1 vol. petit in-8°, avec 799 figures. **16 fr.**

**FÉLIZET.** — *Les Hernies inguinales de l'Enfance*, par le Dʳ G. FÉLIZET, chirurgien de l'hôpital Tenon (Enfants-Malades). 1 vol. grand in-8°, avec 73 figures dans le texte. . . . . . **10 fr.**

**GAUTIER (A.).** — *Cours de Chimie minérale et organique*, par M. ARM. GAUTIER, membre de l'Institut, professeur de chimie à la Faculté de médecine de

Paris. *Deuxième édition*, revue et mise au courant des travaux les plus récents.
2 vol. grand in-8°, avec figures dans le texte.
   I. *Chimie minérale*. 1 vol. grand in-8°, avec 244 figures dans le texte. **16 fr.**
   II. *Chimie organique*. 1 vol. grand in-8°, avec 72 figures. . . . . . . . **16 fr.**
— *Leçons de Chimie biologique normale et pathologique*. *Deuxième édition*, publiée avec la collaboration de M. ARTHUS, professeur de physiologie à l'Université de Fribourg. 1 vol. in-8°, avec 110 figures. . . . . . . . **18 fr.**
— *La Chimie de la cellule vivante*, par M. ARM. GAUTIER. *Deuxième édition*. 1 vol. petit in-8° de l'*Encyclopédie des Aide-Mémoire*. . . . . . . . **2 fr. 50**

GILIS. — *Précis d'Embryologie* adapté aux sciences médicales, par PAUL GILIS, professeur agrégé à la Faculté de médecine de Montpellier, avec préface par M. le professeur DUVAL. 1 vol. in-18 diamant, avec 175 figures. Cartonné toile, tranches rouges. . . . . . . . . . . . . . . . . . . . . **6 fr.**

GLEY. — *Essais de philosophie et d'histoire de la Biologie*, par E. GLEY, professeur agrégé à la Faculté de médecine de Paris, assistant près la chaire de Physiologie générale au Muséum d'Histoire naturelle. 1 vol. in-16. . . **3 fr. 50**

GOUGUENHEIM et GLOVER. — *Atlas de laryngologie et de rhinologie*, par A. GOUGUENHEIM, médecin de l'hôpital Lariboisière. et J. GLOVER, ancien interne de la clinique laryngologique de l'hôpital Lariboisière. 1 vol. in-4°, avec 37 planches en noir et en couleurs, comprenant ensemble 246 figures, et 47 figures dans le texte. Légendes en langue anglaise et en langue française, relié toile. . . . . . . . . . . . . . . . . . . . . **50 fr.**

GRASSET. — *Consultations médicales sur quelques maladies fréquentes*, par le Dr GRASSET, professeur de clinique médicale à l'Université de Montpellier, correspondant de l'Académie de médecine. *Quatrième édition, revue et considérablement augmentée*. 1 vol. in-16, reliure souple, peau pleine. **4 fr. 50**
— *Leçons de Clinique médicale*, faites à l'hôpital Saint-Éloi de Montpellier par le Dr J. GRASSET, professeur de clinique médicale à l'Université de Montpellier, correspondant de l'Académie de médecine, lauréat de l'Institut.
   1re SÉRIE (1886-1890). 1 vol. in-8°, avec 10 planches. . . . . . . . . . . **12 fr.**
   2e SÉRIE (novembre 1890-juillet 1895). 1 fort vol. in-8°, avec une figure dans le texte et 10 planches lithographiées. . . . . . . . . . . . . . . . **12 fr.**
   3e SÉRIE (novembre 1895-mars 1898). 1 vol. in-8° de VII-826 pages, avec 20 planches hors texte, dont 10 en couleurs et 6 en phototypie.. . . . **15 fr.**
— *Traité pratique des maladies du système nerveux*, par le professeur GRASSET, en collaboration avec le Dr RAUZIER. *Quatrième édition*. 2 vol. grand in-8°, avec 33 planches hors texte et 122 figures dans le texte (*Ouvrage couronné par l'Institut : Prix Lallemand*). . . . . . . . . . . . . . . . **45 fr.**

HAYEM. — *Du Sang et de ses altérations anatomiques*, par G. HAYEM, professeur à la Faculté de médecine de Paris, médecin des hôpitaux, membre de l'Académie de médecine. 1 vol. in-8°, avec nombreuses figures noires et en couleurs dans le texte, relié toile à biseaux . . . . . . . . . . . . . . . . **32 fr.**
— *Leçons sur les maladies du sang* (*Clinique de l'hôpital Saint-Antoine*), par Georges HAYEM, recueillies par MM. E. PARMENTIER, médecin des hôpitaux, et R. BENSAUDE, chef du laboratoire d'anatomie pathologique à l'hôpital Saint-Antoine. 1 vol. in-8°, avec 4 planches en couleurs . . . . . . . . . . . **15 fr.**

HÉNOCQUE. — *Spectroscopie biologique*, par le Dr ALBERT HÉNOCQUE, directeur adjoint du laboratoire de physique biologique du Collège de France. 3 vol. petit in-8° de l'*Encyclopédie des Aide-Mémoire*.
   I. *Spectroscopie du sang*. Avec figures dans le texte.
   II. *Spectroscopie des organes, des tissus et des humeurs*. Avec figures dans le texte.
   III. *Spectroscopie de l'urine et des pigments*.
   Chaque volume est vendu séparément . . . . . . . . . . . . . . . . **2 fr 50**

KIRMISSON. — *Leçons cliniques sur les maladies de l'appareil locomoteur* (*os, articulations, muscles*), par le Dr KIRMISSON, professeur agrégé à la Faculté de médecine, chirurgien des hôpitaux, membre de la Société de chirurgie. 1 vol. in-8°, avec figures dans le texte . . . . . . . . . . . . . . . . . . . . . **10 fr.**

— — *Traité des maladies chirurgicales d'origine congénitale*, par le D<sup>r</sup> E. Kirmisson. 1 vol. in-8°, avec 311 figures dans le texte et 2 planches en couleurs. . . . . . . . . . . . . . . . . . . . . . . . . . . . . . . . . **15 fr.**

LACASSAGNE. — *Précis de médecine judiciaire*, par M. A. Lacassagne, professeur à la Faculté de médecine de Lyon. 2<sup>e</sup> édition. 1 volume in-18 diamant, avec 47 figures dans le texte et 4 planches en couleur, cartonné à l'anglaise, tranches rouges . . . . . . . . . . . . . . . . . . . . . . . . . . . . . . . **7 fr. 50**

— *Précis d'hygiène privée et sociale*, par M. A. Lacassagne. 4<sup>e</sup> édition revue et augmentée. 1 vol. in-16 diamant, cartonné à l'anglaise, tranches rouges. . . . . . . . . . . . . . . . . . . . . . . . . . . . . . . . . **7 fr.**

LALESQUE. — *Cure marine de la phtisie pulmonaire*, par le D<sup>r</sup> F. Lalesque, ancien interne des hôpitaux de Paris. 1 vol. in-8° avec planches, dessins, tableaux et graphiques. . . . . . . . . . . . . . . . . . . . . . . . . . . . . . **6 fr.**

LAMY. — *La syphilis des centres nerveux*, par le D<sup>r</sup> Henri Lamy, ancien interne des hôpitaux de Paris. 1 vol. petit in-8° de l'*Encyclopédie des Aide-Mémoire*.. . . . . . . . . . . . . . . . . . . . . . . . . . . **2 fr. 50**

LANGLOIS. — *Le Lait* par P. Langlois, chef du Laboratoire de physiologie à la Faculté de médecine. 1 vol. p. in-8° de l'*Encyclopédie des Aide-Mémoire*. **2 fr. 50**

LANNELONGUE. — *La Tuberculose chirurgicale*, par O. Lannelongue, professeur à la Faculté de médecine de Paris. 1 vol. petit in-8° de l'*Encyclopédie des Aide-Mémoire* . . . . . . . . . . . . . . . . . . . . . . . . . **2 fr. 50**

LAULANIÉ. — *Énergétique musculaire*, par F. Laulanié, professeur de physiologie à l'École vétérinaire de Toulouse; avec une préface de M. Chauveau, de l'Institut. 1 vol. petit in-8° de l'*Encyclopédie des Aide-Mémoire*. . . . **2 fr. 50**

LAUNOIS. — *Manuel d'Anatomie microscopique et d'Histologie*, par MM. P.-E. Launois, professeur agrégé à la Faculté de Paris, médecin des hôpitaux. Préface de M. Mathias Duval, professeur d'histologie à la Faculté, membre de l'Académie de médecine. *Deuxième édition entièrement refondue*. 1 vol. in-16 diamant, cartonné toile. . . . . . . . . . . . . . . . . . . . **8 fr.**

LAVERAN. — *Du Paludisme* et de son hématozoaire, par A. Laveran, membre de l'Académie de médecine, membre correspondant de l'Institut de France. 1 vol. grand in-8°, avec 4 planches en couleur et 2 planches photographiques . **10 fr.**

— *Traité du Paludisme*, par A. Laveran. 1 vol. grand in-8° avec 27 figures dans le texte et une planche en couleurs . . . . . . . . . . . . . . . . . . **10 fr.**

— *Traité d'hygiène militaire* par le D<sup>r</sup> Laveran. 1 vol. in-8°, avec 270 figures. . . . . . . . . . . . . . . . . . . . . . . . . . . . . . . . . . **16 fr.**

LEJARS. — *Leçons de chirurgie* (La Pitié 1893-1894), par le D<sup>r</sup> Félix Lejars, professeur agrégé à la Faculté de médecine de Paris, chirurgien des hôpitaux. 1 vol. grand in-8°, avec 128 figures. . . . . . . . . . . . . . . . . . **16 fr.**

LELOIR ET VIDAL. — *Symptomatologie et anatomie pathologique des maladies de la peau*, par MM. Leloir, professeur à la Faculté de médecine de Lille, et E. Vidal, médecin de l'hôpital St-Louis. Un atlas de 54 planches grand in-8°, tirées en couleur, et accompagnées d'un texte explicatif, relié toile. **70 fr.**

LETULLE. — *L'Inflammation* (Études anatomo-pathologiques), par le D<sup>r</sup> Maurice Letulle, professeur agrégé à la Faculté de médecine de Paris. 1 vol. avec 21 figures et 12 planches en chromolithographie hors texte, relié toile. . **20 fr.**

*Manuel de pathologie externe*, par MM. Reclus, Kirmisson, Peyrot, Bouilly, professeurs agrégés à la Faculté de médecine de Paris, chirurgiens des hôpitaux. Nouvelle édition, illustrée de 720 figures, 4 vol. in-8° avec figures dans le texte . . . . . . . . . . . . . . . . . . . . . . . . . . . . . . . **40 fr.**

I. *Maladies des tissus et des organes*, par le D[r] P. RECLUS. avec figures dans le texte.

II. *Maladies des régions ; Tête et Rachis*, par le D[r] KIRMISSON, entièrement refondue et augmentée, avec figures dans le texte.

III. *Maladies des régions : Poitrine et abdomen*, par le D[r] PEYROT, entièrement refondue et augmentée, avec figures dans le texte.

IV. *Maladies des régions : Organes génito-urinaires*, membres, par le D[r] BOUILLY, avec figures dans le texte.

Chaque volume est vendu séparément. . . . . . . . . . . . . . . . . . . 10 fr.

MARIE. — ***Leçons sur les maladies de la moelle***, par le D[r] PIERRE MARIE, professeur agrégé de la Faculté de médecine de Paris, médecin des hôpitaux. 1 vol. in-8°, avec 244 figures dans le texte. . . . . . . . . . . . . . . . . 15 fr.

— ***Leçons de clinique médicale*** (Hôtel-Dieu 1894-1895), par le D[r] PIERRE MARIE. 1 vol. in-8°, avec 57 figures dans le texte. . . . . . . . . . . . . . . 6 fr.

MAURIAC. — ***Traitement de la syphilis***, par M. CHARLES MAURIAC, médecin de l'hôpital Ricord (Hôpital du Midi). 1 vol. in-8° . . . . . . . . . . . . . 15 fr.

MÉGNIN. — ***La Faune des cadavres***, *application de l'entomologie à la médecine légale*, par M. P. MÉGNIN, membre de l'Académie de médecine. 1 vol. petit in-8° de l'*Encyclopédie des Aide-Mémoire*. . . . . . . . . . . . . . . . . 2 fr. 50

MERKLEN. — ***Examen et séméiotique du cœur***, *signes physiques*, par le D[r] PIERRE MERKLEN, médecin de l'hôpital Laënnec. *Deuxième édition*. 1 vol. petit in-8° de l'*Encyclopédie des Aide-Mémoire*. . . . . . . . . . . 2 fr. 50

METCHNIKOFF. — ***Leçons sur la pathologie comparée de l'inflammation***, faites à l'Institut Pasteur en avril et mai 1891, par ÉLIE METCHNIKOFF, chef de service à l'Institut Pasteur. 1 vol. in-8° avec 65 fig. et 3 pl. en coul. . . 9 fr.

MONOD ET TERRILLON. — ***Traité des maladies du testicule et de ses annexes***. par MM. CH. MONOD et O. TERRILLON, professeurs agrégés à la Faculté de médecine de Paris, chirurgiens des hôpitaux. 1 vol. in-8° avec 92 figures dans le texte. . . . . . . . . . . . . . . . . . . . . . . . . . . . . 16 fr.

MONOD ET VANVERTS. — ***L'Appendicite***, par le D[r] CH. MONOD, professeur agrégé à la Faculté de médecine de Paris, chirurgien de l'hôpital Saint-Antoine, membre de l'Académie de médecine, et J. VANVERTS, interne des hôpitaux de Paris. 1 vol. petit in-8° de l'*Encyclopédie des Aide-Mémoire*. . . . . . 2 fr. 50

OLLIER. — ***Traité expérimental et clinique de la régénération des os*** et de la production artificielle du tissu osseux, par le D[r] OLLIER, chirurgien en chef de l'Hôtel-Dieu de Lyon. Ouvrage qui a obtenu le grand prix de chirurgie. 2 vol. in-8°, avec figures dans le texte et planches en taille-douce.. . . . . . . 30 fr.

— ***Traité des Résections*** et des opérations conservatrices que l'on peut pratiquer sur le système osseux, par le D[r] L. OLLIER, professeur de clinique chirurgicale à la Faculté de médecine de Lyon. 3 volumes grand in-8° avec figures. . . . . . . . . . . . . . . . . . . . . . . . . . . . . . . . . 50 fr.

Tome I. *Introduction. — Résections en général*. 1 vol. in-8° avec 127 figures dans le texte . . . . . . . . . . . . . . . . . . . . . . . . . . . . . . 16 fr.

Tome II. *Résections en particulier. Membre supérieur*. 1 vol. in-8° avec 156 figures . . . . . . . . . . . . . . . . . . . . . . . . . . . . . . . . 16 fr.

Tome III. *Résections en particulier. Résections du membre inférieur, tête et tronc*. 1 vol in-8° avec 224 figures. . . . . . . . . . . . . . . . . . . . 22 fr.

— ***La Régénération des os et les résections sous-périostées***, par le D[r] L. OLLIER. 1 vol. petit in-8° de l'*Encyclopédie des Aide-Mémoire*. . 2 fr. 50

PANAS. — ***Traité des maladies des yeux***, par PH. PANAS, professeur de clinique ophtalmologique à la Faculté de médecine, chirurgien de l'Hôtel-Dieu, membre de l'Académie de médecine, membre honoraire et ancien président de la Société de chirurgie. 2 vol. grand in-8° avec 453 figures et 7 planches en couleurs. Reliés toile. . . . . . . . . . . . . . . . . . . . . . . . . . . . . 40 fr.

**PANAS.** — *Leçons de clinique ophtalmologique, professées à l'Hôtel-Dieu*, par PH. PANAS, recueillies et publiées par le Dʳ A. CASTAN (de Béziers). 1 vol. in-8°, avec figures dans le texte. . . . . . . . . . . . . . . . . . . . . **5 fr.**

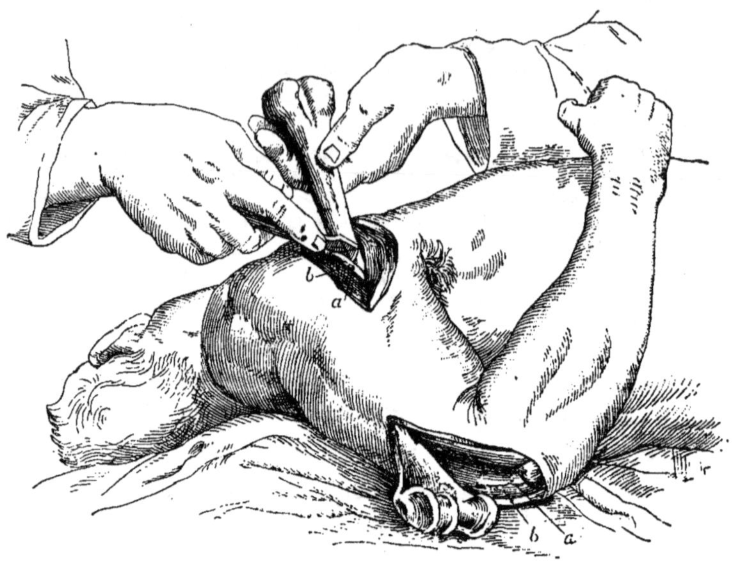

Figure extraite du *Traité des Résections* de M. L. Ollier.

**PANAS ET ROCHON-DUVIGNEAUD.** — *Recherches anatomiques et cliniques sur le glaucome et les néoplasmes intra-oculaires*, par le professeur PANAS et le Dʳ ROCHON-DUVIGNEAUD, ancien chef de clinique de la Faculté. 1 vol. in-8°, avec 41 figures dans le texte. . . . . . . . . . . . . . . . . . . **7 fr.**

**POLIN ET LABIT.** — *Examen des aliments suspects*, par MM. H. POLIN et H. LABIT, médecins-majors de l'armée. 1 vol. petit in-8° de l'*Encyclopédie des Aide-Mémoire*. . . . . . . . . . . . . . . . . . . . . . . . **2 fr. 50**

**PONCET ET BÉRARD.** — *Traité clinique de l'actinomycose humaine. Pseudo-actinomycoses et botryomycose*, par ANTONIN PONCET, professeur de clinique chirurgicale à l'Université de Lyon, ex-chirurgien en chef de l'Hôtel-Dieu, membre correspondant de l'Académie de médecine et LÉON BÉRARD, ex-prosecteur, chef de clinique chirurgicale à l'Université de Lyon, lauréat de l'Académie de médecine. *Ouvrage couronné par l'Académie de médecine et par l'Institut.* 1 vol in-8°, avec 45 fig. dans le texte et 4 planches hors texte en coul. . **12 fr.**

**PONCET ET DELORE.** — *Traité de la cystostomie sus-pubienne chez les prostatiques. Création d'un urèthre hypogastrique. Application de cette nouvelle méthode aux diverses affections des voies urinaires*, par ANTONIN PONCET et XAVIER DELORE, ex-prosecteur, ancien chef de clinique chirurgicale à l'Université de Lyon. 1 vol. in-8° avec 42 figures dans le texte. . . . . . . . **8 fr.**

— *Traité de l'uréthrostomie périnéale dans les rétrécissements incurables de l'urèthre ; création au périnée d'un méat contre nature*, par ANTONIN PONCET et XAVIER DELORE. 1 vol. in-8° avec 11 figures dans le texte . . . . . . **4 fr.**

**PROUST.** — *La Défense de l'Europe contre le choléra*, par M. le professeur PROUST, inspecteur général des services sanitaires, 1 vol. in-8° . . . . . **9 fr.**

— *Douze conférences d'hygiène rédigées conformément aux programmes du*

12 *août* 1890, par A. PROUST, professeur à la Faculté de médecine. Nouvelle
édition. 1 vol. in-18. Cartonné toile. . . . . . . . . . . . . . . . . **2 fr. 50**

— *L'Orientation nouvelle de la politique sanitaire*, par A. PROUST. 1 vol. in-8°,
avec nombreuses figures et plans dans le texte et une carte en couleurs.  **10 fr.**

— *La Défense de l'Europe contre la Peste et la Conférence de Venise
de 1897*, par le professeur PROUST. 1 volume in-8° avec figures et 1 carte
en couleurs . . . . . . . . . . . . . . . . . . . . . . . . . . . . **9 fr.**

PRUNIER. — *Les Médicaments chimiques*, par LÉON PRUNIER, membre de
l'Académie de médecine, pharmacien en chef des hôpitaux de Paris, professeur à
l'Ecole supérieure de pharmacie.
   I. *Composés minéraux*. 1 vol. grand in-8° avec 137 figures dans le texte.  **15 fr.**
   II. *Composés organiques*. 1 volume grand in-8° avec 47 figures, dans le
texte. . . . . . . . . . . . . . . . . . . . . . . . . . . . . . . . **15 fr.**

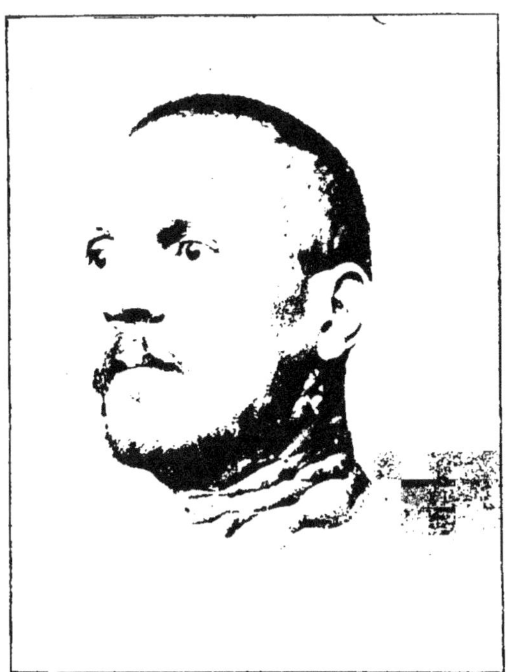

Figure extraite du *Traité clinique de l'actinomycose humaine*,
de MM. A. Poncet et L. Bérard.

RANVIER. — *École pratique des Hautes Études. Laboratoire d'histologie du
Collège de France.* Travaux publiés sous la direction de L. RANVIER, professeur
d'anatomie générale, Membre de l'Institut, avec la collaboration de M. L. MALASSEZ,
directeur adjoint, et des répétiteurs et préparateurs du cours.
   Tomes I à XVII (1784-1899). Chaque vol. in-8° avec pl. hors texte. . . **20 fr.**
   Les tomes V et VIII ne se vendent plus séparément.

— *Traité technique d'histologie.* 2° édition entièrement refondue et corrigée,
par M. L. RANVIER. 1 vol. gr. in-8° de 880 pages, avec 414 gravures dans le texte
et 1 planche en chromo . . . . . . . . . . . . . . . . . . . . . . . **12 fr.**

REDARD. — *Traité pratique des déviations de la colonne vertébrale*, par
P. REDARD, ancien chef de clinique chirurgicale de la Faculté de médecine de

Paris, chirurgien en chef du dispensaire Furtado-Heine, membre correspondant de l'American Ortopédic Association. 1 vol. grand in-8°, avec 231 figures dans le texte . . . . . . . . . . . . . . . . . . . . . . . . . . . . . . . **12 fr.**

REDARD et LARAN. — *Atlas de Radiographie : Chirurgie infantile et orthopédique*, par P. REDARD et F. LARAN. 1 vol. in-4°, contenant 48 planches en photocollographie, avec leur explication, relié toile. . . . . . . . . . . . **25 fr.**

REGNARD. — *La Cure d'altitude*, par le Dr PAUL REGNARD, membre de l'Académie de médecine, professeur de physiologie générale à l'Institut national agronomique, directeur-adjoint du laboratoire de physiologie de la Sorbonne. *Deuxième édition*. 1 fort vol. grand in-8°, avec 29 planches hors texte et 110 figures dans le texte, relié toile pleine. . . . . . . . . . . . . . . . . . . . . . **15 fr.**

RÉNON. — *Étude sur l'Aspergillose chez les animaux et chez l'homme*, par M. RÉNON, ancien interne des hôpitaux de Paris. 1 vol. in-8°, avec figures dans le texte. . . . . . . . . . . . . . . . . . . . . . . . . . . . . . . . . . **5 fr.**

SOLLIER. — *Guide pratique des maladies mentales* (Séméiologie. — Pronostic. — Indications), par le Dr PAUL SOLLIER, chef de clinique adjoint des maladies mentales à la Faculté. 1 vol. in-18 diamant, cartonné toile, tranches rouges.   **5 fr.**

SOULIER (H.). *Traité de thérapeutique et de pharmacologie*, par M. H. SOULIER, professeur à la Faculté de médecine de Lyon, membre correspondant de l'Académie de médecine. *Additionné d'un memento formulaire des médicaments nouveaux* (1901). *Ouvrage couronné par l'Académie des sciences et par l'Académie de médecine*. 2 vol. grand in-8° . . . . . . . . . . . . . . **25 fr.**

TRABUT. — *Précis de Botanique médicale*, par L. TRABUT, professeur d'histoire naturelle médicale à l'École de médecine d'Alger. *Deuxième édition*, entièrement refondue. 1 vol. in-8°, avec 954 figures.. . . . . . . . . . . . . . . . **8 fr.**

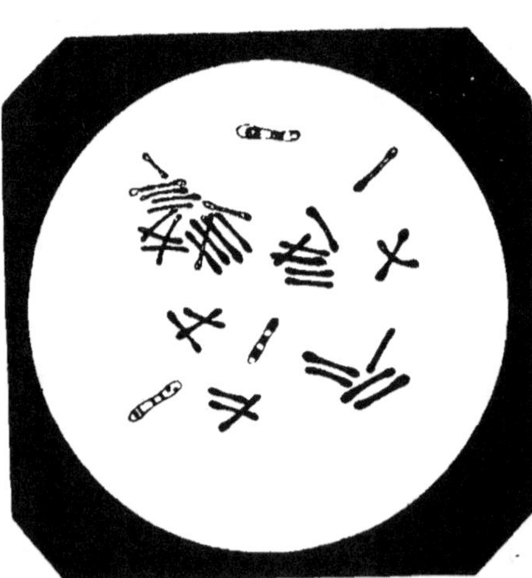


TUFFIER. — *Chirurgie du poumon*, par le Dr TUFFIER, professeur agrégé à la Faculté de médecine de Paris, chirurgien de l'hôpital de la Pitié. 1 vol. in-8°. . . . . . . **6 fr.**

WURTZ (R.). — *Technique bactériologique*, par R. WURTZ, professeur agrégé à la Faculté de médecine de Paris, médecin des hôpitaux. *Deuxième édition*. 1 vol. petit in-8° de l'*Encyclopédie des Aide-Mémoire*. . . **2 fr. 50**

— *Précis de bactériologie clinique*, par le Dr R. WURTZ. *Deuxième édition*, avec tableaux synoptiques et figures dans le texte. 1 vol. in-16 diamant, cartonné à l'anglaise, tranches rouges. . . . . **6 fr.**

ZAMBACO. — *Voyages chez les lépreux*, par le Dr ZAMBACO-PACHA, membre correspondant de l'Académie de médecine de Paris, ex-chef de clinique à la Faculté de médecine. 1 vol. in-8°, avec une carte indiquant les localités lépreuses. . . . . . . . . . . . . . . . . . . . . . . . . . . **8 fr.**

— *Les Lépreux ambulants de Constantinople*, par le Dr ZAMBACO-PACHA, membre associé national de l'Académie de médecine de Paris, membre correspondant de l'Académie de Saint-Pétersbourg, etc. 1 fort vol. in-4°, avec 48 planches hors texte en noir et en couleurs, relié toile . . . . . . . . **90 fr.**

## L'ŒUVRE MÉDICO-CHIRURGICAL
### D<sup>r</sup> CRITZMAN, directeur

# SUITE DE MONOGRAPHIES CLINIQUES
## SUR LES QUESTIONS NOUVELLES
### En Médecine, en Chirurgie et en Biologie

La science médicale réalise journellement des progrès incessants. Les traités de médecine et de chirurgie auront toujours grand'peine à se tenir au courant. C'est pour obvier à ce grave inconvénient que nous avons fondé ce recueil de Monographies, avec le concours des savants et des praticiens les plus autorisés.

*Chaque monographie est vendue séparément*. . . . . . . . . . . . . . . . . . . . . . . . . . **1 fr. 25**

Il est accepté des abonnements pour une série de 10 Monographies consécutives au prix à forfait et payable d'avance de 10 francs pour la France et 12 francs pour l'étranger (port compris).

### MONOGRAPHIES PUBLIÉES (Octobre 1900).

N° 1. **L'Appendicite**, par le D<sup>r</sup> Félix Leguel, chir. des hôp. de Paris (épuisé).

N° 2. **Le Traitement du mal de Pott**, par le D<sup>r</sup> A. Chipault, de Paris.

N° 3. **Le Lavage du sang**, par le D<sup>r</sup> Lejars, prof. agr., chir. des hôp., membre de la Sociéte de chirurgie.

N° 4. **L'Hérédité normale et pathologique**, par le D<sup>r</sup> Ch. Debierre, prof. d'anatomie à l'Université de Lille.

N° 5. **L'Alcoolisme**, par le D<sup>r</sup> Jaquet, privat-docent à l'Université de Bâle.

N° 6. **Physiologie et pathologie des sécrétions gastriques**, par le D<sup>r</sup> A. Verhaegen, assistant à la Clinique médicale de Louvain.

N° 7. **L'Eczéma**, *maladie parasitaire*, par le D<sup>r</sup> Leredde, chef de laboratoire, assistant de consultation à l'hôpital Saint-Louis.

N° 8. **La Fièvre jaune**, par le D<sup>r</sup> Sanarelli, Directeur de l'Institut d'Hygiène expérimentale de Montévidéo.

N° 9. **La Tuberculose du rein**, par le D<sup>r</sup> Tuffier, prof. agr., chir. de l'hôp. de la Pitié.

N° 10. **L'Opothérapie**. *Traitement de certaines maladies par des extraits d'organes animaux*, par A. Gilbert, prof. agr., chef du laboratoire de thérapeutique à la Faculté de médecine de Paris, et L. Carnot, docteur ès sciences, ancien interne des hôpitaux de Paris.

N° 11. **Les Paralysies générales progressives**, par le D<sup>r</sup> M. Klippel, méd. des hôp. de Paris.

N° 12. **Le Myxœdème**, par le D<sup>r</sup> Thibierge, méd. de l'hôp. de la Pitié.

N° 13. **La Néphrite des saturnins**, par le D<sup>r</sup> H. Lavrand, prof. chargé de cours à la Faculté catholique de Lille, lauréat de l'Académie de Paris.

N° 14. **Traitement de la syphilis**, par E. Gaucher, prof. agr. à la Faculté de méd. de Paris, médecin de l'hôpital Saint-Antoine.

N° 15. **Le Pronostic des tumeurs**, *basé sur la recherche du glycogène*, par le D<sup>r</sup> A. Brault, méd. de l'hôp. Tenon, chef des travaux pratiques d'anatomie pathologique à la Faculté.

N° 16. **La Kinésithérapie gynécologique**. *Traitement des maladies des femmes par le massage et la gymnastique (système de Brandt)*, par H. Stapfer, ancien chef de clinique obstétricale et gynécologique de la Faculté de Paris.

N° 17. **De la Gastro-entérite aiguë des nourrissons** (*Pathogénie et étiologie*), par A. Lesage, méd. des hôp. de Paris.

N° 18. **Traitement de l'Appendicite**, par Félix Leguel, prof. agr., chir. des hôp.

N° 19. **Les lois de l'énergétique dans le régime du diabète sucré**, par le D<sup>r</sup> E. Dufourt, ancien chef de clinique médicale à la Faculté de Lyon, méd. de l'hôp. thermal de Vichy.

N° 20. **La Peste** (*Épidémiologie. Bactériologie. Prophylaxie. Traitement*), par le D<sup>r</sup> H. Bourges, chef du laboratoire d'hygiène à la Faculté de médecine de Paris. Auditeur au Comité consultatif d'hygiène publique de France.

N° 21. **La Moelle osseuse à l'état normal et dans les infections**, par MM. G.-H. Roger, prof. agr. à la Faculté de méd. de Paris, méd. des hôp., et O. Josué, ancien interne, lauréat des hôp. de Paris.

N° 22. **L'Entéro-colite muco-membraneuse**, par le D<sup>r</sup> Gaston Lyon, ancien chef de clinique médicale de la Faculté de Paris.

N° 23. **L'Exploration clinique des fonctions rénales par l'élimination provoquée**, par le D<sup>r</sup> Ch. Achard, prof. agr. à la Faculté de méd., méd. de l'hôp. Tenon et J. Castaigne, interne lauréat (médaille d'or) des hôp.

N° 24. **L'Analgésie chirurgicale**, par voie rachidienne (injections sous-arachnoïdiennes de cocaïne), par le D<sup>r</sup> Tuffier, prof. agr. à la Faculté de médecine de Paris, chir. des hôp.

# BIBLIOTHÈQUE
# d'Hygiène thérapeutique

DIRIGÉE PAR

## Le Professeur PROUST

Membre de l'Académie de médecine, Médecin de l'Hôtel-Dieu,
Inspecteur général des Services sanitaires.

Chaque ouvrage forme un volume in-16, cartonné toile, tranches rouges,
et est vendu séparément : **4 fr.**

---

Chacun des volumes de cette collection n'est consacré qu'à une seule maladie ou à un
seul groupe de maladie. Grâce à leur format, ils sont d'un maniement commode. D'un
autre côté, en accordant un volume spécial à chacun des grands sujets d'hygiène thérapeutique, il a été facile de leur donner tout le développement nécessaire.

---

## VOLUMES PARUS :

**L'Hygiène du Goutteux**, par le Professeur PROUST et A. MATHIEU, médecin
de l'hôpital Andral.

**L'Hygiène de l'Obèse**, par le Professeur PROUST et A. MATHIEU.

**L'Hygiène des Asthmatiques**, par E. BRISSAUD, professeur à la Faculté de
Paris, médecin de l'hôpital Saint-Antoine.

**L'Hygiène du Syphilitique**, par H. BOURGES, préparateur au laboratoire
d'hygiène de la Faculté de médecine.

**Hygiène et thérapeutique thermales**, par G. DELFAU, ancien interne des
hôpitaux de Paris.

**Les Cures thermales**, par G. DELFAU, ancien interne des hôpitaux de Paris.

**L'Hygiène du Neurasthénique** (*Deuxième édition*), par le Professeur PROUST
et G. BALLET, professeur agrégé, médecin des hôpitaux de Paris.

**L'Hygiène des Albuminuriques**, par le. Dʳ SPRINGER, chef du laboratoire
de la Faculté de médecine à l'hôpital de la Charité.

**L'Hygiène des Tuberculeux**, par le Dʳ CHUQUET, ancien interne des hôpitaux de Paris, médecin consultant à Cannes, avec une préface du Dʳ DAREM-
BERG, correspondant de l'Académie de médecine.

**Hygiène et thérapeutique des maladies de la bouche**, par le Dʳ CRUET,
dentiste des hôpitaux de Paris, avec une préface du Professeur LANNELONGUE,
membre de l'Institut.

**L'Hygiène des Diabétiques**, par le Professeur PROUST et A. MATHIEU, médecin de l'hôpital Andral.

**L'Hygiène des maladies du cœur**, par le Dʳ VAQUEZ, professeur agrégé à
la Faculté de médecine de Paris, médecin des hôpitaux, avec une préface du
Professeur POTAIN, membre de l'Institut.

**L'Hygiène du Dyspeptique**, par le Dʳ LINOSSIER, professeur agrégé à la Faculté de médecine de Lyon, membre correspondant de l'Académie de médecine,
médecin à Vichy.

## VOLUME EN PRÉPARATION

**L'Hygiène des maladies de la peau**, par le Dʳ THIBIERGE, médecin des
hôpitaux de Paris.

---

44513. — Imprimerie LAHURE, 9, rue de Fleurus, à Paris.